Onco-Nephrology

Onco-Nephrology

Kevin W. Finkel, MD, FACP, FASN, FCCM
Professor and Executive Vice-Chair of Medicine
Director, Division of Renal Diseases & Hypertension
Chief, Section of Critical Care Nephrology
UTHealth Science Center at Houston—McGovern Medical School;
Professor of Medicine
Division of Medicine
Section of Nephrology
University of Texas MD Anderson Cancer Center;
Chief of Nephrology
Memorial Hermann Hospital—Texas Medical Center
Houston, TX

Mark A. Perazella, MD, FACP
Professor of Medicine
Yale University School of Medicine
Section of Nephrology
Department of Internal Medicine
New Haven, CT;
Section of Nephrology
VA Medical Center
West Haven, CT

Eric P. Cohen, MD
Professor of Medicine
University of Maryland School of Medicine
Deputy Director of the Medical Service;
Nephrology Section Chief
Baltimore VAMC
Baltimore, MD

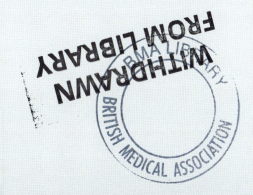

ELSEVIER

Elsevier
Philadelphia, PA

ONCO-NEPHROLOGY, FIRST EDITION   ISBN: 978-0-323-54945-5

Notice

Practitioners and researchers must always rely on their own experience and knowledge in evaluating and using any information, methods, compounds or experiments described herein. Because of rapid advances in the medical sciences, in particular, independent verification of diagnoses and drug dosages should be made. To the fullest extent of the law, no responsibility is assumed by Elsevier, authors, editors or contributors for any injury and/or damage to persons or property as a matter of products liability, negligence or otherwise, or from any use or operation of any methods, products, instructions, or ideas contained in the material herein.

Library of Congress Control Number: 2019937968

Content Strategist: Nancy Anastasi Duffy
Content Development Specialist: Meghan Andress
Publishing Services Manager: Shereen Jameel
Senior Project Manager: Umarani Natarajan
Design Direction: Bridget Hoette

Printed in China

Last digit is the print number: 9 8 7 6 5 4 3 2 1

ELSEVIER

3251 Riverport Lane
St. Louis, Missouri 63043

Working together
to grow libraries in
developing countries

www.elsevier.com • www.bookaid.org

*To my beautiful daughter, Megan, for all her courage
and inspiration.*
–Kevin W. Finkel

*To my family, friends, and colleagues who have been
part of my journey through medicine and my life. In
particular to my parents, Joe and Santina Perazella, who
sacrificed much for me and remain ardent supporters; to
my wife, Donna, who selflessly continues to support my
academic efforts; to my brothers, Joe and Scott, who
make life interesting; and to my boys, Mark and Andrew,
who always make me most proud.*
–Mark A. Perazella

Contributors

Ala Abudayyeh, MD
Internal Medicine
Section of Nephrology
MD Anderson Cancer Center
Houston, Texas

Joseph R. Angelo, MD
Assistant Professor
Renal Services
Baylor College of Medicine/Texas Childrens' Hospital
Houston, Texas

Claude Bassil, MD, FACP, FASN
Assistant Professor
Nephrology;
Program Director
USF Nephrology and Hypertension
University of South Florida;
Renal Coordinator
Onconephrology
H. Lee Moffitt Cancer Center
Tampa, Florida

Vecihi Batuman, MD
Professor of Medicine
Tulane University School of Medicine;
Chief, Nephrology Section
SLVHCS – VA Medical Center
New Orleans, Louisiana

John J. Bissler, MD
Nephrology Division Chief
Pediatrics
University of Tennessee Health Science Center;
Nephrology Medical Director
Nephrology
St. Jude Children's Research Hospital
Memphis, Tennessee

Andrew S. Bomback, MD, MPH
Assistant Professor of Medicine
Department of Medicine
Division of Nephrology
Columbia University Medical Center
New York, New York

Brendan T. Bowman, MD
Associate Professor
Department of Medicine
Division of Nephrology
University of Virginia School of Medicine
Charlottesville, Virginia

Juan C. Calle, MD, FASN
Glomerulonephritis Group
Department of Nephrology and Hypertension
Cleveland Clinic
Cleveland, Ohio

Anthony Chang, MD
Professor
Pathology
University of Chicago
Chicago, Illinois

Sheldon Chen, MD
Associate Professor of Medicine
Section of Nephrology
Division of Internal Medicine
The University of Texas MD Anderson Cancer Center
Houston, Texas

Eric P. Cohen, MD
Professor of Medicine
University of Maryland School of Medicine
Deputy Director of the Medical Service;
Nephrology Section Chief
Baltimore VAMC
Baltimore, Maryland

Laura Cosmai, MD
Department of Internal Medicine and Therapeutics
University of Pavia;
Division of Translational Oncology
IRCCS Istituti Clinici
Scientifici Maugeri
Pavia, Italy

Vidhi Desai
Assistant Professor of Medicine
Division of Hematology/Oncology
Zucker School of Medicine at Hofstra/Northwell
Lake Success, New York

Marcia E. Epstein, MD
Associate Chief Division of Infectious Diseases
Medicine
Northwell
Manhasset, New York

Mohit Gupta
Department of Nephrology and Hypertension
New York-Presbyterian Weill Cornell Medical Center
New York, New York

Kevin W. Finkel, MD, FACP, FASN, FCCM
Professor of Medicine and Director
Division of Renal Diseases & Hypertension
UT Health Science Center at Houston;
Professor of Medicine
Nephrology Section
University of Texas MD Anderson Cancer Center
Houston, Texas

Maurizio Gallieni, MD, FASN
Director
Nephrology and Dialysis Unit
San Carlo Borromeo Hospital, ASST Santi Paolo e Carlo;
Researcher and Adjunct Professor of Nephrology
Dipartimento di Scienze Biomediche e Cliniche "L. Sacco"
University of Milano
Milano, Italy

Pranisha Gautam-Goyal, MD
Assistant Professor
Medicine
Donald and Barbara Zucker School of Medicine
  at Hofstra/Northwell
Manhasset, New York

Ilya Glezerman, MD
Clinical Associate Physician
Renal Service
Memorial Sloan-Kettering Cancer Center;
Associate Clinical Professor
Department of Medicine
Weill-Cornell Medical College
New York, New York

Vijay S. Gorantla, MD, PhD
Clinical Instructor of Pediatrics
Department of Pediatrics
Division of Pediatric Nephrology
University of Tennessee Health Science Center
Memphis, Tennessee

Victoria Gutgarts, MD
Onconephrology Fellow
Renal Service
Memorial Sloan Kettering Cancer Center
New York, New York

Uwe Heemann, Prof.
Chairman
Nephrology
Klinikum Rechts der Isar
Munich, Germany

Leal Herlitz, MD
Director of Renal Pathology
Anatomic Pathology
Cleveland Clinic
Cleveland, Ohio

Sangeeta Hingorani, MD, MPH
Professor
Pediatrics
University of Washington/Seattle Children's Hospital;
Associate Member
Clinical Research Division
Fred Cancer Research Center
Seattle, Washington

Jonathan J. Hogan, MD
Assistant Professor of Medicine
Division of Nephrology
Pereleman School of Medicine
University of Pennsylvania
Philadelphia, Pennsylvania

Jean L. Holley, AB, MD
Clinical Professor of Medicine
Medicine
University of Illinois, Urbana-Champaign;
Carle Physician Group
Urbana, Illinois

Susie L. Hu, MD
Associate Professor of Medicine
Medicine
Division of Kidney Disease and Hypertension
Warren Alpert Medical School of Brown University
Providence, Rhode Island

Colin A. Hutchison, MBChB, PhD
Consultant Nephrologist
Medical Director for the Acute and Medical Directorates
Hawkes Bay DHB
Hastings, HB, New Zealand

Insara Jaffer Sathick, MBBS, MRCP
Assistant Attending Physician
Renal Service
Department of Medicine
Memorial Sloan Kettering Cancer Center
New York, New York

Kenar D. Jhaveri, MD
Professor of Medicine
Nephrology
Zucker School of Medicine at Hofstra/Northwell
Great Neck, New York

Catherine Joseph, MD
Assistant Professor
Renal Services
Baylor College of Medicine/Texas Children's Hospital
Houston, Texas

Jaya Kala, MD
Assistant Professor of Medicine
Division of Renal Diseases and Hypertension
UT Health Science Center at Houston
McGovern Medical School
Houston, Texas

Sabine Karam, MD
Assistant Professor of Clinical Medicine
Department of Medicine
Saint George Hospital University Medical Center
Beirut, Lebanon

Stefan Kemmner
Department of Nephrology
Klinikum Rechts der Isar
Technical University of Munich
Munich, Germany

Sana F. Khan, MD
Assistant Professor
Department of Medicine/Division of Nephrology
University of Virginia Health System
Charlottesville, Virginia

Abhijat Kitchlu, MD, MSc
Clinical Associate Nephrologist
Department of Medicine
Division of Nephrology
University of Toronto
Toronto, Canada

Amit Lahoti, MD
Associate Professor
Section of Nephrology
MD Anderson Cancer Center
Houston, Texas

Benjamin L. Laskin, MD
Assistant Professor
Nephrology
The Children's Hospital of Philadelphia
Philadelphia, Pennsylvania

Sheron Latcha, MD
Physician
Medicine
Memorial Sloan Kettering Cancer Center;
Clinical Instructor
Medicine
Cornell University Medical Center
New York, New York

Wai L. Lau, MD
Instructor of Medicine
Division of Nephrology
Columbia University Medical Center
New York, New York

Randy L. Luciano, MD, PhD
Assistant Professor of Medicine
Internal Medicine
Section of Nephrology
Yale University School of Medicine
New Haven, Connecticut

Niti Madan, MD
Associate Professor of Medicine
Division of Nephrology
Department of Internal Medicine
University of California Davis
Sacramento, California

Prashant Malhotra, MBBS, MD
Assistant Professor
Medicine
Donald and Barbara Zucker School of Medicine
    at Hofstra/Northwell
Manhasset, New York

Peter Mollee, MBBS, FRACP, FRCPA
Associate Professor of Medicine
Clinical Haematology
University of Queensland Medical School
Princess Alexandra Hospital
Southport, Queensland, Australia

Mark A. Perazella, MD, MS
Professor of Medicine
Yale University School of Medicine
Section of Nephrology
Department of Internal Medicine
New Haven, Connecticut

Phillip M. Pierorazio, MD
Associate Professor
Urology and Oncology
Brady Urological Institute and Department of Urology
Johns Hopkins
Baltimore, Maryland

Pierre Delanaye, MD, PhD
Professor
Nephrology Dialysis Transplantation
CHU Sart Tilman
Liege, Belgium

Camillo Porta, MD
Medical Oncology
IRCCS San Matteo University Hospital Foundation
Pavia, Italy

Jai Radhakrishnan, MD, MS
Professor of Medicine
Division of Nephrology
Columbia University Medical Center
New York, New York

Mandana Rastegar, MD, EdM
Assistant Clinical Professor
Department of Medicine
David Geffen School of Medicine at UCLA;
Division of Nephrology
Greater Los Angeles Veterans Health Administration
Los Angeles, California

Robert F. Reilly Jr., MD
Clinical Professor of Medicine
Nephrology
University of Alabama at Birmingham;
Physician
Medical Service
Birmingham VA
Birmingham, Alabama

Danielle L. Saly, MD
Chief Resident, Instructor of Medicine
Internal Medicine
Yale University School of Medicine
New Haven, Connecticut

Joshua A. Samuels, MD, MPH
Pediatrics
University of Texas Medical School at Houston;
Associate Professor
Pediatrics
University of Texas MD Anderson Cancer Center
Houston, Texas

Divya Shankaranarayanan, MBBS
Fellow
Nephrology
Department of Medicine
Weill Cornell/Memorial Sloan
New York, New York

Deirdre Sawinski, MD
Assistant Professor
Renal, Electrolyte and Hypertension Division
Department of Medicine
Hospital of the University of Pennsylvania
Philadelphia, Pennsylvania

Umut Selamet, MD
Clinical Instructor
Department of Medicine, Nephrology
University of California Los Angeles
Los Angeles, California

Anushree C. Shirali, MD
Assistant Professor of Medicine
Internal Medicine
Yale University School of Medicine
New Haven, Connecticut

Ramapriya Sinnakirouchenan, MD
Assistant Professor
Medicine, Nephrology
Medical College of Wisconsin
Milwaukee, Wisconsin

Ben Sprangers, MD, PhD, MPH, MBA
Department of Microbiology and Immunology
Laboratory of Molecular Immunology (Rega Institute)
KU Leuven;
Department of Nephrology, University Hospitals Leuven
Leuven, Belgium

Jyotsana Thakkar, MD
Assistant Professor
Division of Nephrology
Montefiore Medical Center/Albert Einstein College
   of Medicine
Bronx, New York

Jeffrey Turner, MD
Associate Professor of Medicine
Internal Medicine
Section of Nephrology
Yale University
New Haven, Connecticut

Brahm Vasudev, MD
Associate Professor
Division of Nephrology
Medical College of Wisconsin
Milwaukee, Wisconsin

Dia R. Waguespack, MD, FASN
Assistant Professor of Medicine
UTHealth Science Center at Houston- McGovern
   Medical School
Houston, Texas

Rimda Wanchoo, MD
Associate Professor
Medicine
Zucker School of Medicine at Hofstra/Northwell
Great Neck, New York

Brendan M. Weiss, MD
Adjunct Assistant Professor of Medicine
Hematology Oncology Division
Department of Medicine
Perelman School of Medicine
University of Pennsylvania
Philadelphia, Pennsylvania

Robert H. Weiss, MD
Professor
Nephrology
University of California Davis
Davis, California

Germaine Wong, MBBS, MMED, PhD
Associate Professor
Sydney School of Public Health
University of Sydney
Sydney, Australia

Preface

As the discipline of Medicine has advanced, patients and their medical conditions have become significantly more complex and have required physician super-specialization. This realization is especially true in patients with cancer who either develop de novo kidney disease or already have existing impairment of kidney function. Hence, the development of the field of onco-nephrology and the need for this textbook. The growth of onco-nephrology has been stimulated by several coinciding factors: (1) there are numerous kidney disorders unique to cancer patients either caused by underlying malignancy (myeloma cast nephropathy, paraneoplastic glomerulonephritis) or treatment (tumor lysis syndrome, hematopoietic stem cell transplant associated nephropathy); (2) both acute and chronic kidney disease increase mortality and morbidity in cancer patients; (3) chronic kidney disease and renal replacement therapies can affect the availability of certain treatment options for patients or affect the clearance of numerous therapeutic agents; and (4) because cancer patients are surviving longer with newer targeted therapies, there is an increasing need for long-term management of patients who subsequently develop chronic kidney disease. In the past, topics germane to onco-nephrology were haphazardly mentioned in various chapters in textbooks of nephrology or oncology. With this edition of *Onco-Nephrology*, we have attempted to bring together all the relevant issues related to kidney disease in patients with cancer in a single, comprehensive textbook. It is meant to serve as a definitive reference source for all health care providers who care for patients with cancer.

Contents

Onco-Nephrology

Fluid and Electrolyte Disorders in Cancer Patients

1 *Kidney Function*

PIERRE DELANAYE

Introduction

Kidney function in oncologic patients is an important parameter for several reasons. In some specific cases, like urologic cancers, the tumor itself can cause acute or chronic kidney dysfunction. However, the renal function parameter is more frequently followed in oncologic patients because, on one hand, they are likely to get nephrotoxic drugs, and on the other hand, some oncologic patients have chronic kidney disease (CKD) that would necessitate a dosage adaptation for potentially toxic chemotherapies.[1,2] Indeed, excretory renal function plays a fundamental role both in the pharmacokinetics and pharmacodynamics of several drugs. This is particularly the case for water soluble compounds and/or their active metabolites. Even for non-renally-excreted drugs, severe CKD can modify the pharmacokinetics by several mechanisms.[3–6] For this reason, it is now recommended that both pharmacokinetics and pharmacodynamics of every new drug be studied in the context of CKD.[7] Dosage-adjustment according to excretory renal function is required for many medications. However, there is a debate in the literature regarding the best way to estimate excretory function or glomerular filtration rate (GFR) for the purpose of pharmacotherapy.[8–12]

Serum Creatinine

The word "creatinine" was probably used for the first time by Justus von Liebig in 1847. This German chemist was thus describing the product obtained from heating creatine with mineral salts.[13] Nowadays, serum creatinine is one of the most frequently prescribed analysis in Clinical Chemistry. Serum creatinine is the only renal plasma biomarker used in daily clinical practice to estimate GFR.[14,15] However, a good interpretation of the creatinine result remains sometimes problematic, or at least not so simple. To explain these difficulties, there are both physiologic (serum creatinine is not an "ideal" renal marker) and analytical reasons. First, serum creatinine can be measured by two main methods: methods derived from the classical Jaffe reaction on one part, and enzymatic methods on the other part. The Jaffe method is based on a reaction between picrate and creatinine in alkaline milieu that gives a red-orange product.[16] Some components (so-called pseudochromogens) can however also interact with picrate: acetoacetate, pyruvate, ketonic acids, proteins, glucose, and ascorbic acid. These pseudochromogens take part in 15% to 20% of the Jaffe reaction if the serum creatinine is in the normal range. This limitation of Jaffe methods remains even after different technological innovations. The second method is known as the enzymatic and is based on successive enzymatic steps. Different types of reactions have been described, but they all share a higher specificity to measure serum creatinine, compared to Jaffe assays. Enzymatic methods are thus considered as more accurate and precise than Jaffe methods. These methods are recommended even if they are more expensive and not fully free from some interferences.[17] There are two methods to measure creatinine but for each method, there are also several different assays (according to the manufacturers). Until recently, a great heterogeneity was observed between the assays, because of differences in calibration.[15,18–20] Nowadays, several improvements have been done in a quest to standardization, and it is recommended to measure serum creatinine with a standardized, calibrated, and so-called *isotope dilution mass spectrometry* (*IDMS*)-traceable method. This traceability is of the highest importance in the context of creatinine-based equations.[15,18–20]

Beyond analytical issues, there are also physiologic limitations to serum creatinine. The molecular weight of creatinine is 113 Daltons. Creatinine is the anhydric catabolite of creatine and phosphocreatine. Creatinine is a catabolite final product and has no physiologic role. The vast majority of creatine (98%) will be found in muscles where creatine is phosphorylated in phosphocreatine by creatine kinase. Each day, 1% to 2% of the muscle creatine is converted into creatinine.[14,21] It is thus obvious that serum creatinine concentration is highly dependent on muscle mass. If the global creatine concentration is constant in healthy subjects, this concentration will strongly vary notably in muscular pathologies or, from a larger point of view, in all diseases with anorexia and muscle mass decreasing, as it is frequently observed in oncologic diseases. In these situations, serum creatinine will decrease, or will not increase when GFR is decreasing.[14,22,23] The second important limitation is the tubular secretion of creatinine, which explains that creatinine clearance overestimated measured GFR (mGFR). Moreover, even if creatinine clearance, calculated on a 24-hour urine collection, is a relatively simple way to assess GFR, such a clearance also lacks precision, especially because of large errors in urine collection.[24] Therefore creatinine clearance is not recommended for GFR estimation.[25] A last point needs to be underlined: the relationship between serum creatinine and GFR is not linear but hyperbolic (Fig. 1.1).[21,26] To keep this point in mind is fundamental for a good interpretation of a creatinine result. Actually, this hyperbolic relation implies that a little creatinine change will have great consequences in terms of GFR in low creatinine levels, although the same creatinine variation in higher ranges will be negligible in terms of GFR.[14,15,20]

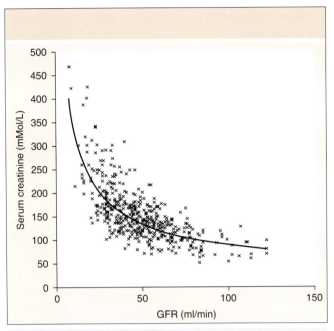

Fig. 1.1 Hyperbolic association between serum creatinine and glomerular filtration rate.

The Creatinine-Based Equations in Oncology

Serum creatinine concentration is dependent on muscular and thus on gender, age, and ethnicity. Moreover, the relationship between serum creatinine and GFR is hyperbolic (see Fig. 1.1). These observations lead authors to propose creatinine-based equations that include simple variables like age, gender, ethnicity and, for some of them, weight.[27–31] Because of the hyperbolic association, a negative exponent is applied to serum creatinine value in these equations, making the association between estimated GFR (eGFR) and mGFR by a reference method, simple and linear. Several equations have been proposed since the 1950s. Before 2000, the Cockcroft and Gault (CG) equation was the most popular and has been used by generations of doctors to estimate GFR.[27] This equation has, however, several limitations, notably a lack of precision caused by the variable weight included in the formula.[32] Today, new equations based on serum creatinine and including only age and gender are recommended and their results can be automatically given by laboratories.[33] These equations are applicable only with IDMS-traceable assays. Among these equations, we can cite the most used, that is, the modification of diet in renal disease (MDRD) equation (most valuable in CKD patients)[28,34] and chronic kidney disease epidemiology (CKD-EPI) equations (also valuable in healthy populations).[29] Recently, some authors have challenged the superiority of these equations both in the general and CKD populations, and proposed new algorithms, known as the *revised Lund-Malmö equation*[31] or the *full age spectrum equations*[30] (Table 1.1). Globally, both in the general or CKD population, one can expect an accuracy around 85% or 90% for creatinine-based equations. This means that results of eGFR equations will be within ±30% of the results of mGFR by a reference method in 85% to 90% of subjects/patients.[35,36] Beyond the experts' discussion to know which equation performs the best, we have to keep in mind that the most important variable in all these equations remains the serum creatinine. Therefore there is no reason to believe that eGFR, by any estimating equations, would be accurate in specific patients or specific populations for who the serum creatinine, in itself, is particularly inadequate.[37] In the context of oncology, it will be particularly relevant in patients with anorexia, loss of weight, and cachexia.[21,38] In these patients, serum creatinine concentration is inaccurate, and can decrease in patients with stable function or remain stable in patients with worsening GFR. Because serum creatinine is inaccurate, eGFR based on serum creatinine will be unable to correctly assess GFR in these patients. In 21 young patients suffering from anorexia nervosa, GFR was measured by a reference method (namely, the ⁵¹Cr-Ethylenediaminetetra-acetic acid (EDTA) plasma clearance). The performance of both the CG and MDRD equations was dramatically poor, with an accuracy within 30% of only 63% and 30%, respectively. Both the MDRD and CKD-EPI equations strongly overestimate mGFR in these specific patients.[22] Redal-Baigorri et al. studied the performances of creatinine-based equations in 185 patients with cancer. GFR was measured by ⁵¹Cr-EDTA plasma clearance before chemotherapy and serum creatinine was IDMS traceable. Majority of patients were suffering from pulmonary cancer (77%). The performance of MDRD and CKD-EPI was acceptable around 89% for both equations, but most of the patients were healthy from a renal point of view, with only 17% of patients with mGFR below 60 mL/min/1.73m².[39] Lauritsen et al. included patients with disseminated germ cell cancer and treated by bleomycin, etoposide, and cisplatin. The GFR was measured by ⁵¹Cr-EDTA single sample plasma clearance in 390 patients, but more than 1600 measurements were obtained with data before and just after chemotherapy, and then after 1, 3 and 5 years. Patients were young with few comorbidities and thus with normal mGFR values. CG, MDRD, and CKD-EPI equations have relatively good performance in estimating GFR before and in the years following chemotherapy (around 85% and 90%). However, values after three cycles of chemotherapy were more disappointing with an accuracy within 30% at 76%, 80%, and 50%, for CG, MDRD, and CKD-EPI, respectively. Actually, mGFR significantly declined during chemotherapy (−9 mL/min/1.73m²) but serum creatinine also decreased (and so eGFR equations increased).[40] Funakoshi et al. also studied the performance of the CKD-EPI equation (both original and Japanese version and de-indexed for body surface area [BSA]) in 50 patients with cancer scheduled for cisplatin therapy (majority had neck and head cancer) before and after treatment. Only subjects with mGFR over 50 mL/min were considered. The accuracy of both CKD-EPI equations was acceptable with an accuracy within 30% of 92% and better than the CG equation (accuracy of 78%) before the therapy. However, a significant decline in accuracy was observed for all equations after the cisplatin cycle: 60%, 68%, and 56% for the original CKD-EPI, the Japanese version, and the CG, respectively. All equations overestimated mGFR, especially in the lower GFR ranges. Moreover, in the

Table 1.1 Creatinine- and Cystatin C-Based Equations to Estimate Glomerular Filtration Rate

Cockcroft and Gault		$((140\text{-age}) \times \text{weight})/(72 \times \text{SCr})$
MDRD		$175 \times \text{SCr}^{-1.154} \times \text{age}^{-0.203} \times [0.742 \text{ if female}] \times [1.212 \text{ if black}]$
CKD-EPI SCr		
women	SCr $\leq$ 0.7 mg/dL	$144 \times (\text{Scr}/0.7)^{-0.329} \times 0.993^{\text{age}} \times [1.159 \text{ if black}]$
	SCr $>$ 0.7 mg/dL	$144 \times (\text{Scr}/0.7)^{-1.209} \times 0.993^{\text{age}} \times [1.159 \text{ if black}]$
men	SCr $\leq$ 0.9 mg/dL	$141 \times (\text{Scr}/0.9)^{-0.411} \times 0.993^{\text{age}} \times [1.159 \text{ if black}]$
	SCr $>$ 0.9 mg/dL	$141 \times (\text{Scr}/0.9)^{-1.209} \times 0.993^{\text{age}} \times [1.159 \text{ if black}]$
CKD-EPI SCys	SCys $\leq$ 0.8 mg/L	$133 \times (\text{Scyst}/0,8)^{-0.499} \times 0.996^{\text{age}} [\times 0.932 \text{ if female}]$
	SCys $>$ 0.8 mg/L	$133 \times (\text{Scys}/0,8)^{-1.328} \times 0.996^{\text{age}} [\times 0.932 \text{ if female}]$
CKD-EPI SCrCys		
women	SCr $\leq$ 0.7 mg/dL and SCys $\leq$ 0.8 mg/dL	$130 \times (\text{SCr}/0.7)^{-0.248} \times (\text{SCyst}/0.8)^{-0.375} \times 0.995^{\text{age}} \times [1.08 \text{ if black}]$
	SCr $\leq$ 0.7 mg/dL and SCys $>$ 0.8 mg/dL	$130 \times (\text{SCr}/0.7)^{-0.248} \times (\text{SCyst}/0.8)^{-0.711} \times 0.995^{\text{age}} \times [1.08 \text{ if black}]$
	SCr $>$ 0.7 mg/dL and SCys $\leq$ 0.8 mg/dL	$130 \times (\text{SCr}/0.7)^{-0.601} \times (\text{SCyst}/0.8)^{-0.375} \times 0.995^{\text{age}} \times [1.08 \text{ if black}]$
	SCr $>$ 0.7 mg/dL and SCys $\geq$ 0.8 mg/dL	$130 \times (\text{SCr}/0.7)^{-0.601} \times (\text{SCyst}/0.8)^{-0.711} \times 0.995^{\text{age}} \times [1.08 \text{ if black}]$
Men	SCr $\leq$ 0.9 mg/dL and SCys $\leq$ 0.8 mg/dL	$135 \times (\text{SCr}/0.9)^{-0.207} \times (\text{SCyst}/0.8)^{-0.375} \times 0.995^{\text{age}} \times [1.08 \text{ if black}]$
	SCr $\leq$ 0.9 mg/dL and SCys $>$ 0.8 mg/dL	$135 \times (\text{SCr}/0.9)^{-0.207} \times (\text{SCyst}/0.8)^{-0.711} \times 0.995^{\text{age}} \times [1.08 \text{ if black}]$
	SCr $>$ 0.9 mg/dL and SCys $\leq$ 0.8 mg/dL	$135 \times (\text{SCr}/0.9)^{-0.601} \times (\text{SCyst}/0.8)^{-0.375} \times 0.995^{\text{age}} \times [1.08 \text{ if black}]$
	SCr $>$ 0.9 mg/dL and SCys $>$ 0.8 mg/dL	$135 \times (\text{SCr}/0.7)^{-0.601} \times (\text{SCyst}/0.8)^{-0.711} \times 0.995^{\text{age}} \times [1.08 \text{ if black}]$
FAS creatinine		$(107.3/\text{SCr}/Q_{\text{creat}}) \times (0.988(\text{Age-40}))$ if $^{\text{age}} > 40$ y
FAS cystatin C		$(107.3/\text{Scyst}/Q_{\text{cyst}}) \times (0.988(\text{Age-40}))$ if $^{\text{age}} > 40$ y
FAS combined		$[107.3/(0.5 \times \text{Scyst}/Q_{\text{cyst}} + 0.5 \times \text{SCr}/Q_{\text{creat}}] \times (0.988^{(\text{Age-40})})$ if $^{\text{age}} > 40$ y
LM	women SCr $<$ 150 μmol/L	$e^{[2.5+0.0121 \times (150\text{-SCr})]-0.0158 \times \text{age}+0.438 \times \text{Ln(age)}}$
	women SCr $\geq$ 150 μmol/L	$e^{[2.5-0.926 \times \text{Ln(SCr/150)}]-0.0158 \times \text{age}+0.438 \times \text{Ln(age)}}$
	men SCr $<$ 180 μmol/L	$e^{[2.56+0.00968 \times (180\text{-SCr})]-0.0158 \times \text{age}+0.438 \times \text{Ln(age)}}$
	men SCr $\geq$ 180 μmol/L	$e^{[2.56-0.926 \times \text{Ln(SCr/180)}]-0.0158 \times \text{age}+0.438 \times \text{Ln(age)}}$
CAPA		$130 \times \text{SCyst}^{-1.069} \times \text{age}^{-0.117} -7$

All equations are in mL/min/1.73m² except the Cockcroft-Gault in mL/min.
CAPA, Equation Caucasian, Asian, pediatric, and adult; *CKD-EPI SCr*, Chronic Kidney Disease-Epidemiology Collaboration based on serum creatinine; *CKD-EPI SCys*, equation CKD-EPI based on cystatin C only; *CKD-EPI SCrCyst*, CKD-EPI equation combining both cystatin C and creatinine; *FAS*, equation Full Age Spectrum; *LM*, equation Lund-Malmö; *MDRD*: Modification of Diet in Renal Disease study equation; *SCr*, serum creatinine (in mg/dL); *SCyst*, cystatine C (in mg/L).

postchemotherapy period, one-quarter of patients with CKD-EPI values over 60 mL/min had actually a measured GFR below 50 mL/min.[41] Lindberg et al. also included 94 patients with advanced head and neck cancer treated by radio-chemotherapy including cisplatin. The GFR was measured by ^{51}Cr-EDTA single sample plasma clearance before the first cycle ($n=94$), after the third cycle of chemotherapy ($n=78$), and after the planned five cycles ($n=35$). The nonindexed BSA result was considered for mGFR and eGFR (CG and CKD-EPI). At baseline, five patients were eventually not treated by cisplatin because mGFR was below 50 mL/min. These five patients had eGFR with CKD-EPI above 50 mL/min (and three with CG). At the end of the treatment, three patients had mGFR below 50 mL/min, but this decline in mGFR was detected by both equations in only one patient. The Bland and Altman analyses showed a relatively acceptable systematic bias between mGFR and CG and a systematic overestimation of mGFR by CKD-EPI, but the precision of both equations was actually poor.[42]

Hingorani et al. measured GFR by iohexol plasma clearance in 50 patients who benefit from a hematopoietic cell transplant at baseline and after 100 days.[43] The authors compared the performance of mGFR with CG (nonindexed for BSA), MDRD, and CKD-EPI (both indexed for BSA). At baseline, all patients were also treated by trimethoprim, which is known to block the tubular secretion of creatinine, leading to an increase in creatinine concentration independently of any change in mGFR.[44] At baseline, CKD-EPI and MDRD underestimated mGFR and CG overestimated it. The accuracies were low for patients with mean normal GFR values. Indeed, accuracy within 30% at baseline was 79%, 70%, and 57% for CKD-EPI, MDRD, and CG equations, respectively. After 100 days, the accuracy observed was similar for CKD-EPI and MDRD and slightly better for CG.[43] All these data in cancer patients compared mGFR by a reference method with eGFR, but the studies share methodologic limitations, notably the samples being relatively limited. However, it appears from these analyses that the accuracy of the equations is, at best, suboptimal in cancer patients. This observation is not fully unexpected as these patients are frequently frail and have decreased muscle mass because of their pathology and/or chemotherapy. In the same vein, the inaccuracy of these equations seems especially important during or after the chemotherapy cycles, which is, once again, not fully unexpected.

The Choice of the Equation in Oncology for Drug Dosage Adaptation

Indexing or not GFR by BSA will impact the GFR results particularly in patients or subjects with extreme height and weight values.[45,46] In the context of drug dosage adaptation, it is fully logical to consider nonindexed GFR. This recommendation is supported by the Food and Drug Administration and the European Medicines Agency (EMA). Indeed, the goal of BSA indexation is to make GFR results from subjects with different body size comparable. However, in the context of drug dosage adaptation, the GFR is considered as the capacity of a given subject to excrete drugs or drugs catabolites. As an example, for an elderly fragile woman with a weight of 45 kg, a height of 160 cm, and a BSA of 1.4 m² who is requiring a cisplatin therapy for ovarian cancer, the antimitotic therapy must be dose-adjusted accordingly to her GFR. If her measured (by a reference method) GFR is 25 mL/min, demonstrating a CKD stage 4, BSA indexing will overestimate the GFR to 31 mL/min/1.73 m², classifying the patient as stage 3 CKD. Which result should be used for dose adjustment of nephrotoxic therapy and what stage of CKD should be ascribed to the patient? It seems more correct to take into account the result of the actual patient's GFR, not the GFR result that the patient could have if her BSA was 1.73 m².[45]

If it is thus widely accepted that non-GFR indexed results must be considered for drug dosage adaptation (even if it is not always applied in clinical practice or research), there is still a huge debate in the literature to know which eGFR equation must be considered for drug dosage adaptation. Several publications have illustrated potential discrepancies in eGFR results and thus in dosage prescription if different equations are used.[8,11,47–59] In the context of oncology, Shord et al. retrospectively studied the dose of carboplatin given to the patient with the Calvert formula (Calvert: Total Dose [mg] = [target Area Under the Curve] × [GFR + 25]).[59] They used the CG equation in the Calvert formula for 186 patients. If they had used MDRD, a discrepant dose of carboplatin (defined as a difference of more than 20%) would have occurred in 48% of patients. Bennis et al. considered 1364 cisplatin cycles in 309 patients and observed a requirement for dose adjustment in 9.7% if the CG was used, but 4.8% if the MDRD would have been considered.[57] For drug dosage adjustment, the sharpest debate consists in choosing between the CG equation,[27] frequently promoted by clinical pharmacologists and geriatricians, and the CKD-EPI equation (or MDRD if CKD patients), promoted by nephrologists.[28,29] From a nephrologic point of view, the superiority of the CKD-EPI over CG equation to estimate GFR is easy to demonstrate.[29,32,37] Moreover, this equation truly estimates GFR, whereas the CG equation estimates creatinine clearance, which in itself, is only a poor estimation of true GFR.[37,60] Finally, *sensu stricto*, the CG equation cannot be used with modern, calibrated, and IDMS-traceable serum creatinine values.[19,61–63] Conversely, there are arguments to support the case for applying the CG equation.[4,64–67] Indeed, the CG equation is the equation that has been used to elaborate drug dosage adjustments for the vast majority of drugs.[49,65–69] Furthermore, the CG equation better predicts the risk of adverse events for several drugs, notably cardiovascular therapies. This may reflect the presence of the variable "body weight" in the CG equation, not in the CKD-EPI equation.[11,65,70] Also the CG equation has been reported to give systematically lower eGFR values than those obtained with CKD-EPI, particularly in the elderly.[7,71,72] This underestimation will lead to a more protective behavior in terms of drug dosage in this frail population.[47,73] In a simulation study, we showed that differences between the two equations are potentially influenced by each variable included in these equations: gender, age, weight, height, and serum creatinine. Among these variables, age and weight are the most important and will systematically impact the results of the equations.[7] As an extreme example, in old frail patients, CG will systematically give lower eGFR results than CKD-EPI, but in young obese subjects, CG will systematically give higher results than CKD-EPI. Because drug dosage adjustment is the quintessence of personalized medicine, one should however be careful in our interpretations of differences between eGFR that are based on population studies and focus on the characteristics of the individual.

Other Biomarkers and Measured Glomerular Filtration Rate

In the general healthy or CKD population, new biomarkers have been largely studied. The most promising biomarker was cystatin C.[74–76] Compared with creatinine, cystatin C is presented as being totally, or at least more, independent to muscular mass.[77,78] However, cystatin C is also influenced by other so-called GFR non-determinants, the most important being thyroid function, inflammation, and obesity.[79] Because of few interactions with muscular mass, cystatin C is potentially of interest in the oncologic population. However, data with this biomarker in such a population are few, lack a reference method for measuring GFR, and/or include too few patients.[77,80,81] Chew-Harris et al. compared creatinine CKD-EPI and combined CKD-EPI equations including both creatinine and cystatin C with mGFR by 99Tc-Diethylenetriaminepenta-acetic acid (DTPA) in 80 cancer patients. They showed that the CKD-EPI combined equation (but not the equation based on cystatin C only) was slightly better than the creatinine-based CKD-EPI equation (accuracy within 30% of 83% vs. 78%).[58] Among the studies we have discussed earlier, Hingorani et al. also considered both cystatin C-based and combined equations. At baseline, only the combined equation showed a slightly better accuracy within 30% (at 89%) compared to creatinine-based equations.[43] Because cystatin C is constantly produced by all nucleated cells, there is also the theoretical possibility that cancer cells produced cystatin C with an increase in cystatin C concentrations without any change in GFR values.[26] However, too few data are available to close the debate.

In oncology, drug dosage adjustment is thus influenced by the choice of the creatinine-based equation, as discussed in the prior paragraph. However, because any eGFR is far from perfect, there is a risk that all equations are inadequate for drug adjustment. A definitive conclusion could only be given by a prospective observational randomized study, where patients would get chemotherapy dosage according to mGFR in one group, and to different eGFR equations in other groups. Efficacy, cancer recurrence, and safety of the chemotherapy could then be compared between the different groups. However, such a study is not available. We have only retrospective data where the dosage of the chemotherapy (calculated with the Calvert formula) obtained with mGFR is compared, by retrospective simulations, with dosage that would have been used if eGFR had been considered instead of mGFR. Several studies performed such an analysis in oncologic patients and all these studies suggest that eGFR (whatever the equation) can lead to significant different dosage than the dosage based on mGFR effectively given to the patient.[49,50,54-56,58] Ainsworth et al. showed data obtained from 660 cancer patients treated by carboplatin. GFR was measured by ^{51}Cr-EDTA. A significant different dose (defined as a difference larger than 20%) was observed in 22% and 32% of cases for CG and MDRD, respectively.[49] In the same type of patients, Craig et al. observed in their 175 subjects that eGFR would have led to a higher dose (> 20%) in 26%, 30%, and 36% of patients with CG, MDRD, and CKD-EPI, respectively.[50] Dooley et al. measured GFR with ^{99}Tc-DTPA in 455 patients treated by carboplatin. They showed a potential discordant dose in 36%, 33%, and 29% of cases for CG, MDRD, and CKD-EPI, respectively, with a high proportion of underdosing with eGFR.[54] Shepherd et al. and Cathomas et al. both studied young patients with seminoma and treated by carboplatin. Both also used the Calvert equation for the dosage adjustment and the dose was determined with GFR measured by ^{51}Cr-EDTA (mixed with ^{99}Tc-DTPA in the Cathomas study).[55,56] Shepherd, in his simulation including 115 patients, showed that, if an error of 20% was considered in the drug dosage, such a difference would have been observed in 33% of patients with (nonindexed) CG (only 1% of underdosing, the rest being overdosing), in 22% with indexed CG (50/50 underdosing and overdosing), 28% with CKD-EPI (6% overdosing and 22% underdosing), and 14% with de-indexed CKD-EPI (11% overdosing and 3% underdosing). If an error of 10% was considered as relevant, the same dose between mGFR and all eGFR equations would have be given in less than 50% of patients.[55] In the Cathomas study, 426 patients were included. A significant overdosing was considered if the difference was over 125% and an underdosing if the difference was less than 90%. Overdosing prevalence would have been 7% and 1% in CG (nonindexed) and CKD-EPI (de-indexed), respectively. Underdosing would have reached 18% and 41%, respectively.[56] Again, all these studies are simulations, but they share the similar key message: using eGFR instead of mGFR for drug dosage adjustment of cis- or carboplatin

would lead to significant different doses. Overdosing can potentially lead to more secondary effects, and thus concerns with safety and underdosing would lead to a significant higher risk of disease recurrence, which is relevant, for example, in young patients treated for seminoma. From these studies, it remains, however, difficult to definitively assert that one equation will lead to overdosing and that another will underdose, because studies are different in their methodologies (different equation considered, serum creatinine IDMS traceable or not, results indexed by BSA or not, use of actual weight or ideal weight in the CG, etc.) and in their populations. If the debate still exists between different eGFR equations for drug adaptation until now, the solution could be, at least in part, in simplified protocols that used measured GFR and reference methods. For this option, it seems that iohexol plasma clearance is certainly the best balance between feasibility and physiology.[82] Of interest, the EMA is now recommending that the manufacturer performs studies with mGFR (and not eGFR) for new therapies that require a dose adjustment according to CKD staging.

Conclusions

Patients with cancer are at high risk of acute or chronic renal failure. Therefore the most exact estimation of GFR is required. Because of the frequently observed anthropometrical characteristics of oncologic patients (declining muscular mass), serum creatinine and thus creatinine-based equations are frequently inaccurate, leading to over- or underdosing of drugs. There is still a debate in the literature about the best creatinine-based equation to be used for drug dosage adjustment. Having said that, there is indirect proof that all equations could be misleading, and some authors argue for using mGFR to adjust drug dosage in cancer patients. No randomized prospective study strongly supports the necessity of mGFR in oncology. However, based on the available literature, we and others would recommend considering mGFR for drug dosage adjustment at least in case of chemotherapy with a potentially nephrotoxic drug and with a narrow therapeutic index, the best example being cis- or carboplatin. In other cases, different eGFR equations can be used and the doctor can calculate the absolute and relative difference between the two equations, flagging up discordant cases (difference of > 10 mL/min or > 10%). If results are concordant, the clinician can reasonably apply drug dosage recommendations available in the literature. If discrepancies occur, it would be important to consider the characteristics of the patients and the safety profile of the drug considered. For highly effective concentration-dependent drugs, the risk of underdosage (and thus risk of cancer recurrence) could be as important as the risk of overdosage, especially if the risk of nephrotoxicity is relatively low. In such cases, it could be more efficient to consider the equation that gives the higher GFR results. Conversely, it could be better to recommend adjusting the dosage of a drug to the equation giving the lower result if the prescription concerns potentially nephrotoxic drugs.[7,66]

Key Points

1. Measuring kidney function is important in patients with cancer to allow appropriate drug dosing and monitoring for development of acute and chronic kidney disease.
2. Serum creatinine is the most widely used test to estimate kidney function despite its limitations.
3. A number of formulae (CKD-EPI, MDRD, CG, etc.) are used to estimate glomerular filtration rate (eGFR), all that have limitations in the individuals studied (because of age, muscle mass, etc).
4. Cystatin C plus creatinine has also been used to calculate eGFR; however, the data are limited at this time, making it premature to draw a conclusion.
5. Measuring GFR (^{99}Tc-DTPA, ^{51}Cr-EDTA, iohexol plasma clearance, etc.) is more cumbersome but is likely the best test to use, when dosing chemotherapeutic agents that are potentially nephrotoxic and have a narrow therapeutic window.

References

1. Izzedine H, Perazella MA. Anticancer drug-induced acute kidney injury. *Kidney Int Rep*. 2017;2:504-514.
2. Malyszko J, Kozlowska K, Kozlowski L, Malyszko J. Nephrotoxicity of anticancer treatment. *Nephrol Dial Transplant*. 2017;32:924-936.
3. Dreisbach AW, Flessner MF. Drug metabolism and chronic kidney disease. In: Kimmel PL, Rosenberg MK, eds. *Chronic Renal Disease*. 1st ed. Elsevier; 2014: 674-681.
4. Verbeeck RK, Musuamba FT. Pharmacokinetics and dosage adjustment in patients with renal dysfunction. *Eur J Clin Pharmacol*. 2009;65:757-773.
7. Delanaye P, Guerber F, Scheen A, et al. Discrepancies between the Cockcroft-Gault and chronic kidney disease epidemiology (CKD-EPI) equations: implications for refining drug dosage adjustment strategies. *Clin Pharmacokinet*. 2017;56:193-205.
9. Park EJ, Wu K, Mi Z, et al. A systematic comparison of Cockcroft-Gault and modification of diet in renal disease equations for classification of kidney dysfunction and dosage adjustment. *Ann Pharmacother*. 2012;46:1174-1187.
10. Bouquegneau A, Vidal-Petiot E, Moranne O, et al. Creatinine-based equations for the adjustment of drug dosage in an obese population. *Br J Clin Pharmacol*. 2016;81:349-361.
13. von Liebig J. Kreatin und kreatinin, bestandtheile des harns der menschen. *Journal für Praktiche Chemie*. 1847;40:288-292.
14. Perrone RD, Madias NE, Levey AS. Serum creatinine as an index of renal function: new insights into old concepts. *Clin Chem*. 1992;38:1933-1953.
15. Delanaye P, Cavalier E, Pottel H. Serum creatinine: not so simple!. *Nephron*. 2017;136:302-308.
17. Panteghini M. Enzymatic assays for creatinine: time for action. *Scand J Lab Invest Suppl*. 2008;241:84-88.
19. Piéroni L, Delanaye P, Boutten A, et al. A multicentric evaluation of IDMS-traceable creatinine enzymatic assays. *Clin Chim Acta*. 2011;412:2070-2075.
20. Delanaye P, Cohen EP. Formula-based estimates of the GFR: equations variable and uncertain. *Nephron Clin Pract*. 2008;110:c48-53.
21. Heymsfield SB, Arteaga C, McManus C, Smith J, Moffitt S. Measurement of muscle mass in humans: validity of the 24-hour urinary creatinine method. *Am J Clin Nutr*. 1983;37:478-494.
22. Delanaye P, Cavalier E, Radermecker RP, et al. Estimation of GFR by different creatinine- and cystatin-C-based equations in anorexia nervosa. *Clin Nephrol*. 2009;71:482-491.
25. Soveri I, Berg UB, Björk J, et al. Measuring GFR: a systematic review. *Am J Kidney Dis*. 2014;64:411-424.
27. Cockcroft DW, Gault MH. Prediction of creatinine clearance from serum creatinine. *Nephron*. 1976;16:31-41.
28. Levey AS, Bosch JP, Lewis JB, Greene T, Rogers N, Roth D. A more accurate method to estimate glomerular filtration rate from serum creatinine: a new prediction equation. Modification of Diet in Renal Disease Study Group. *Ann Intern Med*. 1999;130:461-470.
29. Levey AS, Stevens LA, Schmid CH, et al. A new equation to estimate glomerular filtration rate. *Ann Intern Med*. 2009;150:604-612.
30. Pottel H, Hoste L, Dubourg L, et al. A new estimating glomerular filtration rate equation for the full age spectrum. *Nephrol Dial Transplant*. 2016;31:798-806.
31. Bjork J, Grubb A, Sterner G, Nyman U. Revised equations for estimating glomerular filtration rate based on the Lund-Malmö Study cohort. *Scand J Clin Lab Invest*. 2011;71:232-239.
32. Froissart M, Rossert J, Jacquot C, Paillard M, Houillier P. Predictive performance of the modification of diet in renal disease and Cockcroft-Gault equations for estimating renal function. *J Am Soc Nephrol*. 2005;16:763-773.
33. Levey AS, Stevens LA, Hostetter T. Automatic reporting of estimated glomerular filtration rate–just what the doctor ordered. *Clin Chem*. 2006;52:2188-2193.
37. Delanaye P, Mariat C. The applicability of eGFR equations to different populations. *Nat Rev Nephrol*. 2013;9:513-522.
39. Redal-Baigorri B, Stokholm KH, Rasmussen K, Jeppesen N. Estimation of kidney function in cancer patients. *Dan Med Bull*. 2011;58:A4236.
40. Lauritsen J, Gundgaard MG, Mortensen MS, Oturai PS, Feldt-Rasmussen B, Daugaard G. Reliability of estimated glomerular filtration rate in patients treated with platinum containing therapy. *Int J Cancer*. 2014;135:1733-1739.
41. Funakoshi Y, Fujiwara Y, Kiyota N, et al. Validity of new methods to evaluate renal function in cancer patients treated with cisplatin. *Cancer Chemother Pharmacol*. 2016;77:281-288.
42. Lindberg L, Brødbæk K, Hägerström EG, Bentzen J, Kristensen B, Zerahn B. Comparison of methods for estimating glomerular filtration rate in head and neck cancer patients treated with cisplatin. *Scand J Clin Lab Invest*. 2017;77:237-246.
43. Hingorani S, Pao E, Schoch G, Gooley T, Schwartz GJ. Estimating GFR in adult patients with hematopoietic cell transplant: comparison of estimating equations with an iohexol reference standard. *Clin J Am Soc Nephrol*. 2015;10:601-610.
45. Delanaye P, Krzesinski, JM. Indexing of renal function parameters by body surface area: intelligence or folly? *Nephron Clin Pract*. 2011;119:c289-c292.
49. Ainsworth NL, Marshall A, Hatcher H, Whitehead L, Whitfield GA, Earl HM. Evaluation of glomerular filtration rate estimation by Cockcroft-Gault, Jelliffe, Wright and Modification of Diet in Renal Disease (MDRD) formulae in oncology patients. *Ann Oncol*. 2012;23:1845-1853.
50. Craig AJ, Samol J, Heenan SD, Irwin AG, Britten A. Overestimation of carboplatin doses is avoided by radionuclide GFR measurement. *Br J Cancer*. 2012;107:1310-1316.
51. Hartlev LB, Boeje CR, Bluhme H, Palshof T, Rehling M. Monitoring renal function during chemotherapy. *Eur J Nucl Med Mol Imaging*. 2012;39:1478-1482.
54. Dooley MJ, Poole SG, Rischin D. Dosing of cytotoxic chemotherapy: impact of renal function estimates on dose. *Ann Oncol*. 2013;24:2746-2752.
55. Shepherd ST, Gillen G, Morrison P, et al. Performance of formulae based estimates of glomerular filtration rate for carboplatin dosing in stage 1 seminoma. *Eur J Cancer*. 2014;50:944-952.
56. Cathomas R, Klingbiel D, Geldart TR, et al. Relevant risk of carboplatin underdosing in cancer patients with normal renal function using estimated GFR: lessons from a stage I seminoma cohort. *Ann Oncol*. 2014;25:1591-1597.
57. Bennis Y, Savry A, Rocca M, Gauthier-Villano L, Pisano P, Pourroy B. Cisplatin dose adjustment in patients with renal impairment, which recommendations should we follow? *Int J Clin Pharm*. 2014;36:420-429.
59. Shord SS, Bressler LR, Radhakrishnan L, Chen N, Villano JL. Evaluation of the modified diet in renal disease equation for calculation of carboplatin dose. *Ann Pharmacother*. 2009;43:235-241.
64. Matzke GR, Aronoff GR, Atkinson, Jr., et al. Drug dosing consideration in patients with acute and chronic kidney disease—a clinical update from Kidney Disease: Improving Global Outcomes (KDIGO). *Kidney Int*. 2011;80:1122-1137.

66. Nyman HA, Dowling TC, Hudson JQ, Peter WL, Joy MS, Nolin TD. Comparative evaluation of the Cockcroft-Gault equation and the modification of diet in renal disease (MDRD) study equation for drug dosing: an opinion of the Nephrology Practice and Research Network of the American College of Clinical Pharmacy. *Pharmacother.* 2011;31:1130-1144.

69. Hijazi Z, Hohnloser SH, Oldgren J, et al. Efficacy and safety of dabigatran compared with warfarin in relation to baseline renal function in patients with atrial fibrillation: a RE-LY (Randomized Evaluation of Long-term Anticoagulation Therapy) trial analysis. *Circulation.* 2014;129:961-970.

71. Schaeffner ES, Ebert N, Delanaye P, et al. Two novel equations to estimate kidney function in persons aged 70 years or older. *Ann Intern Med.* 2012;157:471-481.

74. Pottel H, Delanaye P, Schaeffner EE, et al. Estimating glomerular filtration rate for the full age spectrum from serum creatinine and cystatin C. *Nephrol Dial Transplant.* 2017;32:497-507.

75. Inker LA, Schmid CH, Tighiouart H, et al. Estimating glomerular filtration rate from serum creatinine and cystatin C. *N Engl J Med.* 2012;367:20-29.

77. Bretagne M, Jouinot A, Durand JP, et al. Estimation of glomerular filtration rate in cancer patients with abnormal body composition and relation with carboplatin toxicity. *Cancer Chemother Pharmacol.* 2017;80:45-53.

78. Macdonald J, Marcora S, Jibani M, et al. GFR estimation using cystatin C is not independent of body composition. *Am J Kidney Dis.* 2006;48:712-719.

80. Cavalcanti E, Barchiesi V, Cerasuolo D, et al. Correlation of serum cystatin c with glomerular filtration rate in patients receiving platinum-based chemotherapy. *Anal Cell Pathol (Amst).* 2016;2016: 4918325.

81. Schmitt A, Gladieff L, Lansiaux A, et al. A universal formula based on cystatin c to perform individual dosing of carboplatin in normal weight, underweight, and obese patients. *Clin Cancer Res.* 2009; 15:3633-3639.

82. Delanaye P, Ebert N, Melsom T, et al. Iohexol plasma clearance for measuring glomerular filtration rate in clinical practice and research : a review. Part 1: How to measure glomerular filtration rate with iohexol ? *Clin Kidney J.* 2016;9:682-699.

A full list of references is available at Expertconsult.com

2 *Dysnatremias in Cancer*

UMUT SELAMET AND ALA ABUDAYYEH

Hyponatremia

HYPONATREMIA AND CANCER RELATIONSHIP

Hyponatremia is the most common electrolyte abnormality observed in cancer patients. In a retrospective cohort study from a comprehensive cancer center, hyponatremia (serum $Na^+ < 137$ mEq/L) was noted in 47% of hospitalized cancer patients [VO2].[1] In general, hyponatremia is categorized as mild (130–134 mEq/L), moderate (120–129 mEq/L), and severe (< 120 mEq/L), according to serum sodium concentrations.[2] Hyponatremia has been linked to poor prognosis in several types of cancers, which include non-small cell lung cancer, pleural mesothelioma, renal cell carcinoma, gastrointestinal cancer, and lymphoma.[3,4] The risk of mortality increases with more severe hyponatremia.[5] Moreover, low serum sodium concentrations have also been associated with poorer performance status in lung cancer patients.[6] In addition, timely and effective corrections of serum sodium concentrations have been associated with improvement in prognosis for several cancers.[7,8]

SYMPTOMS

Symptoms of hyponatremia are caused primarily by osmotic swelling of brain cells and increased intracranial pressure (ICP).[9] Severity of symptoms usually correlates with the degree of hyponatremia. Most patients with mild to moderate hyponatremia are asymptomatic. Severe hyponatremia, on the other hand, may cause nausea, vomiting, confusion, falls, movement disorders, seizures, and coma. Time course of the development of hyponatremia is another significant factor that determines the severity of symptoms. Chronic hyponatremia (onset > 48 hours) can be asymptomatic whereas acute hyponatremia can manifest as encephalopathy, especially in patients with malnutrition, hypokalemia, alcoholism, or advanced liver disease.[10]

PATHOPHYSIOLOGY

Hyponatremia is the result of imbalance between salt and water concentrations with relatively more total body water (TBW) than salt. Normal kidneys can eliminate up to 20 to 30 L of free water daily.[11] Antidiuretic hormone (ADH) also known as *arginine vasopressin (AVP)* is the major hormone that regulates free water reabsorption by kidney tubules. ADH is a peptide hormone produced by the hypothalamus and transported to the posterior pituitary via nerve axons. It is released into the circulation from the posterior pituitary and binds to V2 receptors at the basolateral side of the collecting tubules in the kidney. Binding of ADH to V2 receptor activates adenylate cyclase and subsequent formation of cyclic adenosine monophosphate (cAMP). This leads to movement and fusion of specific vesicles that contain aquaporin 2 (AQ2) channels in the cytoplasm to the apical membrane of the collecting tubules. Once AQ2 channels are inserted, the apical membrane becomes permeable to water. Water moves from medullary renal space to the apical membrane and is then released into the circulation through the basolateral membrane (Fig. 2.1). ADH release is stimulated by two mechanisms: osmotic and nonosmotic factors. The osmotic regulation of ADH occurs in the anterior hypothalamus as "osmoreceptor cells or osmostat" sense changes in extracellular fluid (ECF) osmolality. This is a tightly controlled system as an increase or decrease in ECF osmolality by 1% stimulates or suppresses ADH release respectively. Nonosmotic stimulation of ADH release occurs in the absence of changes in serum osmolality. Pain, emotional stress, nausea, and reduction in effective arterial blood volume (EABV) are some of the examples of nonosmotic stimuli, which tend to be very common in patients with cancer and those under treatment with various cancer therapies.

APPROACH TO ETIOLOGY OF HYPONATREMIA

Hyponatremia typically develops when there is disruption in the elimination of free water by kidneys, or when water shifts from the intracellular to extracellular space, both of which result in the dilution of extracellular sodium concentration. Several algorithms are considered acceptable when evaluating a patient with hyponatremia. The most commonly used algorithm incorporates both serum osmolality and urine sodium concentrations. We have adopted this approach for specific causes of hyponatremia in cancer patients (Fig. 2.2).

The first step in a patient with hyponatremia is to check serum osmolality. Serum osmolality is normally tightly maintained between 280 to 290 mOsm/L. Using this range, hyponatremia can be classified as hyper-osmolar, iso-osmolar, and hypo-osmolar hyponatremia.

Hyper-Osmolar Hyponatremia

If serum osmolality increases because of an effective osmole other than sodium, then hyper-osmolar hyponatremia develops as the effective osmole causes water shift from intracellular to extracellular space. The most common example of this kind of hyponatremia is caused by hyperglycemia. For each 100 mg/dL increase in plasma glucose, above 150 mg/dL 1.6 to 2.4 mEq/L decrease is observed in serum sodium concentration.[12] Hyperglycemia over time can also stimulate thirst and ADH secretion by causing low EABV secondary to osmotic diuresis.[13]

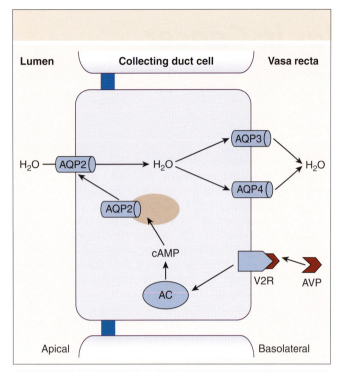

Fig. 2.1 Mechanism of action of arginine vasopressin (AVP) on the collecting tubule. Binding of AVP (aka ADH) to the V2 receptor (V2R) on the basolateral membrane of the collecting duct activates adenylate cyclase (AC) to generate cyclic adenosine monophosphate (cAMP). cAMP signaling induces fusion of intracellular vesicles that contain aquaporin 2 (AQ2) channels into the apical membrane of the collecting tubules. Once AQ2 channels are inserted, the apical membrane becomes permeable to water. Water moves from medullary renal space to intracellular space through AQ2 channels on the apical membrane and is released into the circulation through AQ3 and AQ4 channels located on the basolateral membrane.

Hypertonic mannitol infusion, which is used in the treatment of cerebral edema, or sucrose/maltose carrier used in intravenous immunoglobulin infusions can also increase serum osmolality and subsequent movement of water from intracellular to extracellular space.[14]

Iso-Osmolar Hyponatremia

Hyponatremia in the setting of normal serum osmolality is called *pseudohyponatremia*. Pseudohyponatremia is caused by circulating excessive proteins or lipids, which reduce the water fraction of the serum.[15] Because sodium is restricted to the water phase of the serum, laboratory methods that measure the sodium concentration per unit of total serum give falsely low measurement. However, analyzers that directly measure the sodium concentration or activity in the water phase of serum are not affected by this error. This measurement technique avoids dilution steps and is called *direct potentiometry*. Pseudohyponatremia in cancer patients can be seen with plasma cell dyscrasias (i.e., multiple myeloma, Waldenstrom macroglobulinemia) because of excessive paraproteins or in obstructive jaundice because of increased amount of abnormal lipoprotein, Lipoprotein X.

Another example of iso-osmolar hyponatremia is the use of glycine or sorbitol during hysteroscopy, transurethral resection of the prostate or laparoscopic surgeries as these isosmotic solutions may get systemically absorbed and cause the dilution of the extracellular sodium without changing the serum osmolality.[16]

Hypo-Osmolar Hyponatremia

When serum osmolality is low, ADH release and subsequent hyponatremia can occur through nonosmotic stimuli of ADH. As reduction in EABV is one of the most common reasons of nonosmotic stimuli of ADH, evaluation of hypo-osmolar hyponatremia mandates assessment of volume status to differentiate the underlying causes. This type of hyponatremia can be further classified as *hypervolemic, euvolemic,* and *hypovolemic.*

Hypovolemic Hypo-Osmolar Hyponatremia

Hypovolemic hypo-osmolar hyponatremia is characterized by both TBW and solute loss resulting in low EABV and nonosmotic stimuli of ADH. Solute loss could either be through kidneys or via gastrointestinal tract. Because of low EABV, the renin-angiotensin-aldosterone system is activated and urine sodium (UNa^+) of 20 mEq/L or less is observed as aldosterone mediates renal tubular reabsorption of sodium, to maintain tissue perfusion. However, in the cases of renal solute wasting, UNa^+ is expectedly greater than 20 mEq/L.

In cancer patients, vomiting and diarrhea resulting from chemotherapy are the main causes of gastrointestinal solute loss. On the other hand, renal salt wasting is a well-defined toxicity of platinum-based chemotherapy, especially, cisplatin.[17] Other medications used by cancer patients include loop and thiazide diuretics, which can also cause renal sodium loss.

Another rare cause of hypovolemic hypo-osmolar hyponatremia is an entity described as *cerebral salt wasting (CSW)* syndrome. This is typically seen in patients with central nervous system (CNS) disease, particularly subarachnoid hemorrhage, less commonly CNS metastases. First described by Peters et al. in 1950, CWS syndrome is defined by the development of extracellular volume depletion caused by a renal tubular sodium transport abnormality in patients with intracranial disease and normal adrenal and thyroid functions.[18] CWS has similar features to the syndrome of inappropriate antidiuretic hormone secretion (SIADH) with high urine osmolality and high urine sodium concentration ($UNa^+ > 20$ mEq/L), but the main distinction lies in the volume status: SIADH is characterized by euvolemia, whereas CSW syndrome is a hypovolemic state. Two postulated mechanisms for CSW syndrome are the excess secretion of natriuretic peptides and the loss of sympathetic stimulation to the kidney.[19] It is important to differentiate CSW syndrome from SIADH as treatment of these two conditions is completely different. Treatment of choice for SIADH is free water restriction, whereas it is isotonic fluid replacement in CSW syndrome. Fractional uric acid excretion (FE_{UA}) is one marker suggested to differentiate between CSW and SIADH. Initially, both conditions are associated with a low serum uric acid level and a high fractional excretion of uric acid. However, correction of hyponatremia normalizes FE_{UA} to less than 10% in SIADH but not in CSW syndrome.[19] Also patients with CSW may be hypotensive and orthostatic, whereas patients with SIADH are euvolemic and likely normotensive.

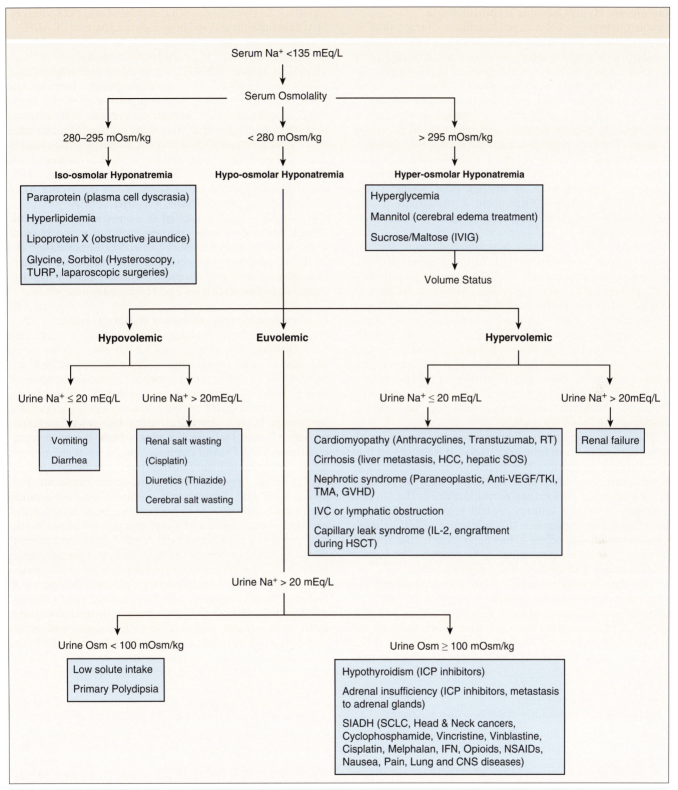

Fig. 2.2 Algorithm for diagnosis of hyponatremia in cancer patients. *CNS,* Central nervous disease; *GVHD,* graft-versus-host disease; *HCC,* hepatocellular carcinoma; *HSCT,* hematopoietic stem cell transplant; *ICP,* immune checkpoint; *IFN,* Interferon; *IL-2,* Interleukin 2; *IVC,* inferior vena cava; *IVIG,* intravenous immunoglobulin; *Na:* sodium; *NSAIDs,* nonsteroidal antiinflammatory drugs; *RT,* radiation therapy; *SCLC,* small cell lung cancer; *SIADH,* syndrome of inappropriate antidiuretic hormone secretion; *SOS,* sinusoidal obstruction syndrome; *TKI,* tyrosine kinase inhibitor; *TMA,* thrombotic microangiopathy; *TURP,* transurethral resection of the prostate, *VEGF,* vascular endothelial factor.

Euvolemic Hypo-Osmolar Hyponatremia

Euvolemic hypo-osmolar hyponatremia is characterized by relatively more TBW than salt. This can be caused by three conditions: low solute intake, increased water intake or diminished water excretion. In euvolemic hypo-osmolar hyponatremia, because EABV is normal to slightly expanded, renin-angiotensin-aldosterone system is suppressed, and so the UNa^+ is always greater than 20 mEq/L. Low solute or salt intake in cancer patients is usually caused by loss of appetite. Primary polydipsia seen in psychogenic disorders is an example of relatively more water intake compared with salt. Because ADH stimulation is not the primary cause of hyponatremia in neither poor solute intake nor primary polydipsia, the urine is maximally diluted in the absence of ADH, and urine osmolality is less than 100 mOsm/kg.

Euvolemic hypo-osmolar hyponatremia can also develop because of excessive ADH. In the presence of ADH, urine cannot be maximally diluted and urine osmolality is 100 mOsm/kg or more. Excessive ADH can be seen in certain endocrinopathies, such as adrenal insufficiency or hypothyroidism. Adrenal insufficiency increases corticotropin-releasing hormone (CRH) mediated secretion of ADH as the inhibitory feedback on CRH by cortisol diminishes.[20] Adrenal insufficiency occurs in cancer patients because of metastatic infiltration of adrenal glands or because of toxicity of cancer drugs, such as seen with immune checkpoint inhibitors promoting an immune response–mediated adrenalitis.

The exact mechanism of hyponatremia observed with hypothyroidism is not fully understood. It is suggested that hypothyroidism induces hyponatremia by impairment of water excretion either by increasing release of ADH or by reduction in glomerular filtration rate.[21] The thyroid hormone normally inhibits central release of ADH, so hypothyroidism diminishes this inhibitory effect. In addition, in an animal study, it has been shown that thyroid hormone deficiency potentiates ADH effect on the kidney tubules by upregulation of AQ2 receptors.[22]

The most common cause of euvolemic hypo-osmolar hyponatremia in a cancer patient is the SIADH. Table 2.1 summarizes common causes of SIADH in cancer patients. SIADH is more frequent in solid tumors, such as small cell lung cancer (SCLC) and head and neck cancers, but it has been associated with many types of malignancies in case reports.[23] In the cases of SCLC and head and neck cancers, SIADH is actually caused by ectopic production of ADH.

Some of the cancer drugs, such as cyclophosphamide and the vinca alkaloids (vincristine, vinblastine) are well known to induce SIADH.[24] These drugs show neurotoxic effects on the paraventricular and supraoptic neurons and alter the normal osmoreceptor control of vasopressin secretion.[25] Cisplatin on the other hand can cause hyponatremia by both potentiating the effect ADH on the kidney tubules and causing renal salt wasting.[17] Cancer patients also frequently use palliative medications, such as antidepressants, antiemetics, opioids, and nonsteroidal antiinflammatory medications that can either stimulate or potentiate ADH, causing a drug-induced form of SIADH.

ADH can also be produced in excess with nonosmotic stimuli because of pain, nausea, infiltrative processes of CNS and lungs with metastasis, infection, or bleeding.[26] All of these conditions are common comorbidities in cancer patients and are likely the most frequent cause of hyponatremia in patients with an underlying malignancy.

Hypervolemic Hypo-Osmolar Hyponatremia

Hypervolemic hypo-osmolar hyponatremia results from both TBW and salt increase, which usually manifest as an edematous state. Urine sodium (UNa^+) concentration is a helpful tool to differentiate between the various causes of hypervolemic hypo-osmolar hyponatremia. In cancer patients, cirrhosis caused by liver metastasis or hepatocellular carcinoma, hepatic sinusoidal obstruction syndrome (venoocclusive disease) following hematopoietic stem cell transplantation (HSCT), and cardiomyopathy from chemotherapy or radiotherapy cardiotoxicity are common causes of hypervolemic hyponatremia. In addition, nephrotic syndrome seen with a number of paraneoplastic syndromes, graft-versus-host disease or because of cancer drugs as well as inferior vena cava and lymphatic compressions by tumor, capillary leak syndrome seen during engraftment phase of HSCT or because of interleukin-2/chimeric antigen receptor T-cell treatment are other examples of edematous hypervolemic hyponatremia with low effective blood volume. These conditions are characterized with UNa^+ of 20 mEq/L or less as the underlying process causing low EABV is the major stimulus for ADH release and renin-angiotensin-aldosterone system stimulation. On the other hand, kidney failure can impair tubular dilution of the

Table 2.1   Common Causes of SIADH in Cancer Patients

Cancers	SCLC, NSCLC, head & neck cancers, breast cancer, mesothelioma, lymphoma, Ewing sarcoma, thymoma, gastrointestinal cancers, urothelial cancers, renal cell carcinoma, prostate cancer, endometrial cancer
Chemotherapy	Vincristine, vinblastine, cyclophosphamide, ifosfamide, cisplatin, melphalan, interferon
Nonchemotherapy drugs	Vasopressin, desmopressin, opiates, SSRIs, TCAs, chlorpropamide, clofibrate, meperidine, barbiturates, carbamazepine, amiodarone, NSAIDs, ACE inhibitors, dopamine agonists, ecstasy
CNS diseases	Infections, mass, bleeding, trauma
Pulmonary diseases	Infections, mass, bleeding, positive pressure intubation, asthma, COPD
Miscellaneous	Pain, nausea

ACE, Angiotensin-converting enzyme; *CNS*, central nervous system; *COPD*, chronic obstructive pulmonary disease; *NSAIDs*, nonsteroidal antiinflammatory drugs; *NSCLC*, non-small cell lung cancer; *SCLC*, small cell lung cancer; *SIADH*, syndrome of inappropriate antidiuretic hormone secretion; *SSRIs*, selective serotonin reuptake inhibitors; *TCAs*, tricyclic antidepressants.

urine and yield hypervolemic hyponatremia. In this case, UNa^+ concentration remains greater than 20 mEq/L.

TREATMENT OF HYPONATREMIA

Treatment of hyponatremia in the cancer patient depends on the etiology, severity, and presence or absence of symptoms. Hyponatremia symptoms develop mainly because of ICP from brain edema. When serum sodium concentration and therefore serum osmolality drops, water shifts from extracellular space to relatively hyperosmolar intracellular space of brain cells. Swelling of brain cells increases intracranial pressure as the skull is a nonexpanding cavity. Increases in intracranial pressure can lead to nausea, vomiting, confusion, ataxia, movement disturbances, seizures, respiratory failure and/or coma. Brain cells quickly adapt to surrounding hypotonicity and extrude solutes, such as sodium, potassium, and chloride in the first couple of hours. This is followed by brain cell extrusion of organic osmoles, such as glutamate, creatinine, and myoinositol to prevent brain edema.[27] Adaptation is usually complete within 48 hours. If hyponatremia persists for more than 48 hours, it is defined as *chronic hyponatremia*, which mandates different therapy than "acute hyponatremia". Rapid correction of chronic hyponatremia results in a life-threatening condition called *osmotic demyelination syndrome* (*ODS*). ODS occurs because regeneration of intracellular organic osmoles takes longer than the correction of extracellular hypo-osmolarity, resulting in further water shift from brain cells and subsequent cell shrinkage and myelin breakdown.[28] It is now common practice to limit the rate of correction of chronic hyponatremia to less than 8 mEq/L in any 24-hour period.[29] This limit is further decreased to 6 mEq/L in 24 hours for patients at high risk of osmotic demyelination.[29] ODS risk is higher in patients with severe hyponatremia (serum $Na^+ \leq 105$ mEq/L), malnutrition, hypokalemia, alcoholism, or advanced liver disease.[29]

In contrast, acute symptomatic hyponatremia (onset < 48 hours) requires immediate correction with much less concern for ODS. Acute hyponatremia in the cancer patient may be seen occasionally following various surgical procedures. Patients during the postoperative period typically have increased ADH activity caused by multiple factors, such as pain, nausea, narcotics, and nonsteroidal antiinflammatory drugs.[13] Nothing per oral status and use of hypotonic intravenous infusions also significantly contribute to hyponatremia during this time.[13] Patients with acute hyponatremia and symptoms of ICP should be treated with a 100-mL bolus of 3% hypertonic saline, followed by up to two additional 100-mL doses (total dose of 300 mL) if symptoms persist over the course of 30 minutes.[29]

Treatment options for chronic hyponatremia in cancer patients vary depending on the etiology. The initial step for deciding on the treatment choice is to evaluate serum osmolality. Hyperosmolar hyponatremia treatment is directed toward eliminating the underlying cause. In the case of hyperglycemia, lowering blood sugar, and in other cases eliminating the hyper-osmolar solute, such as mannitol, sucrose, or maltose corrects hyponatremia. Iso-osmolar hyponatremia, seen in those with plasma dyscrasias, caused by paraproteins, or in obstructive jaundice, caused by Lipoprotein X, does not warrant any specific treatment, as this is pseudohyponatremia caused by the laboratory method of serum sodium measurement.

On the other hand, hypo-osmolar hyponatremia requires treatment, especially when symptomatic (Fig. 2.3). Severe symptomatic cases should be treated aggressively with 3% hypertonic solution for at least the first couple of hours to prevent neurologic complications. In general, 1 mEq/L per hour of increase in serum sodium concentration is targeted with hypertonic saline until symptoms subside. Increase in serum sodium concentration by 4 to 6 mEq/L has been suggested to be sufficient to improve serious symptoms of hyponatremia.[30] This can be approximated by hourly administration of 3% hypertonic saline in the milliliter amount equal to the patient's weight in kilogram (e.g., for a 70-kg patient, 70 mL/h of 3% hypertonic saline).[31] Another formula that is commonly used to calculate the required amount of hourly hypertonic or isotonic saline infused to correct hyponatremia is called *AndrADHogue-Madias formula*, which estimates the effect of 1 L of sodium infusate on serum sodium concentration with the subsequent calculation:[32]

Change in serum sodium = (Infusate Sodium + Infusate Potassium) − Serum Sodium / (Total Body Water + 1)

These equations, however, reflect serum sodium concentration at one cross-section in time, and recently, Chen and Shey suggested the need of a kinetic equation, which integrates time factor with intakes and urinary output when calculating changes in serum sodium concentration.[33] It is important when using any formula to frequently measure serum sodium concentration and to adjust based on the repeat measurement. When symptoms of hyponatremia subside, the treatment plan can be tailored according to the exact etiology of the hypo-osmolar hyponatremia.

Treatment of Hypovolemic Hypo-Osmolar Hyponatremia

Hypovolemic hypo-osmolar hyponatremia is caused by true circulating blood volume and salt loss. Gastrointestinal Na^+ losses from vomiting and diarrhea, renal Na^+ losses from platinum-based chemotherapy, thiazide diuretics, and cerebral salt wasting syndrome are examples of hypovolemic hypo-osmolar hyponatremia. Treatment aims to increase the EABV using isotonic or hypertonic saline infusion, the latter reserved for severe, symptomatic cases. Isotonic normal saline has a higher sodium concentration (154 mEq/L) than the hyponatremic serum, so it slowly increases serum sodium concentration by about 1 mEq/L for each liter of fluid infused. Once hypovolemia is corrected, nonosmotic ADH stimuli disappear, and the rate of correction of hyponatremia accelerates, as free water excretion by the kidneys begins. To avoid rapid correction and ODS, desmopressin acetate (dDAVP) and/or hypotonic solutions, such as dextrose 5% in water, can be administered to re-lower an excessively rapid correction of serum Na^+.[29]

Treatment of Euvolemic Hypo-Osmolar Hyponatremia

The most common cause of euvolemic hypo-osmolar hyponatremia in cancer patients is SIADH, which is characterized

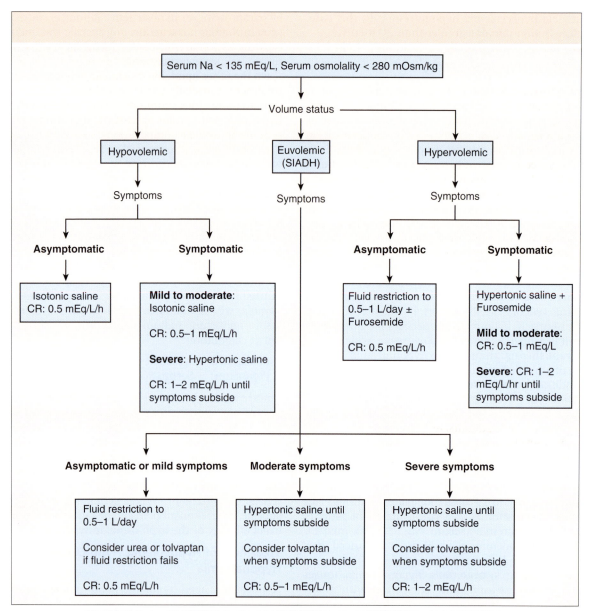

Fig. 2.3 Algorithm for treatment of hypo-osmolar hyponatremia. *CR*, Correction rate; *Na*, sodium.

by increased ADH activity either secondary to augmented production or potentiation of its activity on kidney collecting tubules. The treatment goal in SIADH is to reduce free water in the body. This can be achieved by three ways: restricting free water intake, increasing intake of osmotic solutes to enhance clearance of water, and antagonizing ADH effect on kidney collecting tubules.

Fluid Restriction

Fluid restriction is the first-line therapy for mild to moderate asymptomatic hyponatremia because of SIADH. Fluid restriction includes all fluids consumed per day, not only free water. The main disadvantages of this treatment approach are poor compliance by patients and delayed onset of action. In addition, fluid restriction may not be feasible in patients with active cancer because of required infusion

treatments with chemotherapy. Even normal saline infusion in the patient with SIADH will exacerbate hyponatremia. Furst et al. developed a formula to predict patients who would respond to fluid restriction.[34] This formula evaluates the ratio of urine electrolytes to serum electrolytes (urine sodium + urine potassium/serum sodium). If the ratio is less than 0.5, then fluid restriction can be limited to 1000 mL/day, whereas if the ratio is between 0.5 to 1, fluid restriction needs to be limited to only 500 mL/day. Patients with ratio of 1 or more will not respond to fluid restriction.

Loop diuretics (often with salt tablets) are also shown to be effective in the treatment of SIADH, as they can increase free water excretion by inhibiting medullary concentration ability of the kidneys and replacing renal sodium losses. However, they are not useful in long-term treatment of

SIADH and mainly are used in acute phase of hyponatremia, especially when there is a concern for development of pulmonary edema with the administration of hypertonic saline.

Intake of Osmotic Solutes

Urea is an inexpensive and safe treatment option advocated in Europe to a greater extent than North America for treatment of SIADH. Urea is freely filtered by the glomerulus and excreted in the urine, acting as an osmotic diuretic. Thirty grams of ingested urea provide an additional 500 mOsmol solute intake obligating about 1.25 L of water excretion if urine excretion is considered to be fixed at 400 mOsmol/L (500/400 = 1.25). Recently, urea has been shown to have comparable efficiency to tolvaptan for correcting hyponatremia in chronic SIADH.[35] The major disadvantage of urea is its bitter taste, which lowers patient compliance. However, urea has now been marketed as Urea-Na, which contains urea with a favorable lime flavor and can be mixed in water or juice. Serum urea concentrations can double during the treatment, but this does not reflect true kidney failure.[29]

Antagonizing Antidiuretic Hormone Effect in the Kidneys

Demeclocycline is a tetracycline derivative that induces nephrogenic diabetes insipidus by inhibiting cAMP.[36] It has been historically used in SIADH, especially when it is resulting from chemotherapy. However, it is not a good option for symptomatic patients, as the effect of demeclocycline requires several days of use.[26] In addition, it is also toxic to the liver and kidneys. Nephrotoxicity can be irreversible in some of the cases.[37]

Selective AVP-receptor antagonists for the V2 receptor in the renal collecting ducts are the newer therapeutic options for hyponatremia caused by SIADH. Tolvaptan is an oral V2 receptor antagonist. The Studies of Ascending Levels of Tolvaptan (SALT-1 and SALT-2) in hyponatremia were multicenter, double-blinded randomized control trials, which evaluated 30-day treatment of patients with either euvolemic of hypervolemic hyponatremia with tolvaptan versus placebo.[38] Subgroup analysis of these studies confirmed efficacy of tolvaptan in treating SIADH. Also Salahudeen et al. published a double-blinded randomized placebo-control clinical trial that showed the efficacy and safety of tolvaptan in correcting hyponatremia caused by SIADH in cancer patients.[39] Experts suggest to start tolvaptan in the inpatient setting, and monitor serum sodium levels closely, 4 to 6 hours after the initial dose, and after 24 and 48 hours of treatment.[29] The initial dose of tolvaptan recommended by the manufacturer is 15 mg per day; however, some authors suggest to start it at 7.5 mg dose, if risk of ODS or overcorrection is high.[40] Also patients receiving tolvaptan should not be on fluid restriction, to avoid overcorrection of hyponatremia. The main disadvantages of tolvaptan is the high cost of the drug and potential liver toxicity.

Treatment of Hypervolemic Hypo-Osmolar Hyponatremia

Hypervolemic hypo-osmolar hyponatremia treatment considerations include concern over the possibility of exacerbating hypervolemia when hypertonic saline is used for hyponatremia in symptomatic cancer patients. Thus the initial treatment choice for symptomatic patients is isotonic solution, with or without loop diuretics, with the goal of increasing serum sodium concentration by 1 to 2 mEq/L per hour, until symptoms subside. Once symptoms abate, free water restriction, with or without loop diuretics, is used with a goal serum concentration increase of less than 0.5 mEq/L/h. In contrast, initial treatment of asymptomatic patients is free water restriction and loop diuretics, depending on the severity of hypervolemia and if the patient is getting other sources of intravenous fluids (i.e., medications).

MANAGEMENT OF OVERCORRECTION OF SERUM SODIUM CONCENTRATION

As previously noted, experts recommend a 6 to 8 mEq/L per day increase in serum sodium concentration in severe hyponatremia to avoid ODS. In acute hyponatremia, this correction is done during the initial 6 hours, whereas for chronic hyponatremia it is done over a 24-hour period. Despite the use of sodium correction formulae, patients may develop an excessive rise in serum sodium concentration (overcorrection), which can lead to ODS. In addition to rate and level of serum sodium increase, the etiology of hyponatremia is also a factor that increases risk of overcorrection. In patients with hypovolemic hyponatremia, very low solute intake, psychogenic polydipsia, thiazide-induced hyponatremia, or hyponatremia arising from cortisol deficiency, the rate of rise in serum sodium concentration can be excessively brisk as the underlying conditions are eliminated. As a result, these patients are at higher risk for ODS, and frequent serum sodium testing should be performed in them. A continuous rise above the permitted correction limit can be slowed down using two different approaches. First, infusion of hypotonic solutions, such as dextrose 5% in water can lower serum sodium concentration. Second, administration of dDAVP may be used to stop aquaresis and further increases in serum sodium concentration.[29] The former approach has the disadvantage of requiring large infusion volumes to keep up with the urinary free water loss. There is growing evidence that dDAVP is efficient and generally safe in preventing overcorrection of serum sodium concentration during hyponatremia treatment.[41] The recommended dose of dDAVP is 2 mcg intravenously up to every 8 hours.[29] Again, frequent serum sodium testing is required to avoid under- or overcorrection.

Hypernatremia

Hypernatremia also occurs in patients with cancer and has been associated with increased incidences of morbidity and mortality both in the intensive care units (ICUs) and in the outpatient settings.[42] Thirty-seven percent of ICU patients can develop hypernatremia during their hospital stay.[43] Hypernatremia has been associated with prolonged hospital stay, ICU stay, and the need for renal replacement therapies.[44] The aforementioned outcomes described with hypernatremia are also applicable to the cancer population. In a large Dutch cohort of 80,571 ICU patients, the incidence of hyponatremia nearly halved (47%–25%, $p < .001$), whereas the incidence of hypernatremia (including severe hypernatremia; sodium > 144 mEq/L) nearly doubled (13%–24%, $p < .001$) over a period of years.[45] A recent study in 19,072 adults noted that community-acquired hypernatremia occurred in 21%, hospital-acquired hypernatremia developed in 25.9%, and hospital-aggravated hypernatremia developed in 11.7%. All of these forms of hypernatremia were associated with increased in-hospital mortality, increased length of stay, and need for discharge to a short-/long-term care facility. Patients with hospital-acquired hypernatremia were also more likely to be hospitalized with pneumonia, heart failure, chronic obstructive pulmonary disease, stroke, and sepsis compared with normonatremic patients. In patients with malignancy, 2.5% of the population were observed to develop hospital acquired hypernatremia, which was higher than community-acquired hypernatremia.[46]

In another study, the impact of hypernatremia on 3446 cancer patients, with at least one serum sodium measurement, was specifically examined and noted that 51.4% were eunatremic, 46.0% hyponatremic, and 2.6% hypernatremic.[47] The majority of hypernatremia (90%) was acquired during the hospital stay. Multivariate analysis demonstrated that hypernatremic had a fivefold higher mortality than eunatremic and over twofold higher than hyponatremic patients. The length of hospital stay in hypernatremic patients was twofold higher than in hyponatremic and fourfold higher than in eunatremic patients. The study also highlighted that hypernatremic cancer patients had more frequent critical care unit stays than the nonhypernatremic patients, and that hypernatremia in hospitalized cancer patients was most often acquired in the hospital. Hypernatremia was also more commonly observed in leukemia patients and patients admitted to HSCT service. The cost generated by hypernatremic

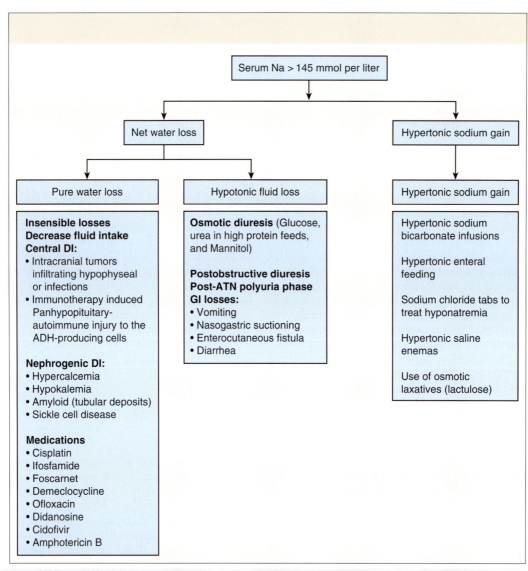

Fig. 2.4 Algorithm for diagnosis of hypernatremia in cancer patients. *ADH*, Antidiuretic hormone; *ATN*, acute tubular necrosis; *DI*, diabetes insipidus; *GI*, gastrointestinal.

patients was also higher (46%) when compared with the eunatremic and hyponatremic patients (37%).[47]

PATHOPHYSIOLOGY

Hypernatremia simply reflects the deficit of water in relation to the body's sodium stores. This can occur with net renal and/or extrarenal water losses or hypertonic sodium loading. The more common etiology would be net water loss, which can be exacerbated by disturbed renal water reabsorption. Sodium loading with intravenous normal saline, along with insensible losses and deficient water intake (hypodipsia, altered sensorium, lack of water access, etc.) occurs more commonly in hospitalized patients requiring various clinical interventions. Hypernatremia is sustained or induced in cancer patients because of insufficient water intake from an impaired thirst mechanism (hypo- or adipsia), altered mental status, and intubation with ventilation or bilevel positive airway pressure. Excessive hypotonic fluid losses occur from chemotherapy and/or malignancy-induced diarrhea, diabetes insipidus induced by chemotherapies, central diabetes insipidus caused by tumor involvement, insensible losses in setting of high fevers, osmotic diuresis in setting of tube feeds, postobstructive diuresis, and the polyuric phase of acute tubular necrosis. When the serum sodium concentration exceeds 160 mEq/L, altered mental status, muscle weakness, confusion, and coma develop and risk other hospital complications. In addition, hypernatremia has been demonstrated to impair cardiac index, insulin-mediated glucose metabolism, hepatic gluconeogenesis, and lactate clearance,[48,49] setting the patient up for worse outcomes. Fig. 2.4 presents an algorithm to assess and diagnose causes of hypernatremia.

MANAGEMENT

Rapid correction of acute hypernatremia (by 1 mEq/L/h) can improve overall prognosis without increasing the risk of cerebral edema, because accumulated electrolytes are rapidly extruded from brain cells.[50] In chronic hypernatremia, reducing the serum sodium concentration at a maximal rate of 0.5 mEq/L per hour prevents cerebral edema and convulsions because the protection afforded by accumulated brain solutes disappears over days.[50]

Summary

Dysnatremias have been studied extensively in cancer population and present a challenge to both oncologist and nephrologist. They have been strongly associated with increased morbidity and mortality. We have presented the common etiologies of dysnatremias that would be applicable to the general population, but also unique ones to cancer patients. Approach to treatment of dysnatremias in cancer patients is similar to our general population, except there is an increase in complexity in setting of severe mucositis and poor oral intake or from or extensive intraabdominal tumor burden that drives increase to ADH. With the algorithms presented, we hope the clinician will be able to address the dysnatremias in cancer patients in a more informed manner, to provide an effective treatment.

Key Points

- The dysnatremias (hyponatremia and hypernatremia) are associated with poor prognosis in cancer patients.
- Hyponatremia in cancer patient is more complex with a more expansive list of etiologies.
- Management of the dysnatremias in the cancer population is similar to noncancer patients, but more challenges are present because of the underlying cancer and its therapy.
- The most common cause of euvolemic hypo-osmolar hyponatremia in a cancer patient is the syndrome of inappropriate antidiuretic hormone secretion (SIADH).
- Use of tolvaptan in hyponatremic cancer patients has been demonstrated to be effective in safely correcting hyponatremia.
- Hypernatremia in cancer patients is caused by both insufficient water intake and excessive hypotonic fluid losses.

References

1. Doshi SM, Shah P, Lei X, Lahoti A, Salahudeen AK. Hyponatremia in hospitalized cancer patients and its impact on clinical outcomes. *Am J Kidney Dis.* 2012;59:222-228.
2. Ghali JK. Mechanisms, risks, and new treatment options for hyponatremia. *Cardiology.* 2008;111:147-157.
3. Ray P, Quantin X, Grenier J, Pujol JL. Predictive factors of tumor response and prognostic factors of survival during lung cancer chemotherapy. *Cancer Detect Prev.* 1998;22:293-304.
4. Kinoshita T, Hotta T, Tobinai K, et al. A randomized controlled trial investigating the survival benefit of dose-intensified multidrug combination chemotherapy (LSG9) for intermediate- or high-grade non-Hodgkin's lymphoma: Japan Clinical Oncology Group Study 9002. *Int J Hematol.* 2004;80:341-350.
5. Waikar SS, Mount DB, Curhan GC. Mortality after hospitalization with mild, moderate, and severe hyponatremia. *Am J Med Sci.* 2009; 122:857-865.
6. Sengupta A, Banerjee SN, Biswas NM, et al. The incidence of hyponatraemia and its effect on the ECOG performance status among lung cancer patients. *J Clin Diagn Res.* 2013;7:1678-1682.
7. Hansen O, Sorensen P, Hansen KH. The occurrence of hyponatremia in SCLC and the influence on prognosis: a retrospective study of 453 patients treated in a single institution in a 10-year period. *Lung Cancer.* 2010;68:111-114.
8. Schutz FA, Xie W, Donskov F, et al. The impact of low serum sodium on treatment outcome of targeted therapy in metastatic renal cell carcinoma: results from the International Metastatic Renal Cell Cancer Database Consortium. *Eur Urol.* 2014;65:723-730.
9. Arieff AI, Llach F, Massry SG. Neurological manifestations and morbidity of hyponatremia: correlation with brain water and electrolytes. *Medicine (Baltimore).* 1976;55:121-129.
10. Verbalis JG. Disorders of body water homeostasis. *Best Pract Res Clin Endocrinol Metab.* 2003;17:471-503.
11. Noakes TD, Wilson G, Gray DA, Lambert MI, Dennis SC. Peak rates of diuresis in healthy humans during oral fluid overload. *S Afr Med J.* 2001;91:852-857.
12. Hillier TA, Abbott RD, Barrett EJ. Hyponatremia: evaluating the correction factor for hyperglycemia. *Am J Med.* 1999;106:399-403.
13. Palmer BF, Clegg DJ. Hyponatremia in the cancer patient. *J Onco-Nephrol.* 2017;1:87-84.
14. Daphnis E, Stylianou K, Alexandrakis M, et al. Acute renal failure, translocational hyponatremia and hyperkalemia following intravenous immunoglobulin therapy. *Nephron Clin Pract.* 2007;106: c143-c148.
15. Weisberg LS. Pseudohyponatremia: a reappraisal. *Am J Med Sci.* 1989;86:315-318.
16. Issa MM, Young MR, Bullock AR, Bouet R, Petros JA. Dilutional hyponatremia of TURP syndrome: a historical event in the 21st century. *Urology.* 2004;64:298-301.

17. Hutchison FN, Perez EA, Gandara DR, Lawrence HJ, Kaysen GA. Renal salt wasting in patients treated with cisplatin. *Ann Intern Med.* 1988;108:21-25.

18. Peters JP, Welt LG, Sims EA, Orloff J, Needham J. A salt-wasting syndrome associated with cerebral disease. *Trans Assoc Am Physicians.* 1950;63:57-64.

19. Palmer BF. Hyponatremia in patients with central nervous system disease: SIADH versus CSW. *Trans Assoc Am Physicians.* 2003;14:182-187.

20. Kalogeras KT, Nieman LK, Friedman TC, et al. Inferior petrosal sinus sampling in healthy subjects reveals a unilateral corticotropin-releasing hormone-induced arginine vasopressin release associated with ipsilateral adrenocorticotropin secretion. *J Clin Invest.* 1996;97:2045-2050.

21. Kimura T. Potential mechanisms of hypothyroidism-induced hyponatremia. *Intern Med.* 2000;39:1002-1003.

22. Chen YC, Cadnapaphornchai MA, Yang J, et al. Nonosmotic release of vasopressin and renal aquaporins in impaired urinary dilution in hypothyroidism. *Am J Physiol Renal Physiol.* 2005;289:F672-F678.

23. Ferlito A, Rinaldo A, Devaney KO. Syndrome of inappropriate antidiuretic hormone secretion associated with head neck cancers: review of the literature. *Ann Otol Rhinol Laryngol.* 1997;106:878-883.

24. Berghmans T. Hyponatremia related to medical anticancer treatment. *Support Care Cancer.* 1996;4:341-350.

25. Sørensen JB, Andersen MK, Hansen HH. Syndrome of inappropriate secretion of antidiuretic hormone (SIADH) in malignant disease. *J Intern Med.* 1995;238:97-110.

26. Berardi R, Rinaldi S, Caramanti M, et al. Hyponatremia in cancer patients: Time for a new approach. *Crit Rev Oncol Hematol.* 2016;102:15-25.

27. Gullans SR, Verbalis JG. Control of brain volume during hyperosmolar and hypoosmolar conditions. *Annu Rev Med.* 1993;44:289-301.

28. Sterns RH, Riggs JE, Schochet SS, Jr. Osmotic demyelination syndrome following correction of hyponatremia. *N Engl J Med.* 1986;314:1535-1542.

29. Verbalis JG, Goldsmith SR, Greenberg A, et al. Diagnosis, evaluation, and treatment of hyponatremia: expert panel recommendations. *Am J Med.* 2013;126:S1-S42.

30. Sterns RH, Nigwekar SU, Hix JK. The treatment of hyponatremia. *Semin Nephrol.* 2009;29:282-299.

31. Verbalis JG, Goldsmith SR, Greenberg A, Schrier RW, Sterns RH. Hyponatremia treatment guidelines 2007: expert panel recommendations. *Am J Med.* 2007;120:S1-S21.

32. Adrogue HJ, Madias NE. Hyponatremia. *N Engl J Med.* 2000;342:1581-1589.

33. Chen S, Shey J. Kinetic sodium equation with built-in rate of correction: aid to prescribing therapy for hyponatremia or hypernatremia. *J Onco-nephrol.* 2017;1:204-212.

34. Furst H, Hallows KR, Post J, et al. The urine/plasma electrolyte ratio: a predictive guide to water restriction. *Am J Med Sci.* 2000;319:240-244.

35. Soupart A, Coffernils M, Couturier B, Gankam-Kengne F, Decaux G. Efficacy and tolerance of urea compared with vaptans for long-term treatment of patients with SIADH. *Clin J Am Soc Nephrol.* 2012;7:742-747.

36. Dousa TP, Wilson DM. Effects of demethylchlortetracycline on cellular action of antidiuretic-hormone invitro. *Kidney Int.* 1974;5:279-284.

37. Curtis NJ, van Heyningen C, Turner JJ. Irreversible nephrotoxicity from demeclocycline in the treatment of hyponatremia. *Age Ageing.* 2002;31:151-152.

38. Schrier RW, Gross P, Gheorghiade M, et al. Tolvaptan, a selective oral vasopressin V2-receptor antagonist, for hyponatremia. *N Engl J Med.* 2006;355:2099-2112.

39. Salahudeen AK, Ali N, George M, Lahoti A, Palla S. Tolvaptan in hospitalized cancer patients with hyponatremia: a double-blind, randomized, placebo-controlled clinical trial on efficacy and safety. *Cancer.* 2014;120:744-751.

40. Kamgar M, Hanna RM, Hasnain H, Khalil D, Wilson JM. Risk of serum sodium overcorrection with V2 antagonists in SIADH and other high risk patients. *J Onco-nephrol.* 2017:143-146.

41. Perianayagam A, Sterns RH, Silver SM, et al. DDAVP is effective in preventing and reversing inadvertent overcorrection of hyponatremia. *Clin J Am Soc Nephrol.* 2008;3:331-336.

42. Güçyetmez B, Ayyildiz AC, Ogan A, et al. Dysnatremia on intensive care unit admission is a stronger risk factor when associated with organ dysfunction. *Minerva Anestesiol.* 2014;80:1096-1104.

43. Lindner G, Funk GC. Hypernatremia in critically ill patients. *J Crit Care.* 2013;28:216.e11-e20.

44. Mendes RS, Soares M, Valente C, Suassuna JH, Rocha E, Maccariello ER. Predialysis hypernatremia is a prognostic marker in acute kidney injury in need of renal replacement therapy. *J Crit Care.* 2015;30:982-987.

45. Oude Lansink-Hartgring A, Hessels L, Weigel J, et al. Long-term changes in dysnatremia incidence in the ICU: a shift from hyponatremia to hypernatremia. *Ann Intensive Care.* 2016;6:22.

46. Tsipotis E, Price LL, Jaber BL, Madias NE. Hospital-associated hypernatremia spectrum and clinical outcomes in an unselected cohort. *Am J Med Sci.* 2018;131:72-82.e1.

47. Salahudeen AK, Doshi SM, Shah P. The frequency, cost, and clinical outcomes of hypernatremia in patients hospitalized to a comprehensive cancer center. *Support Care Cancer.* 2013;21:1871-1878.

48. Lenz K, Gössinger H, Laggner A, Druml W, Grimm G, Schneeweiss B. Influence of hypernatremic-hyperosmolar state on hemodynamics of patients with normal and depressed myocardial function. *Crit Care Med.* 1986;14:913-914.

49. Bratusch-Marrain PR, DeFronzo RA. Impairment of insulin-mediated glucose metabolism by hyperosmolality in man. *Diabetes.* 1983;32:1028-1034.

50. Lien YH, Shapiro JI, Chan L. Effects of hypernatremia on organic brain osmoles. *J Clin Invest.* 1990;85:1427-1435.

3 *Potassium Disorders*

SANA F. KHAN AND BRENDAN T. BOWMAN

Introduction

Potassium abnormalities, both hypo- and hyperkalemia, can occur with significant consequences in patients with malignancies. In addition to typical causes of disturbances in potassium homeostasis, there are unique etiologies within this special cohort including anticancer agent-induced disturbances on potassium excretion, direct effects of malignancies on cellular potassium release or uptake and potassium excretion by the kidneys, as well as artefactual changes more frequently seen in cancer. As the nature of potassium disturbances differ, it is imperative for management strategies to take into account these differences. For example, the clinical entity of tumor lysis syndrome (TLS) (described elsewhere in this text and in Chapter 30) may lead to a prolonged period of intracellular potassium release and potential reduction in potassium excretion if acute kidney injury (AKI) develops. As such, typical short-term hyperkalemia strategies of "stabilize, shift, excrete" used for single episodes may be ineffective. Conversely, chemotherapy-induced proximal tubular damage may lead to prolonged electrolyte wasting, necessitating high doses of potassium and magnesium replacement. Knowledge of the underlying nature of potassium abnormalities in cancer allows the clinician to devise more effective and appropriate treatment plans.

Risk of Potassium Disturbances in Cancer

The risk of a particular patient experiencing potassium disorders during the course of therapy is dependent upon multiple factors including: cancer type and disease burden; cell turnover rate; exposure to anticancer agents associated with electrolyte abnormalities; underlying comorbidities, such as chronic kidney disease (CKD), which may predispose a patient to AKI; and adjunctive therapies, such as nonsteroidal antiinflammatories or antimicrobial agents, which may also induce electrolyte abnormalities. Prevalence of potassium abnormalities among cancer patients is variable depending upon type of cancer, underlying comorbidities and acuity level of the patient—a proxy for risk of worsening renal function/AKI. One review of hypokalemia in hospitalized patients demonstrated that patients with hematologic malignancies were the third most common group to suffer hypokalemia.[1] Hypokalemia is more frequently encountered in the medical literature because of its well-known association with malignancies, such as acute myelogenous leukemia (AML) and in the setting of chemotherapy-induced tubular damage and excessive kaliuresis. Hyperkalemia is more often encountered in the

setting of AKI or in connection with the TLS, or more rarely, adrenal-axis suppression. One small study of more than 600 patients, admitted to a dedicated cancer ward, demonstrated a total of around 2% prevalence of any potassium abnormality, with hypokalemia twice as likely to occur in a broad sample of malignancies.[2] Given the interdisease variability, it is best to consider the risk of potassium abnormalities by patient-related factors and disease-related factors. Whereas solid tumors may be less likely to predispose a patient to potassium disturbances, more than 50% of patients with acute leukemia may suffer multifactorial hypokalemia.[3]

HYPOKALEMIA

Hypokalemia is commonly encountered in cancer patients.[4] Although there are various definitions of hypokalemia, a widely accepted lower limit for a normal potassium concentration is 3.5 mmol/L. A serum potassium concentration of 2.5 to 3.0 mmol/L is considered moderate and a level less than 2.5 mmol/L is regarded as severe hypokalemia.[5] Although the exact prevalence has not been evaluated in large cohorts of cancer patients, one large study showed the rate of hypokalemia to be 12% among hospitalized patients. Hypokalemia was largely of multifactorial etiology, with hematologic malignancy (9%) being a common causative factor. Concomitant hypomagnesemia occurred in 61% of patients.[1] In another cohort of hospitalized patients, hypokalemia was observed in 16.8% of all first-time admissions, and malignancy was noted to be an independent risk factor for hospitalization with hypokalemia.[6] A larger analysis of hospitalized patients revealed that 21% of hospitalized patients developed hypokalemia, with a strong association with malignancy, especially hematologic and gastrointestinal (GI) tract malignancy.[7]

Etiologies

Hypokalemia may result from one of four possible etiologies: pseudohypokalemia; redistribution between cellular compartments; GI losses; and renal losses. In addition, hypomagnesemia is strongly associated with hypokalemia in malignancy, and contributes to kidney losses. Chemotherapy-induced decreased appetite and oral intake further confounds hypokalemia resulting from these losses.[4] Typically, the etiology in cancer patients is largely "multifactorial," and is summarized in Table 3.1.

Workup and diagnosis of "true" hypokalemia are warranted after exclusion of pseudohypokalemia. The most common cause of pseudohypokalemia is acute leukemia, in which there are postphlebotomy transcellular shifts in the large number of abnormal leukocytes, if blood is stored in

Table 3.1 Causes and Mechanisms of Hypokalemia in Cancer Patients

Source of Potassium Loss	Cause	Mechanism
Renal losses	Acute myelogenous leukemia	Lysozymuria (M4/M5)
		Renin secretion
	Chemotherapy agents: cisplatin/ifosfamide	Fanconi syndrome/tubular toxicity
	EGFR inhibitors: cetuximab and panitumumab	Hypomagnesemia/tubular toxicity
	BRAF/MEK inhibitors: vemurafenib and dabrafenib with trametinib	Fanconi syndrome/tubular toxicity
GI losses	Diarrhea/radiation enteritis/GI tumors	Intestinal/colonic BK potassium channel upregulation
Transcellular shifts	Myelopoietic agents	Potassium uptake in rapidly proliferating cells
	Alkalosis	Induced from chemo-associated vomiting or alkaline hydration protocols

BK, Large-conductance calcium-activated potassium channels; *EGFR*, epidermal growth factor receptor; *GI*, gastrointestinal.
Modified from Bowman BT (2017). Electrolyte disorders associated with cancer. *J Onconephrology*, 1, 30–35.

collection vials for prolonged periods, at room temperature. Rapid separation of plasma and storage at 4°C limits this issue.[8]

Transcellular shifts of potassium in cancer patients are associated with malignancy-related medications and their adverse effects. Metabolic alkalosis from chemotherapy-induced vomiting, as well as alkaline volume expansion protocols, cause potassium to move intracellularly, as well as increased aldosterone activity resulting in increased potassium losses by the kidney. In addition, use of myelopoietic growth factors is associated with increased hematopoietic cell production, followed by rapid potassium uptake in the new cells. Similarly, increased production of blast cells in AML can also lead to hypokalemia.[9]

GI losses in malignancy are largely caused by diarrhea that may occur because of chemotherapy, or radiation enteritis. Less commonly, villous adenoma or vasoactive intestinal secreting tumor (VIPoma) are associated with prolonged diarrhea and hypokalemia.[10,11] In addition, certain conditions in malignancy are associated with hypokalemia, secondary to upregulation of colonic/intestinal large-conductance calcium-activated potassium (BK) channels.[12,13] Hypokalemia associated with upper GI losses from vomiting or nasogastric suctioning is minimal, given the low (5–10 mEq/L) concentration of potassium in gastric secretions. The resulting hypokalemia is secondary to a combination of hypovolemia-induced aldosterone release, and increased bicarbonate delivery to the cortical collecting duct. The net effect is increased potassium secretion and urinary potassium wasting.[14]

Potassium losses by the kidney in malignancy are associated with specific cancers and therapeutic agents and will be discussed in detail in the following sections. In addition, it is important to understand the mechanism of hypokalemia with concomitant hypomagnesemia, as it is frequently encountered in hypokalemia of malignancy.[15] Luminal potassium secretion in the cortical collecting duct occurs via apical renal outer medullary potassium (ROMK) channels. Under physiologic conditions, intracellular magnesium binds ROMK and blocks potassium secretion. An increase in ROMK activity from magnesium deficiency (low intracellular magnesium) releases the

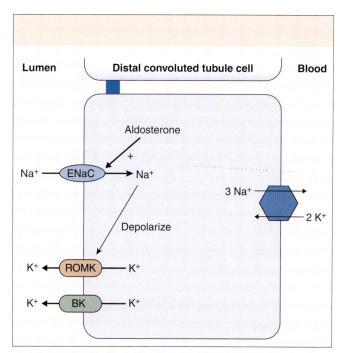

Fig. 3.1 K$^+$ secretion by principal cells. The basolateral Na$^+$K$^+$ ATPase lowers intracellular Na$^+$ concentration, and increases K$^+$ concentration. Entry of Na$^+$ via ENaC channels depolarizes the apical membrane, resulting in K$^+$ efflux via luminal ROMK channels. Flow-induced increases in K$^+$ secretion is mediated by BK channels. *BK*, Large-conductance calcium-activated potassium channels; *ENaC*, epithelial sodium channel; *K$^+$*, potassium; *Na$^+$*, sodium; *ROMK*, renal outer medullary potassium.

magnesium-mediated inhibition of ROMK channels and increases potassium secretion. Additional factors for potassium secretion (distal sodium delivery, increased aldosterone levels) are essential for exacerbating potassium wasting and hypokalemia in magnesium deficiency (Fig. 3.1).[16] Hypomagnesemia in cancer patients may be caused by decreased intake or from increase urinary magnesium wasting. Losses of magnesium by the kidney are largely caused by chemotherapy-mediated injury to the distal nephron.

Hypokalemia Associated With Specific Cancers

Among hematologic malignancies, hypokalemia is the most pronounced electrolyte abnormality in acute leukemia. Hypokalemia has been primarily described in patients with monocytic (M4) and acute myelomonocytic (M5) subtypes. It is mainly attributed to lysozymuria-induced renal tubular injury with kaliuresis.[3,17,18] Lysozyme is an enzyme originating from blood granulocytes and monocytes, as well as tissue macrophages.[19] Lysozyme is normally reabsorbed in the proximal convoluted tubule. Lysozymuria occurring in patients with leukemia has been attributed to proliferation and destruction of lysozyme containing cells. Filtered lysozyme appears to be a direct tubular toxin. In addition, high levels of tubular lysozyme may induce significant kaliuresis and hypokalemia.[20] Lysozymuria leading to profound hypokalemia has also been reported in chronic myelogenous leukemia.[21] There have also been reports of renin-like activity in leukemic cells, stimulating the mineralocorticoid pathways and increasing potassium secretion by the kidney.[18,22]

Additional cancer-specific disorders associated with hypokalemia include disorders of mineralocorticoid excess. Although most adrenal adenomas are nonfunctional, up to 15% can be functional, secreting increased amounts of cortisol, which overwhelm 11-beta-hydroxysteroid dehydrogenase's ability to metabolize cortisol to cortisone. Thus cortisol is able to bind the mineralocorticoid receptor and stimulate potassium excretion via ROMK channels (Fig. 3.2). Adrenal carcinomas are rare and present with signs and symptoms of elevated cortisol levels.[23,24]

Proximal tubular toxicity resulting from κ light chain myeloma, resulting in Fanconi syndrome is an indirect cause of malignancy associated hypokalemia. In dysproteinemias, the degree of filtered light chains exceeds the proximal tubule's resorptive capacity, resulting in light chain proteinuria. Proximal tubule endocytosis of these light chains results in intracellular oxidative stress and cell apoptosis.[25] The resulting proximal tubular disorder is Fanconi syndrome, with bicarbonaturia, glycosuria, aminoaciduria, phosphaturia, hyperuricosuria, and potassium wasting. Hypokalemia in proximal renal tubular acidosis results primarily in cases of supplemental bicarbonate repletion.[5]

Other rare causes of cancer-specific hypokalemia include ectopic adrenocorticotropic hormone (ACTH) producing tumors. These include small-cell lung cancer, bronchial carcinoid tumors, lung adenocarcinomas, thymic tumors, pancreatic tumors and medullary thyroid cancer. Up to 30% of ectopic ACTH syndrome may present as occult tumors.[26]

Hypokalemia Association With Therapeutic Agents

Several drugs commonly used to treat cancer patients are contributory to development of hypokalemia. The mechanisms of common causative antimicrobials will be discussed briefly, before detailed discussions on chemotherapeutic agents.

Common antibiotics causing hypokalemia include aminoglycosides, amphotericin B, and penicillins. Aminoglycoside antibiotics are endocytosed in the proximal tubular cells, causing mitochondrial damage, and proximal tubule dysfunction. This results in a Fanconi-like syndrome, along with distal tubular dysfunction, resulting in hypomagnesemia, and subsequent hypokalemia.[27,28] The aminoglycosides may also cause a Bartter-like syndrome with sodium, potassium, and magnesium wasting. It is thought that these cationic drugs activate the calcium-sensing receptor in the loop of Henle tubular cells, which decreases $Na^+ K^+ 2Cl^-$ transport activity (Fig. 3.3).[29] Similarly, amphotericin B, commonly used in cancer patients for the treatment of fungal infections creates pores in cell membranes, resulting in increased membrane permeability. Increased permeability results in diffusion of potassium ions from distal tubule cells, and subsequent urinary potassium wasting.[30] Lastly, penicillins have also been associated with hypokalemia, because of penicillin being a nonreabsorbable anion present in the distal tubule. The luminal electronegativity results in increased potassium excretion.[31]

Cisplatin is a platinum-based chemotherapeutic agent, causing direct nephrotoxicity, with proximal tubular necrosis and distal tubule apoptosis.[32] The mechanism of cisplatin-induced hypokalemia results mainly from proximal tubular injury and development of Fanconi syndrome, as well as marked hypomagnesemia (Fig. 3.4). Tubular defects from cisplatin use can be permanent in certain cases.[33,34]

Ifosfamide is an alkylating agent used in certain cancers. Nephrotoxicity secondary to ifosfamide includes proximal tubules (Fanconi syndrome), as well as distal tubules (nephrogenic diabetes insipidus, distal renal tubular acidosis). The metabolite chloracetaldehyde is directly toxic to cells, causing glutathione depletion and lipid peroxidation.[35,36]

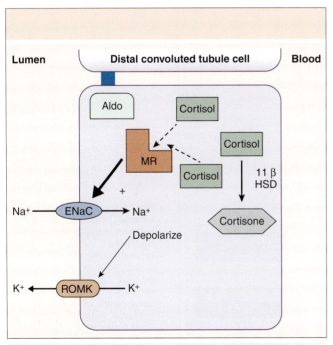

Fig. 3.2 K^+ secretion with adrenal adenomas. Cortisol activates the mineralocorticoid receptor, resulting in increased ENaC, and subsequent ROMK activity. 11 β HSD converts cortisol to cortisone, which does not have mineralocorticoid activity. Increased amounts of cortisol exceed the ability of 11 β HSD to metabolize cortisol. *Aldo,* Aldosterone; *ENaC,* epithelial sodium channel; *K^+,* potassium; *MR,* mineralocorticoid receptor; *Na^+,* sodium; *ROMK,* renal outer medullary potassium; *11 β HSD,* 11 beta hydroxyl steroid dehydrogenase.

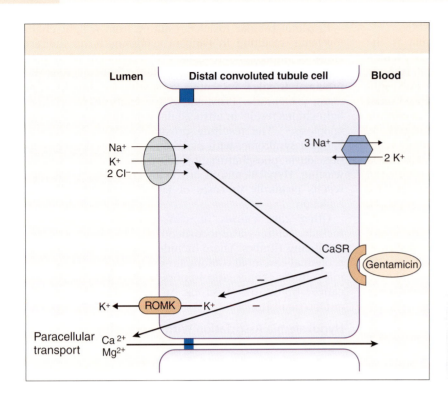

Fig. 3.3 Aminoglycoside induced Bartter-like syndrome, with drug binding to CaSR, resulting in inhibition of NKCC activity, decreased ROMK channel back leak of potassium, with resulting decrease in paracellular Ca^{2+} and Mg^{2+} transport. *Cl$^-$*, Chloride; *CaSR*, calcium sensing receptor; *K$^+$*, potassium; *Na$^+$*, sodium; *ROMK*, renal outer medullary potassium.

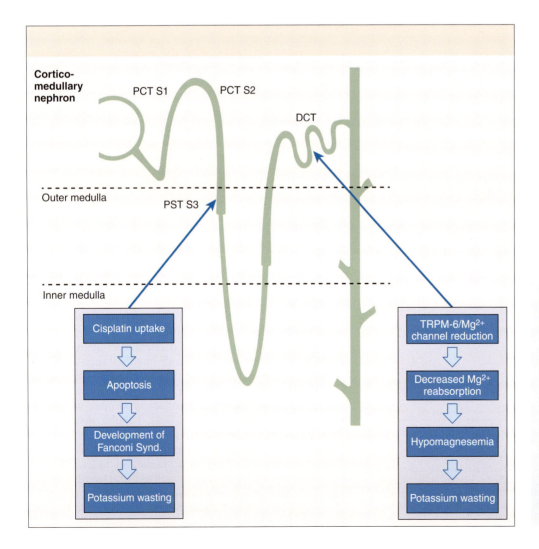

Fig. 3.4 Cisplatin-induced hypokalemia. Cisplatin is taken up by organic ion transporters on the basolateral membrane. High concentrations of intracellular cisplatin lead to cell death and proximal tubular damage concentrated in the S3 segment, and development of a Fanconi-like syndrome. In the distal tubules, TRPM-6 magnesium channels are downregulated (possibly caused by loss of epithelial growth factor) leading to hypomagnesemia and obligate renal potassium wasting. *DCT*, Distal convoluted tubule; *Mg^{2+}*, magnesium; *PCT*, proximal convoluted tubule; *TRPM-6*, transient receptor potential subfamily melastatin.

Adverse effects on kidney function can occur up to 10 years after ifosfamide administration.[37,38]

Epithelial growth factor receptor (EGFR) is a protein, which can be overexpressed by several different tumors: colorectal, lung, breast, pancreas, and head and neck cancers.[39] It is important in modulating several cellular signaling pathways, making it a target for development of chemotherapeutic agents. EGFR monoclonal antibody inhibitors, such as cetuximab and panitumumab, have been shown to cause hypokalemia (up to 14.5% patients) secondary to hypomagnesemia (up to 34% patients).[40] The mechanism of hypomagnesemia is thought to be related to magnesium permeable channels in the distal tubule, mainly transient receptor potential melastatin channel 6 and 7 (TRPM 6 and TRPM 7). EGF and TRPM 6 and 7 are both expressed in the distal convoluted tubule, and magnesium loss results from inhibition of EGF-mediated stimulation of TRPM activity (Fig. 3.5).[41,42]

Targeted melanoma therapy because of inhibition of the oncogenic BRAF V600 molecule, or a downstream signaling partner mitogen activating protein kinase (MAP kinase) has been shown to be effective in melanoma patients with BRAF mutations. Vemurafenib and dabrafenib (BRAF inhibitors) have been shown to be associated with hypokalemia. The mechanism is thought to be secondary to Fanconi syndrome.[43]

Management

Once laboratory measurements confirm the presence of true hypokalemia, two urinary tests are commonly used to assess renal potassium losses. The fractional excretion of potassium (FE_K) and the transtubular potassium gradient (TTKG) may provide insight into the kidney response to hypokalemia: FE_K would have an expected value of less than 2% in hypokalemia, and the TTKG would have an expected value of less than 2 in hypokalemia.[2] More recently, the use of the TTKG has been called into question, and this should not be relied on solely to diagnose hypokalemia.[44] Optimal correction of hypokalemia warrants a diagnosis of the cause and treatment of underlying disorder.

Underlying acid-base disturbances should be investigated and corrected before potassium repletion.

Initial potassium replacement in cancer patients is the same as that in the general population. Given that approximately only 2% of total body potassium is in the extracellular fluid, along with high sensitivity to cellular shifts, serum potassium concentration is not a reliable marker of total body deficits. However, estimates indicate that a serum potassium concentration of less than 3 mmol/L or 2 mmol/L generally indicates deficits of around 200 mmol or 500 mmol respectively.[5] Once the deficit is estimated, potassium supplementation can be administered orally or intravenously, usually as potassium chloride (KCl). Alternatively, potassium citrate can be used, particularly in patients with metabolic acidosis. Given potential GI side effects with oral KCl, cancer patients may possibly require intravenous KCl administration. Moreover, intravenous potassium repletion may be needed, given potential difficulty with oral intake caused by nausea, dysphagia, and mucositis. A rate of 20 mmol/h should not be exceeded, given the risk of rebound hyperkalemia.[5] A recent study noted 16% of hospitalized patients developed hyperkalemia following correction of hypokalemia. The risk of hyperkalemia was associated with hematologic malignancies, as well as administration of total parenteral nutrition, both conditions commonly seen in cancer patients.[1] Potassium sparing diuretics (amiloride, spironolactone, eplerenone, triamterene) can be used for chronic hypokalemia; however, there is an increased risk of hyperkalemia in patients with reduced kidney function, and concomitant administration of nephrotoxic medications. Potassium supplementation is ineffective if hypomagnesemia remains uncorrected, given ongoing potassium losses via ROMK channels.[3] Intravenous magnesium repletion is usually needed because diarrhea is noted to be a dose limiting adverse effect of oral magnesium supplementation. Finally, long-term potassium repletion may be anticipated in some cases. As noted previously, anticancer agents, such as ifosfamide and cisplatin, may lead to persistent or even permanent potassium wasting.

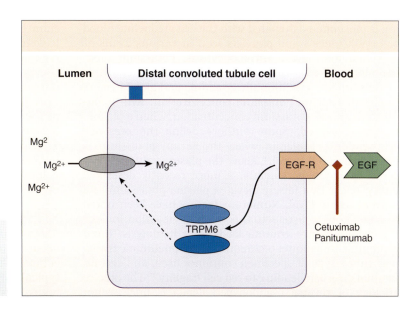

Fig. 3.5 Absorption of magnesium is via EGFR-dependent apical channels, TRPM 6 and 7. This pathway is inhibited by anti-EGFR monoclonal antibodies (cetuximab and panitumumab). *EGF*, Epithelial growth factor; *EGF-R*, epithelial growth factor receptor; *Mg^{2+}*, magnesium; *TRPM6*, transient receptor potential melastatin 6.

Table 3.2 Cancer-Specific Causes of Hyperkalemia

Etiology	Cause	Mechanism
Artefactual potassium elevations	Pseudohyperkalemia	Various: trauma to fragile cell and platelet membranes, often in setting of traumatic venipuncture, fist clenching, tourniquet use, etc.
	Reverse pseudohyperkalemia	Increased cell membrane fragility of cells exposed to heparinized tubes produce intracellular potassium release
Transcellular shifts/ cell lysis	Tumor lysis syndrome	Release of intracellular potassium caused by high rates of tumor cell death
	Posttransplant diabetes mellitus	Hyperglycemic states with osmolar shift of potassium
	Chemotherapy-induced rhabdomyolysis	Often synergistic effect with statin therapy leading to release of intracellular potassium
Low aldosterone state/ adrenal insufficiency	Adrenal metastases	Solid tumors metastases replacing > 90% of adrenal mass or adrenalectomy leading to low Aldosterone state
	Primary adrenal lesions	Primary adrenal lymphoma, adrenal adenocarcinoma replace adrenal tissue leading to adrenal insufficiency or mitotane induced loss of adrenal zona glomerulosa tissue
	Acute leukemia	Idiopathic primary adrenal insufficiency
Direct medication effects	Calcineurin inhibitors	Suppression of principal cell basolateral Na-K-ATPase resulting in decreased Na-K$^+$ exchange
	Thalidomide	Occurs in CKD/ESKD patients via an unclear mechanism
	Hydroxyurea	Rare idiopathic cause of hyperkalemia
	Trimethoprim	Blockade of epithelial sodium channel in distal nephron resulting in decreased Na-K$^+$ exchange/amiloride-like effect

Na-K-ATPase, Sodium potassium ATPase; *CKD*, chronic kidney disease; *ESKD*, end stage kidney disease.

HYPERKALEMIA

Hyperkalemia in cancer patients (Table 3.2) may be encountered because of one or several of the following factors:

- Artefactual hyperkalemia
- Cellular shifts/TLS
- Reduced glomerular filtration rate (GFR) (acute or chronic) with associated decreased potassium clearance (discussed in depth in Sections 7 and 8)
- Hypoaldosteronism/adrenal insufficiency
- Direct medication effect

Artefactual Hyperkalemia

Spurious elevations of potassium in laboratory samples have been generally termed *pseudohyperkalemia*. This finding is most often associated with the elevated white blood cell (WBC) levels and platelets seen in various forms of leukemia and severe thrombocytosis. Potassium measurements may be made using serum, plasma, or whole blood samples. Traditionally, pseudohyperkalemia refers to elevated serum potassium concentration, with a significantly lower potassium concentration, when a plasma test is measured. Some authors define the presence of pseudohyperkalemia when the serum potassium is greater than 0.4 mmol/L above the plasma values.[45] "Reverse" pseudohyperkalemia, a more recently described entity, refers to a falsely elevated plasma potassium and normal serum level. Numerous factors have been noted to contribute to artefactual potassium elevation including: venipuncture trauma leading to hemolysis, hand clenching, tourniquet technique, use of pneumatic transport tubes, type of specimen container used, and certain familial disorders leading to red cell fragility.[46] The precise etiology of reverse pseudohyperkalemia is unclear but

some have suggested the combination of fragile WBCs in disorders, such as chronic lymphocytic leukemia (CLL) and the use of heparinized collection tubes for plasma, which results in potassium leakage/membrane disruption during tube transport and centrifugation.[47] Both types of artefactual potassium elevation have been associated with dialysis initiation and risk of subsequent hypokalemia.[48,49] A study of 57 CLL patients from Katkish and colleagues, in the Veterans Affairs system, described the probability of pseudohyperkalemia occurrence at 8.1% in those with WBC of 100.0×10^9/L or more over 270 patient years of follow-up.[50] Assessing the presence of pseudohyperkalemia requires a high index of suspicion. Many case reports note a surprising lack of electrocardiogram changes despite significantly elevated potassium levels.[46,47] In a series of six patients with various leukemias, Dastych and Cemrakova found that the most reliable method for avoiding artefactual potassium rise was the use of a plasma sample in a heparinized tube (absent separator gel), walked manually to the laboratory. This resulted in a greater than 6.0 mmol/L difference in the potassium of one patient with acute lymphocytic leukemia: 3.9 mmol/L versus more than 10.0 mmol/L.[51] Thus patients with hyperkalemia and hematologic malignancies require judicious interpretation of potassium values to avoid inadvertent initiation of potassium lowering therapies.

Cellular Shifts/Tumor Lysis Syndrome

Short-term (seconds to minutes) potassium management occurs primarily under the influence of insulin and catecholamines, resulting in cellular shifts of potassium, typically into and out of skeletal muscle.[52] Elimination of potassium via renal and GI routes follows in the ensuing hours. In cases of normal renal function, the kidneys excrete around 90% of excess potassium intake and the GI tract excretion handles the remainder. In settings such as CKD or end-stage kidney disease (ESRD), a larger portion of potassium excretion can shift to the GI tract using BK channels, particularly of the colon, for enhanced excretion.[53]

TLS (discussed in detail in Chapter 30) has the potential for rapid rise in plasma potassium levels. Potassium is the major intracellular monovalent cation, and total body stores may equal around 3500 mEq in a 70-kg individual with a distribution of 98% intracellular versus 2% extracellular.[54] The classic description of TLS involves spontaneous or chemotherapy-induced malignant cell lysis with resultant release of high volumes of uric acid, potassium, and phosphorous. Once associated with mainly hematologic malignancies, TLS has been rarely described in solid tumors as well.[55] The large volume of potassium release may overwhelm compensatory mechanisms, particularly in patients with acute disease or CKD. TLS occurring in the setting of preexisting CKD or following TLS-induced AKI may further exacerbate hyperkalemia. If prophylactic and temporizing measures fail, treatment of TLS-associated hyperkalemia may require renal replacement therapy. Given the ongoing release of potassium, prolonged dialysis may be necessary, such as continuous renal replacement therapy (CRRT) or slow low efficiency dialysis.[56] If the initial potassium is markedly elevated, hemodialysis, with its more efficient potassium clearance, is the initial modality, which can then be followed by a period of CRRT—a management plan similar to that used in Lithium ingestion.

Cellular potassium shifts may also occur in the setting of acidosis or hyperglycemic states. Specific to cancer therapies, posttransplant diabetes mellitus (PTDM) may affect up to 30% of hematopoietic stem cell transplant survivors within 2-years posttransplant.[57] This is thought to be mediated, in part, by injury of pancreatic β cells and increased insulin resistance mediated by calcineurin inhibitors, and the use of corticosteroids.[58] Undiagnosed PTDM may present as diabetic ketoacidosis or hyperglycemic hyperosmolar states with accompanying hyperkalemia from osmolar shifts. Tacrolimus, in particular, has been more often associated with the onset of this condition versus cyclosporine in solid organ transplant recipients.[59]

Finally, in addition to TLS, rhabdomyolysis has the potential to release large volumes of potassium from the intracellular stores. Various chemotherapy agents, given alone, in combination, or in combination with synergistic medications, such as statins, have been linked to rhabdomyolysis. For example, abiraterone, a treatment for castration resistant prostate cancer, has been reported to cause rhabdomyolysis, AKI, and hyperkalemia in association with statin use as has the vascular EGF tyrosine kinase inhibitor, pazopanib.[60,61,62] Other agents have also been implicated in cases of rhabdomyolysis and include myeloma therapies lenalidomide and bortezomib, the EGF-receptor inhibitor erlotinib, the tyrosine kinase inhibitors sunitinib and imatinib, and certain combination therapies.[63–68]

Low Aldosterone and Low Aldosterone-Like States

Adrenal metastases are the most common adrenal lesions—far outnumbering primary adrenal cancers. This is attributed to generous sinusoidal blood supply of the adrenal glands. Despite the high prevalence of metastatic disease, clinical symptoms of adrenal insufficiency in these cases are rare. In a single center retrospective review of 464 patients with adrenal metastases over 30 years, only five patients presented with clinical signs/symptoms of adrenal insufficiency (Addison disease).[69] This is attributed to the fact that a large volume of adrenal tissue must be destroyed (90%) before symptoms and laboratory abnormalities develop. Direct metastatic involvement has presented as adrenal insufficiency with hyperkalemia in several cancers including lung, breast, colorectal, and stomach among others.[70–73] Surgical resection of metastatic disease in solid tumor cancers may also induce iatrogenic adrenal insufficiency and hyperkalemia.

In addition to solid tumors, leukemia has also been associated with idiopathic adrenal insufficiency and hyperkalemia. Li, recently reported the case of a 64-year-old man with undiagnosed AML, presenting with the classic electrolyte abnormalities of hyponatremia and hyperkalemia.[74] A Turkish case series of 13 patients, with hyperkalemia and acute leukemia, demonstrated six with adrenal insufficiency of unclear etiology that resolved with disease remission. The authors suggest the presentation of hyperkalemia without an obvious attributable cause in acute leukemia, more often associated with hypokalemia, should prompt screening for adrenal insufficiency. Primary adrenal lymphoma, a rare presentation of extranodal lymphoma, may also produce adrenal insufficiency in more than 60% of patients with resulting hyperkalemia.[75]

As one might expect, the treatment of primary adrenal lesions, such as aldosterone producing adenomas (APA), and the rarer adrenal adenocarcinoma, are often linked with adrenal insufficiency and hyperkalemia. A case series of patients undergoing adrenalectomy for APA reported almost 30% of patients developed hyperkalemia postoperatively.[76] In adrenal adenocarcinoma, the use of mitotane in advanced stage disease has also been associated with adrenal insufficiency and electrolyte abnormalities (17% and 80%, respectively), and early replacement of glucocorticoids and fludrocortisone is recommended to avoid Addisonian crisis and hyperkalemia.[77]

Direct Medication Effects

Although many anticancer agents may result in nephrotoxicities with the widely known complication of hypokalemia, relatively few agents are known to cause hyperkalemia in the absence of associate kidney failure. One example, the immunomodulatory drug thalidomide, gained popularity in the treatment of myeloma in the 1990s and early 2000s. It is still occasionally used in refractory or relapsed cases and has been associated with severe, sometimes fatal, hyperkalemia during the first few weeks of treatment in patients with CKD and ESRD.[78,79] The mechanism of hyperkalemia remains undetermined, but careful monitoring of patients with diminished GFR or on dialysis is warranted when using thalidomide. Hydroxyurea, a long-used medication for many hematologic diseases including polycythemia vera, sickle cell disease, and essential thrombocytosis (among others), has been linked to hyperkalemia in at least one case report.[80] The patient in that case had rapid resolution of hyperkalemia with drug withdrawal and recurrence following reintroduction.

Calcineurin inhibitors (CNIs) prescribed following hematopoietic stem cell transplant (HSCT) have also been directly implicated in hyperkalemia.[81] The mechanism now appears to be threefold. Originally it was thought that afferent arterial vasoconstriction leading to decreased GFR likely reduced clearance of potassium. Caliskan and colleagues, however, described a series of patients with hyperkalemia following allogeneic stem cell transplant despite normal renal function, suggesting an additional etiology.[81] This second proposed mechanism is via disruption of the Na-K$^+$ adenosine triphosphatase (ATPase) on the basolateral membrane of the principal cell.[82] This reduces the gradient for sodium transport through the luminal epithelial sodium channel and leads to decreased distal sodium-potassium exchange. The increased luminal sodium concentration also results in inhibition of proton secretion and resulting acidosis—reminiscent of a "type 4" renal tubular acidosis. Finally, in mouse models, tacrolimus has been shown to increase activation and trafficking of the sodium-chloride channel (NCC) in the distal convoluted tubule. Horn and colleagues determined that the increased NCC activity occurred because of increases in "with no lysine" kinases 3 and 4 as well as the STE20-related kinase. The net effect is increased sodium retention and, in mice fed a high

potassium diet, hyperkalemia. The clinical picture is reminiscent of familial hyperkalemic hypertension.[83] The trimethoprim component of trimethoprim-sulfamethoxazole, used for infection prophylaxis during the high dose steroid treatment of graft-versus-host disease, is another well-documented cause of hyperkalemia. As opposed to the indirect effect of CNIs, trimethoprim directly blocks the epithelial sodium channel in the distal nephron, reducing sodium-potassium exchange in an amiloride-like effect, with resulting hyperkalemia.[84]

Treatment

Like all potassium abnormalities, diagnosis of the underlying cause of hyperkalemia in cancer patients is required for long-term management. In life-threatening scenarios, the usual methods of stabilization of the cardiac membrane, intracellular shifting of potassium, and promoting excretion via renal and GI mechanisms, remain guiding principles (Fig. 3.6). Dialysis is used when necessary for the usual indications. However, there are special considerations in patients with cancer. For example, by definition, TLS is accompanied by hyperkalemia. Various risk prediction scores have been proposed to assess the likelihood of TLS for a particular patient and can allow anticipatory counseling for patients, prophylactic therapy, and early preparations by the oncology and nephrology care teams.[85,86] The usual prophylaxis of enhanced distal sodium delivery via intravenous crystalloid and volume delivery is usually enough to prevent life-threatening hyperkalemia. However, if AKI is encountered with oliguria and hyperkalemia, renal

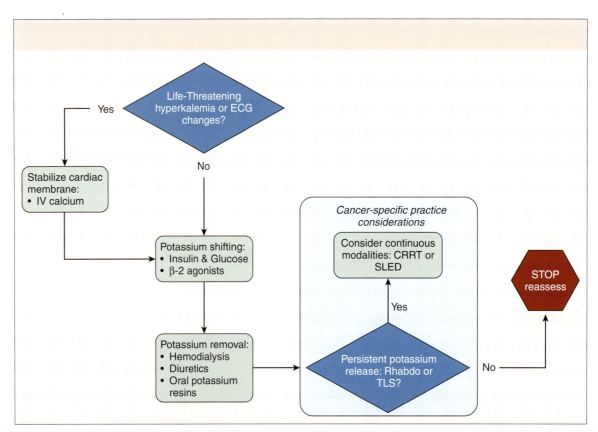

Fig. 3.6 Suggested management algorithm for hyperkalemia in cancer. *ECG*, Electrocardiogram; *CRRT*, continuous renal replacement therapy; *IV*, intravenous; *Rhabdo*, rhabdomyolysis; *SLED*, slow low efficiency dialysis; *TLS*, tumor lysis syndrome.

replacement therapy (RRT) may be indicated. There are no trials to support preemptive RRT in high risk patients; however, the clinician may expect a prolonged period of potassium release (potentially days) in cases of severe TLS. In these situations, intermittent hemodialysis to rapidly clear excess potassium may be indicated along with a period of continuous therapy. Alternately, if potassium has not reached critical levels, but AKI is present, a patient may proceed directly to CRRT until the period of lysis has subsided. Chemotherapy-induced rhabdomyolysis, with sustained potassium release, may also benefit from such an approach.

In the case of medication-induced hyperkalemia, where the offending agent is essential to therapy, such as CNIs following HSCT, conservative therapies, such as dietary modification and judicious use of diuretics may be used. In solid organ transplant recipients, fludrocortisone has been successfully used to treat hyperkalemia.[87] However, improvement in hyperkalemia must be weighed against the risk of worsening hypertension—another side effect of the CNI class.[83] Finally, newer oral potassium binding resins, such as patiromer and sodium zirconium cyclosilicate, approved for the management of CKD-associated hyperkalemia, are now available but have not been studied in cancer-associated hyperkalemia. In general, these novel medications are used to manage the chronic hyperkalemia associated with blockade of the renin-angiotensin-aldosterone system, and are thought easier to tolerate without the potential risk of bowel necrosis associated with sodium polystyrene sulfate.[88] As providers gain more clinical experience, the role of these newer medications will become further defined.

Summary

The presence of potassium abnormalities in cancer varies from the commonly seen hypokalemia of acute leukemia to the rarely experienced hyperkalemia of metastasis-induced adrenal insufficiency. Complicating matters, perhaps more than any other patient population, cancer patients are highly susceptible to inaccurate potassium measurements because of various hematologic perturbations. A familiarity with both the common and obscure etiologies of potassium disorders is essential to the safe management of this complicated patient population.

Key Points

- Potassium abnormalities in patients with cancer result from a confluence of factors including underlying patient characteristics, the specific type of cancer, and patient exposure to various anticancer and associated medications.
- The most commonly occurring potassium disturbance associated with malignancy is hypokalemia in the setting of acute leukemia.
- Cancer patients, particularly those with hematologic malignancies, experience high rates of pseudohyperkalemia and pseudohypokalemia, requiring a high index of suspicion to rule out "laboratory errors" before treatment.

- Potassium abnormalities in cancer, such as medication-induced Fanconi syndrome or chemotherapy-induced rhabdomyolysis, may be persistent and require long-term management strategies.

References

1. Crop MJ, Hoorn EJ, Lindemans J, Zietse, R. Hypokalaemia and subsequent hyperkalaemia in hospitalized patients. *Nephrol Dial Transpl.* 2007;22:3471-3477.
3. Milionis HJ, Bourantas CL, Siamopoulos KC, Elisaf MS. Acid-base and electrolyte abnormalities in patients with acute leukemia. *Am J Hematol.* 1999;62:201-207.
4. Miltiadous G, Christidis D, Kalogirou M, Elisaf M. Causes and mechanisms of acid-base and electrolytes abnormalities in cancer patients. *Eur J Intern Med.* 2008;19:1-7.
6. Jensen HK, Bradbrand M, Vinholt PJ, Hallas J, Lassen AT. Hypokalemia in acute medical patients: risk factors and prognosis. *Am J Med.* 2015;128:60-67.
15. Solomon R. The relationship between disorders of K^+ and Mg^{2+} homeostasis. Semin Nephrol. 1987;7:253-262.
17. Muggia FM, Heinemann HO, Farhangi M, Osserman EF. Lysozymuria and renal tubular dysfunction in monocytic and myelomonocytic leukemia. *Am J Med.* 1969;47:351-366.
18. Perazella MA, Eisen RN, Frederick WG, et al. Renal failure and severe hypokalemia associated with acute myelomonocytic leukemia. *Am J Kidney Dis.* 1993;22:462-467.
19. Patel TV, Rennke HG, Sloan JM, DeAngelo DJ, Charytan DM. A forgotten cause of kidney injury in chronic myelomonocytic leukemia. *Am J Kidney Dis.* 2009;54:159-164.
20. Filippatos TD, Milinoise HJ, Elisaf MS. Alterations in electrolyte equilibrium in patients with acute leukemia. *Eur J Haematol.* 2005;75: 449-460.
21. Evans JJ, Bozdech MJ. Hypokalemia in nonblastic chronic myelogenous leukemia. *Arch Intern Med.* 1981;141:786-787.
22. Wulf GG, Jahns-Streubel G, Strutz F, Basenau D, Hüfner M, Buske C. Paraneoplastic hypokalemia in acute myeloid leukemia: a case of renin activity in AML blast cells. *Ann Hematol.* 1996;73:139-141.
26. Alexandraki KI, Grossman AB. The ectopic ACTH syndrome. *Rev Endocrine Metab Disord.* 2010;11:117-126.
28. Patel R, Savage A. Symptomatic hypomagnesemia associated with gentamicin therapy. *Nephron.* 1979;23:50-52.
29. Chou CL, Chen YH, Chau T, Lin SH. Acquired Bartter-like syndrome associated with gentamicin administration. *Am J Med Sci.* 2005; 329:144-149.
30. Douglas JB, Healy JK. Nephrotoxic effects of amphotericin B, including renal tubular acidosis. *Am J Med.* 1969;46:154-162.
31. Zaki SA, Lad V. Piperacillin-tazobactam-induced hypokalemia and metabolic alkalosis. *Indian J Pharmacol.* 2011;43:609-610.
32. Liamis G, Filippatos TD, Elisaf MS. Electrolyte disorders associated with the use of anticancer drugs. *Eur J Pharmacol.* 2016;777:78-87.
33. Lam M, Adelstein DJ. Hypomagnesemia and renal magnesium wasting in patients treated with cisplatin. *Am J Kidney Dis.* 1986;8: 164-169.
35. Skinner R, Sharkey IM, Pearson AD, Craft AW. Ifosfamide, mesna, and nephrotoxicity in children. *J Clin Oncol.* 1993;11:173-190.
36. Husband DJ, Watkin SW. Fatal hypokalemia associated with ifosfamide/mesna chemotherapy. *Lancet.* 1988;1:1116.
37. Skinner R. Chronic ifosfamide nephrotoxicity in children. *Pediatr Oncol.* 2003;41:190-197.
40. Wang Q, Qi Y, Zhang D, et al. Electrolyte disorders assessment in solid tumor patients treated with anti-EGFR monoclonal antibodies: a pooled analysis of 25 randomized clinical trials. *Tumour Biol.* 2015;36:3471-3482.
41. Schlingmann KP, Weber S, Peters M, et al. Hypomagnesemia with secondary hypocalcemia is caused by mutations in TRPM6, a new member of the TRPM gene family. *Nat Genet.* 2002;31:166-170.
43. Wanchoo R, Jhaveri KD, Deray G, Launay-Vacher V. Renal effects of BRAF inhibitor: a systematic review by the cancer and the kidney international network. *Clin Kidney J.* 2016;9:245-251.
46. Wiederkehr MR, Moe OW. Factitious hyperkalemia. *Am J Kidney Dis.* 2000;36:1049-1053.

47. Mansoor S, Holtzman NG, Emadi A. Reverse pseudohyperkalemia: an important clinical entity in chronic lymphocytic leukemia. *Case Rep Hematol.* 2015;2015:930379.

48. Kellerman PS, Thornbery JM. Pseudohyperkalemia due to pneumatic tube transport in a leukemic patient. *Am J Kidney Dis.* 2005;46:746-748.

50. Katkish L, Rector T, Ishani A, Gupta P. Incidence and severity of pseudohyperkalemia in chronic lymphocytic leukemia: a longitudinal analysis. *Leuk Lymphoma.* 2016;57:1952-1955.

51. Dastych M, Cermáková Z. Pseudohyperkalaemia in leukaemic patients: the effect of test tube type and form of transport to the laboratory. *Ann Clin Biochem.* 2014;51:110-113.

54. Palmer BF, Clegg DJ. Physiology and pathophysiology of potassium homeostasis. *Adv Physiol Educ.* 2016;40:480-490.

56. Wilson FP, Berns JS. Tumor lysis syndrome: new challenges and recent advances. *Adv Chronic Kidney Dis.* 2014;21:18-26.

57. Griffith ML, Jagasia M, Jagasia SM. Diabetes mellitus after hematopoietic stem cell transplantation. *Endocr Pract.* 2010;16:699-706.

59. Shivaswamy V, Boerner B, Larsen J. Post-transplant diabetes mellitus: causes, treatment, and impact on outcomes. *Endocr Rev.* 2016;37:37-61.

60. Rocha NA, Bhargava R, Vaidya OU, Hendricks AR, Rodan AR, et al. Rhabdomyolysis-induced acute kidney injury in a cancer patient exposed to denosumab and abiraterone: a case report. *BMC Nephrol.* 2015;16:118.

67. Penel N, Blay JY, Adenis A. Imatinib as a possible cause of severe rhabdomyolysis. *N Engl J Med.* 2008;358:2746-2747.

69. Lam KY, Lo CY. Metastatic tumours of the adrenal glands: a 30-year experience in a teaching hospital. *Clin Endocrinol (Oxf).* 2002;56:95-101.

74. Li, W, Okwuwa I, Toledo-Frazzini K, Alhomosh A. Adrenal crisis in a patient with acute myeloid leukaemia. *Br Med J Case Rep.* 2013:1-4. pii: bcr2013010426.

75. Mantzios G, Tsirigotis P, Veliou F, et al. Primary adrenal lymphoma presenting as Addison's disease: case report and review of the literature. *Ann Hematol.* 2004;83:460-463.

76. Chiang WF, Cheng CJ, Wu ST, et al. Incidence and factors of post-adrenalectomy hyperkalemia in patients with aldosterone producing adenoma. *Clin Chim Acta.* 2013;424:114-118.

77. Reidy-Lagunes DL, Lung B, Untch BR, et al. Complete responses to mitotane in metastatic adrenocortical carcinoma-a new look at an old drug. *Oncologist.* 2017;22:1102-1106.

78. Harris E, Behrens J, Samson D, Rahemtulla A, Russell NH, Byrne JL. Use of thalidomide in patients with myeloma and renal failure may be associated with unexplained hyperkalaemia. *Br J Haematol.* 2003;122:160-161.

79. Fakhouri F, Guerraoui H, Presne C, et al. Thalidomide in patients with multiple myeloma and renal failure. *Br J Haematol.* 2004;125:96-97.

80. Marusic S, Gojo-Tomic N, Bacic-Vrca V, Bozikov V. Hyperkalaemia associated with hydroxyurea in a patient with polycythaemia vera. *Eur J Clin Pharmacol.* 2011;67:757-758.

81. Caliskan Y, Kalayoglu-Besisik S, Sargin D, Ecder T. Cyclosporine-associated hyperkalemia: report of four allogeneic blood stem-cell transplant cases. *Transplant.* 2003;75:1069-1072.

83. Hoorn EJ, Walsh SB, McCormick JA, et al. The calcineurin inhibitor tacrolimus activates the renal sodium chloride cotransporter to cause hypertension. *Nat Med.* 2011;17:1304-1309.

84. Palmer BF, Clegg DJ. Hyperkalemia. *J Am Med Assoc.* 2015;314:2405-2406.

85. Ejaz AA, Pourafshar N, Mohandas R, Smallwood BA, Johnson RJ, Hsu JW. Uric acid and the prediction models of tumor lysis syndrome in AML. *PLoS One.* 2015;10:e0119497.

87. Ali SR, Shaheen I, Young D. Fludrocortisone-a treatment for tubulopathy post-paediatric renal transplantation: a national paediatric nephrology unit experience. *Pediatr Transplant.* 2018;22(2):1-5

88. Georgianos PI, Agarwal R. Revisiting RAAS blockade in CKD with newer potassium-binding drugs. *Kidney Int.* 2018;93:325-334.

A full list of references is available at Expertconsult.com

4 Calcium and Phosphorus Disorders

ROBERT F. REILLY, JR.

Introduction

Disturbances in calcium and phosphorus homeostasis are commonly encountered when caring for cancer patients. These may result from the malignancy itself or as a complication of the treatment process. A thorough understanding of the pathophysiologic processes, whereby the tumor or its therapy result in abnormalities of calcium and phosphorus balance, is essential to managing cancer patients.

Disorders of Calcium Homeostasis

Disturbances in calcium homeostasis resulting in hypercalcemia in cancer patients can be divided into four types: tumor production of parathyroid hormone related peptide (PTHrP) known as *humoral hypercalcemia of malignancy*, local osteolytic hypercalcemia mediated by cytokine production, tumor production of $1,25(OH)_2$ vitamin D_3, and ectopic parathyroid hormone (PTH) secretion. Hypercalcemia may occur in up to 30% of patients with cancer and is often associated with advanced disease and a poor prognosis.[1]

Hypocalcemia may be the result of osteoblastic metastases, tumor lysis syndrome, hypomagnesemia, chemotherapeutic agents and drugs used to treat hypercalcemia. The incidence of hypocalcemia varies depending on the setting and was 1.6% in outpatients and 10.8% in inpatients.[2,3] In a study of 155 patients with solid tumors and bone metastases, hypocalcemia was present in 5% to 13% depending on the formula used to correct total calcium for serum albumin.[4]

HYPERCALCEMIA

Signs and Symptoms

Clinical signs and symptoms are dependent on severity and rate of rise of the serum calcium concentration.[5] Severe hypercalcemia is associated with significant neurologic and gastrointestinal (GI) symptoms. Neurologic symptoms range from mild confusion to stupor and coma. GI symptoms include constipation, obstipation, nausea, and vomiting, which result from decreased intestinal motility. Epigastric pain may be caused by hypercalcemia-induced pancreatitis. Hypercalcemia leads to extracellular fluid (ECF) volume depletion as a result of several pathophysiologic processes. Hypercalcemia reduces aquaporin 2 expression in the luminal membrane of the collecting duct, resulting in polyuria and potentially hypernatremia.[6] Calcium binds to the calcium-sensing receptor in the basolateral membrane of the thick ascending limb (TAL) and, through multiple second messenger pathways, inhibits the luminal Na-K-2Cl cotransporter leading to natriuresis, with associated volume depletion.[7] In addition, hypercalcemia stimulates afferent arteriolar vasoconstriction and reduces renal blood flow. The combination of the aforementioned leads to prerenal azotemia.

Etiology

Parathyroid Hormone Related Peptide–Mediated

PTHrP overproduction, humoral hypercalcemia of malignancy (HHM), is the cause of hypercalcemia in about 80% of cancer patients. Eight of the first 13 amino acids of PTHrP are identical to PTH, and PTHrP shares many common actions with PTH, including increased calcium reabsorption in the distal convoluted tubule (DCT), and reduced phosphate reabsorption in the proximal convoluted tubule (PCT) that result in hypercalcemia and hypophosphatemia. However, unlike PTH, which stimulates production of $1,25 (OH)_2$ vitamin D_3, PTHrP does not, and as a result, intestinal calcium and phosphorus reabsorption are not increased with PTHrP.[8] It is produced in mammary glands during lactation and by the placenta during pregnancy. It serves several normal regulatory physiologic functions including: uterine blood flow, calcium transport across placenta from mother to fetus, chondrocyte growth and differentiation in long bones, and calcium mobilization from bone into breast milk during lactation. With time, a variety of additional paracrine functions of PTHrP emerged.[9] PTHrP facilitates tooth eruption, promotes branching morphogenesis in mammary glands, and regulates vascular smooth muscle, keratinocyte differentiation, beta cell proliferation, and insulin production.

HHM presents with severe hypercalcemia, serum calcium concentration of 14 mg/dL or more, in a patient with a known malignancy or with a clearly evident malignancy, at time of initial presentation. It portends a poor prognosis. The most common tumors that produce PTHrP are squamous cell carcinomas, most breast cancers, and renal cell carcinoma. In a series of 138 patients with cancer, hypercalcemia and elevated PTHrP levels, solid organ malignancies were seen in 82.6%, hematologic malignancies in 12%, and benign etiologies in 8.7%.[10] The most common solid organ malignancies were squamous cell carcinomas (28.2%) most frequently originating from lung, head and neck, and skin. Adenocarcinomas were almost equally as common (27.5%) with the most common causes adenocarcinoma of unknown primary, breast cancer, renal cell carcinoma, and lung cancer. Other tumors with frequencies above 5% included urothelial and bladder tumors, other non-small cell lung cancers (NSCLC), and non-Hodgkin lymphoma (NHL). In patients with benign disease, 1.4% had community acquired pneumonia and in 7.2% no malignancy was found. Median survival, from the time elevated PTHrP was detected, was 52 days (range 21–132 days). Survival was longer in those with a hematologic etiology, 362 days. In a study at Barnes Jewish Hospital in St. Louis, of patients with a PTHrP level drawn over a 10-year period, evidence of malignancy was found in 242 patients.[11] The most common etiologies were undetermined in 40.5%, HHM in 38%, osteolytic bone lesions in 27.3%, immobilization in 3.3%, and primary hyperparathyroidism in 2.5%.

Patients with adult T-cell leukemia/lymphoma (ATLL) commonly manifest osteolytic bone lesions and hypercalcemia. ATLL results from infection with human T lymphotrophic virus type 1 (HTLV-1). The acute form is resistant to chemotherapy and mean survival is less than a year. In one autopsy series of 18 patients, 72% were hypercalcemic.[12] HTLV-1 infection causes hypercalcemia by several mechanisms. Lymphocytes infected with HTLV-1 produce PTHrP[13] and interleukin (IL)-1.[14] When murine calvaria were exposed to conditioned media from HTLV-1 infected-lymphocytes, increased osteoclast activity was demonstrated that was dependent on receptor activator of nuclear factor kappa-B ligand (RANKL), showing that factors secreted from ATLL cells activate osteoclasts.[15]

Local Osteolytic Metastases and Multiple Myeloma

Hypercalcemia from osteolytic metastases occurs in 20% of patients with cancer-related hypercalcemia and was initially assumed to result from direct physical bone destruction by malignant cells. However, subsequent studies showed that the presence of tumor cells in bone was insufficient to cause hypercalcemia and that bone destruction was mediated by osteoclasts.[16] A variety of osteoclastogenic factors are implicated and discussed later.

About one third of patients with multiple myeloma develop hypercalcemia caused by bone destruction.[17] Lesions occur as a result of local osteoclast stimulation by myeloma cells in their microenvironment. Several cytokines are implicated as possible mediators including: IL-6, IL-1β, tumor necrosis factor (TNF-α), macrophage inflammation protein 1-alpha, and lymphotoxin, but their role in inducing osteolytic bone disease in patients with myeloma is not fully defined. In addition, myeloma cells both express on their surface and secrete RANKL. In multiple myeloma, there is a disturbance in the bone microenvironment, with increases in RANKL and a decrease in osteoprotegerin. Osteoprotegerin competes with RANKL for binding to RANK and prevents receptor activation (Fig. 4.1). Depending on the concentration of RANKL, this may induce osteoclast differentiation or prevent apoptosis. Myeloma cells disturb the balance between osteoprotegerin, a decoy receptor for RANKL, and RANK. The balance between the two plays a key role in maintaining the ratio of osteoclast to osteoblast activity and bone remodeling. When RANKL expression increases and osteoprotegerin decreases, bone resorption is favored. Lytic lesions occur when there is increased osteoclast reabsorption without new bone formation.

Adhesion molecules expressed on the myeloma cell surface also interact with the bone marrow microenvironment

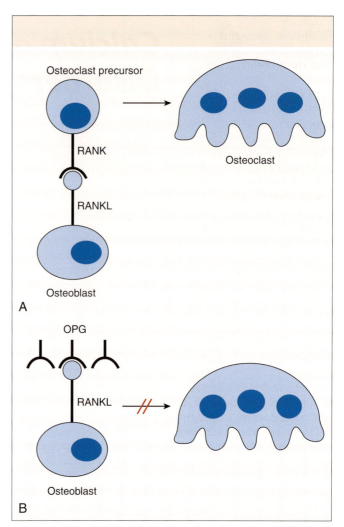

Fig. 4.1 The receptor activator of nuclear factor kappa-B ligand (RANKL)/RANK/osteoprotegerin (OPG) pathway. **A.** RANKL is expressed on the surface of osteoblasts. When it binds RANK expressed on the surface of osteoclast precursors it stimulates osteoclast formation, activation, and survival. **B.** Osteoprotegerin is a decoy receptor for receptor activator of RANKL and prevents its binding to RANK. Osteoprotegerin is secreted by osteoblasts, stromal cells, and B cells. The ratio of RANKL to osteoprotegerin determines the extent of bone resorption.

to stimulate cytokine production and osteoclast formation. In myeloma, osteoblast activity is suppressed. The mechanism is unclear, but several factors were recently implicated including: IL-3, IL-7, blockade of Runx2, and Wnt antagonists.[18] Myeloma cells also induce apoptosis of osteoblasts via the death receptor ligand tumor necrosis factor-related apoptosis-inducing ligand.

Osteolytic metastases from solid tumors also produce cytokines that result in bone calcium release. TNF and IL-1 stimulate osteoclast development from precursors and IL-6 stimulates osteoclast production. Breast cancer cells in bone activate osteoclasts and increase bone resorption. Recent studies showed that a MAP kinase isoform, MAPK11 (p38β), is responsible for bone destruction. p38β upregulates monocyte chemotactic protein-1, which stimulates osteoclast differentiation and activity.[19] PTHrP may play a role locally in bone, in breast cancer metastases.[20] Tumor cells produce PTHrP in the bone microenvironment, which is thought to be mediated by transforming growth factor (TGF)-β. A paracrine loop is established, whereby PTHrP stimulates osteoclast activity, with resultant TGF-β release from the reabsorbed bone.

1,25 (OH)$_2$ Vitamin D$_3$–Mediated

Calcitriol is the major humoral mediator of hypercalcemia in patients with Hodgkin and NHL and accounts for less than 1% of cases of hypercalcemia in cancer patients. Incidence of hypercalcemia in Hodgkin and NHL was reported as 5% and 15%, respectively.[21]

In 38 patients with Hodgkin disease, peak total serum calcium levels ranged from 10.9 to 23.1 mg/dL, median level 14.4 mg/dL.[22] The nodular sclerosing subtype was significantly underrepresented. Most patients had infradiaphragmatic disease and only three had lytic bone lesions. Nearly all patients with hypercalcemia, in which calcitriol levels were measured, were elevated.

In NHL, incidence of hypercalcemia varies with histologic grade from 1% to 2% in low grade, to 23% in high-grade subtypes.[23] In 19 cases of NHL, only one had low-grade histology.[22] In 54 patients with NHL and hypercalcemia, 57.4% had diffuse large B-cell lymphoma.[24] Seventeen of these had both a PTHrP and calcitriol level properly collected, seven (41%) had an elevated calcitriol level, suggesting that in the majority, hypercalcemia was mediated by a noncalcitriol, non-PTHrP mechanism. Intermediate to aggressive histologic features were seen in 83%. In six of seven, peak calcium concentration was less than 14.5 mg/dL. Calcitriol elevation correlated with worse progression-free but not overall survival. Of 345 consecutive patients with NHL, 8.1% were hypercalcemic, 55% had elevated calcitriol levels.[25] In an interesting report, a patient with an intermediate grade B-cell lymphoma confined to the spleen, with hypercalcemia mediated by calcitriol, underwent a splenectomy.[26] Immunochemistry showed 1α-hydroxylase expression in CD68-positive macrophages and not bordering lymphoma cells, suggesting that substances produced by malignant cells stimulated macrophages to produce calcitriol.

There are six case reports of hypercalcemia associated with gastrointestinal stromal tumors (GIST). GIST is the most common mesenchymal tumor in the GI tract but is a very rare tumor with an incidence of 11 to 19.6 per million.[27] In four cases where the mechanism of hypercalcemia was examined, three resulted from calcitriol overproduction and one from PTHrP.[28] There is one case report of calcitriol-mediated hypercalcemia with an ovarian dysgerminoma.[29]

Ectopic Parathyroid Hormone Production

Ectopic PTH production is a rare cause of hypercalcemia of malignancy. There are approximately 25 cases reported. In some, the tumor also secreted PTHrP.[30] Tumors reported to secrete PTH include: squamous cell carcinoma of the tonsil, rhabdoid Wilms tumor, small cell lung cancer, pancreatic carcinoma, ovarian carcinoma, endometrial adenosquamous carcinoma, thymoma, papillary and medullary thyroid cancer, primitive neuroectodermal tumor, hepatocellular carcinoma, transitional cell carcinoma of the bladder, ovarian small cell carcinoma, pancreatic neuroendocrine tumors, nasopharyngeal rhabdomyosarcoma, bronchogenic carcinoma, neuroendocrine neck tumor, gastric carcinoma, and squamous cell carcinoma of the penis.[31]

Treatment

Treatment depends on severity of elevation of serum calcium concentration, and is directed at increasing renal excretion, inhibiting bone resorption, and decreasing intestinal absorption.

Loop diuretics and volume expansion are used to increase renal calcium excretion. Volume expansion and loop diuretics alone may be adequate if serum calcium concentration is less than 12.5 mg/dL. The goal is to maintain a brisk urine output of 200 to 250 mL/min. In theory, this combination ensures adequate sodium delivery to the TAL, and is based on sound physiologic principles. Although this approach is logical, it was recently questioned.[32] The authors argue that furosemide use is largely based on historical practice and not evidence. They recommend saline hydration and bisphosphonates as first line therapy, supplemented in the short-term by calcitonin.

When hypercalcemia is moderate or severe, bone resorption will need to be inhibited. This is done in the short term (hours) with calcitonin at a 4 IU/kg dose. Calcitonin inhibits bone resorption and increases renal calcium excretion. It reduces serum calcium concentration approximately 1 to 2 mg/dL. The main drawback of calcitonin is tachyphylaxis and it has limited use beyond 48 hours. As a result, a second agent to reduce bone resorption should be used concomitantly.[1]

Bisphosphonates are the most commonly used drug class to block bone resorption. They should be dosed simultaneously with calcitonin because of their slow onset of action (48–72 hours) but have a long duration of action (weeks). Zolendronate at a dose of 4 to 8 mg intravenously (IV) over 15 minutes is the most commonly used bisphosphonate to treat hypercalcemia. Bisphosphonates are pyrophosphate analogs that deposit in bone and interfere with osteoclast recruitment, formation, activation, and function. The major renal toxicity of zoledronate is acute kidney injury (AKI) from direct renal tubular epithelial cell toxicity. Zoledronate is contraindicated in patients with an estimated glomerular filtration rate of less than 30 mL/min or AKI. A reduced dose (3.0-3.5 mg) has been recommended for those with a creatinine clearance between 30 and 60 ml/min. Bisphosphonates can also cause osteonecrosis of the jaw with chronic use and this generally occurs after a recent dental procedure. Pamidronate can be used at a dose of 60 to 90 mg IV over 4 hours. Dosage is adjusted based on serum calcium concentration (60 mg < 13.5 mg/dL and 90 mg > 13.5 mg/dL).

In most patients, a combination of fluids, a loop diuretic, calcitonin, and zolendronic acid is sufficient. If hypercalcemia persists, denosumab can be used. In 33 patients with bisphosphonate-resistant hypercalcemia, denosumab lowered calcium levels in 64% within 10 days at a dose of 120 mg subcutaneously on days 1, 8, 15, and 29 and then monthly.[33] Denosumab is a human monoclonal antibody that binds RANKL and inhibits osteoclast function, formation, and survival. Denosumab is preferred over bisphosphonates in patients with advanced renal disease, as it does not require dose reduction and does not appear to be nephrotoxic.

Mithramycin has fallen out of favor with the availability of bisphosphonates because of its side effect profile. It cannot be used in patients with renal or hepatic disease or bone marrow disorders. Side effects include proteinuria, hepatotoxicity, thrombocytopenia, and nausea and vomiting. It has a rapid onset of action, 12 hours, and a peak effect at 48 hours. Dose is 25 μg/kg IV over 4 hours daily for 3 to 4 days.

Gallium nitrate blocks bone resorption through inhibition of acid secretion via the proton adenosine triphosphatase (ATPase) in the osteoclast ruffled membrane. It is administered IV for 5 consecutive days at a dose of 100 to 200 mg/m^2. It is contraindicated if serum creatinine concentration exceeds 2.5 mg/dL. It is not commonly used because of the need for a continuous infusion.

In patients with severe, symptomatic hypercalcemia, especially with associated acute or chronic kidney failure, dialysis can be considered. In one study, calcium removal rates were 682 mg/h with hemodialysis, 124 mg/h with peritoneal dialysis, and 82 mg/h with saline diuresis.[34]

HYPOCALCEMIA

Signs and Symptoms

Rate and degree of decline in serum calcium concentration determines whether symptoms develop.[35] Level of serum calcium at which symptoms occur also depends on serum pH and presence of other electrolyte abnormalities, such as hypokalemia or hypomagnesemia. The most common symptoms are related to increased neuromuscular excitability and include carpopedal spasm, and circumoral and distal paresthesias. Altered mental status and seizures can occur. On physical examination, bradycardia, hypotension, and laryngospasm may be present. There are rare case reports of congestive heart failure with severe hypocalcemia that reverse with calcium repletion. If signs or symptoms are present, one should test for Chvostek and Trousseau's signs.

Etiology

Osteoblastic Metastases

Hypocalcemia caused by osteoblastic metastases and increased bone calcium uptake occurs most commonly in patients with prostate followed by breast cancer. It was reported with lung, thyroid, salivary gland, GI, and neuroendocrine tumors.[36] In bone, metastatic prostate cancer cells produce factors that activate osteoblasts including endothelin-1, platelet derived growth factor, and bone matrix proteins.[37] In 143 patients with bone metastases, 16% had hypocalcemia, with prostate cancer as the most frequent etiology.[38] Tucci et al. reported 210 consecutive patients with hormone-refractory prostate cancer.[39] There was a 26.6% incidence of albumin-corrected hypocalcemia. Hypocalcemia did not adversely affect prognosis. Most cases are mild, but there are reports of severe hypocalcemia requiring prolonged calcium supplementation resembling hungry bone syndrome seen after parathyroidectomy.[40,41] In several reports, hypocalcemia was felt to be exacerbated by bisphosphonate administration.[42,43] There are two possible explanations for this. The first is that bisphosphonate-induced osteoclast suppression leaves osteoblast activity unopposed or it may increase osteoblast maturation and activity in areas of metastasis.

Tumor Lysis Syndrome

Tumor lysis syndrome (TLS) results from rapid tumor cell lysis that occurs spontaneously or from treatment, and is the most common oncologic emergency.[44] Although observed most commonly with hematologic malignancies, it is also seen with solid tumors. Phosphorus, potassium, and nucleic acids are released into the ECF. Purines in nucleic acids are metabolized to uric acid (Fig. 4.2). TLS results when rapid entry of these substances into ECF exceeds the ability of homeostatic mechanisms to remove them.

Hypocalcemia is seen in association with hyperphosphatemia, hyperkalemia, and hyperuricemia. Release of phosphorus into ECF results in hypocalcemia from two potential mechanisms. Mathematic models suggest that a rapid phosphate infusion lowers plasma phosphorus concentration via formation of calcium phosphate complexes.[45] There is also evidence that an acute intravenous phosphate load lowers serum calcium concentration because of reduced calcium efflux from bone.[46]

Patients with malignancies that have high turnover rates, large tumor burdens, and are most sensitive to therapy, such as acute myeloid leukemia (AML), acute lymphoblastic leukemia (ALL), and NHL are at highest risk. TLS occurs in as many as 42% with NHL, 17% with AML, and 8.4% with ALL.[47] Patients with solid tumors often have large tumor burdens. TLS was reported in a wide variety of solid tumors, including metastatic prostate cancer and hepatocellular carcinoma.

There are two commonly used systems to define TLS. To diagnose laboratory-based TLS (LTLS), the Cairo-Bishop system requires a change in two or more laboratory values between 3 days before or 7 days after initial treatment. Criteria include serum concentrations of: uric acid 8 mg/dL or more; potassium 6 mEq/L or more; phosphorus 2.1 mmol/L or more; calcium 1.75 mmol/L or less; or a change in any of these parameters by 25% or more from baseline. Clinical TLS (CTLS) is defined as LTLS plus one of the following: arrhythmia; sudden death; seizure; or serum creatinine 1.5 (or more) times the upper limit of normal.[48] CTLS is less common than LTLS. Limitations of this system are that it does not allow for spontaneous TLS in the absence of treatment and patients with chronic kidney disease (CKD) would meet criteria for CTLS.

The Hande-Garrow system requires a 25% or more change in two of the following five laboratory parameters: a 25% or more increase in blood urea nitrogen; uric acid; potassium; or phosphorus concentration; or a 25% or more decrease in serum calcium concentration.[49]

Patients with preexisting kidney disease are at higher risk for AKI. AKI can occur as a result of uric acid nephropathy, tubular calcium phosphate crystallization, or tumor infiltration of the kidneys and portends a poor prognosis. In 772 patients with AML undergoing induction chemotherapy, 17% developed TLS (5% CTLS, 12% LTLS). Kidney dysfunction was strongly predictive for development of CTLS and LTLS with an odds ratio (OR) in multivariable analysis of 2.9 (95% confidence interval [CI], 1.6–6.8) and 10.7 (95% CI, 4.5–25.1), respectively. In patients with CTLS, oliguria occurred in 83%, and hemodialysis was performed in 13%. CTLS was associated with a statistically significant increase in death rate, 79% versus 23%, and renal failure was a major cause of death.[50] In 63 patients with acute hematologic malignancies and TLS, hospital and 6-month mortality were significantly higher in those with AKI (21% vs. 7%).[51] Presence of AKI was associated with higher in-hospital and 6-month mortality, odds ratio of 10.41 (95% CI, 2.01–19.07) and 5.61 (OR, 1.64–54.66), respectively. Finally, a recent retrospective analysis evaluated the impact of acute hemodialysis on a variety of outcomes in TLS.[52] Acute hemodialysis was carried out in 12% of all TLS hospitalizations. Dialysis for AKI in multivariable analysis was associated with an increased mortality (OR, 1.98; 95% CI, 1.60–2.45), and longer length of stay (19 vs. 14.6 days, $p < .01$). These studies emphasize the importance of risk stratifying patients to identify those at high risk for AKI and to institute prophylactic measures.

Risk stratification systems were developed by several groups. High risk is defined as greater than 5%, intermediate risk 1% to 5%, and low risk less than 1%.[53] For solid tumors and chronic hematologic malignancies, low risk diseases include: most solid tumors except for bulky tumors sensitive to chemotherapy such as small-cell lung cancer, neuroblastomas, and germ-cell tumors; multiple myeloma; chronic myelogenous leukemia (CML) in the chronic phase; and chronic lymphocytic leukemia (CLL) treated with alkylating agents. CLL treated with targeted and/or biologic therapies is intermediate risk. Risk stratification for acute leukemias and lymphomas is more complex and is shown in Tables 4.1 and 4.2. Other patient-related risk factors include: preexisting kidney disease; volume depletion; age; and preexisting hyperuricemia.

Risk stratification allows one to anticipate and prevent TLS via prophylactic measures. An expert consensus panel in the United States and the British Committee for Standards in Hematology developed recommendations for prophylaxis.[53,54] For patients at low risk, monitoring, normal hydration, and withholding prophylaxis for hyperuricemia

Table 4.2 Risk of Tumor Lysis Syndrome in Lymphoma

HODGKIN, SMALL CELL LYMPHOCYTIC, FOLLICULAR, MARGINAL ZONE B CELL, MALT, MANTLE CELL (NON-BLASTOID VARIANTS), CUTANEOUS T CELL

Risk		
low	All cases	

BURKITT LEUKEMIA/LYMPHOMA, LYMPHOBLASTIC

Risk	Stage	LDH
intermediate	early	$< 2 \times$ ULN
high	early	$\geq 2 \times$ ULN
high	advanced	-

ANAPLASTIC LARGE CELL

Risk	Age	Stage
low	adult	-
low	child	I/II
intermediate	child	III/IV

ADULT T CELL LYMPHOMA, DIFFUSE LARGE B CELL, PERIPHERAL T CELL, TRANSFORMED, MANTLE CELL BLASTOID VARIANT

Risk	Age	LDH	Bulky	Stage
low	adult	WNL	-	-
intermediate	adult	> ULN	no	-
high	adult	> ULN	yes	-
low	child	-	-	-
intermediate	child	$< 2 \times$ ULN	-	I/II
high	child	$\geq 2 \times$ ULN	-	III/IV

Renal dysfunction or renal involvement increases risk by one level; serum phosphorus, potassium, or uric acid > ULN increases risk from intermediate to high.
LDH, Lactate dehydrogenase; *MALT*, mucosa-associated lymphoid tissue; *TLS*, tumor lysis syndrome; *ULN*, upper limit of normal; *WNL*, within normal limits.

Table 4.1 Risk of Tumor Lysis Syndrome in Acute Leukemias

ACUTE MYELOGENOUS LEUKEMIA

Risk	WBC per Microliter	LDH
low	< 25,000	$< 2 \times$ ULN
intermediate	< 25,000	$\geq 2 \times$ ULN
intermediate	$\geq 25,000 < 100,000$	-
high	$\geq 100,000$	-

ACUTE LYMPHOCYTIC LEUKEMIA

Risk	WBC per Microliter	LDH
intermediate	< 100,000	$< 2 \times$ ULN
high	< 100,000	$\geq 2 \times$ ULN
high	$\geq 100,000$	-

BURKITT LYMPHOMA/LEUKEMIA

high	-	-

Renal dysfunction or renal involvement increases risk by one level; serum phosphorus, potassium, or uric acid greater than ULN increases risk from intermediate to high.
LDH, Lactate dehydrogenase; *TLS*, tumor lysis syndrome; *ULN*, upper limit of normal; *WBC*, white blood cell count.

were recommended. There should be a low threshold for adding fluids and allopurinol if needed. With bulky or advanced disease, metabolic abnormalities, or a tumor with a high proliferative rate, allopurinol, an inhibitor of xanthine oxidase, is recommended (Fig. 4.2). Patients with intermediate risk disease should be treated with vigorous hydration ($3 L/m^2/day$) with nonbicarbonate-containing isotonic fluids and allopurinol (100–300 mg every 8 hours daily) for up to 7 days. Patients at high risk should be hydrated as mentioned earlier, depending on volume status and presence of AKI, and administered rasburicase (recombinant urate oxidase). Dosage in adults is 0.1 to 0.2 mg/kg, or a fixed dose of 3 mg, with repeat dosing as required. If glucose-6-phosphate deficiency is present, allopurinol is substituted for rasburicase.

Other recommendations include: in patients on rasburicase, urate assays should be sent to the laboratory on ice to avoid falsely low values; rasburicase and allopurinol should not be administered simultaneously because allopurinol may reduce the effectiveness of rasburicase; and urinary alkalinization is not recommended. Patients that were originally classified as low or intermediate risk that develop LTLS should receive rasburicase. Asymptomatic

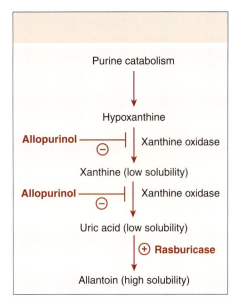

Fig. 4.2 Purine catabolism pathway and mechanism of action of drugs used to treat tumor lysis syndrome. Allopurinol can lead to the accumulation of xanthine, which is poorly soluble in water, and can lead to xanthine nephropathy. Allopurinol can prevent uric acid formation but will not affect uric acid that is already present. Rasburicase (urate oxidase) metabolizes uric acid to the much more soluble allantoin. Urate oxidase is not expressed in humans; as a result uric acid is normally the final endpoint for purine catabolism.

hypocalcemia should not be treated. Symptomatic hypocalcemia can be treated with short calcium gluconate infusions with careful monitoring of serum calcium, phosphorus, and creatinine concentrations. Management of other aspects of TLS are covered in the section on hyperphosphatemia.

Drugs

HYPOMAGNESEMIA-EPIDERMAL GROWTH FACTOR RECEPTOR BLOCKERS. A pooled analysis of six randomized controlled trials (RCTs) that recorded hypocalcemic events showed a 16.8% (95% CI, 14.2%–19.7%) incidence of all-grade hypocalcemia with cetuximab versus 9.9% (95% CI, 8.0%–12.2%) in controls.[55] To standardize adverse drug events in

cancer treatment, the National Cancer Institute developed a system, the Common Terminology Criteria for Adverse Events (CTCAE), for grading severity of hypercalcemia, hypocalcemia, and hypophosphatemia (Table 4.3). There was a 3.8% incidence of grades 3/4 CTCAE hypocalcemia with cetuximab and panitumumab versus 2% in controls. Of three RCTs reporting grades 3/4 hypocalcemia with cetuximab, relative risk (RR) was 2.12 versus controls (95% CI, 1.30–3.45, $p = .003$). Although RR was increased (1.14) with panitumumab versus controls, this increase was not statistically significant. The pathogenesis of hypocalcemia with epidermal growth factor (EGF) receptor inhibitors is unclear. It may be related to the well-known association of cetuximab and hypomagnesemia.[56] The EGF receptor is located on the basolateral membrane of the DCT and its activation increases transient receptor potential channel melastatin subtype 6 (TRPM6) activity and surface expression via sarcoma (Src) kinases and Ras-related C3 botulinum toxin substrate (Rac) 1. TRPM6 is a channel located in the DCT apical membrane that mediates magnesium entry and is the rate limiting step for magnesium reabsorption (Fig. 4.3). Hypomagnesemia can result in end-organ resistance to PTH and impair PTH release from parathyroid gland. End-organ resistance occurs at magnesium concentrations of 1 mg/dL or less, whereas a lower concentration, less than 0.5 mg/dL, is required to reduce PTH secretion.[57] Hypocalcemia will not respond to calcium or vitamin D administration until the magnesium deficit is repleted.

CISPLATIN. Cisplatin is a common antineoplastic agent used to treat a variety of solid tumors. Its major dose limiting side effect is AKI.[58] It is taken up across the basolateral membrane of renal tubular epithelial cells (RTECs) and metabolized to several species, which may play a role in its nephrotoxicity. Cisplatin can injure RTECs via a variety of mechanisms including: oxidative stress; caspase activation; and cytokine and chemokine upregulation. Hypocalcemia can occur secondary to hypomagnesemia. Hypomagnesemia, secondary to renal magnesium wasting, is common with cisplatin. In 23 of 44 patients receiving the drug, hypomagnesemia developed.[59] Hypomagnesemia often occurs with repeated doses administered over time or with exposure to additional drugs, such as aminoglycosides or

Table 4.3   National Cancer Institute Common Criteria for Adverse Events v4.0

Grade	1	2	3	4	5
Hypercalcemia					
TC mg/dL	> ULN–11.5	> 11.5–12.5	> 12.5–13.5	> 13.5	Death
TC mmol/L	> ULN–2.9	> 2.9–3.1	> 3.1–3.4	> 3.4	
iCa mmol/L	> ULN–1.5	> 1.5–1.6	> 1.6–1.8	> 1.8	
		symptoms	Hospitalization indicated	Life threatening	
Hypocalcemia					
TC mg/dL	< LLN–8.0	7– < 8.0	6– < 7.0	< 6	Death
TC mmol/L	< LLN–2.0	< 2.0–1.75	< 1.75–1.50	< 1.5	
iCa mmol/L	< LLN–1.0	< 1.0–0.9	< 0.9–0.8	< 0.8	
		symptoms	Hospitalization indicated	Life threatening	
Hypophosphatemia					
mg/dL	< LLN–2.5	2– < 2.5–2.0	1– < 2.0–1.0	< 1	Death
mmol/L	< LLN–0.8	< 0.8–0.6	< 0.6–0.3	< 0.3	
		symptoms	Hospitalization indicated	Life threatening	

iCa, Ionized calcium; *LLN,* lower limit of normal; *TC,* total serum calcium values corrected for albumin; *ULN,* upper limit of normal.

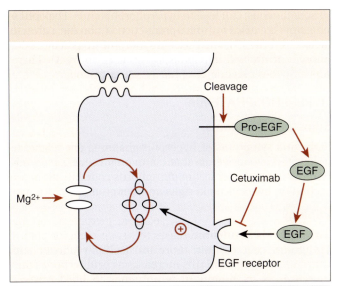

Fig. 4.3 Epidermal growth factor (EGF) regulation of magnesium transport in the distal convoluted tubule (a paracrine pathway). Pro-EGF, a type I membrane protein, is cleaved to EGF, which binds to the EGF receptor. This binding is blocked by EGF receptor antagonists, such as cetuximab. After EGF binds to its receptor, intracellular kinases are activated, and transient receptor protein (TRP) M6 is trafficked to the apical membrane.

amphotericin B, which can also cause renal magnesium wasting. In 66 patients receiving a 5-day combination regimen including cisplatin, hypomagnesemia increased from 41% after one course, to 100% after six cycles.[60] In 35 adults with hypocalcemia, hypokalemia, and hypomagnesemia, the two most common diagnoses were cisplatin and alcoholism.[61]

Cisplatin reduces expression of two important proteins involved in magnesium transport in DCT. The first is the magnesium entry channel, TRPM6, which is expressed in the luminal membrane.[62] Cisplatin also reduces expression of the EGF receptor in the basolateral membrane.[63]

AXITINIB. Axitinib is a VEGF inhibitor. In a phase 2 trial, 52 patients with metastatic or unresectable locally-advanced differentiated or medullary thyroid cancer that was either not amenable or refractory to I-131, there was an 8% incidence of all grade hypocalcemia and a 6% incidence of CTCAE grade 3 (or higher) hypocalcemia.[64] Axitinib was begun at a dose of 5 mg twice daily and titrated to 10 mg twice daily.

5-FLUOROURACIL AND LOW DOSE LEUCOVORIN. The combination of 5-fluorouracil (5-FU) and leucovorin (LV) is used in advanced colorectal cancer. In 25 patients with advanced gastric and colorectal cancer, hypocalcemia occurred in 65%.[65] Patients were treated with LV at 20 mg/m²/day IV before a 1-hour infusion of 5-FU at 425 to 600 mg/m²/day for 5 days at 4 week intervals. In 10 cases, hypocalcemia was CTCAE grade 1 and in five was CTCAE grade 2. Two patients had tetany and two other patients had hiccups, which resolved with calcium supplementation. Five developed hypocalcemia during the first course. Hypocalcemia was associated with a fall in vitamin D levels but no change in PTH. The mechanism for the fall in vitamin D levels is unknown.

ESTRAMUSTINE. Estramustine is a nitrogen mustard linked to estradiol that was used to treat prostate cancer with skeletal metastases after failure of hormonal therapy. There are case reports of profound hypocalcemia with its use.[66] In 90 patients with prostate cancer, 20% developed hypocalcemia (after correction for serum albumin concentration), 44% developed hypophosphatemia, and 40% were hypomagnesemic.[67] Mean calcium level in hypocalcemic patients was 8.06 ± 0.36 mg/dL, range 7.1 to 8.3 mg/dL. Of 18 hypocalcemic patients, eight had concomitant hypophosphatemia and five hypomagnesemia. Hypomagnesemia may have contributed to the hypocalcemia in some patients.

NAB-PACLITAXEL. Nab-paclitaxel is a nanoparticle albumin-bound paclitaxel used to treat lung, breast, and pancreatic cancers. In a phase II trial, 19 patients with pancreatic cancer were treated with nab-paclitaxel 100 mg/m² on days 1, 8, and 15 of a 28-day cycle.[68] CTCAE grades 1 and 2 hypocalcemia was observed in 37%.

HIGH DOSE INTERLEUKIN 2. A combination of high dose IL-2 and entinostat, a histone deacetylase inhibitor, was administered to 47 patients with previously untreated renal cell carcinoma.[69] CTCAE grade 3 and 4 hypocalcemia and hypophosphatemia were noted in 7.2% and 16.4%, respectively.

DRUGS USED TO TREAT HYPERCALCEMIA. The most commonly used drugs to treat hypercalcemia that result in unintended hypocalcemia are bisphosphonates and denosumab. In a metaanalysis of six randomized controlled trials of 7722 patients, denosumab was associated with an increased risk of grade 3 or 4 hypocalcemia versus bisphosphonates (RR, 1.99; 95% CI, 1.11–3.54).[70] Denosumab is often the preferred agent in patients with AKI or advanced CKD (stages 4 and 5). However, caution should be exercised in this setting even though denosumab is not excreted by the kidneys. In four patients with multiple myeloma, refractory hypercalcemia, and renal dysfunction, denosumab was administered at doses from 25 to 60 mg.[71] Serum creatinine ranged from 2.5 to 5.7 mg/dL. The index case was administered 60 mg and developed profound hypocalcemia with total calcium concentration adjusted for albumin of 6.9 mg/dL requiring prolonged intravenous calcium supplementation. With subsequent cases, the dose was adjusted to 0.3 mg/kg and serum calcium concentration normalized in 1 to 5 days with only mild hypocalcemia. The package insert for denosumab does not recommend reduced dosage for renal impairment but does state that risk of hypocalcemia was greater in clinical studies in patients with a creatinine clearance of less than 30 mL/min and those on dialysis.[72]

Bisphosphonates may result in hypocalcemia and hypophosphatemia. In a pooled analysis of two clinical trials comparing zolendronic acid (4 mg) and pamidronate (90 mg) in patients with hypercalcemia of malignancy reported to the U.S Food and Drugs Administration, grade 3/4 hypocalcemia was low with both drugs, 1.2% and 2%, respectively, with all reports being grade 3.[73] However, hypophosphatemia was much more common with grade 3 hypophosphatemia in 51.4% with zolendronic acid, and 33.3% with pamidronate. Grade 4 hypophosphatemia was seen in 1.4% with zolendronic acid, and 4.9% with pamidronate. Risk factors for hypocalcemia include vitamin D deficiency, hypoparathyroidism, hypomagnesemia, and patients with predominantly osteoblastic metastases, such as prostate cancer.[74]

Table 4.4   Oral and Intravenous Calcium Preparations

INTRAVENOUS

Preparation	Ampule Size (mL)	Elemental Calcium (mg)
10% Calcium chloride	10	272
10% Calcium gluconate	10	94
10% Calcium gluceptate	5	90

ORAL

Preparation	Tablet Size (mg)	Elemental Calcium (mg)
Calcium carbonate	500	200
Calcium gluconate	1000	90
Calcium lactate	650	85
Calcium citrate	950	200

Treatment

Choice of oral versus intravenous route of calcium repletion depends on degree of hypocalcemia and whether or not symptoms are present. With life-threatening symptoms. such as hypotension, cardiac arrhythmias, tetany and seizures, calcium should be administered IV, 100 to 200 mg over 10 to 20 minutes.[4] After the initial bolus, an infusion at 0.5 to 1.0 mg/kg/h can be started with frequent monitoring of serum calcium concentration. Intravenous calcium preparations are shown in Table 4.4. As a general rule, intravenous calcium should be used in symptomatic patients, those with a prolonged QT interval, or severe hypocalcemia (serum calcium after correction for albumin less than 7.5 mg/dL). If life-threatening symptoms are not present, but hypocalcemia is severe, a dose of 15 mg/kg of elemental calcium over 4 to 6 hours will generally increase total serum calcium concentration 2 to 3 mg/dL. Calcium chloride should be administered through a large bore IV or a central line to avoid venous sclerosis. Calcium gluconate is preferred when administration is via peripheral vein. With mild hypocalcemia in an outpatient, the oral route should be used. In general, 1 to 2 g of elemental calcium is sufficient. Several oral calcium preparations are available (see Table 4.4). At higher gastric pHs, calcium citrate has higher bioavailability than calcium carbonate. If calcium supplementation alone is insufficient, then a vitamin D preparation may be needed.

Hypomagnesemia is a common cause of hypocalcemia and serum magnesium concentration should be measured and repleted if low. If the patient has an associated metabolic acidosis, the calcium deficit should be corrected first. If acidemia is corrected before hypocalcemia, ionized calcium concentration will decrease, which can potentially convert an asymptomatic patient to a symptomatic one.

Disorders of Phosphorus Homeostasis

One needs to be aware of disorders associated with spurious or pseudo- hypophosphatemia. TLS, whether from treatment or spontaneous, can lead to hyperphosphatemia. Hypophosphatemia is caused by tumor production of fibroblast growth factor 23 (FGF-23), and Fanconi syndrome from drugs, lymphoma, or multiple myeloma. Drugs used to treat cancers may also lower serum phosphorus concentration.

HYPERPHOSPHATEMIA

Signs and Symptoms

Signs and symptoms of hyperphosphatemia are related to associated hypocalcemia that commonly occurs, generally with an acute rise in serum phosphorus concentration (see section on hypocalcemia signs and symptoms).

Etiology

Tumor Lysis Syndrome

Malignant cells contain more intracellular phosphorus than normal cells and this increases as proliferative rates increase, as in malignant lymphomas in blast crisis.[75] When these cells are killed either by chemotherapy, corticosteroids, or radiation therapy, their contents are released into ECF, where hyperphosphatemia and TLS can occur.

The definition, risk factors, risk stratification, pathophysiology, and prophylaxis of TLS were discussed under hypocalcemia. In this section, we will focus on specific aspects of TLS treatment.

Urinary alkalinization is not recommended. Uric acid has low solubility at acidic pH (100 mg/L).[76] It is a weak organic acid with two protons that can dissociate. Only the dissociation of the first proton, which occurs at a pKa of 5.5, is physiologically relevant. At pH less than 5.5, the undissociated acid predominates, whereas at a pH greater than 5.5, the salt sodium urate predominates. Sodium urate is much more soluble in water (1 g/L). From the standpoint of uric acid solubility, alkalinization makes sense. However, as urinary pH rises and approaches the pKa of brushite ($CaHPO_4.2H_2O$), a form of calcium phosphate, calcium phosphate can precipitate in the renal tubular lumen and interstitium, resulting in phosphate nephropathy and AKI. Alkalinization also reduces xanthine and hypoxanthine solubility, which can also precipitate within tubular lumens.

Allopurinol and febuxostat are xanthine oxidase inhibitors that block conversion of xanthine to uric acid (see Fig. 4.3). Allopurinol is converted to oxypurinol, a xanthine analog, which acts as a competitive inhibitor of xanthine oxidase. Allopurinol has several drawbacks. It prevents the formation of uric acid but does not affect existing uric acid. Allopurinol blockade of xanthine oxidase leads to accumulation of xanthine, which is very insoluble in aqueous solution and can lead to xanthine nephropathy.[77] Allopurinol interferes with metabolism of several purine-based therapeutic drugs including azathioprine, 6-mercaptopurine, and high-dose methotrexate. Dosages of these drugs must be reduced in patients on allopurinol. It is contraindicated in patients on cyclophosphamide and other cytotoxic agents due to severe bone marrow suppression.[78] Oxypurinol is renally excreted and dose adjustments are recommended in AKI and advanced CKD. Allopurinol is associated with hypersensitivity reactions that can be life threatening. Febuxostat is a newer xanthine oxidase inhibitor that is metabolized in the liver and not associated with hypersensitivity reactions. It may be a reasonable alternative in those with previous hypersensitivity to allopurinol.

Rasburicase is a recombinant urate oxidase. Urate oxidase is expressed in a variety of species but not humans and converts uric acid to allantoin, which is 5 to 10 times more soluble in water than uric acid. Dosage is 0.2 mg/kg infused over 30 minutes daily for 5 days. It is contraindicated in those with glucose-6-phosphate dehydrogenase deficiency. Rasburicase is very effective in lowering serum uric acid concentration and lowers it much more quickly than allopurinol. In a metaanalysis of four controlled trials and 17 observational studies of 1261 adults with TLS, mean reduction in serum uric acid concentration ranged from 5.3 to 12.8 mg/dL.[79] In the 17 observational studies, 93.4% of patients had a normal uric acid level after rasburicase. There are no studies with hard outcomes that show an advantage of rasburicase over allopurinol. However, clinically rasburicase has several advantages compared with allopurinol. Because it metabolizes existing uric acid, chemotherapy does not need to be delayed in those with a high uric acid level before treatment. Rasburicase is metabolized by peptide hydrolysis and not dependent on hepatic or renal function, so it is not dose adjusted in AKI. It has no significant drug interactions and a low incidence of hypersensitivity reactions.

A historical analysis of patient studies with and without rasburicase showed a marked reduction in need for dialysis with rasburicase. In seven studies with rasburicase, need for dialysis ranged from 0% to 2.8%, whereas in three studies without rasburicase, ranged from 15.9% to 25%.[80] In TLS, AKI can occur via a variety of mechanisms including: (1) precipitation of uric acid or calcium phosphate in the tubular lumen; (2) ureteral obstruction by tumor; (3) tumor infiltration of the kidney; (4) drug-induced renal injury; and (5) sepsis. AKI in TLS is most commonly oliguric. Dialysis indications are no different than other etiologies of AKI. Peritoneal dialysis should not be used because clearances are too low.[54] A variety of dialysis modes were reported including daily hemodialysis,[81] hemodialysis followed by continuous veno-veno hemodialysis (CVVHD),[82] and CVVHD alone.[83] If control of potassium concentration is an issue, hemodialysis has the highest potassium clearance and CVVHD can be used in the interval between hemodialyses. CVVHD should be done with high dialysate and replacement fluid flow rates. In one study, with a dialysate flow rate of 2.5L/h and a replacement fluid rate of 1.5 L/h, clearances of urea, creatinine, uric acid, and phosphorus were 55.8 ± 3.8, 48.9 ± 2.6, 45.1 ± 2.6, and 47.0 ± 3.3, respectively.[83]

Treatment

In the cancer patient, hyperphosphatemia is more likely to be acute than chronic. Renal phosphate excretion can be increased by volume expansion if renal function allows. Some benefit can be obtained by using phosphate binders, especially those with higher binding capacities, such as aluminum hydroxide or lanthanum carbonate. Aluminum hydroxide should not be used beyond 5 to 7 days and avoided in advanced CKD or end-stage renal disease. Dialysis may be required with severe hyperphosphatemia.

Acute hyperphosphatemia often occurs in the setting of TLS. TLS is associated with other fluid and electrolyte abnormalities, such as hyperuricemia and hyperkalemia, which also require treatment. Acute hyperphosphatemia is associated with hypocalcemia. Calcium replacement may worsen calcium phosphate precipitation. Asymptomatic hypocalcemia should not be treated until serum phosphorus concentration is lowered below 6 mg/dL.[84] In the presence of symptoms, where this may not be possible, clinical judgment is required to balance risk and benefits.

HYPOPHOSPHATEMIA

Signs and Symptoms

Clinical consequences vary depending on whether hypophosphatemia is moderate (serum phosphorus concentration 1.0–2.4 mg/dL) or severe ($\leq$ 1.0 mg/dL).[85] In a small number of clinical situations, moderate hypophosphatemia is associated with morbidity. With acute respiratory failure, correction of moderate hypophosphatemia improved measures of diaphragmatic function.[86] The clinical significance of this is unclear, given the lack of a patient centric endpoint. In 321 patients on continuous dialysis, 27% had a serum phosphorus concentration less than 2.0 mg/dL.[87] Hypophosphatemia was associated with increased risk of respiratory failure requiring tracheostomy.

Moderate hypophosphatemia is associated with decreased tissue sensitivity to insulin.[88] The clinical significance of this is unclear. In 16 intensive care unit (ICU) patients with sepsis, 10 were noted to have significant atrial and ventricular arrhythmias.[89] Serum phosphorus concentration was significantly lower in those with (2.8 mg/dL) versus without arrhythmias (3.19 mg/dL). The clinical significance is unclear given the small difference in serum phosphorus concentrations between groups. Mortality was not increased in hypophosphatemic patients. Moderate hypophosphatemia is not associated with impaired myocardial contractility.[90,91]

There is no question that severe hypophosphatemia is associated with significant morbidity. There are many case reports in the 1970s and 1980s of failure to wean from mechanical ventilation until severe hypophosphatemia was corrected.[92] In 566 consecutive patients after open cardiac surgery, severe hypophosphatemia was associated with a statistically significant increase in days on the ventilator (2.1 vs. 1.1 days) and hospital stay (7.8 vs. 5.6 days).[93] Some 34% of 21 malnourished ICU patients developed severe hypophosphatemia after refeeding.[94] Those with hypophosphatemia had a statistically significant prolongation of time on the ventilator (10.5 vs. 7.1 days) and hospital stay (12.1 vs. 8.2 days).

Reversible myocardial dysfunction was described in patients with severe hypophosphatemia. In seven ICU patients, correction resulted in increased mean left ventricular stroke work from 49.57 to 71.71 g-m per beat, which was associated with a fall in pulmonary capillary wedge pressure.[95] The effect was variable between patients. Several other studies showed similar findings with increases in cardiac index of about 20% with correction.[96,97]

Severe hypophosphatemia can increase red cell fragility. Hemolytic anemia has been associated with very low serum phosphate concentrations of 0.1 to 0.2 mg/dL.[98] Red blood cell adenosine triphosphate (ATP) concentration was reduced to very low levels. Severe hypophosphatemia reduces red blood cell 2,3-diphosphoglycerate concentration and shifts the oxygen dissociation curve to the left.[99] This is of unknown clinical significance.

Severe hypophosphatemia can result in rhabdomyolysis in laboratory animals, but this rarely occurs in humans.[100] With a phosphorus concentration less than 0.5 mg/dL, human white cells in vitro show reduced phagocytosis, chemotaxis, and bacterial killing; whether this increases risk of infection is unclear.[101]

Pseudohypophosphatemia

Paraproteinemias are the most common cause of spurious or pseudohypophosphatemia. It was reported with multiple myeloma, Waldenstrom macroglobulinemia, and monoclonal gammopathy of undetermined significance.[102–104] Deproteinizing serum by filtration corrects the problem. When water is used to dilute the sample, immunoglobulin (Ig)M monoclonal proteins will precipitate, causing the blank reading to be erroneously high. When blank absorbance is subtracted from test absorbance, serum phosphorus concentration will be erroneously low.

Spurious hypophosphatemia was also reported in a patient with AML and a severe elevation in white blood cell count (WBC).[105] The WBC was 310,000 cells per microliter and hypophosphatemia, hypokalemia, and hypoxemia were present. When the sample was transported to the laboratory on ice, serum phosphorus, potassium, and partial pressure of oxygen were normal. It was postulated that these abnormalities resulted from metabolic activity of leukocytes in vitro.

Tumor-Induced Osteomalacia

Tumor-induced osteomalacia (TIO) is a paraneoplastic syndrome resulting from overproduction of FGF-23 by mesenchymal tumors.[106] FGF-23 increases endocytosis and reduces expression of sodium-phosphate cotransporters NaPi IIa and c in the luminal membrane, and inhibits 1α-hydroxylase. As a result, the typical laboratory profile in patients with TIO includes hypophosphatemia, normal serum calcium concentration, renal phosphate wasting, elevated alkaline phosphatase, normal PTH, and low or inappropriately normal $1,25(OH)_2$ vitamin D_3 levels.[107] Hypophosphatemia is a potent stimulus for calcitriol production and levels would be expected to be elevated. FGF-23 lowers calcitriol levels by downregulating formation (1α-hydroxylase) and stimulating its breakdown via upregulation of 24-hydroxylase (CYP24a1), converting $1,25(OH)_2$ vitamin D_3 to $24,25(OH)_2$ vitamin D_3 (Fig. 4.4). When FGF-23 is injected into healthy animals, TIO is reproduced.[108]

FGF-23 is secreted by osteocytes, osteoclasts, and osteoblasts in response to hyperphosphatemia and 1,25 vitamin D_3. Full-length FGF-23 is the active form, and when cleaved into N- and C-terminal fragments, is inactive. It can be detected in the circulation of healthy people, indicating that FGF-23 plays a role in normal phosphate homeostasis.

Patients with TIO often present with a long history of muscle and bone pain, weakness and fatigue, and recurrent fractures.[109] Fractures commonly occur in vertebrae, ribs, and long bones with osteomalacia seen on bone histology.

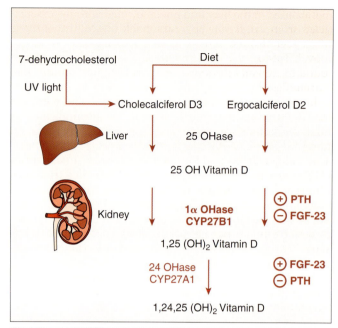

Fig. 4.4 Vitamin D metabolism and its regulation. Parathyroid hormone (PTH) increases $1,25 (OH)_2$ vitamin D levels by increasing its formation by upregulation of 1α-hydroxylase (CYP27B1) and downregulation of 24-hydroxylase (CYP24A1). Fibroblast growth factor (FGF)-23 decreases $1,25 (OH)_2$ vitamin D levels by downregulating 1α-hydroxylase (CYP27B1) and upregulating 24-hydroxylase.

The differential diagnosis includes inherited disorders that can also elevate FGF-23 levels. As a result, one needs to take a good family history. Previously normal serum phosphorus levels are suggestive of an acquired disorder. Inherited disorders tend to present in childhood with one exception, autosomal dominant hypophosphatemic rickets (ADHR).[110] In contrast to other inherited diseases that increase FGF-23 levels, ADHR is characterized by incomplete penetrance and variable expressivity.[111] ADHR is caused by a gain of function mutation at the FGF-23 cleavage site that prevents cleavage into N- and C-terminal fragments, resulting in an increase in intact FGF-23, the biologically active moiety. Patients can present at puberty or in adulthood and are generally women and often iron deficient.[112] Iron deficiency is associated with increased FGF-23 production for unclear reasons. However, cleavage is also increased, and levels do not increase in normals. In ADHR, FGF-23 is resistant to cleavage and levels are elevated.[113] In those with low penetrance and expressivity, iron deficiency during puberty or pregnancy may cause the disease to manifest later.

In a pathologic series of 17 cases of resected tumors causing TIO, four types were identified.[114] The most common type seen in 10 patients was a mixed connective tissue tumor that occurred primarily in soft tissue. It contains prominent hemangiopericytoma-like vascularity, spindle-shaped fibroblasts, and osteoclast-like giant cells, referred to as *phosphaturic mesenchymal tumor*, mixed connective tissue type (PMTMCT). The other three groups occur in bone and were osteoblastoma-like seen in four patients, nonossifying fibroma-like in two, and ossifying fibroma-like in one. In patients with TIO, 70% to 80% of identified tumors are of the PMTMCT subtype, commonly hemangiopericytomas. Less than 5% are malignant.

Causative tumors are not easy to locate. It is often several years from onset of symptoms to diagnosis and several more years from diagnosis to identification and tumor removal. Tumors are often small, slow growing, and can be found in unusual locations, such as the nasal sinuses and extremities.[115]

In most cases, PMTMCT express somatostatin receptors (SSTRs) and can be detected with radiolabeled somatostatin analogs. Initially, this was carried out with ^{111}In-pentatreotide.[116] ^{68}Ga-DOTATOC (1,4,7,10-tetraazacyclodecane-1,4,7,10-tetraacetic acid (DOTA) tyrosine I[3]-octreotide (TOC)) positron emission tomography (PET)/computed tomography (CT) also binds the SSTR and has been used where available. 3 T (Tesla) magnetic resonance imaging and [^{18}F] fluorodeoxyglucose PET/CT have also been reported to detect tumors. Because of the small number of cases, sensitivity and specificity data for these modalities are not available.

More recently, venous sampling of FGF-23 to help identify and localize the causative tumor was reported. In 10 patients with suspected TIO, venous sampling was carried out at 16 to 22 sites.[117] It helped identify the region of the tumor in eight of 10 cases. The authors emphasized that samples could not be collected from the external jugular vein because of technical issues limiting the technique in the head and neck region. They used the vein with the highest FGF-23 value detected as the candidate location. Andreopoulou et al. collected 25 to 49 samples per patient in 14 cases after imaging studies.[118] A ratio of FGF-23 values of 1.6 comparing the tumor bed to the average of the general circulation was considered a positive test. In five patients, imaging identified a single candidate lesion, multiple candidates in four, and no potential source in four. After either biopsy or surgical removal of the tumor, imaging and FGF-23 ratio correctly identified the tumor in seven of 14 cases (true positive). In four of 14, no site was detected on imaging with a negative FGF-23 ratio (true negative). In two of 14, there was a single candidate lesion identified on imaging with a positive FGF-23 ratio with no tumor detected (false positive). Finally, in one of 14, the FGF-23 ratio was negative with a highly suspicious abnormality on scanning (false negative). Sensitivity of venous sampling was 0.87 with a specificity of 0.71. The authors concluded that venous sampling was most helpful when multiple suspicious lesions were seen on imaging but was not helpful in the absence of a candidate lesion on imaging. In a third study, Lee et al. reported venous sampling results in six patients at 10 to 14 sites.[119] Sampling confirmed or detected five of six tumors. Interestingly, in two cases, the tumor was not detected on imaging until 3 years after the positive sampling result. These tumors were located in the mandible and ethmoid sinus, respectively.

Definitive diagnosis is established when the tumor is localized and surgically removed. It is important to remove the tumor with a wide margin to avoid recurrence. After complete resection, biochemical abnormalities disappear within a week. Osteomalacia can take up to a year to resolve. Absent tumor detection, goals of therapy are to improve symptoms, raise serum phosphorus concentration to the lower limit of normal, maintain or achieve a normal PTH and a normal alkaline phosphatase.[115] This is accomplished with phosphorus and calcitriol supplementation.

Calcitriol is given in doses of 1 to 3 μg/day and phosphorus, total of 1 to 4 g/day, in divided doses. The patient must be monitored closely at 3-month intervals with particular attention to avoid hypercalciuria or hypercalcemia. Sustained hypercalcemia and hypercalciuria can lead to nephrolithiasis, nephrocalcinosis, and CKD. Calcitriol improves intestinal phosphorus absorption and minimizes secondary or tertiary hyperparathyroidism that can occur with phosphorus administration alone. Cinacalcet was used in two patients with difficulty tolerating treatment with phosphorus and calcitriol.[120] The authors hypothesized that because PTH promotes phosphaturia and hypothyroid patients are hyperphosphatemic, with elevated serum FGF-23 levels, that a calcium-sensing receptor agonist that reduces PTH might be effective. Treatment with cinacalcet increased serum phosphorus concentration and tubular reabsorption of phosphate, allowing a more tolerable oral phosphorus dose. In one patient awaiting surgery, octreotide was given subcutaneously at 50 μg twice per day (TID) for 5 days and 100 μg TID for 8 days with normalization of serum phosphorus concentration and renal tubular reabsorption of phosphate.[121]

Fanconi Syndrome

Fanconi syndrome is a generalized defect in PCT transport, characterized by variable degrees of impaired reabsorption of amino acids, glucose, calcium, phosphate, potassium, uric acid, and bicarbonate.[122] Adults may manifest glycosuria in the presence of a normal serum glucose concentration, type II renal tubular acidosis, hypophosphatemia, hypokalemia, polyuria, or tubular proteinuria. In addition, children may present with rickets and growth retardation. In cancer patients, it may be secondary to chemotherapeutic agents or hematologic malignancies.

DRUGS

IFOSFAMIDE. Ifosfamide is an alkylating agent and a structural analog of cyclophosphamide. It is used as a first-line agent in treatment of a variety of tumors, primarily in children. Nephrotoxicity can manifest as either glomerular or tubular dysfunction. In 174 children, 41.4% developed tubular dysfunction,[123] whereas 6.3% manifested glomerular damage. Toxicity was severe in 9.2% ($n = 16$), moderate in 9.2% ($n = 16$), and mild in 23% ($n = 40$). Risk factors for severe toxicity were younger age and cumulative dose. Over 5 years of follow-up in a high percentage of cases, tubular dysfunction persisted, seven of 16 in the severe group and four of 16 in the moderate group.

In 62 children, nephrotoxicity was seen in 32.3%.[124] β2-Microglobulinuria, present in all 20, was the most common manifestation. Hypophosphatemia was seen in 10, decreased creatinine clearance in seven, glycosuria in five, and a low serum bicarbonate level in two. In the eight patients with nephrotoxicity followed over a longer period of time (range 3–22 months, median 8 months) after cessation of ifosfamide, all had tubular proteinuria, half had decreased creatinine clearance, five remained hypophosphatemic, glycosuria persisted in 25%, and one continued to have a low serum bicarbonate concentration, indicating that tubular toxicity may persist for a prolonged period of time. Severity was related to cumulative dose and previous cyclophosphamide exposure. Cumulative dose of ifosfamide was the most significant risk factor and a cutoff of 45 g/m^2 was suggested for those with significant previous cyclophosphamide exposure. The authors recommended close monitoring of patients with urinary β_2-microglobulin measurements, which is the most sensitive marker of nephrotoxicity, especially in those with high previous cyclophosphamide exposure ($> 500 \text{ mg/m}^2$).

Not only is β_2-microglobulinuria the most sensitive marker of renal dysfunction, it appears to precede other tubular abnormalities. In 75 patients followed for a median of 31 months, five subjects developed Fanconi syndrome and seven subclinical tubulopathy (not requiring supplementation).[125] Severe impairment of phosphate reabsorption occurred in 17.3%. The cumulative probability of a severe reduction in phosphate reabsorption increased over time with 8% after the first year and 14% after 2 years. Early impairment of PCT phosphate reabsorption predicted subsequent development of Fanconi syndrome. The authors recommend following urinary β_2-microglobulin and phosphate to identify nephrotoxicity early and differentiate those at risk for more severe manifestations.

The mechanism by which ifosfamide damages the PCT is not clear.[122] It is postulated that metabolites, chloracetaldehyde and acrolein, are responsible. Chloracetaldehyde may deplete intracellular glutathione and predispose to oxidative damage.

CHLOROETHYLNITROSOUREAS. The chloroethylnitrosoureas are alkylating agents with activity against a wide variety of tumors. Nephrotoxicity is the most common treatment-limiting side effect. In 106 patients with a wide variety of tumors treated with streptozocin, the most common early manifestations were proteinuria in 28%, reduction in creatinine clearance in 27%, and hypophosphatemia in 13%.[126] With further treatment, hypophosphatemic patients went on to develop renal tubular acidosis. In 24 patients treated with streptozocin, the authors state that reductions in serum phosphorus concentration were common. The average maximal decline was $0.89 \pm 0.65 \text{ mg/dL}$, which occurred on day 7 posttreatment and returned to normal on day 14.[126] Similar results were seen in 52 patients with metastatic islet cell tumors, where 17% developed renal tubular acidosis (type unspecified) and 11% Fanconi syndrome.[127]

AZACITIDINE. Azacitidine is a pyrimidine analog that interferes with deoxyribonucleic acid, ribonucleic acid (RNA), and protein synthesis. Peterson et al. examined the incidence of acid base, fluid, and electrolyte disorders in 22 patients with refractory acute leukemia, after these contributed to the death of two treated patients.[128] Two combination regimens used azacitidine at 200 mg/m^2/day for 5 or 7 days. Twenty of 22 patients developed decreases in serum phosphorus and bicarbonate levels, glycosuria, and polyuria. Hypophosphatemia occurred in 21 of 32 courses (66%), and hypocalcemia in 48%. Fanconi syndrome occurred early and resolved promptly after completion of therapy. The authors recommended close monitoring of all patients receiving azacitidine, as well as aggressive repletion of fluid and electrolyte deficits.

SURAMIN. Suramin is an antiparasitic agent used to treat onchocerciasis and trypanosomiasis that has antitumor activity. In a phase I study, 15 patients received suramin once or twice weekly.[129] Serum phosphorus concentration gradually declined from $4.0 \pm 0.37 \text{ mg/dL}$ at the start of therapy to $3.0 \pm 0.20 \text{ mg/dL}$ at 6 weeks. Two patients treated for longer than 6 weeks both developed absolute hypophosphatemia with a serum phosphorus concentration of 1.5 mg/dL. Both manifested Fanconi syndrome. The second underwent a muscle biopsy 3 weeks after the last dose (received 19.2 g of drug over 14 weeks). Marked changes were noted in morphology and activity of mitochondria. This same group showed that suramin in cell culture acts as an ionophore and respiratory poison. It interferes with ion gradients and disrupts the mitochondrial membrane potential and consequently mitochondrial function.[130,131] Fanconi syndrome occurs likely as a result of generalized mitochondrial dysfunction with reduction in ATP synthesis and Na^+-K^+ ATPase activity disrupting the ion gradients required for secondary active transport in PCT.

LYMPHOMA. Fanconi syndrome was reported in the acute phase of lymphoma either at the time of initial diagnosis or with relapse. In eight patients with lymphoma and Fanconi syndrome, six had ATLL.[132] In one patient with ATLL, Fanconi syndrome resolved with treatment.

MULTIPLE MYELOMA. A variety of tubular defects were reported in multiple myeloma ranging from isolated phosphaturia to complete or incomplete Fanconi syndrome. Full blown Fanconi syndrome is a rare complication.[133] Dash et al. reported two patients with multiple myeloma with severe hypophosphatemia, fractional excretions of phosphorus greater than 100%, with no other explanation for low serum phosphorus concentration other than myeloma.[134] Hypophosphatemia resolved after several weeks of chemotherapy. In some cases, Fanconi syndrome may precede myeloma by several years.[135] In 32 patients with Fanconi syndrome seen at the Mayo Clinic, 44% had monoclonal gammopathy of undetermined significance (MGUS), 19% smoldering multiple myeloma, 6% Waldenstrom macroglobulinemia, and 31% multiple myeloma.[136] At the time of diagnosis, a monoclonal light chain was detected in urine in all patients and blood in 69%. Over an average of 65 months of follow-up only one of 14 with MGUS progressed to multiple myeloma. In 91%, the light chains were kappa. Patients may present with weakness and bone pain that is secondary to osteomalacia from hypophosphatemia resulting from Fanconi syndrome.[137] Renal biopsy classically shows crystals in the cytoplasm of PCT cells.[138] There are reports of Fanconi syndrome resolving with disease treatment.[139] Fanconi syndrome is the result of free light chain (FLC) damage to the PCT and is more commonly caused by kappa light chains.[140] Studies in transgenic mice in which the wild type murine Jκ cluster was replaced with a VκJκ gene segment cloned from a patient with Fanconi syndrome and multiple myeloma attributed the pathogenic effect of Fanconi syndrome-inducing light chains to a short segment in the variable (V) domain, which confers resistance to proteolysis.[141] These mice showed morphologically altered PCT cells, intracellular rhomboid crystals, and impaired reabsorption of uric acid and phosphate, as is seen in humans. Another key study in transgenic mice revealed that reengineered κ light chains accumulated in PCT lysosomes.[142] This accumulation altered the process of lysosomal acidification and proteolytic function and was followed by dedifferentiation of PCT cells and loss of reabsorptive capacity. Receptor-mediated endocytosis was also affected. Mice did not have evidence of intracellular crystal deposition and the authors suggested that the specific light chain toxicity that results in Fanconi syndrome may not be the result of resistance to proteolysis or intracellular crystal deposition. FLCs after endocytosis can also cause cellular injury through oxidative stress and promotion of apoptosis.[143]

Because most patients with FLC-induced Fanconi syndrome have MGUS or smoldering myeloma, chemotherapy is not recommended given the risk of secondary myelodysplastic syndrome and leukemia with alkylating agents.[144] There are no studies evaluating proteasome inhibitors.

Drugs

IMATINIB. Imatinib is a small molecule tyrosine kinase inhibitor that inhibits BCR-ABL, platelet-derived growth factor, and c-kit. It is approved for use in treating chronic myelogenous leukemia (CML) and GIST. In 36 patients with CML, resistant or intolerant to interferon α, hypophosphatemia developed in 39%.[145] The effect was first seen at 3 months, with decreases of 1.0 or more, 1.5 or more, and 2.0 mg/dL or more seen in 39%, 11%, and 2.9%, respectively. Tubular reabsorption of phosphorus was low, indicating renal phosphate wasting. Hypophosphatemia was associated with response to therapy. In phase I and II trials of 403 patients with CML, grade 2 or above, hypophosphatemia was observed in 50% (33% grade 2, 15% grade 3, and 1.5% grade 4).[146] Development of hypophosphatemia was associated with higher doses and younger patient age in a series of 16 patients.[147] Significant hypocalcemia and hypophosphatemia developed in nine patients followed for 2 years; increased PTH was noted and attributed to secondary hyperparathyroidism.[148] Hypophosphatemia may result from either direct tubular toxicity or secondary hyperparathyroidism. There is at least one case report of a partial Fanconi syndrome with imatinib with renal wasting of phosphate and uric acid, suggesting that imatinib causes direct PCT damage.[149]

CERITINIB. Ceritinib is a small molecule, ATP-competitive, tyrosine kinase inhibitor of anaplastic lymphoma kinase (ALK) that can be given orally. It also inhibits the insulin-like growth factor 1 (IGF-1) receptor. A small percentage (5%) of NSCLC have rearrangements of the *ALK* gene. In a phase I study of 130 patients with NSCLC and ALK rearrangements, 3% developed hypophosphatemia.[150] Hypophosphatemia occurred in one of 14 patients receiving 400 mg/day, one of 10 patients receiving 600 mg/day, and two of 81 receiving 750 mg/day, the highest dose used. A study in eight healthy human volunteers showed that IGF-1 increases renal phosphate reabsorption.[151] Perhaps ceritinib results in renal phosphate wasting and hypophosphatemia via inhibition of the IGF-1 receptor.

ERIBULIN-HALICHONDRIN B ANALOG. Eribulin mesylate is a macrocyclic ketone analogue of halichondrin B. Halichondrin B is a natural marine product first isolated from the sponge *Halichondria okadai*.[152] It binds to tubulin and inhibits polymerization, leading to mitotic spindle disruption and inhibition of cell division. Eribulin has activity against a wide variety of tumors. Hypophosphatemia and hypocalcemia were reported in early phase I and II clinical trials. In a phase I study, eribulin mesylate was used in combination with cisplatin to treat 36 patients with advanced solid

tumors.[153] Hypophosphatemia occurred in one of six treated with 1 mg/m² in combination with 60 mg/m² of cisplatin, and in one of six treated with 1.4 mg/m² in combination with 60 mg/m² of cisplatin. It is difficult to interpret these results given that hypophosphatemia is also reported with cisplatin. In a phase I trial of 40 patients with a variety of solid tumors grade 3 hypophosphatemia was reported in one of a subset of 13 patients.[154] In a multicenter phase II trial, 40 patients with recurrent or metastatic squamous cell carcinoma of the head and neck were treated with eribulin mesylate.[155] Hypophosphatemia was not reported; however, one patient was noted to have grade 1 hypocalcemia. Although hypophosphatemia and hypocalcemia are reported with eribulin mesylate, the number of patients is too small to draw any definitive conclusions.

Acute Leukemias

Hypophosphatemia may occur in patients with acute leukemias via a variety of mechanisms. In a large case series of patients with AML ($n = 54$) and ALL ($n = 12$), hypophosphatemia was seen in 35.2% of AML patients and 16.6% of those with ALL.[156] Of 21 patients with hypophosphatemia, 11 had significant renal phosphate wasting; five of the 11 also had hypomagnesemia. Two patients had chronic diarrhea and three had respiratory alkalosis.

There are several case reports of AML associated with hypophosphatemia, hypokalemia, and hypouricemia secondary to PCT dysfunction.[157,158] It has been postulated that PCT dysfunction may be a result of infiltration by leukemic cells or their release of substances that either damage the PCT or compete for tubular reabsorption with normal substrates in the glomerular filtrate.

Acute leukemia can also cause hypophosphatemia because of incorporation of phosphate into white cells. The incorporation can be into a malignant clone of cells[159] or into normal cells after reconstitution of bone marrow after allogeneic peripheral blood stem cell transplantation.[160]

High Dose Estrogens

In the past, patients with metastatic prostate carcinoma were treated with high dose diethylstilbestrol. In 18 patients, serum phosphorus concentration fell from a pretreatment value of 3.7 ± 0.8 mg/dL to 2.6 ± 0.5 mg/dL within the first 3 to 6 weeks.[161] On discontinuation, phosphorus level rapidly returned to normal. No patient had symptoms attributable to hypophosphatemia. The authors postulated that hypophosphatemia resulted from an increase in renal excretion because in short-term studies, a single dose of diethylstilbestrol increased the urinary phosphorus to creatinine ratio. Studies in ovariectomized rats injected with 17β-estradiol or vehicle clarified the molecular mechanism.[162] Estradiol-treated rats showed a decline in serum phosphorus concentration associated with phosphaturia. The decrease in renal phosphate reabsorption was caused by reduced messenger RNA and protein expression of NaPi-IIa, the predominant sodium-phosphate cotransporter in the PCT luminal membrane.

Temsirolimus, Everolimus, Ridaforolimus

Mammalian target of rapamycin (mTOR) inhibitors are commonly used in the treatment of metastatic renal cell carcinoma, advanced neuroendocrine tumors, and some forms of breast cancer. Hypophosphatemia is a common and well-recognized side effect. One review reported an all grade incidence of hypophosphatemia for temsirolimus, everolimus, and ridaforolimus of 13% to 49%, 32% to 37%, and 23%, respectively. Grade 3/4 hypophosphatemia occurred in 13% to 18%, 4% to 6%, and 15% with temsirolimus, everolimus, and ridaforolimus, respectively.[163] Two recent phase II trials of castration-resistant prostate cancer showed a 14% and 18% incidence of hypophosphatemia.[164,165] The mechanism has not been identified.

Data from one study suggested that biologic toxicities are surrogate markers of efficacy.[166] Seventy-five patients from a single institution with renal cell carcinoma were treated with either temsirolimus ($n = 31$) or everolimus ($n = 44$). Longer progression free survival was correlated with each absolute 1% decrease in serum phosphorus concentration.

Treatment

Treatment approach varies depending on degree of hypophosphatemia. There is little evidence that treatment of moderate hypophosphatemia (serum phosphorus concentration 1.0–2.5 mg/dL) is of benefit except in the mechanically ventilated patient. Severe or symptomatic hypophosphatemia (serum phosphorus concentration < 1.0 mg/dL), however, should be treated. One should always replete phosphorus with caution in patients with kidney disease. A supplemental oral dose of phosphorus of up to 1 g per day is enough to replete most patients; however, replacement may be limited by diarrhea. Oral phosphate preparations are listed in Table 4.5.

Because of risk of hypocalcemia or hyperphosphatemia, intravenous phosphate repletion should be reserved for those with either severe hypophosphatemia or who cannot take oral supplements. Sodium phosphate is used unless the patient is hypokalemic. Once serum phosphorus concentration rises above 1.0 mg/dL, the switch is made to the oral route. Blood chemistries should be closely monitored. A variety of aggressive repletion protocols were developed for critically ill patients in the ICU. A small sample of these are shown in Table 4.6.[167–173]

Table 4.5   Phosphate Preparations

Preparation	Contents	Phosphorus	Sodium	Potassium
K-phos original	Monobasic K phosphate	250 mg/tab	13 mEq/tab	1.1 mEq/tab
K-phos neutral	Dibasic Na phosphate Monobasic Na phosphate Monobasic K phosphate	114 mg/tab	-	3.7 mEq/tab
Neutra-phos-K	Monobasic K phosphate Dibasic Na phosphate	250 mg/cap	-	13.6 mEq/cap
Neutra-phos	Monobasic and dibasic Na and K phosphates	250 mg/cap	7.1 mEq/cap	6.8 mEq/cap
Fleets phosphasoda	Monobasic Na phosphate Dibasic Na phosphate	129 mg/mL	4.8 mEq/mL	-
IV Na phosphate	Monobasic Na phosphate	93 mg/mL	4.0 mEq/mL	-
IV K phosphate	Monobasic K phosphate	93 mg/mL	-	4.4 mEq/mL

IV, Intravenous, *cap*, Capsule; *tab*, tablet.

Table 4.6   Rapid Phosphate Infusion Protocols—Critically Ill Patients

Author	Dose	Degree of Hypophosphatemia
Charron (169)	30 mmol over 2–4 hours ([P]: 1.25 mg/dL–2.03 mg/dL) 45 mmol over 3–6 hours ([P]: < 1.25 mg/dL)	Moderate Severe
Kingston (170)	0.25 mmol/kg over 4 hours ([P]: 0.5 mg/dL–1.0 mg/dL) 0.50 mmol/kg over 4 hours ([P]: < 0.5 mg/dL)	Severe
Perreault (171)	15 mmol over 3 hours ([P]: 1.27 mg/dL–2.48 mg/dL) 30 mmol over 3 hours ([P]: < 1.24 mg/dL)	Moderate Severe
Rosen (172)	15 mmol over 2 hours Q6 hours, no > 45 mmol/day total	Moderate
Taylor (173)	10 mmol: 40–60 kg, 15 mmol: 61–80 kg, 20 mmol: 81–120 kg ([P]: 1.8 mg/dL–2.2 mg/dL) 20 mmol: 40–60 kg, 30 mmol: 61–80 kg, 40 mmol: 81–120 kg ([P]: 1.0–1.7 mg/dL) 30 mmol: 40–60 kg, 40 mmol: 61–80 kg, 50 mmol: 81–120 kg ([P]: < 1.0 mg/dL) Infusions given over 6 hours	Mild Moderate Severe
Vannatta (174)	9 mmol Q12 hours for 48 hours	Severe
Vannatta (175)	0.32–0.48 mmol/kg Q12 hours for 48 hours	Severe

IV, Intravenous, *[P]*, serum phosphorus concentration; *Q*, every.

In situations where hypophosphatemia results from renal phosphate wasting, dipyridamole at doses of 75 mg 3 to 4 times a day in both the short- and long-term can reduce renal phosphate losses and result in an increase in serum phosphorus concentration.[174] Eighty percent of patients show a response within 3 months with a maximum effect at 9 months. The mechanism of action is unknown but has been speculated to be the result of a reduction in adenosine uptake in PCT, resulting in a decrease in intracellular cyclic adenosine monophosphate concentration or P-glycoprotein inhibition.

Key Points

- Humoral hypercalcemia of malignancy is associated with a poor prognosis, median survival 52 days.
- Upregulation of a MAP kinase isoform in breast cancer cells stimulates monocyte chemotactic protein-1 and osteoclast activation.
- Hypocalcemia seen with osteoblastic metastases, most commonly in prostate cancer, is exacerbated by bisphosphonates.
- In tumor lysis syndrome, development of acute kidney injury is associated with a 10-fold increase in in-hospital mortality and a fivefold increase in 6-month mortality.
- In the diagnosis of tumor-induced osteomalacia, FGF-23 venous sampling may aid in localizing the tumor, especially when multiple suspicious lesions are detected on imaging.

References

1. Stewart AF. Clinical practice. Hypercalcemia associated with cancer. *N Engl J Med.* 2005;352:373-379.
5. Jain N, Reilly RF. Disorders of serum calcium homeostasis—hypo and hypercalcemia. In: Reilly RF, Perazella MA, eds. *Nephrology in thirty days.* 2nd ed. New York: McGraw Hill; 2013:133-148.
8. Goldner W. Cancer-related hypercalcemia. *J Oncol Pract.* 2016;12:426-432.
9. McCauley LK, Martin TJ. Twenty-five years of PTHrP progress: from cancer hormone to multifunctional cytokine. *J Bone Miner Res.* 2012;27:1231-1239.
10. Donovan PJ, Achong N, Griffin K, Galligan J, Pretorius CJ, McLeod DS. PTHrP-mediated hypercalcemia: causes and survival in 138 patients. *J Clin Endocrinol Metab.* 2015;100:2024-2029.
16. Roodman GD. Mechanisms of bone metastasis. *N Engl J Med.* 2004;350:1655-1664.
17. Roodman GD. Mechanisms of bone lesions in multiple myeloma and lymphoma. *Cancer.* 1997;80:1557-1563.
19. He Z, He J, Liu Z, et al. MAPK11 in breast cancer cells enhances osteoclastogenesis and bone resorption. *Biochimie.* 2014;106:24-32.
22. Seymour JF, Gagel RF. Calcitriol: the major humoral mediator of hypercalcemia in Hodgkin lymphoma and non-Hodgkin lymphoma. *Blood.* 1993;82:1383-1394.
25. Shallis RM, Rome RS, Reagan JL. Mechanisms of hypercalcemia in non-Hodgkin lymphoma and associated outcomes: a retrospective review. *Clin Lymphoma Myeloma Leuk.* 2018;18:e123-e129.
26. Hewison M, Kantorovich V, Liker HR, et al. Vitamin D-mediated hypercalcemia in lymphoma: evidence for hormone production by tumor-adjacent macrophages. *J Bone Miner Res.* 2003;18:579-582.
33. Hu MI, Glezerman IG, Leboulleux S, et al. Denosumab for treatment of hypercalcemia of malignancy. *J Clin Endocrinol Metab.* 2014;99:3144-3152.
35. Penfield J, Reilly RF. The patient with disorders of serum calcium and phosphorus. In: Schrier RW, ed. *Manual of nephrology, diagnosis and therapy.* 8th ed. Boston: Lippincott Williams and Williams; 2015:79-105.
36. Schattner A, Dubin I, Huber R, Gelber M. Hypocalcemia of malignancy. *Neth J Med.* 2016;74:231-239.
37. Ye L, Kynaston HG, Jiang WG. Bone metastasis in prostate cancer: molecular and cellular mechanisms. *Int J Mol Med.* 2007;20:103-111.
39. Tucci M, Lamanna G, Porpiglia F, et al. Prognostic significance of disordered calcium metabolism in hormone-refractory prostate cancer patients with metastatic bone disease. *Prostate Cancer Prostatic Dis.* 2009;12:94-99.
44. Wilson FP, Berns JS. Tumor lysis syndrome: new challenges and recent advances. *Adv Chronic Kidney Dis.* 2014;21:18-26.
47. Burns RA, Topoz I, Reynolds SL. Tumor lysis syndrome risk factors, diagnosis and management. *Pediatr Emerg Care.* 2014;30:571-579.
48. Cairo MS, Bishop M. Tumor lysis syndrome: new therapeutic strategies and classification. *Br J Haematol.* 2004;127:3-11.
52. Garimalle PS, Balakrishnan P, Ammakkanavar NR, et al. Impact of dialysis requirement on outcomes in tumor lysis syndrome. *Nephrology.* 2017;22:85-88.
53. Cairo MS, Coiffer B, Reiter A, Younes A, TLS Expert Panel. Recommendations for the evaluation of risk and prophylaxis of tumor lysis syndrome (TLS) in adults and children with malignant diseases: an expert TLS panel consensus. *Br J Haematol.* 2010;149:578-586.
54. Jones GL, Will A, Jackson GH, et al. Guidelines for the management of tumour lysis syndrome in adults and children with haematological malignancies on behalf of the British Committee for Standards in Haematology. *Br J Haematol.* 2015;169:661-671.
55. Wang Q, Qi Y, Zhang D, et al. Electrolyte disorders assessment in solid tumor patients treated with anti-EGFR monoclonal antibodies: a pooled analysis of 25 randomized clinical trials. *Tumor Biology.* 2015;36:3471-3482.
57. Reilly RF. Disorders of serum magnesium. In: Reilly RF, Perazella MA, ed. *Nephrology in thirty days.* 2nd ed. New York: McGraw Hill; 2013:165-177.
58. Arany I, Safirstein RJ. Cisplatin nephrotoxicity. *Semin Nephrol.* 2003;23:460-464.
70. Menshawy A, Mattar O, Abdulkarim A, et al. Denosumab versus bisphosphonates in patients with advanced cancers-related bone metastasis: systematic review and meta-analysis of randomized controlled trials. *Support Cancer Care.* 2018;26(4):1029-1038.
74. Tanvetyanon T, Stiff PJ. Management of adverse effects associated with intravenous bisphosphonates. *Ann Oncol.* 2006;17:897-907.
76. Reilly RF. Nephrolithiasis. In: Reilly RF, Perazella MA, ed. *Nephrology in thirty days.* 2nd ed. New York: McGraw Hill; 2013:179-193.
78. Coiffier B, Altman A, Pui C-H, et al. Guidelines for the management of pediatric and adult tumor lysis syndrome: an evidence-based review. *J Clin Oncol.* 2008;26:2767-2778.
79. Lopez-Olivio MA, Pratt G, Palla SL, Salahudeen A. Rasburicase in tumor lysis syndrome of the adult: a systematic review and meta-analysis. *Am J Kidney Dis.* 2013;62:481-492.
84. Jain N, Reilly RF. Disorders of serum phosphorus. In: Reilly RF, Perazella MA, eds. *Nephrology in thirty days.* 2nd ed. New York: McGraw Hill; 2013:149-164.
85. Amanzadeh J, Reilly RF. Hypophosphatemia: an evidence based approach to its clinical consequences and management. *Nat Clin Pract Nephrol.* 2006;2:136-148.
107. Clinkenbeard EL, White KE. Heritable and acquired disorders of phosphate metabolism: etiologies involving FGF23 and current therapeutics. *Bone.* 2017;pii:S8756-S3282.
109. Jan de Beur SM. Tumor-induced osteomalacia. *JAMA.* 2005;294:1260-1267.
110. Alizadeh Naderi AS, Reilly RF. Hereditary disorders of renal phosphate wasting. *Nat Rev Nephrol.* 2010;6:657-665.
111. Econs MJ, McEnery PT. Autosomal dominant hypophosphatemic rickets/osteomalacia clinical characterization of a novel renal phosphate-wasting disorder. *J Clin Endocrinol Metab.* 1997;82:674-681.
112. Imel EA, Hui SL, Econs MJ. FGF23 concentrations vary with disease status in autosomal dominant hypophosphatemic rickets. *J Bone Miner Res.* 2007;22:520-526.
113. Wolf M, White KE. Coupling fibroblast growth factor 23 production and cleavage: iron deficiency, rickets, and kidney disease. *Curr Opin Nephrol Hypertens.* 2014;23:411-419.
114. Weidner N, Santa Cruz D. Phosphaturic mesenchymal tumors. A polymorphous group causing osteomalacia or rickets. *Cancer.* 1987;59:1441-1454.
115. Gonciulea AR, Jan de Beur SM. Fibroblast growth factor 23-mediated bone disease. *Endocrinol Metab Clin North Am.* 2017;46:19-39.

122. Izzedine H, Launay-Vacher V, Isnard-Bagnis C, Deray G. Drug-induced Fanconi syndrome. *Am J Kidney Dis.* 2003;41:292-309.

133. Korbet SM, Schwartz MM. Multiple myeloma. *J Am Soc Nephrol.* 2006;17:2533-2545.

138. Herlitz LC, Roglieri J, Resta R, et al. Light chain proximal tubulopathy. *Kidney Int.* 2009;76:792-797.

140. Doshi M, Lahoti A, Danesh FR, et al. Paraprotein-related kidney disease: kidney injury from paraproteins-what determines the site of injury. *Clin J Am Soc Nephrol.* 2016;11:2288-2294.

142. Luciani A, Sirac C, Terryn S, et al. Impaired lysosomal function underlies monoclonal light chain-associated renal Fanconi syndrome. *J Am Soc Nephrol.* 2016;27:2049-2061.

143. Sanders PW. Mechanisms of light chain injury along the tubular nephron. *J Am Soc Nephrol.* 2012;23:1777-1781.

144. Ria R, Dammacco F, Vacca A. Heavy-chain diseases and myeloma-associated Fanconi syndrome: an update. *Mediterr J Hematol Infect Dis.* 2018;10:e2018011.

146. Owen S, Hatfield A, Letvak L. Imatinib and altered bone and mineral metabolism. *N Engl J Med.* 2006;355:627.

156. Milionis H, Bourantos C, Siamopoulos K, et al. Acid-base and electrolyte abnormalities in patients with acute leukemia. *Am J Hematol.* 1999;62:201-207.

163. Soefje S, Karnad A, Brenner A. Common toxicities of mammalian target of rapamycin inhibitors. *Target Oncol.* 2011;6:125-129.

A full list of references is available at Expertconsult.com

5 Volume Disorders and Fluid Resuscitation

JEFFREY TURNER

Introduction

Volume disorders are common in patients with cancer, given the vast array of organ dysfunction that occurs in these patients, as well as the frequent toxicities associated with many of the chemotherapeutics and biologics used for treatment. In healthy physiology, a complex system is in place to preserve volume homeostasis and maintain equilibrium across the major fluid compartments of the body. However, in disease states, several maladaptive changes can occur that disrupt this equilibrium and lead to volume disorders. This chapter describes the volume regulatory apparatus in the body and clinical effects that develop in pathologic cancer states. The various pathways of this system are directly connected to the final common endpoint of alterations in sodium and water handling by the kidneys. The frequent etiologies of hypovolemic and hypervolemic disorders in cancer patients are reviewed, and further discussion is focused on assessing and treating patients with extracellular fluid (ECF) volume contraction.

VOLUME HOMEOSTASIS

Under normal physiologic conditions, the human body tightly regulates fluid volume. This is critical to maintain adequate perfusion of organs and ultimately to provide nutrients to cells and remove waste products. The system for regulating volume is complex, and it consists of a number of afferent sensors and efferent pathways that adapt to fluid changes to maintain homeostasis (Fig. 5.1). Central to volume homeostasis are the kidneys, which regulate salt and water excretion. Additional critical components include the heart, the central nervous system, the vascular tree, and both volume and pressure baroreceptors. Although direct insults to any of these organ components can result in a fluid disorder, so too can insults to nearly any other organ system in the body, irrespective of its primary role in volume homeostasis. As an example, volume disorders are ubiquitous with damage to organs such as the kidneys and heart; however, disease processes involving other organs, such as the intestines, skin, and liver are also commonly associated with significant volume disturbances. For this reason, cancer patients are at significant risk for fluid disorders from a number of different pathologies.

It is important to appreciate that the body does not function like a water-filled balloon, shrinking when water is removed, and expanding when water is added. Rather, the central teaching in volume homeostasis is that there are several key fluid compartments within the body and

adequate distribution of water between these compartments is critical (Fig. 5.2). Total body water volume is roughly equal to 60% of the body weight in men, and 50% of the body weight in women and the elderly. The intracellular fluid (ICF) compartment contains 55% to 65% of total body water, and the ECF compartment contains the remaining 35% to 45%. The ECF compartment is further divided into the interstitial fluid compartment (approximately 75% of the ECF volume) and the intravascular compartment (approximately 25% of the ECF volume). Fluid can readily move across cell membranes, and therefore the volume of both the ICF and the ECF is dependent upon the gradient of effective osmotic agents between these two spaces. Sodium is the predominant osmotic agent in the ECF, and potassium is the predominant osmotic agent in the ICF. The Na^+/K^+ adenosine triphosphatase pump, which is found in the cell membrane of nearly every cell within the body, maintains the distribution of sodium in the ECF compartment and potassium in the ICF compartment. Water will shift across cell membranes to maintain balanced osmolality between the ECF and ICF. Because the body's regulatory mechanisms for sensing volume are mainly present in the ECF, sodium is the major factor that impacts the volume status of the entire body. Excessive sodium intake can lead to increases in ECF fluid volume that clinically manifest as hypertension, edema, and dyspnea. Alternatively, sodium losses can lead to decreases in ECF volume that clinically manifest as hypotension, increased skin turgor, and dizziness.

VOLUME REGULATION

The body's ability to regulate volume is critical to one's survival; as such, a complex set of mechanisms is present to preserve homeostasis. When the body begins to accumulate excess fluid, the fluid will distribute into the ECF and ICF based on the concentration of effective osmolytes within each compartment (predominantly sodium in the ECF and potassium in the ICF). When ECF volume increases, the body's volume regulatory mechanisms will lead to adaptations that ultimately result in an increase in salt and water excretion by the kidneys to reduce the body volume. Alternatively, when ECF volume decreases, regulatory mechanisms will lead to adaptations that result in a decrease in salt and water excretion by the kidneys, in an effort to preserve body volume. The volume sensing components within the body predominantly respond to changes within the intravascular compartment of the ECF. Therefore even though the

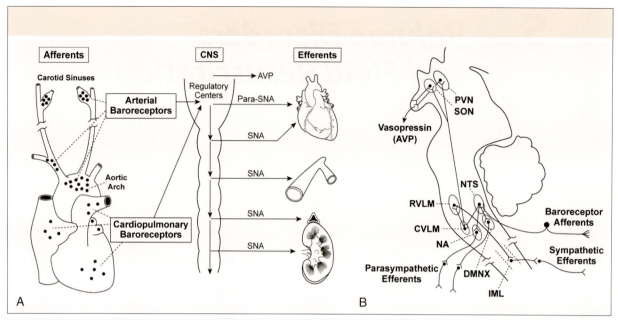

Fig. 5.1 Afferent and efferent pathways for volume regulation. *AVP,* Arginine vasopressin; *CNS,* central nervous system; *CVLM,* caudal ventrolateral medulla; *DMNX,* Dorsal Motor Nucleus of the Vagus Nerve; *IML,* intermediolateral nucleus; *NA,* Nucleus Ambiguus, *NTS,* nucleus of the tractus solitarius; *PVN,* paraventricular nucleus; *RVLM,* rostral ventrolateral medulla; *SON,* supraoptic nucleus; *SNA,* sympathetic nerve activity. Modified from Chapleau MW. Baroreceptor reflexes. In: Robertson D, Biaggioni I, Burnstock G, Phillip A, eds. *Primer on the autonomic nervous system.* 3rd ed. San Diego: Academic Press; 2012:161-165.

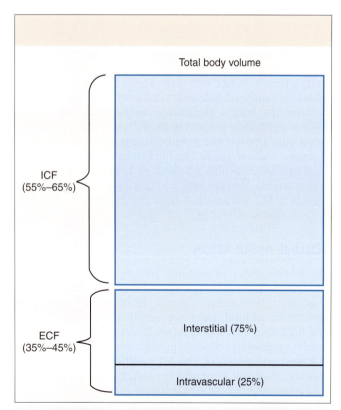

Fig. 5.2 Body fluid compartments. *ECF,* Extracellular fluid; *ICF,* intracellular fluid.

intravascular volume consists of less than 10% of the total body water, its role in regulating body volume is critical. In healthy physiology, the intravascular volume and the ECF are in equilibrium. From a physiologic stand point, the emphasized importance of the intravascular volume, and in particular the arterial vascular volume, makes a lot of sense, as this is what determines organ perfusion and overall survival. The term *effective arterial blood volume* specifically refers to the arterial volume that interacts with the volume sensing components and ultimately drives the response of the kidneys and other vascular mediators.

Integrated Responses to Volume Changes

Changes in ECF volume trigger a number of mechanisms that act to adjust sodium and water excretion by the kidneys (Fig. 5.3). These mechanisms include low pressure receptors in the right atrium and pulmonary blood vessels, as well as baroreceptors in the carotid sinus and aortic arch. In volume depleted states, stretch receptors at these sites upregulate sympathetic nerve activity in the kidneys. This results in a number of effects: (1) reduced glomerular filtration rate (GFR) via afferent arteriole constriction; (2) upregulation of sodium reabsorption in the nephron tubule; and (3) activation of the renin-aldosterone-angiotensin-system (RAAS). In addition, volume depleted states result in a decrease in atrial natriuretic peptide release by the cardiac atria, which further decreases GFR and also promotes sodium and water reabsorption along the nephron, in particular in the collecting duct. Volume overloaded states have the opposite effect on these systems, as they promote sodium and water excretion in the kidney. These integrated responses work together to restore body volume in healthy states. However, in maladaptive states, such as heart failure and cirrhosis, these mechanisms become disassociated from the body volume. More specifically, the ECF and intravascular volumes are no longer in equilibrium. Therefore, elevated ECF volumes are actually worsened because of the coexistence of low effective arterial volumes.

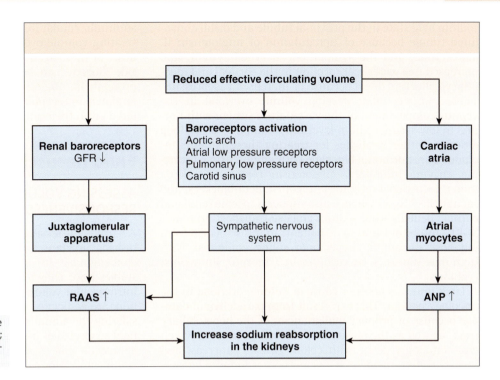

Fig. 5.3 Integrated response to volume regulation. *ANP,* Arial natriuretic peptide; *GFR,* glomerular filtration rate; *RAAS,* renin-aldosterone-angiotensin system.

Volume Disorders in the Cancer Patient

VOLUME DEPLETION

The cancer patient is particularly vulnerable to volume depletion because of disorders of the gastrointestinal tract. Reduced fluid intake is common in cancer patients and etiologies for this include anorexia, mucositis, refractory nausea, and dysfunction of the oropharynx and esophagus. These insults can be direct consequences of the underlying malignancy, as well as the chemotherapeutic agents used to treat the underlying cancer. Despite severe reductions in fluid intake in this setting, the body continues to have unregulated insensible water losses from the skin and respiratory tract, and this can account for up to a liter or more per day. Patients in this scenario tend to develop hypernatremic hypovolemia, or what is more commonly referred to as *dehydration,* given the net loss of more free water than sodium. Another common cause of volume depletion in cancer patients is extensive sodium and water losses from vomiting or diarrhea. Patients may maintain oral hydration in this scenario, but it is often not enough to match the losses, and patients ultimately become volume depleted. The net result in these patients is more sodium loss than water loss, and they typically develop hyponatremic hypovolemia. Patients with substantial vomiting will also be at risk for metabolic alkalosis, given the significant amount of hydrogen and chloride loss in the gastric fluids.[1] This can further promote potassium losses from the kidney because of sodium and bicarbonate delivery to the distal nephron, so called *bicarbonaturia.* On the other hand, in those subjects with diarrhea, a nonanion gap metabolic acidosis typically occurs because of bicarbonate losses from the intestinal fluids.

Polyuria in the setting of diabetes insipidus is another potential cause for volume depletion in patients with cancer. Central diabetes insipidus can result from metastatic tumors in lung cancer, leukemia, and lymphoma.[2] Alternatively, nephrogenic diabetes insipidus can occur in the setting of tumor related obstructive uropathy, hypercalcemia, or ifosfamide and pemetrexed administration.[3,4] These patients present with polyuria and polydipsia, and often times daily urine output will exceed 5 L. Typically, they maintain euvolemia and isonatremia by drinking excess amounts of free water; however, in settings of impaired thirst or when patients are unable to access water because of barriers from changes in mentation or physical barriers, these subjects then develop hypernatremia and hypovolemia.

VOLUME OVERLOAD

Increases in ECF volume are also common in oncology patients and these disorders can often be difficult to manage. Typically, this occurs because of insults to the heart, liver, or kidney, and the etiology can either be directly from the malignancy or from chemotherapeutic treatments. Common cardiac insults include chemotherapeutic-induced cardiomyopathies from anthracyclines (doxorubicin, daunorubicin, and epirubicin) and the human epidermal growth factor receptor 2 (HER2) modulator trastuzumab.[5] In addition, primary malignant tumors of the heart, such as sarcomas, lymphomas, and pericardial malignancies, can also result in severe left ventricular dysfunction, valvular disease, or obstruction.[6] In these scenarios, cardiac output declines and venous congestion occurs, resulting in a reduction of effective arterial volume. This results in neurohormonal changes that leave the kidneys in a sodium avid state in the proximal tubule and distal convoluted tubule because of upregulation of angiotensin II, aldosterone, and the sympathetic nervous system, and increased free water reabsorption in the cortical and medullary collecting ducts because of increased vasopressin.[7] These patients often develop volume overload in the venous compartment of the vasculature system with normal to low serum sodium levels. In addition to using loop diuretics, other strategies for treating these patients include neurohormonal blockade with angiotensin converting enzyme inhibitors, angiotensin receptor blockers, mineralocorticoid receptor antagonist, beta-blockers, and sacubitril.[7,8] New evidence also supports specific renal and cardiac benefits from sodium glucose transport protein 2 SGLT2 inhibitors, and some patients may also benefit from low-dose dopamine, hypertonic saline combined with high dose diuretics, or vasopressin 2 receptor antagonist (vaptans).[9-12]

Liver injury is another cause of volume overload in the oncology patient. This can result from parenchymal damage because of primary malignancies of the hepatobiliary tract, as well as the presence of metastatic tumors, which can commonly occur with colon, gastric, pancreas, and breast cancers. In addition, chemotherapy induced hepatotoxicity can also occur. The state of volume overload in liver injury is typically driven by the distortion in hepatic architecture leading to portal hypertension. This results in nitric oxide and carbon monoxide mediated splanchnic vasodilation, with secondary pooling of blood volume in the splanchnic vessels.[13] In this situation, blood is stolen from other arterial beds, leading to a decrease in effective arterial volume. As a consequence of this, baroreceptor-mediated activation of the RAAS, sympathetic nervous system, and nonosmotic release of antidiuretic hormone occurs in an effort to restore arterial volume.[14] Similar to congestive heart failure, these neurohormonal changes result in sodium and water retention in the kidney, which leads to volume overload. In addition to sodium restriction of less than 200 mg per day, patients with cirrhosis should be managed with diuretics to address volume overload. Guidelines recommend starting with 40 mg of furosemide and 100 mg of spironolactone, with titration upwards maintaining roughly the same ratio.[15]

Kidney failure of any form can result in volume overload given the reduction in sodium and water excretion. This is common in clinical scenarios with a significant reduction in GFR. However, injuries that result in nephrotic-range proteinuria tend to present with more severe degrees of volume overload, even when the GFR is intact or modestly reduced. Recent evidence suggests that this is a result of serine protease activation of the epithelial sodium channel in the collecting duct.[16,17] These injuries are common in patients with cancer and can result as a paraneoplastic syndrome. Membranous nephropathy is the most frequent form of cancer-related nephrotic syndrome, and this occurs in the setting of breast, lung, and colon cancers, but minimal change disease and focal segmental glomerulosclerosis are also well described paraneoplastic lesions.[18] In addition, targeted anticancer agents with antivascular endothelial growth factor properties can also result in proteinuria with volume overload.[19] Agents most likely to cause this include the antiangiogenesis drugs bevacizumab, sorafenib,

sunitinib, vatalanib, and axitinib. Loop diuretics are key to treating volume overload in renal failure, and when high doses of these agents are ineffective, the addition of a thiazide diuretic can be helpful.[20] In states with coexisting proteinuria, angiotensin converting enzyme inhibitors or angiotensin receptor blocking agents should be coadministered given their antiproteinuric effects.

Fluid Resuscitation

ASSESSING VOLUME STATUS AND VOLUME RESPONSIVENESS

Accurately assessing volume status remains an important task for clinicians, and unfortunately one that is particularly challenging.[21] In critically ill, volume depleted patients, studies have shown that both inadequate replacement of intravascular volume, as well as overly aggressive resuscitation, are associated with poorer outcomes.[22-24] When considering the administration of intravenous volume to a patient suspected of having ECF contraction, clinicians should appreciate that the fundamental aim is to increase stroke volume and improve tissue and organ perfusion. It is therefore important to not only assess volume status, but also to anticipate and assess whether the patient is volume responsive, as these variables can be mutually exclusive.

The history and physical examination should be the initial parameters used to assess a patient's need for volume replacement, as these are readily available (Box 5.1). This includes a thorough history inquiring about recent reductions in oral fluid intake, as well as asking about increased fluid losses from vomiting, diarrhea, and bleeding. Routine evaluation of the blood pressure, pulse, and the degree to which these measurements vary with postural changes should also be done. Assessing mentation, capillary refill,

---

Box 5.1   Clinical and Laboratory for Volume Assessment

Vital Signs:

Blood pressure
Pulse
Orthostatic changes of blood pressure and pulse

Physical Examination:

Mentation
Dry mucous membranes and axilla
Capillary refill
Skin turgor
Urine output
Quality of peripheral pulses
Temperature in extremities

Laboratory Findings:

Serum sodium
BUN/Creatinine
Urine sodium
Blood lactate
Brain-natriuretic peptide

BUN, Blood urea nitrogen.

skin turgor, dryness in the axilla and mucosal membranes, temperature in the extremities, and urine output are also part of the basic physical examination to guide fluid management. However, it should be noted that studies have shown poor correlations between physical examination findings and accurate determination of volume status. In fact, data have shown that postural changes in heart rate and blood pressure may be lacking with nonblood loss volume depletion (such as reduced oral intake, vomiting, and diarrhea) or when blood loss is only moderate (< 1 L).[25,26] Therefore clinicians should appreciate the challenge associated with predicting volume status and volume responsiveness based on physical examination findings alone. In many situations, additional testing is performed to further guide fluid management.

Common laboratory testing to assess serum electrolytes, acid base status, and kidney biomarkers should be routinely done in patients suspected of having volume contraction, as these data can be critical to determining the best type of intravenous solution to administer (physiologic vs. chloride rich crystalloid solutions). In addition, several measurement methods are available to assess vascular volumes. The most commonly used techniques are static pressure measurements, which use a catheter to directly determine intravascular and intracardiac pressures. Central venous pressure (CVP) and pulmonary capillary wedge pressures (PCWP) are routinely performed in the intensive care unit. The pressure measurements from these studies provide surrogate markers for intravascular volume and cardiac preload. In clinical practice, many clinicians interpret decreased CVP or PCWP as evidence of intravascular volume depletion and increased levels as volume overload. However, several studies have demonstrated a weak relationship of CVP and PCWP, with both volume status and volume responsiveness.[27–29] This is because of the fact that these variables are not only impacted by volume status, but they are also affected by other factors, such as vascular and cardiac compliance, valvular cardiac disease, and ascites. In addition, there are shortcomings with using CVP and PCWP to predict whether a patient's cardiac output will increase following fluid administration. This is because these methods are unable to determine if a patient's left ventricular function is operating on the steep or flat part of the Frank-Starling curve (Fig. 5.4). In patients functioning on the flat part of the Frank-Starling curve, increasing preload will not positively impact cardiac output, but it will increase risks of worsening tissue edema and acute respiratory distress syndrome. Therefore it is important for clinicians to appreciate these limitations with static pressure measurements and to interpret these studies cautiously.

Recent research has demonstrated that dynamic variables are superior to static pressure measurements for assessing volume responsiveness.[30] Dynamic variables include systolic blood pressure variation, pulse pressure variation, and stroke volume variation. These techniques have been validated in patients who are receiving positive pressure ventilation in the intensive care unit or operating room. They involve measuring the variation in systolic blood pressure, pulse pressure, or calculated stroke volume that occurs during expiration as compared with inspiration. When subjects are on the steep part of the Frank-Starling curve, the

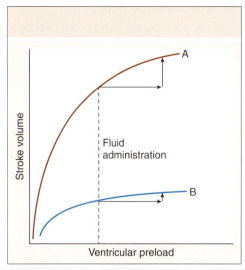

Fig. 5.4 Frank-Starling curve. Reproduced with permission from Kalantari K, Chang JN, Ronco C, Rosner MH. Assessment of intravascular volume status and volume responsiveness in critically ill patients. *Kidney Int.* 2013;83:1017–1028.

variations are more pronounced, and studies support their use for guiding fluid resuscitation.[31,32] In addition, the diameter of the inferior vena cava (IVC) as measured by bedside ultrasound, and the collapsibility of the IVC at positive pressure end inspiration as compared with end expiration, have also been shown to be useful dynamic parameters for predicting fluid responsiveness.[33,34]

RESUSCITATION FLUIDS

When patients are being treated for ECF volume contraction, clinicians must determine the type of fluid to use for volume resuscitation. The ideal resuscitation fluid reliably and predictably increases intravascular volume without accumulation in tissues, is similar in chemical composition to the ECF, does not have adverse effects, and has a favorable cost-benefit ratio.[35] There is no single fluid that meets all these requirements; therefore clinicians must choose which of the clinically available solutions will be the most appropriate for a given clinical scenario. Choices include blood products, physiologic and nonphysiologic crystalloid solutions, and colloid solutions.

Blood Transfusions

In the setting of significant blood loss, packed red blood cells should be given when patients develop severe anemia or if hemodynamic instability from blood loss occurs. Severe anemia is common in cancer patients because of blood loss, destruction with hemolytic anemias (immune and microangiopathic), and underproduction from direct marrow involvement by the malignancy or because of adverse marrow effects of chemotherapy. Current guidelines suggest a conservative strategy for administering blood transfusions.[36] Most patients should receive a transfusion when their hemoglobin is less than 7 g/dL; however, patients undergoing cardiac or orthopedic surgeries, or those with preexisting cardiac disease, should be transfused when their hemoglobin is less than 8 g/dL.

Crystalloid and Colloid Solutions

More commonly, patients are given crystalloid or colloid solutions for fluid resuscitation. Crystalloid solutions contain water soluble molecules, including mineral salts, whereas colloid solutions contain water insoluble molecules that increase intravascular oncotic pressure. Commonly available solutions are listed in Table 5.1. Colloid solutions remain in the intravascular compartment longer than crystalloid solutions, and therefore have a theoretical advantage of more efficiently expanding intravascular volume. However, the cost difference of colloids compared with crystalloids is significant, and certain colloid solutions have been associated with adverse effects, such as acute kidney injury and increased mortality with hydroxyethyl starch.[37–39] Therefore recent research efforts have focused on comparing outcomes of volume resuscitation with crystalloid solutions versus colloid solutions. These data have overwhelmingly concluded that there is no clear benefit of administering colloids over crystalloids, and in fact, mortality has shown to be higher in patients receiving hydroxyethyl starch.[40] Therefore the routine use of colloids for fluid resuscitation in cancer patients should be avoided. Albumin solutions may be considered in specific clinical scenarios, for example when large volumes of crystalloids are being administered; however, the use of hydroxyethyl starch is not recommended.

Sodium chloride is the most frequently used crystalloid solution, as it is inexpensive and commonly familiar to clinicians. Although saline is typically readily available in many areas, there have been several recent periods in which shortages developed in the United States following disruptions in manufacturing.[41] This includes following the devastation in Puerto Rico from hurricane Maria in 2017, as key saline producers were affected. Normal saline contains 0.9% sodium chloride, which is higher than the actual salt concentration in blood of 0.6%, and saline is considered nonphysiologic because it lacks the balance of electrolytes found in the ECF, such as potassium and bicarbonate. When modest and large volumes of normal saline are given, it can result in the development of hyperchloremic metabolic acidosis.[42] The clinical consequences of this include alterations in the immune system leading to inflammation and renal dysfunction.[43,44] Given these risks, controversy exists as to whether patients have better outcomes when physiologic solutions, such as lactated Ringer's solutions or Plasma-Lyte A, are used for volume resuscitation, as opposed to nonphysiologic saline solutions. Recent randomized controlled trials found that both critically ill and noncritically ill hospitalized patients had better renal outcomes when given physiologic crystalloid solutions as compared with normal saline solution.[45,46] Despite these data, there continues to be a lack of consensus on this topic, and wide variability surrounding the choice of crystalloid solution used for resuscitation exists. Choices are often based on institutional protocols, local availability of solutions, and physician familiarity, among other things. Normal saline can and should frequently be used for fluid resuscitation; however, patients should be monitored closely for the development of hyperchloremia with simultaneous decreases in serum bicarbonate, as these findings suggest saline induced metabolic acidosis. In this setting, or in patients with underlying hyperchloremic metabolic acidosis, a physiologic crystalloid solution should be chosen for resuscitation.

Hypotonic and Hypertonic Solutions

Disorders of water homeostasis often occur simultaneously with fluid disorders in cancer patients, and this includes both hyponatremia and hypernatremia (see Chapter 2). These two scenarios represent either an excess (hyponatremia) or deficit (hypernatremia) of free water. The general approach to water disorders is beyond the scope of this chapter, but it is relevant to review management of water disorders that occur in the setting of ECF volume contraction. The central strategy in these scenarios is to balance a patient's free water needs with their need for intravascular expansion. In patients presenting with hypernatremic hypovolemia without signs or symptoms of notable intravascular depletion, a hypotonic solution should be administered to restore the free water deficit. This includes 0.45% saline, 5% dextrose, and hypotonic sodium bicarbonate solution. However, although the administration of hypotonic solutions will expand both the ECF and the ICF, the ICF will be expanded to a greater extent. Therefore in patients with

Table 5.1   Crystalloid and Colloid Solutions

Intravenous Fluid	[Na⁺] mmol/L	[K⁺] mmol/L	[Cl⁻] mmol/L	[Mg²⁺] mmol/L	[HCO₃⁻] mmol/L	Lactate mmol/L	Acetate mmol/L	Dextrose g/L	Osmolality mOsm/L
NONPHYSIOLOGIC CRYSTALLOIDS									
0.9% NaCl	154	0	154						308
0.45% NaCl	77		77						154
3% NaCl	513		513						1026
5% Dextrose								50	252
PHYSIOLOGIC CRYSTALLOIDS									
Ringer's Lactate	131	5.4	2.0			111	29		280.6
Plasma-Lyte A	140	5.0	98	3.0			27		294
COLLOIDS									
5% Albumin	130–160	< 1	130–160						309
25% Albumin	130–160	< 1	130–160						312
6% Hydroxyethyl starch	154		154						310

hypernatremia and notable intravascular depletion, as suggested by hypotension, symptomatic orthostatic changes, cool extremities, or oliguria, an isotonic fluid should still be the initial fluid administered, so as to preferentially expand the intravascular volume and to preserve tissue perfusion. Once the patient has stable hemodynamics, attention should then focus on addressing the free water deficit by administering hypotonic fluid.

The treatment for patients with hyponatremia is a bit more nuanced (see Chapter 2). The pathology in these patients involves nonosmotic stimuli for antidiuretic hormone release, which signals the kidneys to reabsorb more water despite the already present excess of free water in the body. Hypertonic solutions, such a 3% sodium chloride or 1.5% sodium chloride, are indicated only when patients present with severe hyponatremia and related symptoms, such as obtundation, seizures, and comas. Expert guidelines suggest the initial goal should be to achieve a rapid rise in serum sodium of 4 to 6 mEq/L, which is typically adequate to improve or reverse most of the associated symptoms.[47] In patients with volume depletion and asymptomatic hyponatremia, isotonic fluid should be used for resuscitation. With expansion of the intravascular volume, nonosmotic stimulation of vasopressin release will be extinguished, and the kidneys will be able to increase the ratio of free water excretion as compared with isotonic urine excretion, such that the serum sodium concentration will slowly normalize. Oral intake of hypotonic fluids should be restricted in these situations. Finally, close attention should be paid to the rate at which the serum sodium rises irrespective of the solution chosen for treatment. A conservative goal of no more than a 6 to 8 mEq/L rise in serum sodium over 24 hours will prevent osmotic demyelination syndrome, even in high risk patients.

Conclusion

Volume disorders are highly prevalent in patients with cancer, and these abnormalities occur because of a vast spectrum of pathologic mechanisms. The volume regulatory complex includes the kidneys, the heart, the central nervous system, the vascular tree, and both volume and pressure baroreceptors, and this system is critical to maintaining homeostasis. Fluid abnormalities can result from both malignancy and therapy-related insults to one or more of these components, as well as from injury to any other organ system in the body. Clinicians should be diligent in monitoring and assessing the fluid needs in cancer patients, as volume disorders represent an often-treatable component of their illness. Finally, critical thought needs to be given to the assessment of volume status, determining the optimal fluid management strategy, and evaluating the response to this therapy in each individual, to maximize the beneficial impact on clinical outcomes.

Key Points

- Volume disorders are common in cancer patients and can present from a wide range of cancer or therapy related injuries.

- The extracellular fluid compartment and the intracellular fluid compartment are in osmotic equilibrium, and water will distribute within these spaces based on the accumulation of osmotic molecules in each compartment.
- Key regulators of volume homeostasis include the kidneys, heart, brain, vascular tree, and baroreceptors. This system involves multiple mechanisms that lead to a final common pathway of alterations in sodium and water handling within the kidneys.
- Data do not support the routine use of more expensive colloid solutions for volume resuscitation over crystalloid solutions.
- Clinicians should be cautious when administering large amounts of normal saline for volume resuscitation, as this can result in metabolic acidosis and poorer outcomes. In situation in which this occurs, a physiologic solution, such as lactated Ringer's or Plasma-Lyte A, should be chosen.

References

1. Gennari FJ, Weise WJ. Acid-base disturbances in gastrointestinal disease. *Clin J Am Soc Nephrol.* 2008;3:1861-1868.
2. Kimmel DW, O'Neill BP. Systemic cancer presenting as diabetes insipidus. Clinical and radiographic features of 11 patients with a review of metastatic-induced diabetes insipidus. *Cancer.* 1983;52:2355-2358.
3. Negro A, Regolisti G, Perazzoli F, Davoli S, Sani C, Rossi E. Ifosfamide-induced renal Fanconi syndrome with associated nephrogenic diabetes insipidus in an adult patient. *Nephrol Dial Transplant.* 1998;13:1547-1549.
4. Stavroulopoulos A, Nakopoulou L, Xydakis AM, Aresti V, Nikolakopoulou A, Klouvas G. Interstitial nephritis and nephrogenic diabetes insipidus in a patient treated with pemetrexed. *Ren Fail.* 2010;32:1000-1004.
5. Higgins AY, O'Halloran TD, Chang JD. Chemotherapy-induced cardiomyopathy. *Heart Failure Reviews.* 2015;20:721-730.
6. Natale LA, Agostino M. Non-ischemic acquired heart disease. In: *Grainger and Allison's diagnostic radiology.* 6th ed. New York: Churchill Livingstone; 2015:447-500.
7. Mullens W, Verbrugge FH, Nijst P, Tang WHW. Renal sodium avidity in heart failure: from pathophysiology to treatment strategies. *Eur Heart J.* 2017;38:1872-1882.
8. McMurray JJ, Packer M, Desai AS, et al. Angiotensin-neprilysin inhibition versus enalapril in heart failure. *N Engl J Med.* 2014;371:993-1004.
9. Zinman B, Wanner C, Lachin JM, et al. Empagliflozin, cardiovascular outcomes, and mortality in type 2 diabetes. *N Engl J Med.* 2015;373:2117-2128.
10. Tuttolomondo A, Pinto A, Parrinello G, Licata G. Intravenous high-dose furosemide and hypertonic saline solutions for refractory heart failure and ascites. *Semin Nephrol.* 2011;31:513-522.
11. Konstam MA, Gheorghiade M, Burnett JC, et al. Effects of oral tolvaptan in patients hospitalized for worsening heart failure: the EVEREST Outcome Trial. *JAMA.* 2007;297:1319-1331.
12. Chen HH, Anstrom KJ, Givertz MM, et al. Low-dose dopamine or low-dose nesiritide in acute heart failure with renal dysfunction: the ROSE acute heart failure randomized trial. *JAMA.* 2013;310:2533-2543.
13. Martell M, Coll M, Ezkurdia N, Raurell I, Genescà J. Physiopathology of splanchnic vasodilation in portal hypertension. *World J Hepatol.* 2010;2:208-220.
14. Schrier RW, Arroyo V, Bernardi M, Epstein M, Henriksen JH, Rodés J. Peripheral arterial vasodilation hypothesis: a proposal for the initiation of renal sodium and water retention in cirrhosis. *Hepatology.* 1988;8:1151-1157.
15. Runyon BA, AASLD. Introduction to the revised American Association for the Study of Liver Diseases Practice Guideline management of adult patients with ascites due to cirrhosis 2012. *Hepatology.* 2013;57:1651-1653.
16. Siddall EC, Radhakrishnan J. The pathophysiology of edema formation in the nephrotic syndrome. *Kidney Int.* 2012;82:635-642.

17. Svenningsen P, Bistrup C, Friis UG, et al. Plasmin in nephrotic urine activates the epithelial sodium channel. *J Am Soc Nephrol.* 2009; 20:299-310.

18. Humphreys BD, Soiffer RJ, Magee CC. Renal failure associated with cancer and its treatment: an update. *J Am Soc Nephrol.* 2005;16:151-161.

19. Hayman SR, Leung N, Grande JP, et al. VEGF inhibition, hypertension, and renal toxicity. *Current Oncology Reports.* 2012;14:285-294.

20. Agarwal R, Sinha AD. Thiazide diuretics in advanced chronic kidney disease. *J Am Soc Hypertens.* 2012;6:299-308.

21. Eisenberg PR, Jaffe AS, Schuster DP. Clinical evaluation compared to pulmonary artery catheterization in the hemodynamic assessment of critically ill patients. *Crit Care Med.* 1984;12:549-553.

22. Rivers E, Nguyen B, Havstad S, et al. Early goal-directed therapy in the treatment of severe sepsis and septic shock. *N Engl J Med.* 2001;345: 1368-1377.

23. Vincent JL, Sakr Y, Sprung CL, et al. Sepsis in European intensive care units: results of the SOAP study. *Crit Care Med.* 2006;34:344-353.

24. Investigators RRTS, Bellomo R, Cass A, et al. An observational study fluid balance and patient outcomes in the Randomized Evaluation of Normal vs. Augmented Level of Replacement Therapy trial. *Crit Care Med.* 2012;40:1753-1760.

25. McGee S, Abernethy WB, 3rd, Simel DL. The rational clinical examination. Is this patient hypovolemic? *JAMA.* 1999;281: 1022-1029.

26. Stéphan F, Flahault A, Dieudonné N, Hollande J, Paillard F, Bonnet F. Clinical evaluation of circulating blood volume in critically ill patients–contribution of a clinical scoring system. *Br J Anaesth.* 2001;86: 754-762.

27. Marik PE, Baram M, Vahid B. Does central venous pressure predict fluid responsiveness? A systematic review of the literature and the tale of seven mares. *Chest.* 2008;134:172-178.

28. Gödje O, Peyerl M, Seebauer T, Lamm P, Mair H, Reichart B. Central venous pressure, pulmonary capillary wedge pressure and intrathoracic blood volumes as preload indicators in cardiac surgery patients. *Eur J Cardiothorac Surg.* 1998;13:533-539.

29. Michard F, Teboul JL. Predicting fluid responsiveness in ICU patients: a critical analysis of the evidence. *Chest.* 2002;121:2000-2008.

30. Kalantari K, Chang JN, Ronco C, Rosner MH. Assessment of intravascular volume status and volume responsiveness in critically ill patients. *Kidney Int.* 2013;83:1017-1028.

31. Berkenstadt H, Margalit N, Hadani M, et al. Stroke volume variation as a predictor of fluid responsiveness in patients undergoing brain surgery. *Anesth Analg.* 2001;92:984-989.

32. Marik PE, Cavallazzi R, Vasu T, Hirani A. Dynamic changes in arterial waveform derived variables and fluid responsiveness in mechanically ventilated patients: a systematic review of the literature. *Crit Care Med.* 2009;37:2642-2647.

33. Yanagawa Y, Nishi K, Sakamoto T, et al. Early diagnosis of hypovolemic shock by sonographic measurement of inferior vena cava in trauma patients. *J Trauma.* 2005;58:825-829.

34. Sefidbakht S, Assadsangabi R, Abbasi HR, Nabavizadeh A. Sonographic measurement of the inferior vena cava as a predictor of shock in trauma patients. *Emerg Radiol.* 2007;14:181-185.

35. Myburgh JA, Mythen MG. Resuscitation fluids. *N Engl J Med.* 2013;369: 1243-1251.

36. Carson JL, Guyatt G, Heddle NM, et al. Clinical practice guidelines from the AABB: red blood cell transfusion thresholds and storage. *JAMA.* 2016;316:2025-2035.

37. Zarychanski R, Abou-Setta AM, Turgeon AF, et al. Association of hydroxyethyl starch administration with mortality and acute kidney injury in critically ill patients requiring volume resuscitation: a systematic review and meta-analysis. *JAMA.* 2013;309:678-688.

38. Finfer S, Bellomo R, Boyce N, et al. A comparison of albumin and saline for fluid resuscitation in the intensive care unit. *N Engl J Med.* 2004;350:2247-2256.

39. Myburgh JA, Finfer S, Bellomo R, et al. Hydroxyethyl starch or saline for fluid resuscitation in intensive care. *N Engl J Med.* 2012;367: 1901-1911.

40. Perel P, Roberts I, Ker K. Colloids versus crystalloids for fluid resuscitation in critically ill patients. *Cochrane Database Syst Rev.* 2013;2: CD000567.

41. Mazer-Amirshahi M, Fox ER. Saline shortages - many causes, no simple solution. *N Engl J Med.* 2018;378:1472-1474.

42. Morgan TJ, Venkatesh B, Hall J. Crystalloid strong ion difference determines metabolic acid-base change during acute normovolaemic haemodilution. *Intensive Care Med.* 2004;30:1432-1437.

43. Kellum JA, Song M, Li J. Science review: extracellular acidosis and the immune response: clinical and physiologic implications. *Crit Care Med.* 2004;8:331-336.

44. Hadimioglu N, Saadawy I, Saglam T, Ertug Z, Dinckan A. The effect of different crystalloid solutions on acid-base balance and early kidney function after kidney transplantation. *Anesth Analg.* 2008;107: 264-269.

45. Self WH, Semler MW, Wanderer JP, et al. Balanced crystalloids versus saline in noncritically ill adults. *N Engl J Med.* 2018;378:819-828.

46. Semler MW, Self WH, Wanderer JP, et al. Balanced crystalloids versus saline in critically ill adults. *N Engl J Med.* 2018;378:829-839.

47. Verbalis JG, Goldsmith SR, Greenberg A, et al. Diagnosis, evaluation, and treatment of hyponatremia: expert panel recommendations. *Am J Med.* 2013;126:S1-42.

Paraprotein-Related Kidney Diseases

6 Paraproteins

VECIHI BATUMAN

Introduction

This section of the book focuses on paraprotein-related kidney disorders. In this chapter, we describe a general overview of paraproteins and their adverse effects on the kidneys with emphasis on proximal tubule disorders. In the following chapters, detailed discussions on other types of paraprotein-mediated kidney disorders, including cast nephropathy, monoclonal immunoglobulin light chain (AL) amyloidosis, light and heavy chain diseases, etc., are provided.

Paraprotein Basics

Paraproteins are monoclonal light chains (LCs), heavy chains, or intact immunoglobulins detected in the serum or urine in abnormal quantities. The majority of the paraproteinemia-associated kidney disorders result from free monoclonal light chains (FLC), as these immunoglobulin fragments have relatively unrestricted access to kidneys and kidney tubules. There is an expanding spectrum of kidney disorders caused by either direct effects of FLCs on kidney cells or by deposition of intact immune globulins or their fragments in the glomeruli or along the kidney tubules (Box 6.1).[1]

Paraproteins are produced by plasma cells or B cells, and their presence in blood or urine indicates clonal proliferation of either of these cell lines, that is, multiple myeloma (plasma cells), or lymphomas (B cells).[2] Thus paraproteinemias are typically associated with cancer of these cell lines. In some cases, however, the workup for their clonal origin may not meet the criteria for cancer and there may be no overt kidney disorder, a condition referred to as *monoclonal gammopathy of unknown significance* (MGUS).[3] Upon closer scrutiny, many MGUS cases are found to have renal abnormalities, although without an obvious cancer identifiable as their source. Such conditions are termed *monoclonal gammopathy of renal significance* (MGRS).[3–5] In most cases of MGRS, the initial diagnosis is suspected when a kidney disorder is diagnosed in the presence of monoclonal gammopathy, or when a kidney biopsy is reported to show monoclonal immunoglobulin deposition, and when clonal workup fails to meet the criteria for the diagnosis of overt multiple myeloma or a B cell tumor.[4,6,7] Paraproteins, whether produced by a cancer, such as myeloma, lymphoma, or leukemia, or by a small clone that does not meet the criteria for cancer, often affect the kidneys by various mechanisms that include disruption of transport systems,[8–14] triggering inflammatory reactions in the kidney,[1,8,10,15–20] cast formation,[21,22] or kidney deposition of organized or unorganized monoclonal proteins.[5,16,23–27] Renal involvement in paraproteinemia always implies a worse prognosis.[1,28–30]

Historical Background

The earliest association of a paraprotein with the kidney dates back to 1845 when Dr. William Macintyre found a unique nonalbumin protein in the urine of his patient Thomas Alexander McBean diagnosed with "mollities and fragilitas ossium," now known as *multiple myeloma*. The significance of this finding with respect to kidney involvement and the source of this protein were not clearly understood. Both Dr. Macintyre and Dr. Thomas Watson, a consultant on the same case, sent a urine sample from the patient to Dr. Henry Bence Jones, a recognized clinical pathologist of his time. Dr. Watson in his letter to Bence Jones described the sample as containing a large amount of "animal matter" that precipitated when nitric acid was added, became clear when heated, and reappeared upon cooling.[31] Bence Jones confirmed the physical properties of this "animal matter," which he thought was "hydrated deutoxide of albumen," and recommended that the presence of this protein to be looked for in the urine of patients with 'mollities and fragilitas ossium.'[32,33] This may possibly be the first instance of designating a urinary biomarker for a kidney disorder associated with a systemic disease, multiple myeloma. This protein later came to be known as "*Bence Jones protein*," although Bence Jones himself was not aware of its source or its significance for kidney disease.[31–34]

After the first characterization of plasma cells in 1895 by Marschalko, in 1900, Wright defined the "gelatiniform substance" found in the bones of patients with mollities as a tumor consisting of plasma cells.[31] Korngold and Lipari, in 1956, 111 years after the first demonstration of Bence Jones protein, using Ouchterlony technique, identified two distinct antigenic types of Bence Jones proteins, and also demonstrated the presence of the same proteins in the sera of multiple myeloma patients. These two antigenic types were later named kappa (κ) and lambda (λ) LCs honoring Korngold and Lipari.[31,35] Edelman and Gally showed in 1962 that LCs derived from a patient with immunoglobulin G myeloma in the serum had the same amino acid sequence with the Bence Jones protein in the urine and share the same heat properties, finally solving the mystery of Bence Jones proteins.[31] With precise characterization of the monoclonal proteins associated with multiple myeloma and other tumors, and the demonstration that myeloma proteins are toxic to kidneys,[14,36,37] it became possible to investigate kidney disorders associated with paraproteinemias and explore therapies for such disorders.

Proximal Tubule Disorders

Proximal tubule disorders are very common in myeloma and may be present with or without cast formation in the distal tubules.[1,10,38–40] The paraproteins responsible for proximal tubule disorders are almost exclusively immunoglobulin LCs. Although tubular involvement is sometimes present in AL amyloidosis or other paraprotein deposition disorders, they are rare, and do not usually feature as prominent components of the underlying disorders. These disorders are discussed in the following chapters; here we will focus on proximal tubule disorders associated with immunoglobulin LCs.

LCs are approximately 210 to 220 amino acid polypeptide subunits of immunoglobulins, smaller than albumin, and are relatively positively charged compared with albumin. Monomeric LCs are approximately 22 to 25 kDa and most κ-FLCs exist in monomeric state whereas λ-FLCs tend to form approximately 44 kDa dimers. Either way, FLCs are relatively unhindered in the glomerulus, and based on an estimated glomerular sieving coefficient of approximately .09, significant quantities are filtered and presented to the renal tubule.[9,10,41] In normal healthy individuals 100 to 600 mg of polyclonal FLCs may be filtered in the glomerulus, and only minute quantities, no more than 2 to 3 mg per day, is excreted in the urine, implying near complete reabsorption in the renal tubule.[10,15] It is now clear that FLCs reabsorption takes place in the proximal tubules mostly via receptor-mediated endocytosis, after binding to the tandem endocytic receptors megalin/cubilin; most of the internalized FLCs are catabolized into their amino acid constituents through the action of lysosomal enzymes in the lysosomes.[8,10,42–44]

In myeloma and in other clonal proliferative disorders, the overproduction of monoclonal LCs overwhelms the proximal tubules' capacity to process all the filtered FLCs and overflow proteinuria ensues. In such situations, there is always evidence of stress on the endocytic apparatus of the kidney, often seen as droplets or cytoplasmic (vacuolar) inclusion of monoclonal FLCs demonstrated by immunofluorescence, or electron microscopy (Fig. 6.1).[45] Some myeloma patients have been observed to excrete up to 20 g per day of FLCs with minimal albuminuria with a dipstick test negative for proteinuria[46]—a situation that often results in delayed diagnosis. Electron microscopically, the FLCs appear in the lysosomes and the clinical picture reflects lysosomal dysfunction, such as Fanconi syndrome (FS).[47] Thus

the kidney's abnormalities seen in myeloma patients are related to the renal handling of FLCs and both proximal and distal tubule disorders are common.[16] Although most of the distal tubule disorders are related to cast formation because of the interaction of FLCs with unique amino acid sequence, in their CDR 3 domain with Tamm-Horsfall proteins (discussed separately),[1,21,22,48,49] proximal tubule disorders range from subtle tubule transport disorders to tubule cell death—apoptosis or necrosis, acute kidney injury, and tubulointerstitial nephritis (Box 6.2).[8,15,38,39,45]

There is a broad range of renal disorders associated with FLC-proteinuria and significant variability exists in the structure, mostly in the variable region, V_L, of the involved FLCs. These disorders display marked heterogeneity ranging from subtle functional abnormalities to severe kidney failure. Some patients may have a modest degree of monoclonal gammopathy along with asymptomatic FLC proteinuria—often referred to as *MGUS*. Detailed investigations of such patients frequently reveal some renal abnormalities involving either the tubules or sometimes the glomeruli, a condition referred to as *MGRS*.[50] Many of these patients on long-term follow-up develop overt myeloma.[5,51,52] The variability in both the type and the severity of the FLC-associated renal disorders can be linked to the specific sequences in the V_L of the involved FLCs;[47,53] however, these disorders also require overproduction of a clone of FLCs.

The most common proximal tubule disorder associated with monoclonal FLCs, whether in the setting of overt myeloma or MGRS, is proximal tubular acidosis (type 2) that may be accompanied by one or a combination of sodium-dependent transport abnormalities, such as bicarbonaturia (along with renal potassium wasting), glycosuria, aminoaciduria, phosphaturia, and hyperuricosuria; that is, partial or complete FS.[1,8–10,16,28,47,53] Although the observations that FLCs inhibit sodium-dependent amino acid, glucose, and phosphate transports in renal brush border membrane vesicles and kidney proximal tubule cells in vitro imply a direct effect by possibly membrane-bound FLCs,[10,12,13] cytoplasmic deposition of crystalline or noncrystalline FLCs is often present in proximal tubule cells of patients with FS and FLC-proteinuria. FLC-associated FS is most frequently caused by κ-LCs restricted to the Vk I subgroup, often with extensive crystal formation in the proximal tubule cells (PTCs) (see Fig. 6.1), and is linked to the variable domain of the monoclonal LC, which interestingly, is also associated with resistance to proteolysis.[54] There are also reports of FS associated with λ-FLCs, and again the expression of FS is linked to the V region of the involved FLCs.[55–60] Sometimes FS can occur without any discernible FLC deposition, crystalline or noncrystalline, in the proximal tubule cells, and conversely, not all patients with crystalline deposition always have FS. The patients with FS generally display various degrees of acute tubule injury, a condition referred to as *light chain proximal tubulopathy*, which may be associated with overt or smoldering myeloma, occasionally with MGRS, and rarely with other neoplasms elaborating monoclonal FLCs.[15,45]

Animal experiments in vivo and studies in vitro have shown that some FLCs induce extensive apoptosis in proximal tubules, which may be a mechanism contributing to acute tubule injury.[8,17,53] Proximal tubule cells exposed to tubulopathic FLCs, isolated from patients with myeloma, elicit a range of cytotoxic and inflammatory responses,

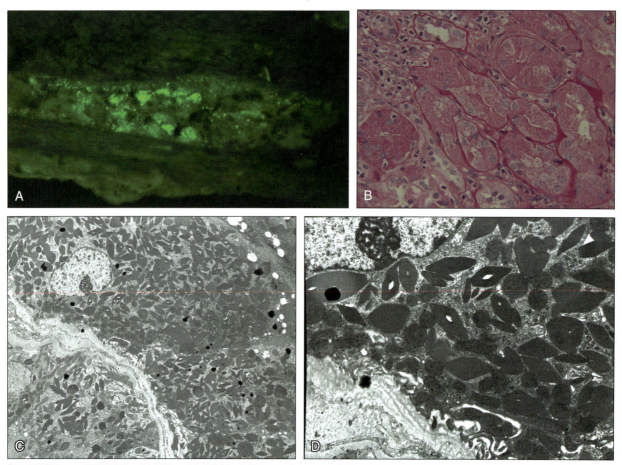

Fig. 6.1 Kappa light chain proximal tubulopathy in a patient with monoclonal κ-FLC gammopathy diagnosed as monoclonal gammopathy of renal significance (patient did not meet criteria for multiple myeloma). **A.** Immunofluorescence demonstrates intracellular crystals staining for κ-light chain within the tubular epithelial cytoplasm. Staining for all other immune reactants was negative. **B.** Periodic acid-Schiff staining shows the proximal tubular epithelia are laden with intracellular crystalline inclusions. Magnification 600×. **C.** Electron microscopy demonstrating abundant electron-dense intracellular crystals within the cytoplasm of proximal tubular epithelium. **D.** Electron microscopy-higher magnification of the intracellular crystals, most of them larger than the adjacent mitochondria.

Box 6.2 Proximal Tubule Disorder Associated With Monoclonal Gammopathies

- Asymptomatic light chain proteinuria
- Urinary concentration and/or dilution defects
- Fanconi syndrome (partial or complete)
- Light chain proximal tubulopathy with crystalline or noncrystalline cytoplasmic deposits
- Acute kidney injury (acute tubular necrosis variant)
- Proximal tubulopathy associated with inflammatory reaction (acute tubulointerstitial variant)
- Chronic tubulointerstitial nephritis (tubule atrophy, interstitial fibrosis)
- Lysosomal impaction ("indigestion/constipation")

---

such as generation of reactive oxygen species, activation of the transcription factors, nuclear factor-κB, leading to transcription and release to medium of inflammatory cytokines (interleukins 6, 8, monocyte chemoattractant protein-1, tumor necrosis factor-α, transforming growth factor-β1, etc.), mediated through phosphorylation of mitogen-activated protein kinases (MAPK), especially p38

MAPK.[8,10,16,19] FLC-exposed proximal tubule cells also undergo morphologic changes that include disruption of cytoskeletal organization, extensive vacuolization, and cell death (apoptosis and necrosis).[11] Furthermore, the tubulopathic FLCs can induce phenotypical changes in proximal tubule epithelium, inducing loss of epithelial cell marker E-cadherin and acquisition of myofibroblast marker α-smooth muscle actin (i.e., epithelial-to-mesenchymal transformation (EMT)),[8] suggesting that this phenomenon may contribute to the extensive tubulointerstitial fibrosis frequently seen in patients with myeloma, although EMT is difficult to identify in human kidney biopsies. Most of these cytotoxic or inflammatory responses associated with monoclonal FLCs appear to require their internalization in the cell, and could be prevented by maneuvers that inhibit FLC endocytosis, such as disrupting the clathrin-coated pathway, inhibiting vacuolar acidification, or knocking down megalin and cubilin expression in proximal tubule epithelia,[8,19,20,61,62] although the studies with brush-border membrane vesicles also suggest direct toxic effects by FLCs at the membrane level.[10,61]

Proximal tubular disorders seen in the setting of FLC paraproteinemia may exhibit many additional structural lesions other than crystalline and noncrystalline cytoplasmic deposition in the proximal tubule cells. Such lesions generally have not attracted much attention until recently. However, the recent biopsy studies suggest that proximal tubule findings are common.[38,39,45] For example, Ecotiere et al. reviewed kidney biopsies of 70 patients with myeloma, and observed varying degrees of interstitial fibrosis, tubule atrophy, and interstitial inflammation in more than 50% of biopsies.[38] In a systematic review of 5410 kidney biopsies, Herrera reported that 2.5% had kidney lesions related to monoclonal gammopathies, and 46% of these demonstrated significant histopathologic changes in the proximal tubules. Herrera classified these lesions into four categories (see Box 6.1): (1) proximal tubulopathy without cytoplasmic inclusions (acute tubular necrosis, ATN variant); (2) tubulopathy associated with inflammatory reaction (acute tubular interstitial nephritis variant); (3) proximal tubulopathy associated with intracytoplasmic inclusions; and (4) proximal tubulopathy associated with "lysosomal indigestion/constipation."[39]

In summary, tubule abnormalities are very common in patients with FLC paraproteinemia and comprise functional and morphologic changes that range from subtle transport abnormalities, including FS, to acute kidney injury, as well as inflammatory responses that contribute to renal interstitial fibrosis and chronic kidney disease. These disorders can be seen in patients with overt myeloma, or sometimes in cases with monoclonal gammopathy that cannot be linked to a cancerous clone (MGRS). The proximal tubule changes are always associated with overproduction of FLCs, and the type and severity of the lesions are determined by the V region of the involved FLCs. The majority of these disorders also require FLC endocytosis by the proximal tubule cells, and appear potentially reversible if their endocytosis can be prevented.[8,10,19,20,61,62]

Other Paraprotein-Associated Kidney Lesions

Among many types of kidney disorders associated with paraproteinemias, the most common is myeloma cast nephropathy (MCN).[1,30] Of note, MCN is predominantly a tubulointerstitial disease and the extent of cast formation in kidney biopsies from patients with myeloma is highly variable. In myeloma patients who present with acute kidney injury, cast formation is usually extensive.[21,29,48] However, in other patients who are diagnosed after a slow-progressing indolent course, casts may be less extensive and chronic tubulointerstitial lesions, such as interstitial fibrosis, tubule atrophy, and occasionally inflammatory cell infiltration may be the prominent features.[1,38,39] It is plausible that FLC-induced inflammatory responses in the proximal tubule epithelial cells are instrumental in the pathogenesis of these lesions.[1,8–10,18–20] Beyond the proximal tubular disorders discussed here, there is a broad range of kidney disorders with paraproteins, including LC and heavy chain immunoglobulin deposition diseases, AL amyloidosis, fibrillary glomerulonephritis, cryoglobulinemia, paraprotein-associated C3 glomerulonephritis, and proliferative glomerulonephritis with monoclonal immunoglobulin depositions disease (see Box 6.1).[2,7,23,25,27,28,48,52,63–65] In-depth discussion on these disorders are presented in the following chapters (see Chapters 7–10).

Key Points

- Paraproteins are monoclonal heavy chains, light chains, or intact immunoglobulins present in the blood or urine produced by a clone of plasma cells or B cells.
- Paraproteins can cause kidney disease through a variety of mechanisms because of the intrinsic properties of the involved paraproteins, including direct toxicity to kidney cells, deposition of organized or unorganized paraproteins in glomerular or tubular cells.
- In recent years, an increasing number of paraprotein-associated kidney disorders have been identified in which a clonal workup may fail to reveal a discernible cancer, and these disorders are now classified as *monoclonal gammopathy of renal significance* (MGRS).
- Immunoglobulin light chains are among the most common paraproteins associated with kidney lesions, which include myeloma cast formation, proximal tubulopathies, and AL amyloidosis.
- Basic research has revealed that excessive endocytosis of immunoglobulin light chains in the proximal tubule cells induce cell stress responses including activation of inflammatory pathways, epithelial-to-mesenchymal transformation, and apoptosis and necrosis. These mechanisms contribute to both acute renal injury as well as chronic tubulointerstitial disease frequently seen in patients with multiple myeloma or with free light chain producing MGRs.

References

1. Doshi M, Lahoti A, Danesh FR, Batuman V, Sanders PW, American Society of Nephrology Onco-Nephrology Forum. Paraprotein-related kidney disease: kidney injury from paraproteins-what determines the site of injury? *Clin J Am Soc Nephrol.* 2016;11:2288-2294.
2. Perazella MA, Finkel KW, American Society of Nephrology Onco-Nephology Forum. Paraprotein-related kidney disease: attack of the killer M proteins. *Clin J Am Soc Nephrol.* 2016;11:2256-2259.
3. Glavey SV, Leung N. Monoclonal gammopathy: the good, the bad and the ugly. *Blood Rev.* 2016;30:223-231.
4. Hogan JJ, Weiss BM. Bridging the divide: an onco-nephrologic approach to the monoclonal gammopathies of renal significance. *Clin J Am Soc Nephrol.* 2016;11:1681-1691.
5. Leung N, Bridoux F, Hutchison CA, et al. Monoclonal gammopathy of renal significance: when MGUS is no longer undetermined or insignificant. *Blood.* 2012;120:4292-4295.
6. Bridoux F, Leung N, Hutchison CA, et al. Diagnosis of monoclonal gammopathy of renal significance. *Kidney Int.* 2015;87:698-711.
7. Vignon M, Cohen C, Faguer S, et al. The clinicopathologic characteristics of kidney diseases related to monotypic IgA deposits. *Kidney Int.* 2017;91:720-728.
8. Batuman V. The pathogenesis of acute kidney impairment in patients with multiple myeloma. *Adv Chronic Kidney Dis.* 2012;19:282-286.
9. Nakhoul N, Batuman V. Role of proximal tubules in the pathogenesis of kidney disease. *Contrib Nephrol.* 2011;169:37-50.
10. Batuman V. Proximal tubular injury in myeloma. *Contrib Nephrol.* 153:87-104.
15. Hutchison CA, Batuman V, Behrens J, et al. The pathogenesis and diagnosis of acute kidney injury in multiple myeloma. *Nat Rev Nephrol.* 2011;8:43-51.
16. Sanders PW. Mechanisms of light chain injury along the tubular nephron. *J Am Soc Nephrol.* 2012;23:1777-1781.
17. Khan AM, Li M, Balamuthusamy S, Maderdrut JL, Simon EE, Batuman V. Myeloma light chain-induced renal injury in mice. *Nephron Exp Nephrol.* 2010;116:e32-e41.
18. Li M, Hering-Smith KS, Simon EE, Batuman V. Myeloma light chains induce epithelial-mesenchymal transition in human renal proximal tubule epithelial cells. *Nephrol Dial Transplant.* 2008;23:860-870.

19. Sengul S, Zwizinski C, Batuman V. Role of MAPK pathways in light chain-induced cytokine production in human proximal tubule cells. *Am J Physiol Renal Physiol.* 2003;284:F1245-1254.

20. Sengul S, Zwizinski C, Simon EE, Kapasi A, Singhal PC, Batuman V. Endocytosis of light chains induces cytokines through activation of NF-kappaB in human proximal tubule cells. *Kidney Int.* 2002;62: 1977-1988.

21. Ying WZ, Allen CE, Curtis LM, Aaron KJ, Sanders PW. Mechanism and prevention of acute kidney injury from cast nephropathy in a rodent model. *J Clin Invest.* 2012;122:1777-1785.

23. Leung N, Drosou ME, Nasr SH. Dysproteinemias and glomerular disease. *Clin J Am Soc Nephrol.* 2018;13:128-139.

24. Ravindran A, Go RS, Fervenza FC, Sethi S. Thrombotic microangiopathy associated with monoclonal gammopathy. *Kidney Int.* 2017;91: 691-698.

26. Mahmood U, Isbel N, Mollee P, Mallett A, Govindarajulu S, Francis R. Monoclonal gammopathy of renal significance triggering atypical haemolytic uraemic syndrome. *Nephrol.* 2017;22:15-17.

27. Leung N, Drosou ME, Nasr SH. Dysproteinemias and glomerular disease. *Clin J Am Soc Nephrol.* 2017;13:128-139.

28. Rosner MH, Edeani A, Yanagita M, Glezerman IG, Leung N, American Society of Nephrology Onco-Nephrology Forum. Paraprotein-related kidney disease: diagnosing and treating monoclonal gammopathy of renal significance. *Clin J Am Soc Nephrol.* 2016;11:2280-2287.

29. Zand L, Nasr SH, Gertz MA, et al. Clinical and prognostic differences among patients with light chain deposition disease, myeloma cast nephropathy and both. *Leuk Lymphoma.* 2015;56:3357-3364.

30. Nasr SH, Valeri AM, Sethi S, et al. Clinicopathologic correlations in multiple myeloma: a case series of 190 patients with kidney biopsies. *Am J Kidney Dis.* 2012;59:786-794.

31. Kyle RA, Rajkumar SV. Multiple myeloma. *Blood.* 2008;111:2962-2972.

32. Kyle RA. Henry Bence Jones–physician, chemist, scientist and biographer: a man for all seasons. *Br J Haematol.* 2001;115:13-18.

33. Kyle RA. Multiple myeloma: an odyssey of discovery. *Br J Haematol.* 2000;111:1035-1044.

34. Steensma DP, Kyle RA. A history of the kidney in plasma cell disorders. *Contrib Nephrol.* 2007;153:5-24.

35. Korngold L, Lipari R. Multiple-myeloma proteins. III. The antigenic relationship of Bence Jones proteins to normal gammaglobulin and multiple-myeloma serum proteins. *Cancer.* 1956;9:262-272.

38. Ecotière L, Thierry A, Debiais-Delpech C, et al. Prognostic value of kidney biopsy in myeloma cast nephropathy: a retrospective study of 70 patients. *Nephrol Dial Transplant.* 2016;31:64-72.

39. Herrera GA. Proximal tubulopathies associated with monoclonal light chains: the spectrum of clinicopathologic manifestations and molecular pathogenesis. *Arch Pathol Lab Med.* 2014;138:1365-1380.

40. Sengul S, Li M, Batuman V. Myeloma kidney: toward its prevention—with new insights from in vitro and in vivo models of renal injury. *J Nephrol.* 2009;22:17-28.

42. Klassen RB, Allen PL, Batuman V, Crenshaw K, Hammond TG. Light chains are a ligand for megalin. *J Appl Physiol.* 2005;98:257-263.

43. Batuman V, Verroust PJ, Navar GL, et al. Myeloma light chains are ligands for cubilin (gp280). *Am J Physiol.* 1998;275, F246-F254.

44. Batuman V, Guan S. Receptor-mediated endocytosis of immunoglobulin light chains by renal proximal tubule cells. *Am J Physiol.* 1997;272: F521-530.

45. Stokes MB, Valeri AM, Herlitz L, et al. Light chain proximal tubulopathy: clinical and pathologic characteristics in the modern treatment era. *J Am Soc Nephrol.* 2015;27:1555-1565.

47. Luciani A, Sirac C, Terryn S, et al. Impaired lysosomal function underlies monoclonal light chain-associated renal fanconi syndrome. *J Am Soc Nephrol.* 2016;27:2049-2061.

48. Finkel KW, Cohen EP, Shirali A, Abudayyeh A, American Society of Nephrology Onco-Nephrology Forum. Paraprotein-related kidney disease: evaluation and treatment of myeloma cast nephropathy. *Clin J Am Soc Nephrol.* 2016;11:2273-2279.

49. Huang ZQ, Sanders PW. Biochemical interaction between Tamm-Horsfall glycoprotein and Ig light chains in the pathogenesis of cast nephropathy. *Lab Invest.* 1995;73:810-817.

50. Kyle RA, Rajkumar SV. Monoclonal gammopathy of undetermined significance and smoldering multiple myeloma. *Hematol Oncol Clin North Am.* 2007;21:1093-1113.

51. Kyle RA, Larson DR, Therneau TM, et al. Clinical course of light-chain smouldering multiple myeloma (idiopathic Bence Jones proteinuria): a retrospective cohort study. *Lancet Haematol.* 2014;1: e28-e36.

52. Sethi S, Fervenza FC, Rajkumar SV. Spectrum of manifestations of monoclonal gammopathy-associated renal lesions. *Curr Opin Nephrol Hypertens.* 2016;25:127-137.

53. Sirac C, Herrera GA, Sanders PW, et al. Animal models of monoclonal immunoglobulin-related renal diseases. *Nat Rev Nephrol.* 2018;14: 246-264.

54. Sirac C, Bridoux F, Carrion C, et al. Role of the monoclonal kappa chain V domain and reversibility of renal damage in a transgenic model of acquired Fanconi syndrome. *Blood.* 2006;108:536-543.

55. Yao Y, Wang SX, Zhang YK, Wang Y, Liu L, Liu G. Acquired Fanconi syndrome with proximal tubular cytoplasmic fibrillary inclusions of lambda light chain restriction. *Intern Med.* 2014;53:121-124.

56. Isobe T, Kametani F, Shinoda T. V-domain deposition of lambda Bence Jones protein in the renal tubular epithelial cells in a patient with the adult Fanconi syndrome with myeloma. *Amyloid.* 1998;5: 117-120.

57. Bate KL, Clouston D, Packham D, Ratnaike S, Ebeling PR. Lambda light chain induced nephropathy: a rare cause of the Fanconi syndrome and severe osteomalacia. *Am J Kidney Dis.* 1998;32:E3.

58. Leboulleux M, Lelongt B, Mougenot B, et al. Protease resistance and binding of Ig light chains in myeloma-associated tubulopathies. *Kidney Int.* 1995;48:72-79.

61. Sengul S, Erturk S, Khan AM, Batuman V. Receptor-associated protein blocks internalization and cytotoxicity of myeloma light chain in cultured human proximal tubular cells. *PLoS One.* 2013;8:e70276.

62. Li M, Balamuthusamy S, Simon EE, Batuman V. Silencing megalin and cubilin genes inhibits myeloma light chain endocytosis and ameliorates toxicity in human renal proximal tubule epithelial cells. *Am J Physiol Renal Physiol.* 2008;295:F82-F90.

65. Motwani SS, Herlitz L, Monga D, Jhaveri KD, Lam AQ, American Society of Nephrology Onco-Nephrology Forum. Paraprotein-related kidney disease: glomerular diseases associated with paraproteinemias. *Clin J Am Soc Nephrol.* 2016;11:2260-2272.

A full list of references is available at Expertconsult.com

7 Cast Nephropathy

COLIN A. HUTCHISON AND PETER MOLLEE

Introduction

Acute kidney injury (AKI) remains a common presentation of multiple myeloma (MM). Depending on the definition of AKI used, between 18% and 56% of patients with MM are affected. It is not infrequent that myeloma is first identified during the workup of a patient with unexplained AKI. When this AKI is severe, it has historically been associated with a limited chance of renal recovery and a greatly reduced survival for individuals with MM compared with those with no renal impairment.

Paraproteins, or M-proteins, are associated with many patterns of renal injury within the nephron, and in turn these different pathologies are associated with a diverse range of clinical presentations. In 2012 the International Kidney and Monoclonal Gammopathy Research Group (IKMG) introduced the classification, monoclonal gammopathy of renal significance (MGRS), to capture some of the rarer renal pathologies associated with small paraproteins in individuals who do not meet the diagnostic criteria for MM. Cast nephropathy does not fit into this diagnostic classification, as patients with cast nephropathy always meet the criteria for MM.

With the combination of improved diagnostic techniques and modern chemotherapy agents, the kidney and overall outcomes for patients with cast nephropathy have greatly improved in recent years.

Epidemiology

MM is a hematologic malignancy characterized by the clonal expansion of malignant plasma cells in the bone marrow and end organ dysfunction. MM accounts for 1% of all malignancies and 12% to 15% of hematologic malignancies.[1] The annual age adjusted incidence is 5.6 cases per 100,000 persons in Western countries with a median age at presentation of 70 years.[2] Renal impairment at diagnosis remains common with an incidence that ranges from 20% to 50%.[3]

The development of AKI reduces 1-year survival in patients with MM, with recovery of renal function more predictive of survival than hematologic response.[4] According to the European Renal Association-European Dialysis and Transplant Association registry study, the incidence rate of end-stage kidney disease (ESKD) secondary to complications of MM in Europe increased from 0.7 per million population (pmp) from 1986 to 1990 to 2.52 pmp between 2001 and 2005.[5] The incidence rate was observed to be higher in the United States at 4.3 cases per million per year between 2001 and 2010.[6] The mortality rates for patients with ESKD secondary to MM were significantly higher in comparison to patients without myeloma: 86.7, 41.4, and 34.4 per 100 person-years in the first 3 years of renal replacement therapy (RRT) compared with 32.3, 20.6, and 21.3, respectively.[6] The overall adjusted hazard ratio for death was 2.5 in patients with ESKD caused by myeloma versus other causes.

Pathophysiology

Although there are diverse potential causes of AKI in patients with MM, the majority of individuals affected have the tubulointerstitial pathology of cast nephropathy, also known as *myeloma kidney*.[7] In biopsy series, cast nephropathy accounts for between 66% and 100% of the pathologic diagnoses. This tubulointerstitial pathology is a direct consequence of the very high concentrations of monoclonal free light chains (FLC) present in the circulation of individuals with MM. These middle-molecular weight proteins are freely filtered at the glomeruli and pass with the ultrafiltrate into the proximal and then distal tubules.

POLYCLONAL FREE LIGHT CHAINS AND BENCE-JONES PROTEINS

About 500 mg of polyclonal FLCs are produced daily by the normal lymphoid system and catabolized by the proximal tubule. This system is highly efficient and only 1 to 10 mg of polyclonal FLCs normally appear in the urine each day.[8] However, in the setting of a plasma cell dyscrasia, FLC production increases considerably, producing circulating levels of monoclonal FLCs that can be hundreds of fold higher than normal.[9] When this increase occurs, the capacity of the multiligand endocytic receptor complex of the proximal tubule is quickly exceeded, and high concentrations of FLCs appear in the tubular fluid and finally in the urine. The FLCs that appear in the urine are traditionally termed *Bence-Jones proteins (BJP)*.[8] Before the advent of serum assays for the measurement of monoclonal FLCs, the identification of BJP was a critical element of the workup of patients with suspect myeloma.

MECHANISMS OF INJURY

Monoclonal FLCs are known to induce isolated proximal tubular injury, cast nephropathy, or a combination of both. FLC interaction with proximal tubule cells (PTCs) can activate inflammatory cascades that lead to tubulointerstitial fibrosis, a major feature of myeloma kidney. Similarly, FLC interaction with Tamm-Horsfall proteins (THPs; also known as *uromodulin*) and cast formation in the distal tubule can block glomerular flow and produce tubular atrophy and contribute to interstitial fibrosis.

Proximal Tubule Cell Injury

FLCs can exert direct toxic effects on PTCs, the most abundant cell type in the kidney, and many of the renal consequences of myeloma involvement of the kidney are related to proximal tubular injury.[10–18] Studies have shown that FLCs purified from the urine of myeloma patients without glomerular disease inhibited substrate transport in isolated brush border membrane vesicles, cultured PTCs in vitro, and in perfused proximal tubules in rats in vivo.[19–21]

Although FLCs can be directly toxic to PTCs by blocking transport of glucose, amino acids, or phosphate, and by activating redox signaling upon contact with PTCs, most of the toxicity is mediated after endocytosis of FLCs, through the tandem endocytic receptors cubilin and megalin.[22,23] Excessive FLC endocytosis can induce a spectrum of inflammatory effects that include activation of redox pathways and expression of nuclear factor κB and mitogen-activated protein kinases, leading to transcription of inflammatory and profibrotic cytokines, such as interleukin (IL)-6, C-C motif chemokine 2 (also known as *monocyte chemoattractant protein*), IL-8, and transforming growth factor β1. Excessive FLC endocytosis can also trigger apoptotic pathways and alter the phenotype of PTCs towards a fibroblastic one through epithelial–mesenchymal transition in vitro and in vivo.[24,25] Studies have shown that blocking FLC endocytosis, either by inhibition of endocytosis or by silencing the endocytic receptors cubilin and megalin, abrogates cytotoxicity. These observations support the principle that endocytosis is a prerequisite for these inflammatory processes and are the basis of three potential therapeutic strategies to prevent tubular injury: first, to eliminate or reduce the FLC burden in myeloma patients with renal involvement; second, to block the inflammatory pathways that are activated as a result of FLC toxicity; and third, to potentially block FLC endocytosis.

Cast Nephropathy

In addition to this proximal tubule injury, the major mechanism of FLC-mediated tubule damage is intratubular obstruction from precipitation of FLCs in the lumen of the distal nephron (Figs 7.1A and B), which leads to interstitial inflammation and fibrosis.[26] The clinical relevance of cast formation was initially revealed by an eloquent series of studies that infused nephrotoxic human FLCs in rats. These studies demonstrated that infusion of these FLCs resulted in increased proximal tubule pressure and simultaneously decreased single-nephron glomerular filtration rate. Intraluminal protein casts were identified in these rat kidneys.[27] Persistence of intraluminal casts in vivo reduces single-nephron glomerular blood flow to the obstructed nephron and results in atrophy of the nephron proximal to the obstruction.[28,29] When infused directly into the rat nephron in vivo, monoclonal FLCs from patients with cast nephropathy produced dose-dependent intraluminal obstruction by precipitating in the distal nephron; casts were not observed before the tip of the loop of Henle.[30] Obstruction was accelerated by the presence of furosemide. Pretreatment of rats with colchicine decreased urinary levels of THP and prevented intraluminal cast formation and obstruction.[30] Additional studies demonstrated an integral relationship between monoclonal FLCs and THPs in cast formation and the associated kidney injury. In humans, casts are generally observed in the distal portion of the nephron, although

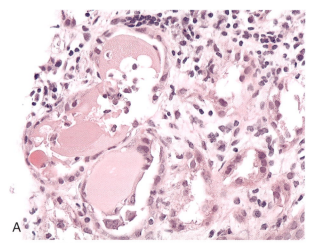

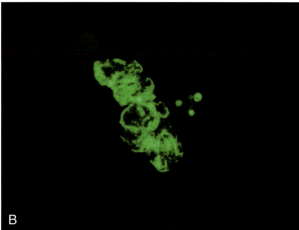

Fig. 7.1 Cast Nephropathy. A, Atypical casts show irregular shapes with fracture lines on light microscopy. Cells are often see coating light chain casts and this "cellular reaction" is one of the features that differentiates these casts from other proteinaceous casts. Hematoxalyn and Eosin, 400x. **B,** Strong immunofluorescence positivity for kappa light chains with corresponding negative staining for lambda light chains (not shown) supports the diagnosis of light chain cast nephropathy. (Images provided by Leal Herlitz, MD, Department of Pathology, Cleveland Clinic Foundation.)

they have also been found in proximal tubular segments and even in glomeruli in renal biopsy specimens.[31] However, these casts also contained THP, suggesting intraluminal reflux of coprecipitated THP and FLC into the proximal nephron.[31]

Cast formation in vivo is a complex process that is dictated by multiple variables, including the ionic composition of the tubule fluid, tubule fluid flow rates, the concentration of THP and FLC, the strength of binding interaction between THP and FLC, and the presence of furosemide. These observations have direct clinical relevance as many of these factors (except the intrinsic binding interaction between THP and FLC) can be modified with current treatment modalities.

IDENTIFYING NEPHROTOXIC LIGHT CHAINS

Not all monoclonal FLCs are nephrotoxic. Although the risk of AKI in patients with MM is increased when FLC proteinuria reaches 2 g per day, some patients do not develop kidney disease despite high FLC urine concentrations.[32] Because no tool to predict toxicity of a given FLC is currently available, preventive measures and removal of precipitating factors are mandatory.

The mechanisms involved in the renal pathogenic effects of individual monoclonal FLCs remain incompletely understood. Nephrotoxicity appears to be an intrinsic property of some FLCs, as indicated by the recurrence of similar renal lesions after kidney transplantation, and by animal studies that have specifically reproduced human FLC-related nephropathies using injections of purified human FLCs, intraperitoneal injections of transfected plasmacytomas secreting a pathogenic human FLC,[33,34] or gene-targeted insertion.[35] Growing evidence shows that the pattern of renal injury is governed by both structural peculiarities of monoclonal FLCs, particularly of the variable (V) domain, and is influenced by environmental factors, such as pH, urea concentration, or local tissue proteolysis. In addition, intrinsic host factors are likely to have an important role in determining both the type and severity of any renal response to a given FLC.

Pathogenic FLCs purified from patients' urine are characterized by their propensity to form high-order aggregates or polymers in vitro, which differ according to the sequence variability of the V domain.[36] The peculiarities of the V domain are observed in many types of renal disease induced by light chains. Myeloma-associated Fanconi syndrome, for example, is characterized by proximal tubule dysfunction secondary to FLC reabsorption and crystallization within the lysosomal compartment of PTCs. FLCs associated with Fanconi syndrome are nearly always of the Vκ1 subgroup and are derived from only two germ line genes, immunoglobulin kappa variable *(IGKV)1-39* and *IGKV1-33*. In immunoglobulin light chain (AL) amyloidosis and light chain deposition disease, the pathogenic role of V regions is suggested by overrepresentation of the Vλ6 and Vκ462 subgroups, respectively, N-glycosylation of the V region, and substitutions of key amino acids induced by somatic mutations that might account for the propensity of certain FLCs to aggregate and influence tropism of deposition.[37–41] FLCs associated with light chain deposition disease are characterized by cationic isoelectric points, whereas the isoelectric point profile of FLCs involved in AL amyloidosis is heterogeneous. This observation suggests that fibrillar amyloid deposits form by electrostatic interaction between oppositely charged polypeptides, whereas granular deposits in light chain deposition disease result from the binding of cationic polypeptides to anionic basement membranes.

The role of the molecular characteristics of FLCs in myeloma kidney is less clear. In high-mass myeloma, the capacity of the proximal tubule to reabsorb and degrade FLCs is rapidly overwhelmed by the dramatic increase in the burden of filtered FLCs. Large amounts of FLCs reach the distal tubule lumen where they interact with THP. Huang and Sanders identified a binding domain for FLCs on THP, which consisted of nine amino acids and was termed *light chain binding domain*. Importantly, all FLCs tested bound to this FLC-binding domain. In turn, the CDR 3 domain in the variable region of both κ and λ FLCs interacted with THP. The binding affinities of FLCs for THP are related to the amino acid composition of the CDR 3 domain.

Despite our growing understanding of the pathogenic mechanisms by which immunoglobulin (Ig) FLCs induce renal injury, there are currently no clinically relevant tools for identifying the potential nephrotoxicity of a specific monoclonal FLC.

Diagnostic Approach to Myeloma Kidney

Myeloma kidney should be high on the differential diagnosis list for patients with unexplained AKI across a wide spectrum of ages. Although frequently considered a disease of the elderly, myeloma kidney has been reported in early to mid-adult life and should be particularly considered in the setting of a severe AKI with an acellular urine. When approaching these patients, there are two key considerations: (1) is there a monoclonal protein present, which can be responsible for the renal injury? and (2) are the criteria for MM met? With the advent of the serum free light chain assays (FLC) this diagnostic workup can be undertaken rapidly at little cost.[42]

Identifying Monoclonal Free Light Chains by Immunoassays

During the assessment of an individual with AKI, it is often appropriate and necessary to screen for the presence of a potentially nephrotoxic monoclonal FLC (Fig. 7.2). In such cases, it is essential that the nephrologist and laboratories work together to minimize diagnostic delays to enable the rapid initiation of disease-specific treatment. In patients with AKI, the most rapid way to assess for a monoclonal protein of renal significance is by the quantitative measurement of FLC in the serum by nephelometric immunoassays.[43,44] These immunoassays provide a quantitative measurement of both κ and λ FLCs; an overproduction of one of these monoclonal FLCs will lead to a ratio of the two FLCs that deviates outside the normal range (0.26–1.65).[45] Use of these assays as a screening tool can help overcome

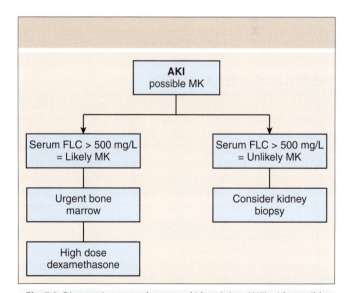

Fig. 7.2 Diagnostic approach to acute kidney injury (AKI) with possible myeloma kidney. A serum free light chain (FLC) level of less than 500 mg/L makes myeloma kidney unlikely diagnosis and a kidney biopsy should be considered to identify the cause of AKI. A serum FLC level of more than 500 mg/L in the context of AKI makes myeloma kidney the most likely diagnosis and confirmation of the diagnosis of multiple myeloma becomes the most important priority, by a rapid bone marrow biopsy, which will then enable early initiation of high dose dexamethasone. *AKI*, Acute kidney injury; *MK*, myeloma kidney.

logistic delays and analytic inaccuracies associated with other laboratory methods used for the identification of monoclonal FLCs (such as serum and urine protein electrophoresis and immunofixation).[46]

In an assessment of 1877 patients with plasma cell dyscrasias, Katzmann et al. found that serum protein electrophoresis and a quantitative serum FLC assay identified 100% of patients with MM and macroglobulinemia, 99.5% of patients with smoldering MM, 96.5% of patients with AL amyloidosis, and 78% of patients with light chain deposition disease.[47] International guidelines now recommend that screening of serum alone (with serum protein electrophoresis and a quantitative serum FLC assay) for plasma cell dyscrasias is a viable alternative to urinary assessment.[48,49] Despite the accumulation of serum polyclonal FLCs in renal impairment, the assay remains useful in patients with renal failure, but absolute values are raised and the normal range for the FLC ratio is changed from that in the general population to 0.37 to 3.17.[50] By using this renal range in a dialysis-dependent AKI population, the number of false positives was reduced.[44] In addition to these diagnostic advantages, the FLC immunoassays offer the ability to monitor clonal disease response,[48] which has particular relevance in patients with myeloma kidney in whom an early reduction in serum FLC concentrations is associated with renal recovery.

Diagnostic Assessment for Multiple Myeloma

Once MM has been suspected, a targeted hematologic assessment should be undertaken. This should include: full assessment of the paraprotein (serum FLC, serum protein electrophoresis and immunofixation; urinary assessment is optional); skeletal survey (magnetic resonance imaging or low dose computed tomography are now recommended opposed to plain film); bone marrow aspirate and biopsy; full blood count; and serum calcium.

THE ROLE OF A RENAL BIOPSY

The utility of a renal biopsy in suspected myeloma kidney remains undetermined. Advocates argue that undertaking a renal biopsy in patients with a paraprotein is safe, when ultrasound guidance is used with no significant increased risk of a major hemorrhagic complication, compared with the population without a paraprotein.[51] The biopsy clarifies the diagnosis of AKI in patients with MM, when it is secondary to a pathology other than cast nephropathy. The review of the renal histology also allows the chronicity of the process to be determined, potentially guiding how aggressive therapy should be.

However, in a patient with severe AKI and a high serum FLC concentration (greater than 500 mg/L), the biopsy in the vast majority of patients will reveal myeloma kidney or an associated acute tubular necrosis secondary to the FLCs without casts. In this setting undertaking a renal biopsy puts the patient at unnecessary risk and potentially delays more relevant hematologic investigations and early treatment.

Although both approaches have merit, the most important consideration is time. A rapid diagnosis allows early disease specific treatment to be started and potentially prevents irreversible tubulointerstitial fibrosis, which can occur over a short time frame.[52] Therefore in centers where same day, or very rapid FLC results, are available, the combination of a high serum FLCs and a significant AKI makes myeloma kidney the most likely diagnosis. In this setting, the focus should then be on clarifying the diagnosis of MM by bone marrow biopsy as quickly as possible. However, in centers where there is potentially a significant delay in FLC results being available, then a renal biopsy can provide rapid light microscopy to confirm the presence or absence of casts. This should be undertaken whenever there is a high clinical index of suspicion of myeloma kidney causing AKI, when serum FLCs are not rapidly available.

Technical Considerations for Processing the Biopsy

The most common renal findings seen in patients with circulating monoclonal FLC and AKI are tubulointerstitial lesions. FLC cast nephropathy is most frequent and is well recognized by pathologists. However, there are two other principal abnormalities that are not always correctly identified. These include proximal tubulopathy (also referred to as *acute tubular necrosis* or *acute tubulopathy*) and an inflammatory tubular interstitial process without casts that has morphologic features identical to those seen in classic acute tubulointerstitial nephritis. Although the main pathologic processes seen in the latter two entities may be recognized by pathologists in renal biopsy samples, the association of those lesions with an underlying plasma cell dyscrasia is frequently missed.

Even in the diagnosis of FLC cast nephropathy, there is currently a need to define definitive criteria as to how many distal nephron casts are needed to make a diagnosis, with the understanding that sampling can have an important role in this situation. Carefully controlled studies are therefore required to define parameters in renal biopsy samples that correlate with recovery or irreversibility of renal damage although some parameters, such as the degree of interstitial damage, are intuitive.

Other renal lesions related to monoclonal light and heavy chains, such as AL amyloidosis, heavy chain (AH) amyloidosis, or light/heavy chain deposition disease, tend to present less acutely, but can also exhibit (or mimic) AKI and need to be considered in the differential diagnosis of AKI in patients with monoclonal gammopathies. It is not uncommon that more than one pathology can be present at the same time.

Evaluation of renal biopsy samples must include staining for κ and λ FLCs and careful examination of the Ig stains. This approach will help to determine isotype restriction for light and/or heavy chains and enable the morphologic manifestations to be directly related to the underlying plasma cell dyscrasia. Heavy chains have not been documented to be involved in tubulointerstitial pathology although, in rare cases, a coexisting FLC can result in a cast nephropathy. The evaluations must carefully assess not only immunofluorescence, but also ultrastructural findings and correlate these with the light microscopic features.

Immunofluorescence evaluation is key in defining the presence of monoclonal light or heavy chain deposition in the renal biopsy sample to make a definitive diagnosis. However, available commercial antibodies do not detect some of the abnormal monoclonal Igs that may be deposited in the various renal compartments, and that are directly responsible for renal dysfunction. This lack of recognition is caused by the fact that the monoclonal proteins can be quite abnormal physiochemically or truncated to such an extent that the epitopes recognized by routine polyclonal antibodies are no longer present.

Timing of Later or Repeat Biopsies

In selected cases, a late or repeat kidney biopsy should be considered when a patient is not responding to treatment as expected, for example, a good clonal response but ongoing significant kidney dysfunction. The results from a biopsy sample can establish therapeutic response and whether additional therapy is recommended. In this situation, a renal biopsy can provide evidence of improvement (or lack thereof) by comparing the findings in the initial biopsy sample with repeat biopsies. This approach has been documented in the literature primarily in patients with plasma cell dyscrasias and glomerular lesions.[53,54] A renal biopsy may also provide evidence that further treatment may be of no, or rather limited, value as the renal parenchymal damage is deemed to be extensive and/or irreversible.[55]

Treatment Options in Myeloma Kidney

SUPPORTIVE THERAPY IN PATIENTS WITH MYELOMA KIDNEY

As with all causes of AKI, the importance of generalized supportive therapies cannot be overstated. Stopping nephrotoxins, and early correction of hypercalcemia and dehydration can reduce the precipitation of FLCs with Tamm-Horsfall protein. Nonsteroidal antiinflammatory drugs and loop diuretics are both associated with the formation of casts and should be stopped on suspicion of myeloma kidney. Hypercalcemia is independently associated with cast formation and early correction should occur following local guidelines, potentially using steroids and bisphosphonates. Replacement fluids, for patients who are intravascularly depleted, should be approached with caution. Although a high urine output will reduce the rate of cast formation, by simply dilution of the urine, increased distal delivery of sodium with the use of normal saline has been associated with cast formation.[56] Historically, there has been interest in the alkalization of the urine to reduce the rate of cast formation. However, this approach has not been validated in robust clinical trials.

Once these simple measures have been undertaken, focus must then be on achieving an early rapid reduction in the serum concentrations of the monoclonal FLCs, which has been demonstrated to be directly related to kidney outcomes. To enable this, effective treatment of the underlying plasma cell clone is required.

TREATMENT OF THE PLASMA CELL CLONE IN PATIENTS WITH MYELOMA KIDNEY

The treatment of MM has progressed considerably over recent decades. Complete response (disappearance of all detectable monoclonal component from the serum and urine,

as well as < 5% bone marrow plasmacytosis) rates have improved from less than 5% with melphalan and prednisolone[57–59] to more than 80% with combination novel agent approaches.[60] These improved responses have led to prolonged disease control and improved overall survival in clinical trials, as well as population-based studies.[61] Alkylation-based regimens have been replaced by novel agent combinations including the proteasome inhibitors (bortezomib, carfilzomib, ixazomib), immunomodulatory agents (thalidomide, lenalidomide, pomalidomide), histone deacetylase inhibitors (panobinostat), monoclonal antibodies (daratumumab, elotuzumab, isatuximab), and numerous other agents and immunotherapies in clinical development.

The treatment of the plasma cell clone in patients with myeloma kidney differs in a number of respects from the treatment of patients with normal renal function. Firstly, because of the importance of renal recovery to avoid the long-term complications of end-stage renal failure, therapies that produce rapid hematologic responses are vital. Secondly, given the setting of renal impairment, chemotherapeutics with minimal renal excretion have particular advantages. Thirdly, renal impairment increases the toxicity profile of most therapies and needs to be considered when making treatment decisions.

There is good evidence from prospective clinical trials conducted specifically in patients with myeloma kidney that recovery of renal function following chemotherapy is predicted by the achievement of hematologic response.[62] This equates to a reduction in the monoclonal Ig or the difference between the involved and uninvolved FLCs of at least 90%.[63] The goal of any antimyeloma chemotherapy therefore is the achievement of such responses, as quickly as possible. The best evidence to date comes from prospective randomized trials, which included patients with mild to moderate renal impairment. In these studies, renal recovery and survival were superior in the bortezomib containing arms.[64,65] Recent prospective studies of bortezomib-based regimens show renal recovery rates in patients, initially dialysis-dependent, are approximately 60%.[62] Because of its pharmacokinetics, bortezomib can be used at full doses in patients with renal impairment and numerous studies have shown that bortezomib is safe and effective in this population. On the basis of these data, bortezomib is the agent recommended in current consensus guidelines addressing myeloma-related renal impairment.[66] There is also retrospective evidence that three drug proteasome inhibitor-based regimens result in improved response rates when compared with two drug regimens.[67] All such regimens include a corticosteroid, typically dexamethasone, which has pronounced antiplasma cell activity. The third drug may be a traditional chemotherapeutic agent, such as cyclophosphamide, which has been used extensively in patients with renal disease, and in one randomized study was associated with improved responses compared with adriamycin in patients with myeloma and mild renal impairment.[68] Bendamustine, a chemotherapeutic with both alkylating and antimetabolite actions, does not accumulate in end-stage renal failure and has been combined with bortezomib and prednisolone to successfully treat patients with myeloma kidney. Bortezomib and dexamethasone may also be combined with an immunomodulatory agent, such as thalidomide in the Velcade, Thalidomide, Dexamethasone (VTD) regimen, which has been successfully used in renal impairment.[67] Thalidomide's pharmacokinetics are unaltered by renal impairment and no dose modification is required. Such bortezomib-based triplets are now the cornerstone of management of newly diagnosed myeloma presenting with AKI.

Treatment options for myeloma kidney are not limited to bortezomib-based regimens, particularly in the relapsed setting where the underlying plasma cell clone may be resistant to bortezomib. The other proteasome inhibitors, carfilzomib[69] and ixazomib,[70] appear safe in patients with renal impairment, but more data are required before their routine use as initial therapy of myeloma kidney can be recommended. Of the immunomodulatory agents, lenalidomide is renally excreted, requires dose modification in renal impairment,[71] and there is some evidence that its antimyeloma activity is blunted in this setting.[72] Pomalidomide appears not to require dose modification in severe renal impairment or dialysis.[73] The monoclonal antibodies daratumumab, isatuximab, and elotuzumab have not been specifically studied in patients with renal impairment, but given their lack of renal elimination should be able to be used safely. The ability of daratumumab to achieve faster hematologic responses with minimal additional toxicity, when combined with bortezomib-based chemotherapy,[74] makes it an attractive option to further improve outcomes in myeloma kidney.

AUTOLOGOUS STEM CELL TRANSPLANTATION IN PATIENTS FOLLOWING A PRESENTATION WITH MYELOMA KIDNEY

Autologous stem cell transplantation, following high-dose melphalan, is standard consolidation therapy in younger patients with myeloma. Several different conditioning regimens and doses have been compared over time, but intravenous melphalan at a dose of 200 mg/m^2 has been confirmed as the optimal conditioning before stem cell reinfusion, in patients with normal renal function.[75] Such transplants were initially shown to improve myeloma control and overall survival when compared with multiagent chemotherapy and, more recently, has been shown to provide the best long-term disease control in randomized comparisons to bortezomib, lenalidomide, or combined bortezomib-lenalidomide regimens.[76–78] These trials excluded patients over 65 years of age, as well as patients with more severe degrees of renal impairment. In the three most recent randomized studies, the lower limit of allowed renal function was a creatinine clearance of 15, 20, and 50 mL/min, respectively. To date, none of these studies has reported outcomes specifically for the subgroup of patients with reduced creatinine clearance, and thus we have no high-level evidence to support the use of autologous stem cell transplantation in patients with renal impairment.

In retrospective studies, it appears that transplantation is associated with an increased risk of morbidity and mortality in patients with renal impairment compared with patients with normal renal function. Transplant related mortality ranges from 0% to 38% in this setting; however, the most recent and largest study from an international transplant registry found a transplant related mortality rate of 0%, for transplants performed in severe renal impairment, including patients on dialysis at the time of transplantation. Because of melphalan's predominant renal clearance,[79] the standard 200 mg/m^2 dose results in excess nonhematologic toxicity in patients with renal impairment. An initial report found a melphalan dose of 140 mg/m^2 reduced toxicity without compromising efficacy among 21 patients with a creatinine greater than 2 mg/dL.[80] Subsequent retrospective studies have suggested that the standard melphalan dose of 200 mg/m^2 can be used in patients with a creatinine clearance greater than 30 mL/min whereas those with creatinine clearance less than 30 mL/min or on dialysis should be treated with a dose of 140 mg/m^2.[81]

There is likely to be a fair degree of patient selection in these retrospective studies and so it is debatable how generalizable these findings are to all patients with myeloma kidney who may otherwise be transplant candidates. Balancing the limitations of these data with the known importance of autologous stem cell transplantation in younger patients, with myeloma kidney, is a challenge. As the transplant procedure becomes safer with better renal function, it is important to maximize the chance of renal recovery before transplantation by using the most effective pretransplant induction therapy. If the patient maintains good performance status with minimal comorbidity, then the available evidence would suggest that consolidation with autologous stem cell transplantation is not unreasonable, albeit with a reduced melphalan dose of 140 mg/m^2 for those with severe renal impairment at the time of transplantation.

DIRECT REMOVAL OF FREE LIGHT CHAINS IN MYELOMA KIDNEY

Although the pathophysiology of myeloma kidney is clear, with the high concentrations of monoclonal FLCs undoubtedly being responsible for the AKI, the role for the removal of these pathogenic molecules remains in debate. In 2005 the Canadian Apheresis Group appeared to publish the definitive study to demonstrate that FLC removal by plasma exchange did not provide clinical benefit to patients with severe AKI secondary to MM.[82] This large randomized clinical trial evaluated standard chemotherapy plus plasma exchange or standard chemotherapy alone for patients with severe AKI in the setting of MM. The trial showed no benefit to patients in terms of renal outcomes or overall survival. Future discussions identified limitations of the study in terms of lack of a kidney biopsy to clarify the diagnosis and questioned whether the dose of FLCs removed by plasma exchange was clinically relevant.[83] A series of studies then explored methods by which an increased dose of FLC removal could be given using high cut-off hemodialysis.

High cut-off hemodialysis uses a conventional hollow-fiber dialyzer with a higher molecular weight cut-off, allowng the removal of all large middle-molecules including FLCs. Pilot studies demonstrated that both κ at 22.5 kDa and λ at 45 kDa were effectively cleared into the dialysate using these membranes, with reduction ratios of up to 80% per dialysis session. Early single-center pilot studies showed high rates of renal recovery from dialysis-dependent AKI when these dialyzers were used in patients with AKI secondary to MM. However, these studies also demonstrated that use of these dialyzers was associated with a significant degree of albumin loss with potential adverse consequences.

Interest in this new treatment culminated in two multicenter European studies exploring FLC removal by high cut-off hemodialysis in patients with AKI secondary to myeloma kidney.[62,84] The now reported French study

Multiple Myeloma and Renal Failure due to Myeloma Cast Nephropathy (MYRE) shows high cut-off hemodialysis resulted in improved renal outcomes for patients at 6 and 12 months. In comparison, The European Trial of Free Light Chain Removal by Extended Hemodialysis in Cast Nephropathy (EuLITE) study showed no definitive patient benefit.[62,84] Analysis of the full results will be required to fully understand why there is a difference in results, but likely explanations will be in relation to the studies being underpowered and differences in enrollment criteria. Unfortunately, when both studies were being designed, the only renal outcome data available to power the studies were from historical studies, where chemotherapy was based around thalidomide or older generations of chemotherapy. With the advent of bortezomib-based chemotherapy, renal recovery rates more than doubled, thus fundamentally changing the numbers of patients who were required in these studies.

In 2016 a further "next generation" of hemodialysis membrane became available that may be of relevance to the treatment of patients with myeloma kidney. Like the high cut-off membranes, these new "medium cut-off" membranes have a molecular weight cut-off that enables the effective removal of both κ and λ FLCs, but because the pores in these membranes are more uniform, there is limited albumin loss. This may be of particular relevance in this setting, as the high degree of albumin loss seen with the high cut-off membranes could potentially have led to adverse outcomes, through reduced efficiency of chemotherapy or higher rates of infections. Early studies are just starting to report patient outcomes with these medium cut-off membranes, and future clinical studies should assess their use in combination with effective chemotherapy.

At this stage, we can conclude that bortezomib-based chemotherapy, in combination with dexamethasone, remains the standard of care for severe AKI in patients with MM. FLC removal by high cut-off hemodialysis may complement the use of this effective chemotherapy, but evidence is currently contradictory.

LONG-TERM SURVEILLANCE AND FOLLOW-UP OF PATIENTS IN REMISSION

Once hematologic and hopefully renal response has been achieved, patients with myeloma kidney require careful long-term monitoring. As a generalization, in myeloma the pattern of relapse is similar to the initial clinical presentation.[85] As such, patients who present with myeloma kidney are at particular risk for developing AKI at relapse, as their pathologic FLC has already displayed a predilection for combining with Tamm-Horsfall protein, leading to cast nephropathy. These patients need close monitoring every 1 to 3 months (more frequently in the early posttreatment period), which must include FLC and creatinine measurement in addition to the other modalities of myeloma assessment. In relation to FLC measurement, biochemical relapse is defined as a 25% increase in the difference between involved and uninvolved FLC levels (absolute increase must be > 100 mg/L) but salvage treatment in myeloma is not always indicated at the first sign of biochemical relapse. In fact, the International Myeloma Working Group has suggested that treatment is indicated when there is either a clinical relapse (reoccurrence of end-organ damage) or a significant and quick paraprotein increase (doubled monoclonal protein within 2 months, with an increase in the absolute levels of monoclonal protein of 1 g/dL or more in serum or of 500 mg or more per 24 hours in urine confirmed by two consecutive measurements). However, in the presence of a high-risk clinical feature, such as prior light chain-induced renal impairment, it would seem reasonable that treatment should be commenced at the stage of biochemical relapse before renal injury develops.

Myeloma Kidney Outcome

Historically, the prognosis for patients presenting with severe AKI secondary to MM was very poor and perceived by many to be a palliative care situation. Rates of renal recovery were as low as 20% when patients were dialysis dependent and overall survival was measured in months.[39] The glimmer of hope in this bleak outlook was the kidney biopsy, which frequently showed what appeared to be little chronic damage and the potential for renal recovery. Since the advent of "novel chemotherapies," with first thalidomide then bortezomib, the outcomes for this cohort of patients has continued to improve and improve. Renal recovery rates are now consistently above 50% even for patients presenting with dialysis-dependent AKI and when an early renal recovery occurs, the survival of these patients is restored back to that of the general myeloma population.[41,42] Once sufficient renal recovery has occurred to enable dialysis independence, 95% of patients will remain dialysis independent through long-term follow-up.

Summary

AKI occurs commonly in patients with MM and is most often caused by precipitation of FLCs with Tamm-Horsfell protein in the distal tubules resulting in cast nephropathy. The development of cast nephropathy is associated with poorer 1-year survival rates compared with patients with MM and normal renal function. Renal recovery is more predictive of survival than hematologic response. Recovery of renal function, including discontinuation of hemodialysis, is achievable in 50% of patients treated with bortezomib-based chemotherapy. The role of high cuff-off hemodialysis as an adjunct to chemotherapy in treating cast nephropathy is still unsettled despite the report of two recent randomized controlled trials.

Key Points

- Acute kidney injury is common in patients with multiple myeloma.
- The most common cause of AKI is cast nephropathy.
- Rapid reduction in serum free light chain concentrations is associated with renal recovery.
- Bortezomib-based chemotherapy has significantly improved renal recovery rates compared with older chemotherapeutic regimens.
- The role of high cuff-off hemodialysis in the treatment of cast nephropathy is still unclear.

References

1. Finkel KW, Cohen EP, Shirali A, Abudayyeh A. Paraprotein-related kidney disease: evaluation and treatment of myeloma cast nephropathy. *Clin J Am Soc Nephrol.* 2016;11:2273-2279.
2. Altekruse SF, Kosary CL, Krapcho M, et al. *SEER cancer statistics review, 1975-2007.* Bethesda, MD: National Cancer Institute; 2010. Available from http://seer.cancer.gov/csr/1975_2007/index.html.
3. Korbet SM, Schwartz MM. Multiple myeloma. *J Am Soc Nephrol.* 2006;17:2533-2545.
4. Eleutherakis-Papaiakovou V, Bamias A, Gika D, et al. Renal failure in multiple myeloma: incidence, correlations, and prognostic significance. *Leuk Lymphoma.* 2007;48:337-341.
5. Tsakiris DJ, Stel VS, Finne P, et al. Incidence and outcome of patients starting renal replacement therapy for end-stage renal disease due to multiple myeloma or light chain deposit disease: an ERA-DETA registry study. *Nephrol Dial Transplant.* 2010;25:1200-1206.
7. Hutchison CA, Batuman V, Behrens J, et al. The pathogenesis and diagnosis of acute kidney injury in multiple myeloma. *Nat Rev Nephrol.* 2011;8:43-51.
8. Berggård I, Peterson PA. Polymeric forms of free normal κ and λ chains of human immunoglobulin. *J Biol Chem.* 1969;244:4299-4307.
9. Mead GP, Carr-Smith HD, Drayson MT, Morgan GJ, Child JA, Bradwell AR. Serum free light chains for monitoring multiple myeloma. *Br J Haematol.* 2004;126:348-354.
10. Batuman V, Guan S, O'Donovan R, Puschett JB. Effect of myeloma light chains on phosphate and glucose transport in renal proximal tubule cells. *Ren Physiol Biochem.* 1994;17:294-300.
11. Li M, Hering-Smith KS, Simon EE, Batuman V. Myeloma light chains induce epithelial-mesenchymal transition in human renal proximal tubule epithelial cells. *Nephrol Dial Transplant.* 2008;23:860-870.
12. Pote A, Zwizinski C, Simon EE, Meleg-Smith S, Batuman V. Cytotoxicity of myeloma light chains in cultured human kidney proximal tubule cells. *Am J Kidney Dis.* 2000;36:735-744.
13. Sengul S, Zwizinski C, Batuman V. Role of MAPK pathways in light chain-induced cytokine production in human proximal tubule cells. *Am J Physiol Ren Physiol.* 2003;284:F1245-F1254.
23. Batuman V. Proximal tubular injury in myeloma. *Contrib Nephrol.* 2007;153:87-104.
24. Sengul S, Li M, Batuman V. Myeloma kidney: toward its prevention—with new insights from in vitro and in vivo models of renal injury. *J Nephrol.* 2009;22:17-28.
26. Sanders PW, Herrera GA, Kirk KA, Old CW, Galla JH. Spectrum of glomerular and tubulointerstitial renal lesions associated with monotypical immunoglobulin light chain deposition. *Lab Invest.* 1991;64:527-537.
32. Woodruff R, Sweet B. Multiple myeloma with massive Bence Jones proteinuria and preservation of renal function. *Aus N Z J Med.* 1977;7:60-62.
33. Khamlichi AA, Rocca A, Touchard G, Aucouturier P, Preud'homme JL, Cogné M. Role of light chain variable region in myeloma with light chain deposition disease: evidence from an experimental model. *Blood.* 1995;86:3655-3659.
34. Decourt C, Rocca A, Bridoux F. Mutational analysis in murine models for myeloma-associated Fanconi's syndrome or cast myeloma nephropathy. *Blood.* 1999;94:3559-3566.
35. Sirac C, Bridoux F, Carrion C, et al. Role of the monoclonal κ chain V domain and reversibility of renal damage in a transgenic model of acquired Fanconi syndrome. *Blood.* 2006;108:536-543.
36. Myatt EA, Westholm FA, Weiss DT, Solomon A, Schiffer M, Stevens FJ. Pathogenic potential of human monoclonal immunoglobulin light chains: relationship of in vitro aggregation to in vivo organ deposition. *Proc Natl Acad Sci USA.* 1994;91:3034-3038.
37. Cogné M, Preud'homme JL, Bauwens M, Touchard G, Aucouturier P. Structure of a monoclonal kappa chain of the V kappa IV subgroup in the kidney and plasma cells in light chain deposition disease. *J Clin Invest.* 1991;87:2186-2190.
38. Stevens FJ. Four structural risk factors identify most fibril-forming kappa light chains. *Amyloid.* 2000;7:200-211.
42. Cockwell P, Hutchison CA. Management options for cast nephropathy in multiple myeloma. *Curr Opin Nephrol Hypertens.* 2010;19:550-555.

44. Hutchison CA, Plant T, Drayson M, et al. Serum free light chain measurement aids the diagnosis of myeloma in patients with severe renal failure. *BMC Nephrol.* 2008;9:11.
48. Durie BG, Harousseau JL, Miguel JS, et al. International uniform response criteria for multiple myeloma. *Leukemia.* 2006;20:1467-1473.
49. Dispenzieri A, Kyle R, Merlini G, et al. International Myeloma Working Group guidelines for serum-free light chain analysis in multiple myeloma and related disorders. *Leukemia.* 2009;23:215-224.
50. Hutchison CA, Harding S, Hewins P, et al. Quantitative assessment of serum and urinary polyclonal free light chains in patients with chronic kidney disease. *Clin J Am Soc Nephrol.* 2008;3:1684-1690.
51. Fish R, Pinney J, Jain P, et al. The incidence of major hemorrhagic complications after renal biopsies in patients with monoclonal gammopathies. *Clin J Am Soc Nephrol.* 2010;5:1977-1980.
52. Basnayake K, Cheung CK, Sheaff M, et al. Differential progression of renal scarring and determinants of late renal recovery in sustained dialysis dependent acute kidney injury secondary to myeloma kidney. *J Clin Pathol.* 2010;63:884-887.
53. Montseny JJ, Kleinknecht D, Meyrier A, et al. Long-term outcome according to renal histological lesions in 118 patients with monoclonal gammopathies. *Nephrol Dial Transplant.* 1998;13:1438-1445.
56. Sanders PW. Pathogenesis and treatment of myeloma kidney. *J Lab Clin Med.* 1994;124:484-488.
57. San Miguel JF, Schlag R, Khuageva NK, et al. Bortezomib plus melphalan and prednisone for initial treatment of multiple myeloma. *N Engl J Med.* 2008;359:906-917.
58. Facon T, Mary JY, Hulin C, et al. Intergroupe Francophone du Myélome. Melphalan and prednisone plus thalidomide versus melphalan and prednisone alone or reduced-intensity autologous stem cell transplantation in elderly patients with multiple myeloma (IFM 99-06): a randomised trial. *Lancet.* 2007;370:1209-1218.
59. Hulin C, Facon T, Rodon P, et al. Efficacy of melphalan and prednisone plus thalidomide in patients older than 75 years with newly diagnosed multiple myeloma: IFM 01/01 trial. *J Clin Oncol.* 2009;27:3664-3670.
60. Korde N, Roschewski M, Zingone A, et al. Treatment with carfilzomib-lenalidomide-dexamethasone with lenalidomide extension in patients with smoldering or newly diagnosed multiple myeloma. *JAMA Oncol.* 2015;1:746-754.
61. Liwing J, Uttervall K, Lund J, et al. Improved survival in myeloma patients: starting to close in on the gap between elderly patients and a matched normal population. *Br J Haematol.* 2014;164:684-693.
62. Bridoux F, Carron PL, Pegourie B, et al. Effect of high-cutoff hemodialysis vs conventional hemodialysis on hemodialysis independence among patients with myeloma cast nephropathy: a randomized clinical trial. *JAMA.* 2017;318:2099-2110.
63. Kumar S, Paiva B, Anderson KC, et al. International Myeloma Working Group consensus criteria for response and minimal residual disease assessment in multiple myeloma. *Lancet Oncol.* 2016;17:e328-e346.
64. Scheid C, Sonneveld P, Schmidt-Wolf IG, et al. Bortezomib before and after autologous stem cell transplantation overcomes the negative prognostic impact of renal impairment in newly diagnosed multiple myeloma: a subgroup analysis from the HOVON-65/GMMG-HD4 trial. *Haematologica.* 2014;99:148-154.
81. Mahindra A, Hari P, Fraser R, et al. Autologous hematopoietic cell transplantation for multiple myeloma patients with renal insufficiency: a center for international blood and marrow transplant research analysis. *Bone Marrow Transplant.* 2017;52:1616-1622.
82. Clark WF, Stewart AK, Rock GA, et al. Plasma exchange when myeloma presents as acute renal failure: a randomized, controlled trial. *Ann Intern Med.* 2005;143:777-784.
83. Hutchison CA, Cockwell P, Reid S, et al. Efficient removal of immunoglobulin free light chains by hemodialysis for multiple myeloma: in vitro and in vivo studies. *J Am Soc Nephrol.* 2007;18:886-895.
84. Hutchison CA, Cook M, Heyne N, et al. European trial of free light chain removal by extended haemodialysis in cast nephropathy (EuLITE): a randomised control trial. *Trials.* 2008;9:55.
85. Fernández de Larrea C, Jiménez R, Rosiñol L, et al. Pattern of relapse and progression after autologous SCT as upfront treatment for multiple myeloma. *Bone Marrow Transplant.* 2014;49:223-227.

A full list of references is available at Expertconsult.com

8 Systemic Light Chain Amyloidosis

RAMAPRIYA SINNAKIROUCHENAN

Introduction

Systemic amyloidoses encompass a group of diseases characterized by deposition of abnormal, insoluble, misfolded, β-pleated protein fibrils in different organs. Amyloid protein positively stains with Congo red and demonstrates apple-green birefringence under polarized light. The deposition of the β-pleated amyloid fibrils causes disruption of tissue architecture and thereby results in organ dysfunction and eventually organ failure. The kidneys, heart, gastrointestinal tract, peripheral nerves, and liver are most commonly involved organs. Many different proteins can form amyloid fibrils and to date, 36 different proteins have been recognized to form amyloid fibrils in vivo.[1] The different amyloidogenic proteins form the basis of classification of systemic amyloidosis. Systemic light chain (AL) amyloidosis (formerly known as *primary amyloidosis*) is the most common type of systemic amyloidosis in the United States. AL amyloidosis may affect five to 12 people per million per year[2] and the incidence may be higher based on autopsy results. Among 474 patients seen at the Mayo Clinic, 60% of patients were between 50 and 70 years of age and only 10% were under 50 years of age.[3] Approximately 70% of patients with amyloidosis have kidney involvement at the time of presentation with 4% to 5% requiring dialysis.[4] The precursor amyloidogenic protein in AL amyloidosis is a monoclonal immunoglobulin (Ig) light chain or its fragment produced by a clone of plasma cells in the bone marrow. The clonal plasma cell burden in the bone marrow is less than 10% in 50% of patients with AL amyloidosis[4] and occurs in association with multiple myeloma in 10% to 15% of patients.[3] The disease has an insidious onset with an extensive clinical heterogeneity. Therefore a high level of clinical suspicion is necessary to avoid a delay in diagnosis and initiation of therapy before irreversible organ damage develops.

Pathogenesis

Reduced folding stability is a unifying feature of amyloidogenic proteins. Polypeptide chains are synthesized in the endoplasmic reticulum, enter a funnel-like pathway, in which the conformational intermediates become progressively more organized as they merge, resulting in the most stable native state.[4] Mutations result in destabilization of these polypeptides and in the extracellular environment, the mutant polypeptides change from a fully folded state to a partially folded state and then retrace the final part of the folding pathway, ultimately forming either a native

or misfolded protein. Some of the extracellular influences that affect the fate of the mutated proteins and direct them toward the pathologic pathway include temperature, pH, metal ions, oxidation, and proteolysis. The partially folded proteins have high propensity to aggregate and form oligomers and eventually fibrils that are insoluble. The deposition of these insoluble fibrils in the extracellular space alters tissue architecture and causes amyloidosis.

The Ig light chain is the amyloidogenic precursor in AL amyloidosis. Solomon et al. used an in vivo animal model to investigate the nephrotoxic potential of Bence-Jones proteins from patients with AL amyloidosis or multiple myeloma. They could reproduce kidney lesions in mice similar to that observed in patients from whom the light chains were purified.[5] The clonal plasma cells producing the amyloidogenic light chains undergo antigen driven selection resulting in a highly mutated Ig light chain variable (VL) domain. It is now believed that the alterations in the amino acid sequences in the Ig VL domain are responsible for the structure, stability, predisposition to aggregation, localization of deposits, and distinct ultrastructural organization of the fibrils. This explains the structural heterogeneity of the fibrils and the protean nature of the disease. Although definitive common structural motif has not yet been identified, both germline sequences of VL domain and acquired amino acid replacements during somatic mutations are thought to be involved in the reduction of the folding stability of the amyloidogenic light chains.[6]

Intense research is currently being conducted on the physiochemical properties of amyloid fibrils to understand amyloidogenesis in the kidneys. Pathogenic light chains can affect the tubulointerstitium or the glomerulus. About 70% of the pathogenic light chains are deposited in the tubulointerstitial compartment and are called tubulopathic light chains, whereas the remainder of the pathogenic light chains are deposited in the mesangium and are called glomerulopathic light chains. The term *AL amyloidosis* was coined in 1970 by Glenner and colleagues, when he showed that light chains formed a type of amyloid.[7] In 1981 Gise observed and documented glomerular amyloidosis begins in the mesangium.[8] Mesangial cells of the kidneys play a key role in the pathogenesis of AL amyloidosis. They phenotypically transform as macrophages in the presence of pathogenic AL amyloidosis light chains and aid in the generation of more amyloid fibrils.[9] In contrast, in light chain deposition disease, they have a phenotype similar to myofibroblasts. Ting et al. validated the pathogenesis of AL amyloidosis in vivo using an animal model, where mice were injected with amyloidogenic light chains purified from the urine of patients with biopsy-proven, light-chain associated glomerular amyloidosis.[10] The sequential steps involved are internalization of the amyloidogenic light chains by mesangial cells using caveolae followed by trafficking to the mature lysosomal compartment where they aggregate because of their thermodynamic instability and form fibrils through proteolysis. The fibrils are then extruded into the extracellular space where they accumulate and disrupt normal mesangium. Increasing evidence is emerging that the precursor amyloidogenic proteins also have direct cytotoxicity and contribute to disease manifestations.[11] Oligomers or protofibrils may mediate cellular toxicity through a mechanism that activates apoptosis in the cells of target tissues.

Although in the normal bone marrow there is a greater proportion of Kappa (κ) than Lambda (λ) expressing clonal plasma cells, λ isotype plasma cells are more commonly associated with amyloidosis (λ:κ is 3:1) and the λ VI light chains have shown to be those most frequently linked to amyloidosis in the kidneys.[12] This association may be related to specific amino acid sequences in the Ig VL domain and hence λ VI light chains are associated with kidney involvement, κ with hepatic involvement, and λ VIII with soft tissue deposits.

Clinical Presentation

AL amyloidosis initially presents with vague clinical features, such as generalized fatigue and weight loss. Suspicion arises only when it affects a specific organ system. The most frequently involved organ systems at the time of diagnosis include the kidneys and the heart presenting as nephrotic syndrome, with or without kidney dysfunction and congestive heart failure, respectively. However, AL amyloidosis can involve any organ system other than the central nervous system. The peripheral nervous system and gastrointestinal tract are also commonly involved.

KIDNEYS

Nearly 45% to 50% of patients with AL amyloidosis have dominant involvement of the kidneys.[13] It is predominantly a glomerular lesion presenting as nephrotic syndrome except in a small proportion of patients (< 10%), where the amyloid deposition occurs in the kidney vasculature and tubulointerstitium, causing kidney dysfunction without nephrotic syndrome.[14] Considerable albuminuria in the setting of multiple myeloma, as opposed to isolated Bence-Jones proteinuria, should alert the physician to investigate for AL amyloid. Clinical signs and symptoms are like that of any nephrotic syndrome and include peripheral edema, fatigue, pericardial effusions, pleural effusions, and edema/anasarca. Nearly 20% of patients with kidney involvement will require dialysis after a median interval of 13 to 14 months.[15] The amount of proteinuria and the degree of kidney dysfunction at the time of diagnosis predicts the need for dialysis in the future.

HEART

Cardiac amyloidosis causes concentric ventricular wall thickening, impaired cardiac filling, and restrictive cardiomyopathy resulting in rapidly progressive heart failure associated with a poor prognosis. Low voltage QRS complexes in the standard leads of an electrocardiogram (EKG) are found in a high proportion of patients and may precede clinical manifestations. Echogenic hypertrophy on echocardiogram is characteristic. Cardiac silhouette appears normal in a chest x-ray. Clinical signs and symptoms are the result of right-sided heart failure and include elevated jugular venous pressure, peripheral edema, hepatomegaly, arrhythmias, and signs of low cardiac output state, such as orthostatic hypotension.

PERIPHERAL AND AUTONOMIC NEUROPATHY

Neural involvement gives rise to a varied range of nonspecific clinical symptoms frequently resulting in a long delay from presentation to diagnosis. Peripheral symmetrical sensory neuropathy is common and presents as paresthesia and numbness that can progress to motor neuropathy. Compression lesions, such as carpal tunnel syndrome, is very common and may precede other symptoms by more than a year. Autonomic neuropathy is severely debilitating by causing severe postural hypotension, bladder and erectile dysfunction, or gastrointestinal motility disorders.

GASTROINTESTINAL AND HEPATIC INVOLVEMENT

Gastrointestinal symptoms depend on the site and extent of amyloid deposition. Hepatomegaly is present in about 25% of patients and could be caused by either direct amyloid infiltration or hepatic congestion from amyloid cardiomyopathy. Hepatomegaly from amyloid infiltration is usually massive, rock hard, and nontender. Substantial elevation of alkaline phosphatase, as compared with transaminases, is a typical trait of hepatic amyloid as the infiltration involves the sinusoids.[16] Features of gastrointestinal amyloid include early satiety, diarrhea, chronic nausea, malabsorption, weight loss, gut perforation, and rectal bleeding. Some of the symptoms, such as early satiety and explosive postprandial diarrhea, may be related to gastrointestinal motility disorders from autonomic neuropathy. Macroglossia is a hallmark feature of AL amyloidosis, although found in only about 10% of patients and may lead to airway obstruction, sleep apnea, and difficulty eating.

HEMOSTATIC ABNORMALITIES

Amyloidosis manifests with hemorrhage and an abnormal clotting screen at some point during the disease in about one-third of patients. Periorbital purpura presenting as raccoon eyes is characteristic. The mechanism is thought to be caused by vascular endothelial wall friability caused by amyloid deposits, increased fibrinolysis, reduced conversion of fibrinogen to fibrin, circulating anticoagulants, and loss of vitamin K dependent clotting factors via binding to amyloid deposits in the spleen causing a warfarin-like effect.[17] Factor X deficiency is most common, affecting up to 9% of the patients. Although purpura is the most common presenting symptom of hemorrhage, serious life-threatening bleeding can also occur after diagnostic liver or kidney biopsy.

OTHER ORGAN SYSTEMS

Additional clinical findings include skin nodules, carpal tunnel syndrome, alopecia, nail dystrophy, splenomegaly, lymphadenopathy, and painful seronegative arthropathy. Endocrinopathies, such as hypothyroidism and hypoadrenalism, have been reported but are rare. Hoarseness of voice may occur because of infiltration of the vocal cords with amyloid deposits. Bone involvement can also occur resulting in lytic lesions and bone pain; pathologic fractures are rare in contrast to multiple myeloma. Localized AL amyloidosis happens infrequently in the upper respiratory and urogenital tracts.

Diagnosis

Because AL amyloidosis presents with a wide array of clinical features and has an insidious onset, physicians should have a high index of clinical suspicion for its timely diagnosis. Delay in diagnosis results in advanced organ dysfunction at the time of diagnosis, when the response to therapy and prognosis remain poor. AL amyloidosis should be suspected in any patient who presents with nondiabetic nephrotic syndrome, hepatomegaly with elevated alkaline phosphatase and normal liver on imaging, heart failure with preserved ejection fraction or nonischemic cardiomyopathy with normal cardiac silhouette on chest x-ray and hypertrophy on echocardiography, polyneuropathy with monoclonal protein, or monoclonal gammopathy of unknown significance (MGUS) with unexplained fatigue, weight loss.[18] As a next step, electrophoresis and immunofixation of serum and urine, and serum-free light chain (FLC) assays should be performed. Amyloidosis is a histologic diagnosis. If a monoclonal protein is detected, then a bone marrow biopsy and abdominal fat pad aspiration are recommended next. Noninvasive fine needle aspiration of abdominal fat pad in combination with bone marrow biopsy may reveal amyloid deposits in more than 70% of patients. Other organs where noninvasive biopsies can be performed to aid diagnosis are salivary gland, rectum, gingiva, and skin. Bone marrow biopsy aids to determine the type and burden of plasma cells and rule in or out other plasma cell disorders, such as multiple myeloma and Waldenstrom macroglobulinemia. Negative bone marrow biopsy and fat pad aspiration do not rule out amyloidosis. Biopsy of the affected organ is often necessary to establish the diagnosis of amyloidosis in cases of high clinical suspicion. However, presence of amyloid deposits alone does not confirm the diagnosis of AL amyloidosis, because several other forms of amyloid deposition have been described that are caused by other proteins besides light chains. These non-AL amyloid proteins include transthyretin (senile amyloidosis) and serum amyloid A (AA amyloidosis).[19] Therefore it is crucial for histologic diagnosis to be followed by identification of the type of amyloid fibril and the extent of organ involvement, because chemotherapy is contraindicated in non-AL amyloidosis. Identification of the amyloid protein may be accomplished by using immunohistochemistry, deoxyribonucleic acid (DNA) analysis, or protein sequencing and mass spectrometry. However, protein sequencing through mass spectrometry is considered gold standard. See Fig. 8.1 for the diagnostic algorithm of AL amyloidosis.

HISTOLOGY

Amyloid is usually diagnosed by biopsy of an affected organ and staining with Congo red dye. Amyloid deposits stain positive with Congo red dye (Fig. 8.2A) and give a pathognomonic apple-green birefringence under polarized light microscopy (Fig. 8.2B). Observation of the amyloid deposits through electron microscopy reveals the presence of haphazardly arranged nonbranching fibrils, with a diameter in the range of 8 to 10 nm and 30 to 1000 nm long (Fig. 8.3A). They may also be present as organized parallel bundles of nonbranching fibrils (Fig. 8.3B). Each fibril is composed of two twisted 3 nm filaments, with an antiparallel β-pleated sheet configuration stabilized by covalent bonding. Glycosaminoglycans and serum amyloid-P component (SAP) provide additional stabilization to the fibrils.[20]

IMMUNOHISTOCHEMISTRY AND DNA ANALYSIS

Immunohistochemical staining for Ig light chain has less than 60% sensitivity and hence diagnosis is made by exclusion of hereditary types of amyloidosis through DNA sequencing and of AA and transthyretin types through immunohistochemical staining. The low sensitivity to detect Ig light chain may be caused by light chain epitopes that interact with antisera to κ, and λ light chains are lost during processing of the specimen or during fibril formation. It is imperative that immunohistochemical staining be performed in experienced laboratories, as it is very common to have false negative or positive results.[21] Immunohistochemical staining is rarely possible in an abdominal fat specimen, so kidney or gastrointestinal tract specimens are preferred for this purpose.

Certain types of hereditary amyloidosis have clinical features that mimic AL amyloidosis and seem to occur much more frequently, making diagnosis challenging. Hereditary fibrinogen A α-chain amyloidosis and hereditary transthyretin amyloidosis need mention in this context. A family history of amyloidosis is often absent because of variation in penetrance. Hereditary fibrinogen A α-chain amyloidosis presents with exclusive kidney involvement and has a characteristic kidney biopsy pattern with extensive glomerular involvement in the absence of significant extraglomerular amyloid.

PROTEIN SEQUENCING AND MASS SPECTROMETRY

Amino acid sequencing and mass spectrometry confirms the amyloid protein composition and is the definitive method of identifying the protein subunits of the amyloid deposits.[22] It can also identify genes involved in hereditary amyloidosis. The technique can be applied to any tissue type and can detect both light and heavy chains. Mass spectrometry is considered superior to immunohistochemistry in typing the protein subunits.

IMAGING AND OTHER TESTS

Imaging of amyloid deposits is challenging, and progress has been very slow. A comprehensive assessment of the

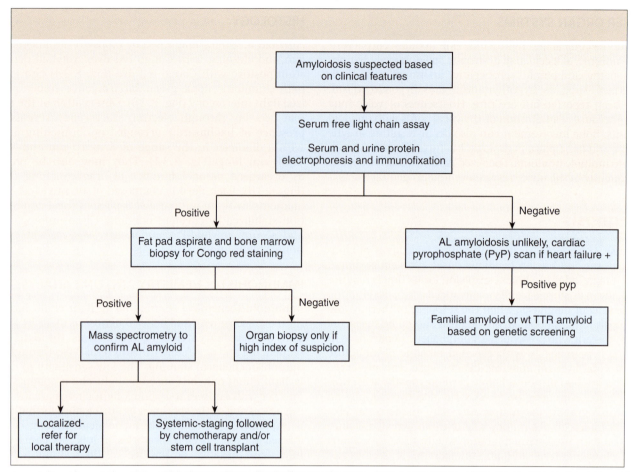

Fig. 8.1 Diagnostic algorithm for systemic light chain (AL) amyloidosis.

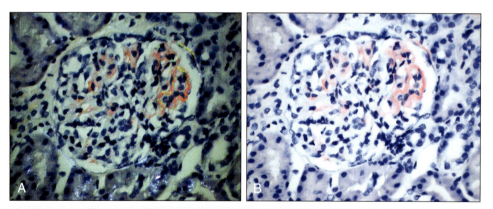

Fig. 8.2 A. Congo red stain: Congo red positive acellular material is present in mesangial regions, segmentally along capillary walls, and in Bowman's capsule. **B.** This figure shows apple-green birefringence under polarized light microscopy, confirming the presence of amyloid. Original magnification 600×. (From Christine Vanbeek, MD).

extent of organ involvement can be done by performing the SAP scanning when feasible. SAP is involved in the stabilization of all amyloid fibrils and this is the basis of a novel disease assessment tool called the *SAP scintigraphy*. Radiolabeled 123I-SAP scintigraphy localizes amyloid deposits rapidly and specifically in proportion to the amount of deposits.[23] SAP scintigraphy is useful for diagnosis and quantification of amyloid deposits, although cardiac and nerve amyloid are poorly visualized. Treatment effects and the

extent of organ involvement can be monitored using the SAP scintigraphy. However, the technical complexity of the procedure has limited its wider usability outside expert centers.

Extent of cardiac involvement is a major determinant of amyloidosis outcome. Although histologic diagnosis is the gold standard, it is not always feasible in cardiac amyloid, as endocardial biopsy is a technically challenging and high-risk procedure. Cardiac imaging is the preferred

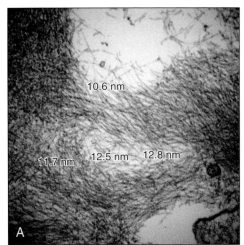

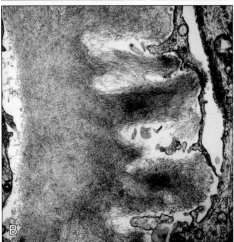

Fig. 8.3 A. Electron microscopy: amyloid deposits are typically composed of haphazardly arranged fibrils with average diameters approximately in the range of 8 to 12 nm (original magnification 80,000×). **B.** Electron microscopy: occasionally, amyloid fibrils in subepithelial locations (underlying podocytes) may become organized into parallel bundles, which are perpendicular to the glomerular capillary basement membrane (original magnification 30,000×). (From Christine Vanbeek, MD).

Box 8.1 Diagnostic Tests Used in the Evaluation of Systemic Light Chain Amyloidosis

Screening Tests

Serum and urine electrophoresis and immunofixation
Serum-free light chains and their ratio

Imaging Tests

Cardiac – CXR, EKG, ECHO, cardiac MRI
Radionuclide – SAP scintigraphy, PYP scan, DPD scan, florbetapir PET

Histology

Bone marrow biopsy and fat pad aspirate
Organ biopsy
Mass spectrometry and protein sequencing

Other Tests

24-hour urine for albumin
Complete blood count, basic chemistry profile, alkaline phosphatase
cTnT and NT-proBNP levels
Nerve conduction studies
Autonomic function tests

cTnT, Cardiac troponin T; *CXR*, chest x-ray; *DPD*, 3,3-diphosphono-1, 2-propanodicarboxylic acid; *ECHO*, echocardiogram; *EKG*, electrocardiogram; *MRI*, magnetic resonance imaging; *NT-proBNP*, N-terminal pro-brain natriuretic peptide; *PYP*, pyrophosphate; *SAP*, serum amyloid protein.

Treatment and Prognosis

MARKERS OF PROGNOSIS AND TREATMENT RESPONSE

Deeper understanding of the pathogenesis and organ involvement in AL amyloidosis has led to major advances in risk stratification, disease monitoring, and expanding therapeutic strategies. It is promising that the treatment outcomes and long-term survival rates are improving because of this advancement.[26] However, the 1-year survival rate continues to be low, likely because of delayed diagnosis.[27] As previously mentioned, the extent of cardiac involvement is the major determinant of prognosis of AL amyloidosis. N-terminal pro-brain natriuretic peptide (NT-proBNP) alone or in conjunction with serum troponin T are strong predictors of survival.[28] Assessment of serum FLC burden is also a key prognostic indicator.[29] High sensitivity cardiac troponin T assays at presentation, and reduction in serum FLC burden and NT-proBNP post chemotherapy are strong predictors of long-term outcome.[30] Recent studies reveal that low differences between amyloidogenic (involved) and nonamyloidogenic (uninvolved) FLC levels (< 50 mg/L) have lower rates of cardiac involvement and increased rates of kidney involvement and thereby have a more favorable prognosis and outcome.[31] The staging system for AL amyloidosis based on cardiac biomarkers is shown in Table 8.1.[32] This system was proposed over a decade ago and was later revised to include the difference between involved and uninvolved FLCs

modality of diagnosis in such situations. Echocardiogram, EKG, chest x-ray, cardiac magnetic resonance imaging (MRI) (an emerging gold standard), 99m Tc-labelled 3,3-diphosphono-1,2-propanodicarboxylic acid (99m Tc-DPD) scintigraphy, and 99m Tc-labelled pyrophosphate (99m Tc-PYP) scintigraphy are used for cardiac amyloid imaging. Cardiac MRI is especially useful in differentiating amyloidosis induced left ventricular hypertrophy/thickening from other causes, such as hypertension. Late gadolinium enhancement is highly characteristic of cardiac amyloid. Radionuclide imaging with 99m Tc-DPD and 99m Tc-PYP helps differentiate between AL cardiac amyloidosis (no uptake) and Transthyretin (TTR) or senile cardiac amyloidosis (2+ or greater uptake).[24] More recently, positron emission tomography tracers (18F-florbetapir) used in the diagnosis of Alzheimer disease are used to study cardiac and extracardiac involvement of amyloidosis.[25] Nerve conduction studies, and autonomic function tests, should be performed if neuropathy is suspected. Box 8.1 provides a list of the diagnostic tests used in the evaluation of AL amyloidosis.

Table 8.1 Staging System for Systemic Light Chain Amyloidosis Based on Cardiac Biomarkers Cardiac Troponin T and N-Terminal Pro-Brain Natriuretic Peptide

Criteria[a]	Staging
Both markers below threshold	I
One marker above threshold	II
Both markers above threshold	III

[a]Threshold values of NT-proBNP and cTnT are < 332 ng/L, and < 0.035 µg/L, respectively.

cTnT, Cardiac troponin T; *NT-proBNP*, N-terminal pro-brain natriuretic peptide.

Table 8.2 Internationally Validated Response Criteria for Use in Systemic Light Chain Amyloidosis to Assess Treatment Response at 3 or 6 Months After Treatment Initiation

HEMATOLOGIC RESPONSE	
Complete response (CR)	Negative serum and urine immuno-fixation and normal FLC ratio
Very good partial response (VGPR)	dFLC < 40 mg/L
Partial response (PR)	dFLC decrease > 50% compared with baseline
Low dFLC response	dFLC < 10 mg/L
CARDIAC RESPONSE	
Pretreatment NYHA class III or IV	At least 2 points decrease of NYHA class
Pretreatment NT-proBNP ≥ 650 ng/L	Decrease of NT-proBNP by > 30% and 300 ng/L
RENAL RESPONSE	
Pretreatment proteinuria > 0.5 g/24 hours	At least 30% decrease in proteinuria or drop below 0.5 g/24 hours, in the absence of renal progression defined as drop in eGFR by > 25%

dFLC, Difference between uninvolved and involved free light chain; *eGFR*, estimated glomerular filtration rate; *FLC*, free light chain; *NT-proBNP*, N-terminal pro-brain natriuretic peptide; *NYHA*, New York Heart Association.

(dFLC). Scores are calculated by assigning one point for each of the following: cardiac troponin T greater than 0.025 ng/mL, NT proBNP greater than 1800 pg/mL, and dFLC levels greater than 180 mg/L.[33] This provides a staging system of I, II, III, IV based on the number of points assigned (0,1,2,3). In patients with kidney dysfunction, BNP is preferred over NT-proBNP because of less effects on serum levels by reduced glomerular filtration rate (GFR).[34] Concomitant presence of multiple myeloma confers an adverse prognosis. The degree of nephrotic range proteinuria and kidney dysfunction at presentation, along with response to chemotherapy, determine the long-term need for dialysis in patients with kidney involvement.[35] Overall, the presence of kidney involvement is associated with longer survival mainly because of lower proportion of patients with cardiac involvement.[36] Based on the estimated GFR (< 50 mL/min/1.73 m²) and 24-hour proteinuria (> 5 g/day) at presentation, a staging system has been validated to distinguish three groups for risk stratification of dialysis requirement.[37] Both values below cut-off is stage I, one value above cut-off is stage II, and both values above cut-off is stage III with 1%, 12%, and 48% risk of dialysis at 2 years, respectively. Kastritis et al. also validated this staging system and identified the ratio of 24-h proteinuria to estimated GFR, as a sensitive marker of kidney risk and progression to dialysis.[38] λ Light chains are known to be more nephrotoxic than the κ type and have worse outcomes.[39] Response to therapy criteria have been established for uniform reporting, and to monitor disease activity and therapeutic outcomes (Table 8.2).

TREATMENT

Treatment of AL amyloidosis is complex because it not only involves the amyloidogenic precursor proteins and the plasma cells producing them, but also the different organ systems where the proteins are deposited. There is no current standard of care for the treatment of AL amyloidosis and hence treatment should be individualized based on risk assessment and organ involvement. For this reason, patients should be referred to specialized centers and involved in clinical trials when possible.

THERAPY TARGETING PLASMA CELLS

Targeting the amyloidogenic plasma cell clone remains to be mainstay of therapy in AL amyloidosis. Chemotherapy against amyloidogenic plasma cells was first introduced in

1972 in the form of melphalan and prednisone.[40] Only a small proportion of patients responded to this chemotherapy and therapy remained the same until the institution of autologous stem cell transplantation (ASCT) in 1996. Early on, the mortality associated with ASCT was high, but with the development of eligibility criteria and risk stratification, this has drastically reduced in recent years.[41] Eligibility criteria vary from center to center and include but are not limited to troponin T less than 0.06 µg/L, NT-proBNP less than 5000 pg/mL, cardiac ejection fraction greater than 45%, systolic blood pressure greater than 90 mmHg, age younger than 65 years, and estimated GFR greater than 50 mL/min per 1.73 m².[42] Based on these criteria, only about 20% to 25% patients are eligible for ASCT. They are the low-risk patients. However, induction with bortezomib (proteasome inhibitor) before transplant can turn initially transplant ineligible to eligible patients capable of undergoing ASCT.[43] There is also evidence that the outcomes associated with bortezomib induction followed by ASCT is superior to ASCT alone.[44] When ASCT is done at specialized centers following appropriate selection criteria and induction, the outcomes are excellent, with hematologic response in 71% of patients and complete response (CR) in approximately 35% of patients.[45] Hematologic response is the strongest predictor of outcome and translates to longer survival.[46]

Transplant ineligible patients should be treated with systemic chemotherapy directed against the amyloidogenic plasma cells. This includes steroids (dexamethasone, prednisone), alkylating agents (melphalan, cyclophosphamide), immunomodulatory drugs (thalidomide, lenalidomide), and proteasome inhibitors (bortezomib). See Box 8.2 for list of available chemotherapy. Until recently, the typical treatment for these patients consisted of melphalan plus dexamethasone (MDex).[47] This regimen extended survival with minimum toxicity resulting in a hematologic response of

Box 8.2 Systemic Chemotherapy Options for Systemic Light Chain Amyloidosis

Current Options

Melphalan-dexamethasone (MDex)
Cyclophosphamide-thalidomide-dexamethasone (toxicity profile limits usage)
Melphalan-lenalidomide-dexamethasone
Bortezomib-dexamethasone (less neurotoxicity)
Cyclophosphamide-bortezomib-dexamethasone (CyBorD)
Lenalidomide-cyclophosphamide-dexamethasone

Novel Alternate Agents

Plasma Cell-Directed Therapy

Pomalidomide—second generation immunomodulatory drug
Carfilzomib—second generation proteasome inhibitor, limited use because of cardiotoxicity
Ixazomib—third generation proteasome inhibitor, trial ongoing
Daratumumab—anti-CD38 antibody
Venetoclax—inhibitor of antiapoptotic protein BCL-2
Bendamustine—alkylating agent, trial ongoing

Light Chain Directed Therapy—Future Therapy Options

Doxycycline—trial ongoing
Epigallocatechin-3-gallate
Monoclonal antibody therapy
- NEOD001—antibody binding to unique epitope on abnormal light chain; trial stopped as of April 2018
- 11-1F4—chimeric fibril reactive monoclonal antibody, binds to a conformational epitope
- Miridesap—small molecule drug, competitive inhibitor of circulating SAP
- Dezamizumab—monoclonal antibody against SAP

SAP, Serum amyloid protein.

76% and CR of 31% in patients who received the full dose dexamethasone. The availability of the proteasome inhibitor bortezomib has changed this practice. The amyloidogenic plasma cells produce proteasomes and are vulnerable to proteasome inhibition in the presence of amyloidogenic light chains. The intermediate risk patients are likely to take the greatest advantage from the addition of bortezomib to MDex,[48] because there is no difference in outcome for the low-risk groups. The combination of cyclophosphamide, bortezomib, and dexamethasone (CyBorD) also produces rapid and complete hematologic response and is currently the standard induction regimen in several specialized centers.[49,50] Bortezomib is contraindicated in patients with peripheral neuropathy. CyBorD or bortezomib plus dexamethasone is preferred in patients with potentially reversible contraindications to ASCT or in patients with kidney failure. Melphalan has poor outcome with gain1q21 and bortezomib has poor outcome with t(11;14).[51–53] The choice of best combination, such as CyBorD or bortezomib plus MDex or bortezomib plus dexamethasone, or only MDex should consider clonal and patient characteristics. High-risk patients constitute about 15% of patients with AL amyloidosis and have poor response to chemotherapy because of advanced cardiac disease. These patients are treated with low-dose combinations and weekly dose escalations, based on tolerability of side effects under intense monitoring.

Relapsed patients either have a repeat of the initial therapy or switch to second-line therapy. Immunomodulatory drugs form the foundation of second-line therapy. Lenalidomide can overcome resistance to bortezomib, thalidomide, and alkylating agents, and when used with dexamethasone, acts as a good salvage therapy in refractory AL amyloidosis.[54] However, it can worsen kidney function and increase NT-proBNP levels and hence close monitoring is recommended. Most plasma cell-directed therapies used in treating multiple myeloma are being investigated in AL amyloidosis as well.[55] The proteasome inhibitor carfilzomib achieves good hematologic response, but the associated cardiac toxicity limits its use. The oral proteasome inhibitor ixazomib is being tested in relapsed/refractory patients and may allow for an oral drug regimen. Daratumumab, an anti-CD 38 monoclonal antibody directed against the plasma cells, appears to be one of the most promising novel therapies in refractory AL amyloidosis. It is a highly effective agent that produced rapid and deep hematologic responses without unexpected toxicity in a cohort of heavily pretreated patients with AL amyloidosis.[56] Clinical trials assessing use of daratumumab in the treatment of AL amyloidosis are underway. Bendamustine is an alkylating agent used in several lymphoproliferative disorders. Bendamustine was recently studied in a group of 122 patients by Milani et al.,[57] and was shown to have a survival advantage especially in pretreated AL amyloidosis patients.[58] Venetoclax is an orally bioavailable inhibitor of antiapoptotic protein, BCL-2. It induces cell death in plasma cells, particularly in those harboring t(11;14), which express high levels of BCL-2. With encouraging results seen in t(11;14) multiple myeloma[59] and with more than 50% of AL amyloidosis patients with t(11;14), venetoclax seems to be a potential opportunity to improve outcomes in heavily pretreated AL amyloidosis.

FUTURE DIRECTIONS—THERAPY INTERFERING WITH AMYLOIDOGENESIS AND TARGETING AMYLOID DEPOSITS

Although antiplasma cell chemotherapy remains the cornerstone of treatment in AL amyloidosis, the disadvantage of this therapy is that it has no effect on the abnormal protein that has already been deposited. Novel therapeutics are being developed to target the abnormal amyloid protein already deposited and thereby reverse organ failure and improve organ function. These therapeutic agents are either given along with chemotherapy or postchemotherapy after hematologic response. Therapeutic drugs targeting the existing amyloid deposits are the future of AL amyloidosis therapy development. Doxycycline, by effect of its inhibition of matrix metalloproteinases, was able to disrupt amyloid fibrils in transgenic mouse models of systemic amyloidosis.[60] Doxycycline, when used as post-ASCT antibacterial prophylaxis, improved survival in patients with AL amyloidosis and has a low toxicity profile.[61] A phase III clinical trial testing chemotherapy with or without doxycycline is being designed and a single center, open label phase 2 study is ongoing.[62] Polyphenols, such as epigallocatechin-3-gallate, can redirect amyloidogenic polypeptides into unstructured, off pathway oligomers and induce their aggregation.[63,64]

Miridesap, a small molecule drug that competitively inhibits SAP binding to amyloid fibrils, depletes circulating SAP in the blood, so that the monoclonal SAP antibody, dezamizumab, administered afterwards can access the amyloid in the tissues.[65] NEOD001 and 11-1F4 are monoclonal antibodies against unique epitopes in the amyloid protein. 11-1F4 is a murine monoclonal antibody that recognizes a confirmation epitope on the amyloid fibril. It showed promising organ response rates in a phase I clinical trial.[66] NEOD001 is a humanized murine monoclonal antibody 2A4 that binds to a unique epitope on the abnormal light chain protein. NEOD001 was being evaluated in two randomized, placebo-controlled trials, but they were terminated because primary and secondary endpoints were not met.[67,68]

SUPPORTIVE THERAPY

Supportive therapy is a key component of the therapeutic regimen in AL amyloidosis. This includes treatment of end-organ dysfunction, as well as managing the side effect profile of ongoing chemotherapy. This becomes complex in the setting of heart failure, nephrotic syndrome, and autonomic dysfunction. Hypotension caused by autonomic neuropathy hampers diuretic treatment of heart failure and nephrotic syndrome. Heavy urinary protein losses and high catabolic rate result in hypoalbuminemia and worsen peripheral edema. Significant peripheral edema and volume overload warrant dietary sodium restriction, daily weights, and an aggressive diuretic regimen that needs constant titration. Hyperlipidemia and venous thromboembolism can occur as consequences of nephrotic syndrome. Anticoagulation may be necessary if other procoagulant factors are present. Intradialytic hypotension, caused by cardiac and autonomic system involvement, is a common complication in patients requiring renal replacement therapy. Cardiac or renal transplantation can be offered to patients who have achieved remission, but have persistent severe heart failure or are dialysis dependent.

Key Points

- Delayed diagnosis remains a major challenge to initiate therapy timely and effectively. Physicians should have a high index of clinical suspicion to avoid delay in the diagnosis of AL amyloidosis.
- AL amyloidosis is a histologic diagnosis and hence requires confirmation through biopsy. Bone marrow biopsy and abdominal fat pad aspirate can detect more than 70% of amyloidosis without the need for invasive organ biopsy. Organ biopsy is indicated if the aforementioned tests are negative and there is a high suspicion for amyloidosis.
- It is mandatory to confirm the type of amyloid fibril because of the common coexistence of different types of amyloidosis. Mass spectrometry and protein sequencing is considered the gold standard for this purpose.
- Late gadolinium enhancement in cardiac magnetic resonance imaging is the emerging gold standard for the diagnosis of cardiac amyloid. Radionuclide imaging such as serum amyloid-P component, 99m Tc-labelled

3,3-diphosphono-1,2-propanodicarboxylic acid and 99m Tc-labelled pyrophosphate scintigraphy, and 18F-florbetapir positron emission tomography can also detect amyloidosis but are not widely available for use.

- The cardiac biomarkers, N-terminal pro-brain natriuretic peptide and troponin T along with serum uninvolved free light chain levels, form the basis of prognostication in AL amyloidosis and their use is critical in risk stratification. Cardiac involvement is the strongest predictor of outcome.
- Once amyloidosis is confirmed to be of light chain origin, risk stratification should be performed and eligibility for autologous stem cell transplantation (ASCT) determined. High-dose melphalan followed by ASCT is the treatment of choice in AL amyloidosis.
- Hematologic response is the strongest predictor of treatment outcomes.
- In transplant ineligible patients, systemic chemotherapy should be tried. Plasma cell-directed therapy remains the backbone of chemotherapy for this disease.
- Since bortezomib-based therapy has emerged, response rates have improved in the intermediate risk group.
- Several novel therapeutic agents are available and seem promising for refractory or relapsing AL amyloidosis. These are either plasma cell-directed therapies or directed against amyloid light chains.
- Drug combinations and doses should be individualized and based on clonal and patient characteristics.
- Overall, significant advancements have occurred in the therapeutic world of amyloidosis providing an opportunity for an optimistic future for this disease.

References

1. Sipe JD, Benson MD, Buxbaum JN, et al. Amyloid fibril proteins and amyloidosis: chemical identification and clinical classification International Society of Amyloidosis 2016 Nomenclature Guidelines. *Amyloid.* 2016;23(4):209-213.
2. Kyle RA. Amyloidosis. Introduction and overview. *J Intern Med.* 1992;232(6):507-508.
3. Kyle RA, Gertz MA. Primary systemic amyloidosis: clinical and laboratory features in 474 cases. *Semin Hematol.* 1995;32(1):45-59.
4. Dobson CM, Karplus M. The fundamentals of protein folding: bringing together theory and experiment. *Curr Opin Struct Biol.* 1999;9(1):92-101.
5. Solomon A, Weiss DT, Kattine AA. Nephrotoxic potential of Bence Jones proteins. *N Engl J Med.* 1991;324(26):1845-1851.
6. Bellotti V, Mangione P, Merlini G. Review: immunoglobulin light chain amyloidosis—the archetype of structural and pathogenic variability. *J Struct Biol.* 2000;130(2-3):280-289.
7. Glenner GG, Ein D, Eanes ED, Bladen HA, Terry W, Page DL. Creation of "amyloid" fibrils from Bence Jones proteins in vitro. *Science.* 1971;174(4010):712-714.
8. von Gise H, Christ H, Bohle A. Early glomerular lesions in amyloidosis. Electron microscopic findings. *Virchows Arch A Pathol Anat Histol.* 1981;390(3):259-272.
9. Keeling J, Teng J, Herrera GA. AL-amyloidosis and light-chain deposition disease light chains induce divergent phenotypic transformations of human mesangial cells. *Lab Invest.* 2004;84(10):1322-1338.
10. Teng J, Turbat-Herrera EA, Herrera GA. An animal model of glomerular light-chain-associated amyloidogenesis depicts the crucial role of lysosomes. *Kidney Int.* 2014;86(4):738-746.
11. Brenner DA, Jain M, Pimentel DR, et al. Human amyloidogenic light chains directly impair cardiomyocyte function through an increase in cellular oxidant stress. *Circ Res.* 2004;94(8):1008-1010.
12. Solomon A, Frangione B, Franklin EC. Bence Jones proteins and light chains of immunoglobulins. Preferential association of the V lambda VI subgroup of human light chains with amyloidosis AL (lambda). *J Clin Invest.* 1982;70(2):453-460.

13. Kyle RA. Primary systemic amyloidosis. *J Intern Med*. 1992;232 (6):523-524.
14. Dember LM. Emerging treatment approaches for the systemic amyloidoses. *Kidney Int*. 2005;68(3):1377-1390.
15. Gertz MA, Kyle RA O'Fallon WM. Dialysis support of patients with primary systemic amyloidosis. A study of 211 patients. *Arch Intern Med*. 1992;152:2245-2250.
16. Park MA, Mueller PS, Kyle RA, Larson DR, Plevak MF, Gertz MA. Primary (AL) hepatic amyloidosis: clinical features and natural history in 98 patients. *Medicine (Baltimore)*. 2003;82(5):291-298.
17. Choufani EB, Sanchorawala V, Ernst T, et al. Acquired factor X deficiency in patients with amyloid light-chain amyloidosis: incidence, bleeding manifestations, and response to high-dose chemotherapy. *Blood*. 2001;97(6):1885-1887.
18. Perfetto F, Moggi-Pignone A, Livi R, Tempestini A, Bergesio F, Matucci-Cerinic M. Systemic amyloidosis: a challenge for the rheumatologist. *Nat Rev Rheumatol*. 2010;6(7):417-429.
19. Comenzo RL, Zhou P, Fleisher M, Clark B, Teruya-Feldstein J. Seeking confidence in the diagnosis of systemic AL (Ig light-chain) amyloidosis: patients can have both monoclonal gammopathies and hereditary amyloid proteins. *Blood*. 2006;107(9):3489-3491.
20. Merlini G, Bellotti V. Molecular mechanisms of amyloidosis. *N Engl J Med*. 2003;349(6):583-596.
21. Linke RP, Oos R, Wiegel NM, Nathrath WB. Classification of amyloidosis: misdiagnosing by way of incomplete immunohistochemistry and how to prevent it. *Acta Histochem*. 2006;108(3):197-208.
22. Vrana JA, Gamez JD, Madden BJ, Theis JD, Bergen HR III, Dogan A. Classification of amyloidosis by laser microdissection and mass spectrometry-based proteomic analysis in clinical biopsy specimens. *Blood*. 2009;114(24):4957-4959.
23. Hawkins PN, Lavender JP, Pepys MB. Evaluation of systemic amyloidosis by scintigraphy with 123I-labeled serum amyloid P component. *N Engl J Med*. 1990;323(8):508-513.
24. Harb SC, Haq M, Flood K, et al. National patterns in imaging utilization for diagnosis of cardiac amyloidosis: a focus on Tc99m-pyrophosphate scintigraphy. *J Nucl Cardiol*. 2017;24(3):1094-1097.
25. Wagner T, Page J, Burniston M, et al. Extracardiac (18)F-florbetapir imaging in patients with systemic amyloidosis: more than hearts and minds. *Eur J Nucl Med Mol Imaging*. 2018;45(7):1129-1138.
26. Muchtar E, Gertz MA, Kumar SK, et al. Improved outcomes for newly diagnosed AL amyloidosis between 2000 and 2014: cracking the glass ceiling of early death. *Blood*. 2017;129(15):2111-2119.
27. Kumar SK, Gertz MA, Lacy MQ, et al. Recent improvements in survival in primary systemic amyloidosis and the importance of an early mortality risk score. *Mayo Clin Proc*. 2011;86(1):12-18.
28. Palladini G, Campana C, Klersy C, et al. Serum N-terminal pro-brain natriuretic peptide is a sensitive marker of myocardial dysfunction in AL amyloidosis. *Circulation*. 2003;107(19):2440-2445.
29. Kourelis TV, Kumar SK, Gertz MA, et al. Coexistent multiple myeloma or increased bone marrow plasma cells define equally high-risk populations in patients with immunoglobulin light chain amyloidosis. *J Clin Oncol*. 2013;31(34):4319-4324.
30. Palladini G, Lavatelli F, Russo P, et al. Circulating amyloidogenic free light chains and serum N-terminal natriuretic peptide type B decrease simultaneously in association with improvement of survival in AL. *Blood*. 2006;107(10):3854-3858.
31. Dittrich T, Bochtler T, Kimmich C, et al. AL amyloidosis patients with low amyloidogenic free light chain levels at first diagnosis have an excellent prognosis. *Blood*. 2017;130(5):632-642.
32. Dispenzieri A, Gertz MA, Kyle RA, et al. Serum cardiac troponins and N-terminal pro-brain natriuretic peptide: a staging system for primary systemic amyloidosis. *J Clin Oncol*. 2004;22(18): 3751-3757.
33. Kumar S, Dispenzieri A, Lacy MQ, et al. Revised prognostic staging system for light chain amyloidosis incorporating cardiac biomarkers and serum free light chain measurements. *J Clin Oncol*. 2012;30(9): 989-995.
34. Palladini G, Foli A, Milani P, et al. Best use of cardiac biomarkers in patients with AL amyloidosis and renal failure. *Am J Hematol*. 2012; 87(5):465-471.
35. Gertz MA, Leung N, Lacy MQ, et al. Clinical outcome of immunoglobulin light chain amyloidosis affecting the kidney. *Nephrol Dial Transplant*. 2009;24(10):3132-3137.
36. Milani P, Merlini G, Palladini G. Novel therapies in light chain amyloidosis. *Kidney Int Rep*. 2017;3(3):530-541.
37. Palladini G, Hegenbart U, Milani P, et al. A staging system for renal outcome and early markers of renal response to chemotherapy in AL amyloidosis. *Blood*. 2014;124(15):2325-2332.
38. Kastritis E, Gavriatopoulou M, Roussou M, et al. Renal outcomes in patients with AL amyloidosis: prognostic factors, renal response and the impact of therapy. *Am J Hematol*. 2017;92(7):632-639.
39. Sidiqi MH, Aljama MA, Muchtar E, et al. Light chain type predicts organ involvement and survival in AL amyloidosis patients receiving stem cell transplantation. *Blood Adv*. 2018;2(7):769-776.
40. Jones NF, Hilton PJ, Tighe JR, Hobbs JR. Treatment of "primary" renal amyloidosis with melphalan. *Lancet*. 1972;2(7778):616-619.
41. Gertz MA, Lacy MQ, Dispenzieri A, et al. Refinement in patient selection to reduce treatment-related mortality from autologous stem cell transplantation in amyloidosis. *Bone Marrow Transplant*. 2013;48(4): 557-561.
42. Palladini G, Merlini G. What is new in diagnosis and management of light chain amyloidosis? *Blood*. 2016;128(2):159-168.
43. Cornell RF, Zhong X, Arce-Lara C, et al. Bortezomib-based induction for transplant ineligible AL amyloidosis and feasibility of later transplantation. *Bone Marrow Transplant*. 2015;50(7):914-917.
44. Huang X, Wang Q, Chen W, et al. Induction therapy with bortezomib and dexamethasone followed by autologous stem cell transplantation versus autologous stem cell transplantation alone in the treatment of renal AL amyloidosis: a randomized controlled trial. *BMC Med*. 2014;12:2.
45. D'Souza A, Dispenzieri A, Wirk B, et al. Improved outcomes after autologous hematopoietic cell transplantation for light chain amyloidosis: a Center for International Blood and Marrow Transplant Research Study. *J Clin Oncol*. 2015;33(32):3741-3749.
46. Gertz MA, Lacy MQ, Dispenzieri A, et al. Effect of hematologic response on outcome of patients undergoing transplantation for primary amyloidosis: importance of achieving a complete response. *Haematologica*. 2007;92(10):1415-1418.

A full list of references is available at Expertconsult.com

Monoclonal Immunoglobulin Deposition Disease

LEAL HERLITZ AND JUAN C. CALLE

Introduction

Monoclonal immunoglobulin deposition disease (MIDD) is characterized by the deposition of monoclonal light and/or heavy chains within glomerular, tubular, and vessel wall basement membranes. Three subtypes of MIDD have been described and they are subdivided according to the composition of monoclonal protein deposited. The most common form of MIDD is light chain deposition disease (LCDD), where either kappa or lambda light chains are deposited in tubular, glomerular, and vessel wall basement membranes. Much less common than LCDD are heavy chain deposition disease (HCDD) and light and heavy chain deposition disease (LHCDD), which show basement membrane accumulation of a monoclonal immunoglobulin heavy chain, either with a corresponding monoclonal light chain (LHCDD) or without an accompanying light chain (HCDD).[1,2] In contrast to the fibrils seen in amyloidosis, the deposits of MIDD lack substructure. In the past, the term *monoclonal immunoglobulin deposition disease* has been used as a generic term to encompass a wide variety of paraprotein-related diseases including light chain amyloid and cast nephropathy. In this chapter, we restrict ourselves to the currently accepted narrower usage of the term as defined earlier, or what has been historically called *Randall-type monoclonal immunoglobulin deposition disease*. For much of the chapter we combine our discussion of patients with LCDD, LHCDD, and HCDD, referring to them as patients with MIDD. Notable differences between subtypes of MIDD are pointed out where appropriate and summarized in Table 9.1.

Epidemiology of Monoclonal Immunoglobulin Deposition Disease

MIDD is a relatively rare disease. The incidence of pure MIDD (MIDD in the absence of light chain cast nephropathy or amyloidosis) in native kidney biopsies has been reported to range from 0.32% in a study from Columbia University Medical Center in New York[1] up to 0.7% of renal biopsies processed at the Mayo Clinic.[2] Overall, MIDD appears to be approximately half as common as amyloidosis. In an autopsy series of patients with multiple myeloma

(MM), LCDD was found in 5% of patients, whereas amyloid was detected in 11%.[3] Similarly, out of the 1078 biopsies studied at Columbia University between 2000 and 2014 with paraprotein deposition in the kidney, pure MIDD was identified in 209 (19%), compared with amyloidosis in 451 (41%), and light chain proximal tubulopathy in only 54 (5%).[4]

The association of MIDD with underlying hematologic conditions has varied across different studies as our understanding of plasma cell dyscrasias has evolved and new definitions of MM have emerged.[5] In a recent report by Kourelis et al., 57% of patients with MIDD had either smoldering MM or MM.[6] The literature indicates that MM is present in roughly half of patients with LCDD and LHCDD,[7] but the percentage has been reported as high as 58% to 65% for those with LCDD.[1,2,8] In contrast, HCDD has a much lower reported incidence of MM compared with LCDD and LHCDD, with reports ranging from 19% to 33%.[2,9,10] After the introduction of the term *monoclonal gammopathy of renal significance* (MGRS), virtually all patients with MIDD have been shown to have a plasma cell dyscrasia.[2,6,9–11]

Patient characteristics of those diagnosed with MIDD are notable for mean age, typically in the late 50s, although ages have ranged from patients in their 20s to patients over 90 years.[1,2,6–8,12] In the series by Nasr et al., approximately one-third of patients with MIDD were under 50 years of age.[2] In patients with LCDD, there appears to be a male predominance, with approximately twice as many men as women. This is in contrast to HCDD, where men and women appear to be equally affected.[1,2,7–10,12–14] Race is not reported in all studies; however, in those large case series where it was, patients were white in more than 80% of the cases.[2,9,12] Of interest, the only study with a significant number of black patients (22%) was from a single institution in New York, and four of five of those patients had either HCDD or LHCDD.[1] The only large case series from Asia, reported to date by Li et al., examined 48 patients, all of whom were Chinese, and age and gender data were similar to the trends described previously.[15] It is difficult to draw meaningful conclusions regarding any differences in racial involvement, given that most of the reports have come from geographic areas where there is not a wide range of racial diversity and the majority of patients studied were white.

Table 9.1 Notable Clinical and Histopathologic Contrasts Between Light Chain Deposition Disease and Heavy Chain Deposition Disease

	LCDD	HCDD
CLINICAL FEATURES		
Gender	Male:Female of 2:1	Male:Female of 1:1
Hypocomplementemia	uncommon	Occurs in approximately 30% Very common in patients with IgG1 and IgG3 heavy chains
Nephrotic range proteinuria	~40%	~60%
% with multiple myeloma	~50%	~20–30%
% with hypertension	~50%	~100%
HISTOPATHOLOGIC FEATURES		
Nodular sclerosis	~60%	~100%
Crescent formation	~10%	More common than LCDD, crescents in 2/3 cases of HCDD with IgA heavy chains
Mesangial deposits	~60%	More common than LCDD
Type of monoclonal protein	~80% kappa, 20% lambda	~80% IgG heavy chains, 20% IgA, rare cases of IgM or IgD
Key pathogenic features of the paraprotein	N-glycosylation site promotes basement membrane deposition Hydrophobic surface residues favoring tissue deposition	CH1 deletion causing premature secretion without a light chain Hydrophobic surface residues favoring tissue deposition

HCDD, Heavy chain deposition disease; *Ig*, immunoglobulin; *LCDD*, light chain deposition disease.

Clinical Manifestations of Monoclonal Immunoglobulin Deposition Disease

Whereas MIDD can present as a multisystem disease, renal manifestations typically predominate. More than 83% of the patients reported with MIDD and kidney disease had renal insufficiency based on serum creatinine greater than 1.2 mg/dL or chronic kidney disease (CKD) stage 2/3. Many patients experience a rapid decline in renal function.[2,6–8,10,16] Proteinuria is present in almost all patients with MIDD, and about 40% to 50% of patients will have nephrotic range proteinuria.[2,15,17] The prevalence of nephrotic range proteinuria and nephrotic syndrome seems to be higher in those with HCDD.[9] In contrast to amyloidosis, hypertension is widely present at the time of diagnosis in patients with MIDD, with two large series reporting hypertension in approximately 80% of patients.[1,2] However, reports of hypertension in LCDD[7,18] may be closer to 50%, whereas patients with HCDD have a higher incidence with nearly 100% of them being affected.[1,2,9,10] Incidence of microscopic hematuria is reported to range from 60% to 90% of the cases of MIDD and also appears to be somewhat more common in patients with HCDD.[2,12,18] Hypocomplementemia was absent in all 12 patients with LCDD reported by Lin et al., but was present in three of six of their HCDD patients.[1] Bridoux et al. reported low C3 in five of their 15 patients with HCDD; four of these patients had γ1-HCDD and the other had γ3-HCDD, correlating with the known complement fixing abilities of immunoglobulin (Ig)G subtypes 1 and 3.[9]

Of note, a recent report from China did show C3 hypocomplementemia in up to one-third of patients with LCDD.[15]

Whereas renal manifestations in MIDD typically predominate, extrarenal involvement in multiple organ systems is well described. From the first descriptions of LCDD by Randal et al. in the 1970s, it was demonstrated that visceral deposition in multiple organs was a feature of the disease.[19] LCDD has been described to involve the heart, liver, lungs, pancreas, thyroid, skin, lymph nodes and spleen, muscles, and the gastrointestinal and neurologic systems. As reported by Ganeval et al., when extrarenal manifestations were specifically evaluated for, they were found in all MIDD patients. Light chain deposits were found in the blood vessels walls of most organs.[20] Heart and liver involvement are the most commonly described extrarenal sites of MIDD involvement.[21] Heart disease is reported in up to 80% of cases with LCDD; however, whether the etiology of the cardiac disease can be attributed to MIDD is unknown, because most patients do not undergo heart biopsy or have evidence of an infiltrative process in the heart. A significant portion of the cardiac disease in MIDD patients may relate to confounding factors, specifically age and renal impairment.[2,22,23] In the past, cardiac involvement may have been historically underdiagnosed because of lack of usage of immunohistologic and electron microscopic methods in endomyocardial biopsies.[24] Lack of uniformity in nomenclature also hampers our ability to estimate cardiac involvement because in the cardiac literature, some studies refer only to cardiac nonamyloidotic immunoglobulin deposition disease (CIDD), light-chain cardiomyopathy, or simply describe cases as cardiomyopathies with light chain deposition disease.[25] Toor et al. reported the experience of one MM referral center where less than 2% of the patients referred for evaluation of MM underwent cardiac biopsy. Of those, 20% (six patients) had CIDD. In total, eight cases were analyzed but four of eight patients also had proven concomitant amyloidosis in other organs. Interestingly, none of the patients had any symptoms related to heart failure. The median age for these patients at presentation and diagnosis was somewhat earlier (median age of 49.5 years, range 40–64 years).[26] In general, in patients with cardiac manifestations, the most common clinical features include congestive heart failure, usually with a restrictive pattern, arrhythmias, and conduction anomalies. In two series in which echocardiography was reported, 10/13 patients had left ventricular hypertrophy.[22,26]

In one of the earliest case series, liver deposits were found in almost all of the patients who underwent hepatic tissue analysis.[20] Hepatomegaly and moderate abnormalities in liver function tests are often observed; however, more rarely, cases of portal hypertension, hepatic insufficiency, and death from fulminant liver failure have also been described. Histologic features of liver involvement include abnormal chromophilic material along sinusoids, in vascular walls, and in basement membranes of biliary ductules under light microscopy. Portal areas were enlarged by fibrosis and usually contained abnormal material. The distribution of lesions varied from patient to patient.[20,27] The burden of deposits in liver biopsies has been described as moderate to severe, but mild lesions with nearly normal sinusoids are also seen.[20,28]

Pulmonary symptoms and involvement of the respiratory system are less common. Respiratory symptoms can be heterogeneous, involving multiple sites including the large airways. Pulmonary involvement can be very indolent and patients may remain asymptomatic for several years,[29] although severe cases requiring lung transplant have been reported.[30] Histologically, pulmonary involvement can be characterized by either diffuse involvement or a more nodular distribution.[31] Newer images with high resolution computed tomography scans show that almost all patients with pulmonary involvement have thin-walled cysts, usually with pulmonary nodules.[32]

Neurologic involvement in MIDD is common, with up to 20% to 30% of patients having peripheral neuropathy caused by deposits along the nerve fibers.[23,33,34] Central nervous system involvement is rare likely because of limited crossing of paraproteins through the blood-brain barrier. However, "aggregomas"—a term coined by Rostagano et al., and described as localized tumoral masses of Congo-red-negative monoclonal nonfibrillar Ig light chain, have also been reported.[35,36] Isolated "aggregomas" without evidence of any plasma cell dyscrasia and presenting with large, intracerebral lesions exerting significant mass effect have been recently reported.[37,38]

Histopathologic Features of Renal Involvement

The light microscopic findings in LCDD, LHCDD, and HCDD overlap considerably. Whereas earlier series describe nodular

sclerosing glomerulopathy as essentially universal in all forms of pure MIDD,[1] subsequent series have found nodular sclerosis in only 61% of cases, with the remaining cases showing only mild or no mesangial sclerosis.[2] Notably, in HCDD, nodular mesangial sclerosis appears to be more universal than in LCDD or LHCDD.[2,9] Cases of MIDD with nodular sclerosis often show mild mesangial hypercellularity and some segmental membranoproliferative features (Fig. 9.1). Less common is the finding of cellular crescent formation, seen in 9% of MIDD in one series.[2] Crescent formation (also called *extracapillary proliferation*) was observed in two of three cases of alpha-HCDD.[9] The deposits of MIDD are periodic-acid Schiff-positive and can cause ribbon-like thickening of tubular basement membranes and vessel wall myocyte basement membranes, but glomerular basement membrane thickening is uncommon.[1,2] Congo red staining is negative in pure forms of MIDD, although concurrent amyloidosis was described in three of 23 patients in one series.[1] Light chain cast nephropathy is also seen in a subset of patients with MIDD. In the series by Lin et al., 11 of 34 cases of MIDD were accompanied by cast nephropathy. Among the 11 patients with MIDD and cast nephropathy, only two showed the characteristic nodular sclerosis of MIDD, two showed mild

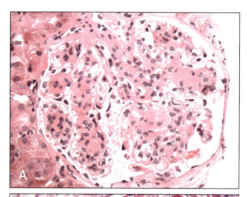
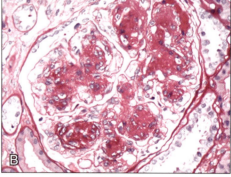

Fig. 9.1 Light microscopic findings of monoclonal immunoglobulin deposition disease (MIDD). Nodular sclerosis is the most common appearance of glomeruli in patients with MIDD and is encountered in approximately 60% of light chain deposition disease and virtually all heavy chain deposition disease. **A.** (Hematoxylin and Eosin, ×400 original magnification) highlights the mesangial nodules, along with the mesangial hypercellularity that is often seen. Periodic-acid Schiff (PAS) staining (**B.** ×400 original magnification) highlights nodular mesangial expansion by PAS-positive material. In contrast to diabetic nephropathy, where glomerular basement membranes are usually quite thick, glomerular basement membranes in MIDD are usually normal in thickness. Segmental double contours of the glomerular basement membrane (membranoproliferative features) are also highlighted with PAS staining.

mesangial sclerosis, and the remaining seven had normal appearing glomeruli.[1]

Immunofluorescence is critical for the diagnosis of MIDD. Linear basement membrane staining for a monotypic light and/or heavy chain is a central criterion for the diagnosis of MIDD (Fig. 9.2). Staining of tubular basement membranes (TBMs) appears to be essentially universal with the vast majority of cases also showing linear deposits in the glomerular basement membrane (GBM) deposits, myocyte basement membrane, vessel walls, and mesangium.[1,2,8] Immunofluorescence allows for the subclassification of MIDD cases into LCDD, LHCDD, and HCDD, depending on the staining profile of the monoclonal protein. In cases of LCDD, kappa staining predominates over lambda staining, with series showing between 68% and 91% kappa LCDD.[1,2,8] The largest series of HCDD to date shows that most HCDD is gamma-HCDD, which accounted for 12 of 15 cases in the series. The remaining cases were composed of alpha-HCDD.[9] Cases of HCDD caused by IgM[39] and IgD[40] heavy chains have also been reported. Notably, HCDD cases composed of IgG3 or IgG1 heavy chains also often have C3 deposition detected by immunofluorescence, correlating with the established ability of IgG subtypes 1 and 3 to effectively fix complement.[9]

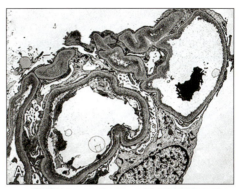

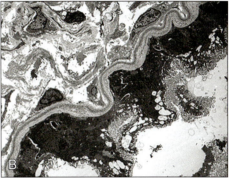

Fig. 9.3 Ultrastructural features of monoclonal immunoglobulin deposition disease (MIDD). **A.** (×5800 original magnification) shows the powdery, punctate electron dense deposits of MIDD involving glomerular basement membranes. Within glomeruli, the deposits are usually most prominent along the subendothelial aspect of the glomerular basement membrane. **B.** (×5800 original magnification) shows a tubular basement membrane with powdery electron dense deposits. Note that in tubular basement membranes, the deposits are most prominent along the outer aspect of the membrane, closest to the interstitium.

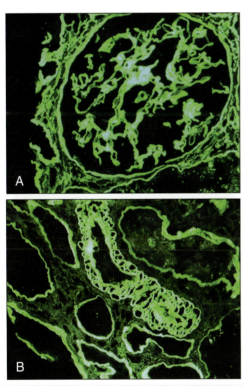

Fig. 9.2 Immunofluorescence staining in monoclonal immunoglobulin deposition disease (MIDD). All renal basement membranes can show the characteristic linear deposits of MIDD. **A.** (×400 original magnification) highlights strong glomerular basement membrane staining for kappa in a patient with light chain deposition disease (LCDD). Notably, prominent nodular sclerosis and mesangial deposits are not seen in this case, a finding which is not uncommon in LCDD, but would be uncharacteristic of heavy chain deposition disease. Note that Bowman's capsule and the surrounding tubular basement membranes are also showing strong linear staining. **B.** (×400 original magnification) highlights the strong tubular basement membrane linear staining, that is a nearly universal feature of MIDD. A vessel is also pictured, and linear staining of the vessel wall myocyte basement membranes is also prominent in this image.

Electron microscopy of MIDD cases reveals highly electron dense, punctate, powdery deposits within renal basement membranes (Fig. 9.3). TBM deposits are typically located along the outer aspect of the TBM, whereas GBM deposits are concentrated along the inner aspect of the lamina densa. Granular mesangial deposits may also be seen, a finding more commonly seen in HCDD than LCDD.[1,2] Lin et al. described a subset of cases where LCDD and cast nephropathy were coexistent by immunofluorescence, but the characteristic electron dense deposits of MIDD were not present. These cases were labeled as LCDD "by immunofluorescence only" and were hypothesized to represent nonspecific trapping of the monoclonal light chain in basement membranes, reflecting high circulating serum levels.[1] The series reported by Nasr et al. required the presence of characteristic deposits by electron microscopy as one of the two diagnostic criteria, along with monoclonal protein deposition along GBMs and TBMs in immunofluorescence.[2]

Pathogenesis of Monoclonal Immunoglobulin Deposition Disease

As is true with many forms of dysproteinemia related renal disease, the disease phenotype depends in large part of the physiochemical properties of the deposited monoclonal protein. Although LCDD, LHCDD, and HCDD share many morphologic findings, such as nodular sclerosis, basement membrane thickening, and powdery deposits in renal basement membranes, there are distinct structural characteristics that promote deposition of light chains and heavy chains.

In LCDD, approximately 80% of the cases are caused by kappa light chains,[23] which is notably different than the lambda predominance seen in light chain amyloidosis.[7] Congé et al. published the first complete primary structure of a light chain causing LCDD.[41] Notable findings included an overall normal kappa light chain structure with a variable domain composed of the *VkappaIV* gene along with the *Jkappa1*. The *VkappaIV* sequence had several point mutations, including one resulting in an N-glycosylation site. Protein glycosylation and the development of diabetic nephropathy, which shows strikingly similar nodular sclerosis and basement membrane thickening to LCDD, has been recently investigated in a rat model of diabetic nephropathy.[42] It is possible that the N-glycosylation in some kappa chains that cause LCDD could promote their deposition in basement membranes and cause nodular sclerosis in a similar fashion to what is seen in diabetic nephropathy. Although the VkappaIV variable region subgroup is found in approximately 7% of monoclonal kappa light chains, it appears to be disproportionately overrepresented in LCDD.[43] Study of additional primary structures of cases of LCDD revealed multiple hydrophobic residues exposed at the molecule surface, including along complementarity determining regions (CDR). The presence of surface hydrophobic residues can have a significant influence on light chain conformation. The location of hydrophobic residues along the CDR, which is the portion of the light chain molecule responsible for contacting an antigen, suggests that there may be a specific tropism for extracellular structures, such as components of basement membranes, which appear "antigen-like" to these light chains.[7,44] A mouse model, in which a human LCDD VkappaIV chain was secreted, showed that the amino acid changes in the V region were sufficient to produce deposits that were similar in distribution to those observed in patients with LCDD.[45] The increase in hydrophobicity of the light chains in LCDD may favor precipitation into tissue, because they would be less soluble in an aqueous environment. The combination of glycosylation and hydrophobicity appear to be important to the pathogenic potential of the light chains in LCDD.

In HCDD, the overarching structural abnormality found in the heavy chain is the deletion of the first constant domain CH1. Moulin et al. demonstrated CH1 deletion in four cases of gamma HCDD.[46] The CH1 domain is essential for nascent heavy chains to interact with heavy chain binding protein in the endoplasmic reticulum. When this interaction is prevented, incompletely assembled heavy chains are prematurely secreted, without an associated light chain.[47] Although CH1 deletion appears to be necessary for HCDD, by itself it is not sufficient. The variable regions in HCDD heavy chains commonly show mutated amino acid residues in the CDR and framework regions that result in formation of large hydrophobic regions and a positive charge at physiologic pH. This combination of charge and hydrophobicity is hypothesized to favor tissue deposition in the anionic sites of renal basement membranes.[9] This is in comparison with

heavy chain disease (HCD), which is characterized by circulating heavy chains without accompanying light chains. In contrast to HCDD, the heavy chains in HCD are not deposited in tissues. Similar to HCDD, these heavy chains frequently show CH1 deletions, allowing them to be prematurely secreted in a truncated form. In contrast, however, the variable region of the heavy chains in HCD are either fully or partially deleted, suggesting that an intact variable region is essential for tissue deposition.[48]

Structural alterations of the light and heavy chains described earlier help explain their deposition in renal basement membranes, but the development of nodular sclerosis requires more than simple deposition of a monoclonal protein. The nodules in MIDD are largely composed of the same constituents encountered in nodular diabetic glomerulosclerosis, including type IV collagen, fibronectin, laminin, and heparin sulfate proteoglycan.[49] The large oligomeric protein tenascin has also been found to be an essential component of the matrix accumulation in MIDD. In the normal kidney, tenascin expression is limited to the mesangial matrix, but expression becomes more widespread in a variety of pathologic conditions.[50] An in vitro model of mesangial cells, grown in three-dimensional matrices, and incubated with light chains from patients with LCDD, showed a significant increase in tenascin-C expression, centrally located within the newly formed mesangial nodules.[51] These in vitro experiments also showed that transforming growth factor-β (TGF-β) overexpression results in an increased production of extracellular matrix components and that platelet derived growth factor-β is largely responsible for the proliferation of mesangial cells.[51–53]

Treatment and Outcomes

Treatment of plasma cell dyscrasias has changed significantly since the first reported cases of MIDD, thanks to advancements in treatment for MM and amyloidosis. The primary goal of therapy is to decrease the production of the monoclonal Ig to prevent ongoing paraprotein deposition in tissue and stabilize or improve the function of affected organs.[20] Similar to the many other rare diseases which lack large studies and randomized clinical trials, there is no standardized treatment for MIDD. Introduction of proteasome inhibitors (PI), and autologous stem cell transplantation in the treatment of MM, amyloidosis and subsequently MIDD, has dramatically changed outcomes.

If left untreated at presentation, patients who present with compromised renal function will almost invariably progress to end-stage kidney disease (ESKD) with progression taking as little as 2 months or up to 2 years in the series by Ganeval et al., in which long-term follow-up was available.[20] In a more recent series by Li et al., all seven patients with MIDD who presented with renal disease and did not receive treatment for their underlying hematologic disorder progressed to ESKD.[15] Alkylating agents (mainly melphalan) and prednisone were advocated as initial therapies in early series.[17,20] Using intermittent administration of melphalan and prednisone, a series by Heilman et al. showed overall[51–53] 5-year survival and renal survival rates of 70% and 37%, respectively. This is in contrast to untreated patients who show inevitable progression to ESKD. In addition, there was improvement in proteinuria in approximately one-third of patients receiving melphalan and prednisone and renal function either stabilized or improved in approximately two-thirds of patients with serum creatinines of less than 4.0 mg/dL. In patients with serum creatinine over 4 mg/dL, over 80% progressed to ESKD despite therapy. Duration of therapy in this series ranged from 3 months to 42 months and the best results were seen in the nine patients out of 19 who received more than a year of treatment.[17] Results in an early study by Pozzi et al. showed lower rate of response, albeit this case series had more aggressive hematologic malignancies with 11 of 19 patients meeting criteria for MM (vs. five of 19 patients with MM in the Heilman series).[17,34] In the Pozzi series, almost 80% of patients died within 37 months of observation despite all of the patients but one being treated with high-dose steroids and cytotoxic medications. Those with concomitant MM had worse outcomes.[34] Plasma exchange has been used as coadjuvant, but there is no consensus regarding its benefit and its usage has declined, perhaps driven by current recommendations on management in patients with MM.[40] In the early Pozzi series, plasma exchange did not appear to show benefits in the seven patients treated with plasma exchange and chemotherapy, because six of seven died within the first year.[34] In a later study from the same group, the use of chemotherapy plus plasma exchange was found to be a poor prognostic factor in terms of renal and overall survival.[8]

Recently, there have been major changes in our approach to treating MM, amyloidosis, and subsequently MIDD. Success using stem cell transplantation along with chemotherapy was reported in sporadic case reports, but a group from Italy reported five MIDD patients treated with stem cell transplantation and only one reached symptomatic renal failure during a median follow-up of 44 months; none of the five patients died over that period.[8] In 2004 Royer et al. published a retrospective study of 11 patients with LCDD or LHCDD in which patients were treated with high-dose therapy with the support of autologous stem cell transplant.[54] The protocol for mobilization of stem cells and the subsequent therapeutic protocol varied somewhat in the 11 patients based on when they were treated (before and after 1995) but in all cases, high-dose therapy was supported by the reinfusion of at least 2×10^6/kg CD34-positive cells. In eight of 10 patients who initially had a monoclonal gammopathy, high-dose therapy and autotransplantation produced a decrease in the level of monoclonal immunoglobulin. All three patients with nephrotic syndrome experienced remission. Within a median follow-up of 51 months, three patients were re-treated because of MM relapse; one died 93 months posttransplant because of progressive myeloma and one required hemodialysis.[54] Weichman et al., also reported encouraging results with high-dose melphalan and autologous stem cell transplant. In five cases with LCDD, during a median follow-up of 12 months (range 4–29 months), all patients remained alive and well. Complete hematologic response was achieved in 83% of the cases, and the median percentage reduction in proteinuria was 75.3% (range 38.7–89.3). All patients had normalization of their serum free light chain assays. In addition, there were no major side effects (Grade 4 toxicities) related to the therapy.[55] Firkin et al. described a patient with LCDD and incipient dialysis dependency who showed sustained improvement in renal function

resulting in discontinuation of dialysis after myeloablative melphalan and autologous stem cell transplant. This improvement in renal function and proteinuria was noted despite a repeat renal biopsy performed at 7 months after transplantation that did not show any diminution of the kappa light chain deposits. At 20 months after transplant, creatinine clearance had increased from 14 mL/min to 44 mL/min.[56] Series by Hassoun et al.[57] and Lorenz et al.[58] provided additional experience confirming the efficacy of high-dose chemotherapy and autologous stem cell transplant, and in both of these series, kidney transplantation was performed in a patient with ESKD who had achieved hematologic remission, with good follow-up results. With respect to potential toxicity of these regimens, one of these series reported the death of one patient caused by multiorgan failure at 26 days postautologous stem cell transplant.[58] Renal transplantation, although a viable consideration in patients with ESKD who have achieved hematologic remission, should not be considered in patients without the elimination of light chain production based on the experience at the Manchester Royal Infirmary and the Mayo Clinic.[59,60]

More recently, bortezomib is gaining an increased role in the treatment of MIDD. Bortezomib has multiple mechanisms with the potential to improve outcomes in patients with MIDD. Bortezomib both suppresses production of the responsible paraprotein and also inhibits the nuclear factor kappa-light-chain-enhancer of activated B cells pathway that appears to be involved in mesangial cell proliferation and mesangial sclerosis.[61–63] Bortezomib has also been shown to decrease levels of TGF-β1 levels, which are profibrotic and have been implicated in the pathogenesis of nodule formation in MIDD.[51–53] Bortezomib may also have a role in downregulating collagen and tissue inhibitor of metalloproteinases 1 production.[64] Thus bortezomib may decrease the progression of glomerulosclerosis, improve glomerular filtration rate, and reduce proteinuria by interrupting this cascade of events.[61] Bortezomib along with dexamethasone was shown to have excellent results in four patients in whom two of them were treatment naïve. There was complete hematologic response in two patients, whereas the others had a decrement in their free light chains of greater than 50%. Three of these patients later underwent autologous stem cell transplant and were disease free after 10 to 18 months of follow-up.[62] Another group reported on three patients with LCDD induced with bortezomib in combination with cyclophosphamide and dexamethasone. Because of severe side effects, the authors recommended a less aggressive approach with patients with LCDD than patients with MM.[65] In patients with recurrence of MIDD after renal transplantation, bortezomib (plus dexamethasone or lenalidomide and dexamethasone) has shown the ability to salvage the allograft with excellent long-term results, including continuing function for at least 10 years.[66] In patients with HCDD, bortezomib-based therapy seems to show encouraging results, with a recent series showing 70% of patients in reaching hematologic response and 90% with renal response.[9]

There is still significant variability in the treatments chosen for patients with MIDD, specifically in patients with LCDD as shown in the recent report by Sayed et al., in which multiple cytotoxic and immunomodulatory agents were used (thalidomide, lenalidomide, bortezomib, alkylator based, melphalan plus autologous stem cell transplant, and steroids alone). Nonetheless, complete remission (CR) was achieved more frequently in patients treated with bortezomib.[12] Similar success with bortezomib was reported in series by Cohen et al. and Kourelis et al. Regimens included bortezomib plus dexamethasone; bortezomib plus lenalidomide plus dexamethasone; bortezomib plus thalidomide plus dexamethasone; cyclophosphamide plus bortezomib plus dexamethasone; and high-dose melphalan followed by autologous stem cell transplant.[6,67] In the largest series to date with MIDD treated with bortezomib (49 patients of which 35 had LCDD; 12 HCDD; and 12 LHCDD), 25 were only treated with bortezomib. The overall hematologic response rate was 91%. With a median follow-up of 54 months, of 38 patients treated with bortezomib as first-line of therapy, only one had renal relapse after almost 53 months. Of the total cases, 53% of them achieved renal response with estimated glomerular filtration rate (eGFR) improvement of 35% and proteinuria decreasing from a median of 1.5 to 0.2 g/day.[67] Similarly, in the largest case series of patients with MIDD described, patients receiving autologous stem cell transplant or PI-based therapies were more likely to achieve CR or very good partial remission (VGPR) compared with those receiving other therapies (66% vs. 2%, $p < .0001$). In those patients achieving CR/VGPR, renal survival at 5 years was 77% compared with 54% of those achieving partial response (PR) or no response.[6]

Autologous stem cell transplant has a peritransplant mortality (within the first 100 days of engraftment) of less than 10%.[6,12] In the study by Sayed et al., among 11 patients not requiring dialysis, median eGFR before autologous stem cell transplant was 24 mL/min, which had increased among the 10 surviving patients to 38 mL/min by end of follow-up. Thirteen of 15 patients who survived autologous stem cell transplant achieved a hematologic CR and two achieved PR. Patients with CKD 5 not on dialysis did have worse outcomes.[12] In the study by Kourelis et al., overall outcomes were better in patients who underwent autologous stem cell transplant compared with those with PI and other treatments and were more likely to achieve at least a CR/VGPR: 77% for autologous stem cell transplant versus 56% for PI-based therapies versus 6% for other treatments, ($p < .0001$). Patients who achieved hematologic CR were more likely to achieve renal response as well.[6] In a retrospective study of four patients with MIDD on dialysis, high-dose melphalan and autologous stem cell transplant were analyzed. All of them underwent kidney transplant at a median of 2.6 years after the stem cell transplant and all patients were alive by the time of publishing in 2018. It was suggested by the authors that this therapy was feasible and toxicity and mortality seemed to be acceptable even in selected patients with ESKD secondary to MIDD.[68] The treatment of patients with MIDD should therefore have a multidisciplinary approach with both nephrologists and hematologists involved.

As presented previously, outcomes in MIDD are dependent to a large extent on the therapy provided. One subset of MIDD patients that merits specific mention is those who present with MIDD and coexisting light chain cast nephropathy. Patients with coexisting cast nephropathy have a significantly worse prognosis, both in terms of progression to ESKD and overall patient survival, compared with those without cast nephropathy.[1,18] When comparing outcomes,

especially when using some of the early literature, effort needs to be made to separate cases of "pure" MIDD from cases of MIDD with cast nephropathy. In general, patients with severe cardiac disease have worse prognosis as well.[16] Patients with pulmonary presentation, in whom a nodular pattern is observed, tend to have better prognosis compared with those with diffuse pulmonary LCDD.[31] Low hemoglobin at presentation is also associated with worse ESKD prognosis and worse survival,[2] and patients who present with more advanced renal failure tend to have a less robust renal response to therapy.[6,67]

Conclusions

MIDD is a relatively uncommon form of dysproteinemia related renal disease, appearing to occur at approximately half the rate of amyloidosis. Like amyloidosis, it can be a multisystem disease with cardiac, pulmonary, and liver involvement, although renal manifestations typically predominate. The most common histologic finding is that of nodular glomerulosclerosis with characteristic deposition of light and/or heavy chains along renal basement membranes. Whether MIDD develops in the setting of plasma cell dyscrasia appears to be largely dictated by the physiochemical properties of the light and heavy chains produced. N-glycosylation sites in light chains, CH1 deletion in heavy chains, and hydrophobic surface residues in both heavy and light chains appear to favor tissue deposition characteristic of MIDD. Therapy and prognosis have evolved considerably over the last several decades and the most successful current approaches appear to involve bortezomib and/or autologous stem cell transplant.

Key Points

- Monoclonal immunoglobulin deposition disease (MIDD) is characterized by the deposition of monoclonal light and/or heavy chains within glomerular, tubular, and vessel wall basement membranes. Nodular glomerulosclerosis is the most common histologic appearance of MIDD, but nodular sclerosis may be seen in only 60% of light chain deposition disease (LCDD), in contrast to virtually 100% of heavy chain deposition disease (HCDD).
- LCDD is approximately half as common as light chain amyloidosis, and in contrast to light chain amyloid, most LCDD (~ 80%) is caused by kappa light chains.
- Compared with LCDD, HCDD is more likely to present with nephrotic range proteinuria and hypocomplementemia and is less likely to be associated with multiple myeloma.
- Physiochemical alterations in paraproteins that cause MIDD include the addition of N-glycosylation sites, prominent surface hydrophobic residues that favor tissue deposition, and deletion of the CH1 domain in heavy chains of HCDD.
- Optimal treatment for MIDD remains to be determined, but the use of proteasome inhibitors and autologous stem cell transplantation has shown encouraging results with regards to both hematologic remission and improvement in renal function.

References

1. Lin J, Markowitz GS, Valeri AM, et al. Renal monoclonal immuno-globulin deposition disease: the disease spectrum. *J Am Soc Nephrol.* 2001;12:1482-1492.

2. Nasr SH, Valeri AM, Cornell LD, et al. Renal monoclonal immuno-globulin deposition disease: a report of 64 patients from a single insti-tution. *Clin J Am Soc Nephrol.* 2012;7:231-239.

3. Iványi B. Frequency of light chain deposition nephropathy relative to renal amyloidosis and Bence Jones cast nephropathy in a necropsy study of patients with myeloma. *Arch Pathol Lab Med.* 1990;114:986-987.

6. Kourelis TV, Nasr SH, Dispenzieri A, et al. Outcomes of patients with renal monoclonal immunoglobulin deposition disease. *Am J Hematol.* 2016;91:1123-1128.

7. Ronco P, Plaisier E, Mougenot B, Aucouturier P. Immunoglobulin light (heavy)-chain deposition disease: from molecular medicine to pathophysiology-driven therapy. *Clin J Am Soc Nephrol.* 2006;1:1342-1350.

8. Pozzi C, D'Amico M, Fogazzi GB, et al. Light chain deposition disease with renal involvement: clinical characteristics and prognostic factors. *Am J Kidney Dis.* 2003;42:1154-1163.

9. Bridoux F, Javaugue V, Bender S, et al. Unravelling the immunopatho-logical mechanisms of heavy chain deposition disease with implications for clinical management. *Kidney Int.* 2017;91:423-434.

10. Oe Y, Soma J, Sato H, Ito S. Heavy chain deposition disease: an over-view. *Clin Exp Nephrol.* 2013;17:771-778.

12. Sayed RH, Wechalekar AD, Gilbertson JA, et al. Natural history and outcome of light chain deposition disease. *Blood.* 2015;126:2805-2810.

13. Alexander MP, Nasr SH, Watson DC, Méndez GP, Rennke HG. Renal crescentic alpha heavy chain deposition disease: a report of 3 cases and review of the literature. *Am J Kidney Dis.* 2011;58:621-625.

14. Kambham N, Markowitz GS, Appel GB, Kleiner MJ, Aucouturier P, D'Agati VD. Heavy chain deposition disease: the disease spectrum. *Am J Kidney Dis.* 1999;33:954-962.

15. Li XM, Rui HC, Liang DD, et al. Clinicopathological characteristics and outcomes of light chain deposition disease: an analysis of 48 patients in a single Chinese center. *Ann Hematol.* 2016;95:901-909.

16. Buxbaum JN, Chuba JV, Hellman GC, Solomon A, Gallo GR. Monoclo-nal immunoglobulin deposition disease: light chain and light and heavy chain deposition diseases and their relation to light chain amy-loidosis. Clinical features, immunopathology, and molecular analysis. *Ann Intern Med.* 1990;112:455-464.

17. Heilman RL, Velosa JA, Holley KE, Offord KP, Kyle RA. Long-term follow-up and response to chemotherapy in patients with light-chain deposition disease. *Am J Kidney Dis.* 1992;20:34-41.

18. Zand L, Nasr SH, Gertz MA, et al. Clinical and prognostic differences among patients with light chain deposition disease, myeloma cast nephropathy and both. *Leuk Lymphoma.* 2015;56:3357-3364.

20. Ganeval D, Noël LH, Preud'homme JL, Droz D, Grünfeld JP. Light-chain deposition disease: its relation with AL-type amyloidosis. *Kidney Int.* 1984;26:1-9.

22. Buxbaum JN, Genega EM, Lazowski P, et al. Infiltrative nonamyloid-otic monoclonal immunoglobulin light chain cardiomyopathy: an underappreciated manifestation of plasma cell dyscrasias. *Cardiology.* 2000;93:220-228.

23. Ronco PM, Alyanakian MA, Mougenot B, Aucouturier P. Light chain deposition disease: a model of glomerulosclerosis defined at the mo-lecular level. *J Am Soc Nephrol.* 2001;12:1558-1565.

28. Bedossa P, Fabre M, Paraf F, Martin E, Lemaigre G. Light chain deposi-tion disease with liver dysfunction. *Hum Pathol.* 1988;19:1008-1014.

31. Bhargava P, Rushin JM, Rusnock EJ, et al. Pulmonary light chain de-position disease: report of five cases and review of the literature. *Am J Surg Pathol.* 2007;31:267-276.

34. Pozzi C, Fogazzi GB, Banfi G, Strom EH, Ponticelli C, Locatelli F. Renal disease and patient survival in light chain deposition disease. *Clin Nephrol.* 1995;43:281-287.

36. Skardelly M, Pantazis G, Bisdas S, et al. Primary cerebral low-grade B-cell lymphoma, monoclonal immunoglobulin deposition disease, cerebral light chain deposition disease and "aggregoma": an update on classification and diagnosis. *BMC Neurol.* 2013;13:107.

39. Liapis H, Papadakis I, Nakopoulou L. Nodular glomerulosclerosis secondary to mu heavy chain deposits. *Hum Pathol.* 2000;31:122-125.

40. Royal V, Quint P, Leblanc M, et al. IgD heavy-chain deposition disease: detection by laser microdissection and mass spectrometry. *J Am Soc Nephrol.* 2015;26:784-790.

41. Cogné M, Preud'homme JL, Bauwens M, Touchard G, Aucouturier P. Structure of a monoclonal kappa chain of the V kappa IV subgroup in the kidney and plasma cells in light chain deposition disease. *J Clin Invest.* 1991;87:2186-2190.

43. Denoroy L, Déret S, Aucouturier P. Overrepresentation of the V kappa IV subgroup in light chain deposition disease. *Immunol Lett.* 1994;42:63-66.

44. Déret S, Chomilier J, Huang DB, Preud'homme JL, Stevens FJ, Aucou-turier P. Molecular modeling of immunoglobulin light chains impli-cates hydrophobic residues in non-amyloid light chain deposition disease. *Protein Eng.* 1997;10:1191-1197.

45. Khamlichi AA, Rocca A, Touchard G, Aucouturier P, Preud'homme JL, Cogné M. Role of light chain variable region in myeloma with light chain deposition disease: evidence from an experimental model. *Blood.* 1995;86:3655-3659.

46. Moulin B, Deret S, Mariette X, et al. Nodular glomerulosclerosis with deposition of monoclonal immunoglobulin heavy chains lacking C(H)1. *J Am Soc Nephrol.* 1999;10:519-528.

47. Hendershot L, Bole D, Köhler G, Kearney JF. Assembly and secretion of heavy chains that do not associate posttranslationally with im-munoglobulin heavy chain-binding protein. *J Cell Biol.* 1987;104:761-767.

48. Cogné M, Silvain C, Khamlichi AA, Preud'homme JL. Structurally abnormal immunoglobulins in human immunoproliferative disor-ders. *Blood.* 1992;79:2181-2195.

49. Bruneval P, Foidart JM, Nochy D, Camilleri JP, Bariety J. Glomerular matrix proteins in nodular glomerulosclerosis in association with light chain deposition disease and diabetes mellitus. *Hum Pathol.* 1985;16:477-484.

50. Truong LD, Pindur J, Barrios R, et al. Tenascin is an important com-ponent of the glomerular extracellular matrix in normal and patho-logic conditions. *Kidney Int.* 1994;45:201-210.

51. Keeling J, Herrera GA. An in vitro model of light chain deposition disease. *Kidney Intl.* 2009;75:634-645.

52. Russell WJ, Cardelli J, Harris E, Baier RJ, Herrera GA. Monoclonal light chain—mesangial cell interactions: early signaling events and subse-quent pathologic effects. *Lab Invest.* 2001;81:689-703.

53. Zhu L, Herrera GA, Murphy-Ullrich JE, Huang ZQ, Sanders PW. Patho-genesis of glomerulosclerosis in light chain deposition disease. Role for transforming growth factor-beta. *Am J Pathol.* 1995;147:375-385.

54. Royer B, Arnulf B, Martinez F, et al. High dose chemotherapy in light chain or light and heavy chain deposition disease. *Kidney Int.* 2004;65:642-648.

55. Weichman K, Dember LM, Prokaeva T, et al. Clinical and molecular characteristics of patients with non-amyloid light chain deposition disorders, and outcome following treatment with high-dose melpha-lan and autologous stem cell transplantation. *Bone Marrow Trans-plant.* 2006;38:339-343.

56. Firkin F, Hill PA, Dwyer K, Gock H. Reversal of dialysis-dependent renal failure in light-chain deposition disease by autologous periph-eral blood stem cell transplantation. *Am J Kidney Dis.* 2004;44:551-555.

57. Hassoun H, Flombaum C, D'Agati VD, et al. High-dose melphalan and auto-SCT in patients with monoclonal Ig deposition disease. *Bone Marrow Transplant.* 2008;42:405-412.

58. Lorenz EC, Gertz MA, Fervenza FC, et al. Long-term outcome of au-tologous stem cell transplantation in light chain deposition disease. *Nephrol Dial Transplant.* 2008;23:2052-2057.

59. Leung N, Lager DJ, Gertz MA, Wilson K, Kanakiriya S, Fervenza FC. Long-term outcome of renal transplantation in light-chain deposition disease. *Am J Kidney Dis.* 2004;43:147-153.

61. Jimenez-Zepeda VH. Light chain deposition disease: novel biological insights and treatment advances. *Int J Lab Hematol.* 2012;34:347-355.

62. Kastritis E, Migkou M, Gavriatopoulou M, Zirogiannis P, Hadjikonstantinou V, Dimopoulos MA. Treatment of light chain deposition disease with bortezomib and dexamethasone. *Haemato-logica.* 2009;94:300-302.

63. Keeling J, Herrera GA. The mesangium as a target for glomerulopathic light and heavy chains: pathogenic considerations in light and heavy chain-mediated glomerular damage. *Contrib Nephrol.* 2007;153:116-134.

64. Fineschi S, Reith W, Guerne PA, Dayer JM, Chizzolini C. Proteasome block-ade exerts an antifibrotic activity by coordinately down-regulating type I collagen and tissue inhibitor of metalloproteinase-1 and up-regulating metalloproteinase-1 production in human dermal fibroblasts. *FASEB J.* 2006;20:562-564.

65. Minarik J, Scudla V, Tichy T, et al. Induction treatment of light chain deposition disease with bortezomib: rapid hematological response with persistence of renal involvement. *Leuk Lymphoma.* 2012;53:330-331.

66. Kuppachi S, Holanda D, Thomas CP. Light chain deposition disease after kidney transplantation with long graft survival: case report. *Transplant Proc.* 2016;48:255-258.

67. Cohen C, Royer B, Javaugue V, et al. Bortezomib produces high hema-tological response rates with prolonged renal survival in monoclonal immunoglobulin deposition disease. *Kidney Int.* 2015;88:1135-1143.

68. Batalini F, Econimo L, Quillen K, et al. High-dose melphalan and stem cell transplantation in patients on dialysis due to immunoglobulin light-chain amyloidosis and monoclonal immunoglobulin deposition disease. *Biol Blood Marrow Transplant.* 2018;24:127-132.

A full list of references is available at Expertconsult.com

10 Fibrillary and Immunotactoid Glomerulonephritis

WAI L. LAU AND ANDREW S. BOMBACK

Fibrillary Glomerulonephritis

OVERVIEW AND EPIDEMIOLOGY

Fibrillary glomerulonephritis (FGN) was first described in 1977. It is a rare disease, with incidence of less than 1% of native kidney biopsies. It is mostly a disease of Caucasians, with more than 90% of patients in the two largest series self-identified as white. Clinically, the patient with FGN can present with hypertension, proteinuria (full nephrotic syndrome [NS] in up to 50% of patients), hematuria, and renal insufficiency. The mean age of presentation is 55 to 60 years of age.

DIAGNOSIS

Currently, a diagnosis of FGN can only be made via kidney biopsy. On light microscopy, the patterns of injury include mesangioproliferative, membranoproliferative, diffuse proliferative, membranous, diffuse sclerosing, and crescentic forms of glomerulonephritis, although the crescentic variant is only rarely encountered (Fig. 10.1A). Congo red staining is negative. On immunofluorescence, immunoglobulin (Ig)G (most cases are polyclonal), kappa and lambda light chains, and complement are present and often have a "smudgy" appearance. On electron microscopy, randomly arranged fibrillary deposits, 16 to 24 nm in diameter (larger than amyloid), are seen in the mesangium and capillary walls (Fig. 10.1B).[1-3]

ETIOLOGY

Laser microdissection and mass spectrometry have provided further information on the composition of the classic fibrillary deposits of FGN. This process involves the extraction of glomerular protein, digestion, and identification of the protein constituents via amino acid sequencing. Apoprotein E, serum amyloid P, and Ig heavy/chain C region are some of the identifiable proteins that can help distinguish amyloidosis from FGN from immunotactoid glomerulonephritis (ITGN).[4] The recent discovery of DNAJB9 in the glomeruli of FGN patients by mass spectrometry and use of anti-DNAJB9 antibodies for immunofluorescence/immunohistochemistry will likely transform the diagnosis of this disease and allow for potential therapeutic targets. DNAJB9 is a member of a family of cochaperones to heat shock proteins, which play an important role in the proper folding/unfolding/translocation/degradation of key cellular protein constituents.[5,6] All these tools are particularly useful since the recent finding of congophilic cases of fibrillary GN. Eighteen of such scenarios were described by the Mayo clinic- this accounted for about 4% of the fibrillary GN cases there.[7]

Most FGN cases at this time are considered idiopathic. In a series of 66 FGN cases from the Mayo Clinic, 15 (23%) were associated with malignancy (mostly carcinomas, including six with multiple myeloma). Ten (15%) were associated with autoimmune disease (Crohn, systemic lupus erythematosus, Graves disease, idiopathic thrombocytopenic purpura, primary biliary cholangitis, ankylosing spondylitis, scleroderma, and Sjögren). Two patients (3%) were hepatitis C positive.[3] A series of 42 FGN patients (26% black) from the University of North Carolina included seven of 26 (27%) testing positive for hepatitis C with no detectable cryoglobulinemia. These patients had the poorest outcome, with all but one proceeding to end-stage renal disease (ESRD). They did not receive antiviral therapy or rituximab.[8] There is one reported case of FGN associated with tuberculosis-related osteomyelitis.[9]

TREATMENT

Aside from treating an underlying disorder in secondary cases, immunosuppressive (IS) agents including corticosteroids (CS), cyclophosphamide (CYT), mycophenolate, cyclosporine (CyA), azathioprine, and rituximab (RTX) have been used with limited success in the largest series in the literature from the Mayo Clinic. Creatinine at presentation was 2.1 mg/dL, and 29/61 patients were treated with IS: complete/partial renal response (CR/PR) were seen in less than 10%, and at least 40% had "persistent renal dysfunction" or went on to ESRD.[3] In a French series of 27 FGN cases in which 13 received IS, there were six PRs (decrease of proteinuria by at least 50% with stable glomerular filtration rate [GFR]): five with RTX and one with CYT.[10] A case series from Columbia, reporting 12 FGN patients with mean creatinine 2.1 (GFR 39 mL/min) treated with RTX, found only four of 12 had no progression of disease. These nonprogressors had the mildest disease at the time of RTX treatment by clinical parameters (i.e., highest estimated GFR and lowest proteinuria).[11] In an earlier Columbia series of 61 FGN patients, the majority of subjects did not respond to IS (CS, CYT, CyA), although it is noted that the mean presenting

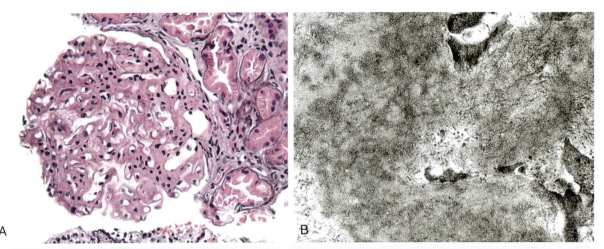

Fig. 10.1 Fibrillary glomerulonephritis. A, A glomerulus showing infiltration by eosinophilic material, which is expanding mesangial areas and segmentally infiltrating glomerular capillaries. The proliferative pattern in this case is predominantly mesangial. Mesangial areas and glomerular basement membranes typically stain black with a silver stain. In this case, the native matrix has been largely infiltrated and replaced by fibrillary deposits, which are also involving glomerular basement membranes. Jones silver stain, 400x. **B,** Electron microscopy shows an admixture of fibrils and more granular electron dense deposits. The fibrils are randomly oriented with mean diameter typically ranging from 16-24 nm, typically larger than amyloid fibrils. Electron Microscopy, 68000x. (Images provided by Leal Herlitz, MD, Department of Pathology, Cleveland Clinic Foundation.)

creatinine was 3.1 mg/dL.[2] In a series of eight reported crescentic FGN cases treated with CS and CYT, six of eight (75%) patients went on to ESRD.[12] Hence the overall prognosis is guarded at best.

TRANSPLANTATION

The reported incidence of FGN recurrence in the allograft is varied. In the Mayo series, five of 14 (36%) recurred.[3] In a more recent series from Australia and New Zealand, only one of 13 (8%) patients had recurrence.[13] In an older series of 12 FGN patients who underwent kidney transplantation, reduced allograft and patient survival was observed in those with untreated concomitant monoclonal gammopathy.[14]

Immunotactoid Glomerulonephritis

OVERVIEW AND EPIDEMIOLOGY

ITGN is tenfold less common than FGN, representing only 0.06% of all native kidney biopsies. Patients with ITGN can present with proteinuria (NS in up to 70%), microscopic hematuria, renal insufficiency, and hypertension. The average age of presentation is 60 years.

DIAGNOSIS

The diagnosis of ITGN requires a kidney biopsy. On light microscopy, the patterns of injury seen include membranoproliferative, diffuse proliferative, and membranous glomerulonephritis. Immunofluorescence staining shows the presence of IgG or IgM (often monoclonal), kappa and lambda light chains, and complement. On electron microscopy, there are glomerular microtubules measuring 30 to 50 nm in diameter (larger than FGN or amyloidosis) in parallel arrangement, located predominantly in the subepithelial and subendothelial space (Fig. 10.2). Cryoglobulin

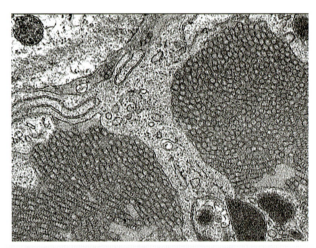

Fig. 10.2 Immunotactoid glomerulonephritis. Electron microscopy of glomerulus showing the more organized, microtubular substructure (30-50 nm) of immunotactoid glomerulonephritis. This contrasts the smaller, haphazard fibrils seen in fibrillary glomerulonephritis. Electron Microscopy, 60000x. (Image provided by Leal Herlitz, MD, Department of Pathology, Cleveland Clinic Foundation.)

deposits on electron microscopy can be indistinguishable from ITGN and must be excluded clinically.[17]

ETIOLOGY

The cause of ITGN is unclear. It was once thought that FGN and ITG were related entities. But compared with FGN, there is greater likelihood of hypocomplementemia, monoclonal gammopathy (63% vs. 17% in the Mayo series), and lymphoproliferative disease (especially chronic lymphocytic leukemia) in ITGN.[15] A few cases of ITGN have been associated with human immunodeficiency virus (HIV) (+/-hepatitis C).[16] Also of note is the absence of DNAJB9 protein in ITG disease.

TREATMENT

Given the high association with hematologic disorders, chemotherapy directed against the underlying lymphoproliferative disorder, if identified, is paramount. In the French series of 14 ITGN patients (mean presenting creatinine 1.5 mg/dL), seven were found to have a B cell hematologic disorder. Chemotherapy with or without a stem cell transplantation led to "NS remission" in five of seven patients.[18] Even a partial remission of the hematologic disease has led to complete renal remission.[19] In the Mayo series of 12 ITGN patients with mean baseline creatinine of 1.5 and follow-up of 4 years, six of 12 patients treated with CS/chemotherapy for hematologic condition/RTX/CYT/velcade achieved CR/PR. The overall prognosis for ITGN appears better than for FGN in the two Mayo series. At 48 months, 17% of ITGN patients progressed to ESRD versus 44% FGN group at 52 months follow-up.[3,15] The few cases of reported HIV-positive ITGN patients have showed variable responses to antiretroviral therapy, CS, and angiotensin-converting enzyme inhibitor.[16]

TRANSPLANTATION

Data on allograft fate after kidney transplantation are sparse given the rarity of disease. Recurrence has ranged from 25% in the Australia and New Zealand series[10] to 50% in another small report from the United States.[20]

Key Points

- Fibrillary and immunotactoid glomerulonephritis are rare forms of glomerular disease that can be associated with malignancy, including monoclonal gammopathies.
- Fibrillary glomerulonephritis can present with hypertension, proteinuria (full nephrotic syndrome [NS] in up to 50% of patients), hematuria, and renal insufficiency. Diagnosis is made by kidney biopsy.
- Fibrillary glomerulonephritis is treated with immunosuppressive agents including corticosteroids, cyclophosphamide, mycophenolate, cyclosporine, azathioprine, and rituximab with limited success.
- Patients with immunotactoid glomerulonephritis can present with proteinuria (NS in up to 70%), microscopic hematuria, renal insufficiency, and hypertension. Diagnosis requires a kidney biopsy.
- Given the high association of immunotactoid glomerulonephritis with hematologic disorders, chemotherapy directed against the underlying lymphoproliferative disorder, if identified, is paramount.

References

1. Motwani, SS, Helitz L, Monga D, Jhaveri KD, Lam AQ, American Society of Nephrology Onco-Nephrology Forum. Paraprotein related kidney disease: glomerular disease associated with paraproteinemias. *Clin J Am Soc Nephrol.* 2016;11:2260-2272.
2. Rosenstock JL, Markowitz GS, Valeri AM, Sacchi G, Appel GB, D'Agati VD. Fibrillary and immunotactoid glomerulonephropathy. Distinct entities with different clinical and pathological features. *Kidney Int.* 2003;63:1450-1461.
3. Nasr SH, Valer AM, Cornell LD, et al. Fibrillary glomerulonephropathy: 66 cases from single institution. *J Am Soc Nephrol.* 2011;6:775-784.
4. Sethi S, Theis JD, Vrana JA, et al. Laser microdissection and proteomic analysis of amyloidosis, cryoglobulin glomerulonephritis, fibrillary and immunotactoid glomerulonephritis. *Clin J Am Soc Nephrol.* 2013;8:915-921.
5. Nasr SH, Vrana JA, Dasari S, et al. DNAJB9 is a specific immunohistochemical marker for fibrillary glomerulonephritis. *Kidney Int Rep.* 2018;1:56-64.
6. Andeen NK, Yang HY, Dai DF, MacCoss MJ, Smith KD. DNAJ homolog subfamily B member 9 is a putative autoantigen in fibrillary GN. *J Am Soc Nephrol.* 2018;29:231-239.
7. Alexander MP, Dasari S, Vrana JA, et al. Congophilic fibrillary glomerulonephritis: a case series. *Am J Kidney Dis.* 2018;72(3):325-336.
8. Payan Schober F, Jobson MA, Poulton CJ, et al. Clinical features and outcomes of a racially diverse population in fibrillary glomerulonephropathy. *Am J Nephrol.* 2017;45:248-256.
9. Lui X, Liu H, Zhao Z, Zhang Z, Ding X. Fibrillary glomerulonephritis complicated by membranous nephropathy in a patient with tuberculosis. *Int Urol Nephrol.* 2013;45:1501-1504.
10. Javaugue V, Karras A, Glowacki F, et al. Long-term kidney disease outcomes in fibrillary glomerulonephritis: case series of 27 patients. *Am J Kidney Dis.* 2013;62:679-690.
11. Hogan J, Restivo M, Canetta PA, et al. Rituximab treatment in fibrillary glomerulonephritis. *Nephrol Dial Transplant.* 2014;29:1925-1931.
12. Shah HH, Thakkar J, Pullman JM, Mathew AT. Fibrillary glomerulonephritis presenting as crescentic glomerulonephritis. *Indian J Nephrol.* 2017;27:157-160.
13. Mallett A, Tang W, Hart G, et al. End stage kidney disease due to fibrillary glomerulophritis and immunotactoid glomerulonephritis: outcomes in 66 ANZ data registry consecutive cases. *Am J Nephrol.* 2015;42:177-184.
14. Czarnecki PG, Lager DJ, Leung N, Dispenzieri A, Cosio FG, Fervenza FC. Long-term outcomes of kidney transplantation in patients with fibrillary glomerulonephritis or monoclonal gammopathy with fibrillary deposits. *Kidney Int.* 2009;75:420-427.
15. Nasr SH, Cornell LD, Leung N, et al. Immunotactoid glomerulonephritis. *Nephrol Dial Transplant.* 2012;27:4137-4146.
16. Chen C, Jhaveri KD, Hartono C, Seshan SV. An uncommon glomerular disease in an HIV patient. *Clin Nephrol.* 2011;75:80-88.
17. Alpers CE, Kowalewska J. Fibrillary and immunotactoid glomerulonephritis. *J Am Soc Nephrol.* 2008;19:34-37.
18. Bridoux F, Hugue V, Coldefy O, et al. Fibrillary and immunotactoid glomerulonephropathy are associated with distinct immunologic features. *Kidney Int.* 2002;62:1764-1775.
19. Witzens-Harig M, Waldherr R, Beimler J, et al. Long-term remission of paraprotein induced immunotactoid glomerulonephropathy after high dose therapy and autologous blood stem cell transplantation. *Ann Hematol.* 2007;86:927-930.
20. Korbet BF, Rosenberg BF, Schwartz MM, Lewis EJ. Course of renal transplantation in immunotactoid glomerulophritis. *Am J Med.* 1990;89:91-95.

Hematopoietic Stem Cell Associated Kidney Disease

11 Hematopoietic Cell Transplant Associated Kidney Injury

CATHERINE JOSEPH, JOSEPH R. ANGELO, BENJAMIN L. LASKIN, AND SANGEETA HINGORANI

Kidney Injury in Graft Versus Host Disease

INTRODUCTION

Hematopoietic cell transplant (HCT) is a commonly used procedure to treat both malignant and nonmalignant conditions. As transplant methods have improved, the overall survival of patients following HCT has also improved. However, morbidities associated with HCT remain a significant problem, and acute kidney injury (AKI) and chronic kidney disease (CKD) occur frequently after transplant, affecting between 10% and 70% of transplant recipients.[1] Multiple risk factors and exposures contribute to the onset of kidney injury after HCT, including preconditioning chemotherapy, calcineurin inhibitors, other potentially nephrotoxic medications, radiation nephritis, and sinusoidal obstruction syndrome. Endothelial injury is a pathophysiologic pathway leading to post-HCT kidney injury, and kidney involvement in the setting of graft-versus-host disease (GVHD) has been proposed as a potential mechanism of both AKI and chronic kidney injury.

There can be significant overlap with several of these processes contributing to multifactorial mechanisms of kidney injury and clear distinction of the underlying cause can be difficult in the clinical setting. Related to this, there is some controversy regarding the direct involvement of GVHD in AKI and chronic kidney injury. However, there is evidence in both animal models and humans that GVHD can involve the kidney and is a significant contributing factor to AKI and CKD.[2] In addition, thrombotic microangiopathy (TMA) has become an established mechanism of kidney injury after HCT, but diagnosis requires a high index of suspicion because the signs and symptoms of TMA can overlap with other common complications of HCT, such as anemia and thrombocytopenia. TMA now replaces an older term, "*bone marrow transplant nephropathy*," which described an entity characterized by late occurrence of renal insufficiency post-HCT, anemia, and hypertension (HTN), and with pathologic findings of mesangial hypercellularity, mesangial matrix expansion, mesangiolysis, widening of the subendothelial space, red blood cell (RBC) trapping, and fibrosis.[3,4]

As further details of the varied pathophysiologic mechanisms of kidney injury after HCT are being elucidated, the importance of more explicitly defining the underlying cause of this injury has become clear so that prevention and treatment approaches can target these specific pathways. This chapter will focus on the contribution of GVHD and TMA to the kidney injury seen after HCT.

GRAFT-VERSUS-HOST DISEASE PATHOPHYSIOLOGY

(GVHD is a potentially life-threatening complication of HCT and occurs commonly after transplant. GVHD occurs when immunocompetent donor T-cells recognize recipient tissue antigens resulting in immune activation and subsequent cytolytic destruction of target antigen bearing cells.[5] Classically, the epithelial tissue of the skin, liver, and gastrointestinal (GI) tract have been considered the major target organs in GVHD. However, there is evidence that the kidney is a target in GVHD and that similar cellular and molecular processes in the kidney drive the initiation and progression of kidney GVHD.[6] In addition, there can be overlap between other causes of kidney injury with the pathologic changes seen in GVHD, potentially indicating a link between GVHD and the common clinical presentations of kidney disease seen post-HCT, such as glomerulonephritis and TMA.

T-cells are considered the traditional effectors in GVHD and T-cell involvement in GVHD has been shown in animal models. In these models, histologic evaluation shows infiltration of the kidney with CD3+, CD4+, C8+, and FoxP3+ T-cells along with associated endarteritis, interstitial nephritis, tubulitis, and glomerulitis.[7] In a rat model of acute GVHD, similar histologic findings were seen, as well as elevated levels of serum blood urea nitrogen and urinary N-acetyl-β-D-glucosaminidase, indicators of kidney dysfunction.[8] There is evidence that alterations in expression of major histocompatibility complex molecules and increased presentation of such antigens by antigen presenting cells are involved in the pathogenesis of GVHD.[9,10] In addition, recruitment of T-cells to the endothelium of target organs by chemokines and adhesion molecules can be involved in initiating GVHD.[11] In a study comparing expression of genes related to T-cell associated pathways in GVHD, similar genes were seen to be expressed in both the liver, a classic target of GVHD, and the kidney.[12]

In addition to direct T-cell mediated damage, proinflammatory cytokines have also been implicated in the pathogenesis of GVHD. Although the diffuse nature of GVHD with multiple organs targeted suggests that this is a systemic inflammatory process, there is evidence that the kidney produces a localized inflammatory environment, which promotes both acute and chronic changes within the kidney. This is supported by the presence of elevated gene expression and urinary levels of cytokines such as tumor necrosis factor (TNF)-α, interleukin (IL)-1, IL-2, IL-6, and IL-10, and other markers of local tissue inflammation, such as elafin, which has been shown to be marker of GVHD and is elevated in the urine of patients with AKI and chronic kidney injury post-HCT.[13,14] Beyond the acute period, histologic signs of inflammation associated with chronic kidney damage including tubular atrophy, peritubular capillary loss, and interstitial fibrosis have been reported.[15] Clinically, the presence of GVHD has been associated with CKD.[16]

Finally, B-cells are also involved in the pathogenesis of GVHD. Supporting this is the identification of both auto- and alloantibodies in patients with chronic GVHD.[17,18] From a kidney GVHD standpoint, kidney biopsies from patients after HCT have shown positive staining for C4d in peritubular capillaries, which is a marker for antibody mediated rejection in kidney transplantation.[19,20] This finding suggests that there is a humoral component in GVHD, and that the kidney might have specific antigenic targets that trigger GVHD within the kidney.

Together, these data provide evidence for the idea that kidney involvement in GVHD is not only related to the generalized processes of systemic inflammation and diffuse endothelial damage in multiple organs, but also more specifically related to changes within the kidney itself that can drive local changes, resulting in AKI and chronic kidney injury. In addition, many of the GVHD-associated pathways seen in the kidney are similar to those seen in other organs thought to be major targets of GVHD, suggesting that the kidney may also be a primary focus where GVHD can occur. Although the pathophysiology of kidney GVHD clearly has overlap with other etiologies of post-HCT kidney injury, such as TMA, these findings also suggest that some of the pathologic changes seen in kidney GVHD are unique, potentially indicating that kidney GVHD is a distinct entity. Consideration of kidney GVHD in this more specific way could allow for targeted diagnostic and treatment approaches.

Graft-Versus-Host Disease Risk Factors

Although a detailed review of systemic GVHD risk factors is beyond the scope of this chapter, a brief overview is important to understanding the association between GVHD and kidney injury. In addition, there is overlap between the risk factors for GVHD and for kidney injury after HCT, further linking GVHD and kidney disease in the setting of HCT. Risk factors for acute GVHD include the degree of human leukocyte antigen (HLA) mismatch, receipt of a transplant from an unrelated donor, female donor for a male recipient, the use of peripheral blood stem cell grafts, and the intensity of the conditioning regimen.[21] Risk factors for chronic GVHD, defined by the presence of GVHD beyond 100 days post-transplant, include a prior episode of acute GVHD, receipt of peripheral blood stem cell grafts, grafts from female donors to male recipients, HLA disparity, older age of either recipient or donor, and a primary diagnosis of chronic myeloid leukemia.[21] Identification of individuals at increased risk for GVHD provides an opportunity for heightened awareness of kidney injury in these patients allowing for closer monitoring and early intervention.

Kidney Manifestations of Graft-Versus-Host Disease

Scoring systems for severity of GVHD typically focus on the three main target organs: skin, liver, and GI tract. However, as alluded to previously, GVHD has been shown to be an independent risk factor for AKI and chronic kidney injury. Clinically, GVHD can present as various forms of kidney disease including AKI, nephrotic syndrome (NS), glomerulonephritis, and TMA.

The most commonly accepted manifestation of kidney GVHD is as NS, characterized by a high degree of proteinuria, hypoalbuminemia, and edema. Among those presenting with NS the most common underlying pathology is membranous nephropathy (MN), with approximately 60% to 80% of patients having this diagnosis.[22,23] Histologic findings of MN post-HCT are similar to those seen in MN in other settings, including subepithelial deposits made up of antigen-antibody complexes. Minimal change associated with NS is the next most common pathology seen in patients after HCT.[24] Less commonly reported pathologic findings in post-HCT NS patients are membranoproliferative, glomerulonephritis, focal segmental glomerulosclerosis, and immunoglobulin A nephropathy.[1,24,25] The typical timeframe for presentation of NS is 6 to 12 months post-transplant.[26] Of note, the timing of the appearance of NS post-HCT is temporally associated with the discontinuation of prophylaxis for GVHD.[27] This is somewhat in contrast to the previous idea that "Bone Marrow Transplant (BMT) associated nephropathy" was strictly a multifactorial process that included renal toxicity related to calcineurin inhibitor exposure. In addition, NS post-HCT rarely occurs without the presence of GVHD, and also can occur in the absence of GVHD in other sites, suggesting kidney specific targeting in the setting of GVHD.[28] Regarding MN, a case report by Cho et al. examined patients, all with GVHD, presenting with MN-associated NS following HCT for serum antiphospholipase A2 receptor, an antibody that has been associated with both primary and secondary MN.[29] None of the seven MN patients had detectable levels of the antibody.[30] Such findings suggest that although overlap may exist between NS seen post-HCT and the development of NS in other settings, there may be unique aspects of these processes associated with GVHD.

TMA is also a common clinical presentation after HCT. Several risk factors for TMA have been identified, including total body irradiation (TBI), exposure to calcineurin inhibitors, combined use of tacrolimus and sirolimus, HCT-associated infections, performance of HCT for nonmalignant conditions, and transplantation of peripheral blood stem cells.[31] In addition, GVHD has been independently associated with TMA.[32] Because endothelial damage is a primary feature of TMA, one hypothesis linking TMA and GVHD is that, similar to other organ systems, the vascular endothelium is a target in GVHD.[33] Lending further support to this are previously mentioned findings in the renal capillaries, including C4d and cytotoxic T-cells, and evidence of complement activation, all suggesting immune targeting of the recipient endothelium by donor graft cells is involved in the pathophysiology of posttransplant TMA.[20,34] As with TMA in other clinical settings, activation of the TMA cascade then results in AKI and, subsequently, the potential for chronic kidney changes as the acute inflammation progresses to fibrosis with loss of functional glomeruli and renal tubules.

Although the development of CKD post-HCT is likely multifactorial owing to exposure to TBI and nephrotoxic medications, such as calcineurin inhibitors, infections and sepsis, and recurrent episodes of AKI, GVHD has also been shown to be independently associated with CKD. The triggering of multiple inflammatory pathways following immunologic targeting of the kidney in the setting of GVHD ultimately can lead to fibrosis and irreversible kidney damage.[1,16] This is particularly true when GVHD is chronic and therefore immune-mediated renal damage occurs over a prolonged time course.

GVHD is a common secondary effect of HCT and can cause significant detrimental kidney outcomes, emphasizing the importance of pursuing a detailed investigation for the clinical effects of GVHD on the kidney.

Evaluation

As noted, GVHD is a multisystem condition characterized by symptoms reflecting damage to each of the major organs involved, including maculopapular rash, hyperbilirubinemia, cholestasis, jaundice, nausea, abdominal pain, diarrhea, vomiting, and anorexia.[5] Although the kidney is not classified as a major target of GVHD, and kidney disease is not included in the grading of GVHD, as previously noted, the presence of GVHD in other organs is a risk factor for the development of kidney GVHD. Therefore the presence of systemic GVHD should raise suspicion for involvement of the kidney as well. Similar to other clinical scenarios, when evaluating for kidney injury, initial laboratory results should include markers of kidney function with serum creatinine (SCr) and serum electrolytes. Because there are many factors that can affect the accuracy of SCr as a measure of glomerular filtration rate (GFR) in this patient population, such as relatively poor nutrition or decreased muscle mass, cystatin C has also been proposed as an additional marker of GFR and formulas exist to use SCr and cystatin C in conjunction to provide a more accurate estimate of GFR.[14,35,36]

Urinary studies should include a urinalysis and urine microalbumin to urine creatinine ratio for the presence of hematuria and proteinuria. Microalbuminuria is defined as 30 to 299 milligrams of albumin to grams of creatinine in a spot urine sample. Macroalbuminuria is defined as a urinary albumin-to-creatinine level of more than 300 mg/g Cr. If patients are able to accurately collect a sample for 24 hours, a 24-hour urine for urinary albumin levels can also help better define the degree of albuminuria. This does require more effort on the part of patients and can be challenging to accurately obtain in some groups, such as small children. Recent consensus guidelines suggest monitoring for albuminuria at day +80 post-HCT and then annually. For patients with macroalbuminuria on initial screening, more frequent monitoring at intervals of 3 to 6 months is suggested.[37] Other important measures are determination of active TMA markers, including complete blood count, lactate dehydrogenase (LDH), haptoglobin, and peripheral blood smear for schistocytes.

When investigating for GVHD-related kidney damage, markers of endothelial and glomerular dysfunction, such as urinary albumin, can be important to determine the underlying etiology and to predict long-term outcomes. The presence of microalbuminuria and macroalbuminuria in the first 100 days after HCT have both been associated with increased risk of death at 1 year posttransplant. Similarly, the presence of albuminuria during this period has also been associated with increased risk of progression to CKD.[38]

HTN is another common complication of HCT, with as many as 70% of patients developing HTN in the first 2 years following transplant.[39,40] It is relatively easy to diagnose and, like albuminuria, has been associated with negative long-term outcomes, including CKD and increased risk of death.[30,39,41] Monitoring for HTN should be performed during the period that patients are admitted post-HCT, then at each outpatient clinic visit. Twenty-four hour ambulatory blood pressure monitoring (ABPM) should also be used to more accurately measure blood pressure and evaluate for white coat and masked HTN. The importance and utility of 24-hour ABPM has been emphasized recently in the clinical guidelines for screening for HTN in children and adolescents, and ABPM provides similar advantages in the adult population.[42] The presence of chronic HTN can have significant effects on kidney and cardiovascular health and therefore early diagnosis is important.

Although there can be risks in the post-HCT population, a kidney biopsy should be strongly considered for those patients with signs of kidney injury after transplant. A kidney biopsy may support evidence of kidney involvement in GVHD and will also provide information about other etiologies of posttransplant kidney disease, such as TMA and viral infections. Most importantly, diagnosis of the underlying cause of kidney disease allows for a treatment plan that more accurately targets the specific pathology. Because many of the processes in the kidney after HCT are inflammatory in nature, early identification and treatment to quiet disease activity can reduce the amount of fibrosis that forms because of prolonged inflammation and therefore decrease the risk of developing irreversible chronic kidney injury. A kidney biopsy can provide information that is not otherwise obtainable and is an invaluable tool in caring for patients following HCT.

Treatment

Treatment of GVHD-associated renal disease starts with prevention and treatment of systemic GVHD. Typical immunosuppressive medications used for GVHD prophylaxis include the calcineurin inhibitors (CNI) cyclosporine and tacrolimus, which target transcription factors involved in IL-2 production, reducing IL-2 levels and, thereby, blocking the activation of T-cells. Methotrexate, a folate antagonist, is often used in conjunction with CNI, and the combination of these two drugs has been shown to decrease the incidence of both acute and chronic GVHD.[43] Other drugs targeting T-cell activation include cyclophosphamide and the mammalian target of rapamycin (mTOR) inhibitor rapamycin. Both of these drugs work by inhibiting the expansion of or depleting conventional T-cells with relatively less activity against regulatory T-cells.[44,45] In addition to T-cell inhibitory strategies, T-cell depleting therapies, such as rabbit antithymocyte globulin (ATG), are used to reduce the development of GVHD and have been shown to be effective when used in conjunction with standard prophylaxis.[46,47]

Cell-based therapies, which aim to reduce donor T-cell immune activity by generating a more regulatory T-cell milieu, have also been investigated.[48]

In spite of prophylaxis, GVHD can still occur. In this case glucocorticoids represent first-line therapy and responsiveness to steroids is an important prognostic marker for patients with GVHD. Those with glucocorticoid resistant GVHD have increased mortality risk. Although there is no standardized second-line therapy for glucocorticoid resistant GVHD, other immunomodulatory therapies have been investigated, including antibodies directed against T-cell antigens, such as gavilimomab.[5]

A key component in the treatment of patients that develop kidney injury after HCT is symptomatic control of proteinuria and HTN. Angiotensin-converting enzyme inhibitors (ACE-I) or angiotensin receptor blockers (ARB) are ideally suited to address both of these problems, because they are not only effective in treating HTN, but also have antiproteinuric properties.[38] In addition, there is evidence that ACE-I or ARB have long-term renoprotective effects, which slow progression of CKD. Specific to the NS seen post-HCT, this effect has been shown to be particularly effective in proteinuric nephropathies.[49,50]

An important consideration in the prevention and treatment of GVHD related to the kidney is that markers of disease activity can be monitored. As noted, urinary albumin excretion, HTN, and serum markers of kidney function have been shown to be good markers of kidney disease following HCT. These indicators are relatively easy to obtain and may help guide duration of prophylaxis and possibly allow for earlier initiation of treatment. In this way, monitoring of kidney changes can provide additional data regarding the onset and activity of GVHD in other organs.

Owing to the complexity of its pathophysiology, the prevention and treatment of GVHD require a multifaceted approach that targets a variety of pathways involved in the process of GVHD. Reducing the incidence of GVHD could provide protection to the kidney after HCT, therefore reducing the occurrence of AKI and chronic kidney injury posttransplant.

Conclusion

There are many potential mediators of kidney injury after HCT, and interactions between them adds significant complexity. GVHD is one factor that has been shown to generate injury within the kidney and has been associated with acute kidney disease and CKD after HCT. This relationship highlights the importance of pretransplant evaluation and close monitoring of patients posttransplant for markers of kidney damage. Transplant providers and nephrologists must be cognizant of the potential for kidney disease and work closely together to provide a multidisciplinary approach to care for patients after HCT.

Transplant Associated-Thrombotic Microangiopathy

INTRODUCTION

Transplant-associated thrombotic microangiopathy (TA-TMA) is a potentially lethal complication of HCT that is characterized by endothelial dysfunction, leading to microangiopathic hemolytic anemia, thrombocytopenia, and dysfunction of multiple organs, notably the kidney, lung, central nervous system, and GI tract. Endothelial cell dysfunction is thought to play a central role in the pathogenesis of this disorder. Diagnosis and treatment remain challenging. This section will review the pathophysiologic mechanisms and diagnostic criteria of TA-TMA and provide an overview of therapeutic options.

Epidemiology

The reported incidence of TA-TMA is quite variable and ranges between 0.5% to 64%. This is partly owing to the difficulty in detection of the condition and variations between centers in diagnostic criteria applied.[51] An older retrospective study by Iacopino et al.,[52] conducted in 4334 patients via questionnaire between 1985 and 1995, yielded a 0.5% incidence rate. More recent studies estimate incidence between 12% and 35%.[53] A prospective study by Jodele et al. showed a 39% incidence of TA-TMA, of which 18% had severe TMA.[31] Shayani et al. published a series of 177 patients, of whom 22% were diagnosed with likely or probable TA-TMA, based on their institutional criteria.[54] Another factor that has contributed to varied incidence are changes in the pretransplant conditioning regimens, which have changed the risk of development of TMA following HCT. At this time, further studies using standardized definitions are still needed to understand the true epidemiology of TA-TMA.

Risk Factors

TA-TMA is more often associated with allogeneic transplant but can occur with autologous transplant as well. Other risk factors that are thought to play a role include HCT from unrelated donors, nonmyeloablative transplants, HLA mismatch, female gender, and advanced recipient age.[51,53]

CNI are thought to contribute to the development of TA-TMA.[55] Possible mechanisms include increased thromboxane A2 and endothelin levels and direct CNI-related endothelial injury. In addition, decreased nitric oxide and prostacyclin levels related to CNI exposure may play a role.[56,57] CNI use in combination with mTOR inhibitors causes increased concentration of CNI in the kidney, resulting in lower vascular endothelial growth factor levels and, thereby, increasing risk of TA-TMA.[58,59]

High-dose conditioning chemotherapy used for myeloablative transplants, such as busulfan, fludarabine, cisplatin, and radiation, are associated with an increased risk of TA-TMA.[60] The mechanism is thought to be direct endothelial damage.

Viral infections, such as cytomegalovirus, parvovirus, adenovirus B19, human herpes virus 6, and BK, have also been associated with the development of TA-TMA. The exact mechanisms for this are unclear.[61,62] However, it has been postulated that these lymphotropic viruses affect monocytes and lymphocytes that then cause release of mediators of endothelial injury, such as TNF-α and IL-1.[51]

GVHD has been shown to be a risk factor for TA-TMA in several studies. In a study conducted by Changsirikulchai et al., a fourfold higher risk of developing TA-TMA associated with GVHD was shown independent of the CNI levels or dosing regimen.[32] Higher grades of acute GVHD are associated with higher risk of TA-TMA.[63] As noted previously, GVHD is thought to produce vascular endothelial injury, which is the fundamental process in TA-TMA. A recent study noted an association of GVHD, both acute and chronic, in seven patients who developed TA-TMA post-HCT. These authors noted that the histopathology in the kidney demonstrated glomerular and tubular inflammation along with renal arteriolar complement (C4d) deposition, similar to acute rejection after kidney transplant, which favors a role of GVHD in the pathogenesis of TA-TMA.[63] C4d deposition is a well-known marker of complement activation and endothelial injury.[31] Some arguments against a direct association between GVHD and TA-TMA are that both of these complications can occur independently of each other, and that TA-TMA develops in patients with autologous HCT and allogeneic HCT. Although there is not a clear causal link between GVHD and TA-TMA, they share endothelial injury as a common denominator and often overlap clinically in post-HCT patients.

Pathophysiology

Endothelial injury is thought to be a key factor in the pathogenesis of TA-TMA. All of the risk factors outlined in the previous section lead to damage of endothelium directly or via upregulation of T-cell and an increase in inflammatory mediators such as IL-1 and TNF-α. These mediators increase expression of plasminogen activator inhibitor 1 (PAI-1) and tissue factor (TF).[64] Exposure of the injured endothelium promotes binding of von Willebrand factor and glycoprotein (GP)1a, which in turn activates platelets through GP1b. There is concomitant TF activation, which complexes with Factor 7a and 10a to form thrombin. The platelet aggregation along with fibrin forms a thrombus. RBCs are mechanically sheared by fibrin-rich thrombi, resulting in the typical microangiopathic hemolytic anemia, in addition to thrombocytopenia caused by consumption during thrombi formation.[53]

Neutrophil Extracellular Traps

Neutrophil extracellular traps (NETS) are lacy structures composed of activated neutrophils that extrude their granular proteins, such as myeloperoxidase, neutrophil elastase, and lactoferrin along with their chromatin. They are a component of innate antimicrobial immunity and can kill a wide variety of pathogens. NETS are known to activate complement by both alternative and classic pathways.[15,65] They are thought to be an important component of autoimmune processes and thrombotic events. NETS levels have been noted to be elevated in patients with TMA.[65,66] In a more recent study in 103 pediatric patients post-HCT, the authors attempted to find a causal link between endothelial injury and TA-TMA. They found that serum double stranded deoxyribonucleic acid (DNA), a known surrogate marker for NETS, levels peaked around engraftment and with occurrence of TA-TMA and GVHD within 100 days post-HCT. Thus NETS provide a possible link between complement-mediated endothelial injury and disease processes, including TA-TMA and GVHD post-HCT.[67]

Complement Dysregulation

Perhaps the most intriguing aspect of the pathogenesis of TA-TMA in recent years has been the elucidation of the role of complement dysregulation. The complement system is composed of more than 30 proteins and serves to provide host immunosurveillance. Among the three pathways of the complement system, the persistent activation of the alternative pathway is the most important mediator of endothelial injury. This has been well studied in other thrombotic microangiopathies, such as atypical hemolytic uremic syndrome (aHUS). In aHUS, defects in complement regulatory proteins, either genetic or acquired, lead to unchecked complement activation and formation of membrane attack complex (MAC) on the surface of endothelial cells, resulting in endothelial injury and the clinical findings of TMA. In addition, the complement staining pattern of TA-TMA in kidney tissue on biopsy is similar to that in aHUS with C4d deposition localized to glomeruli and arterioles.[20] There are published data from Jodele et al. regarding complement pathway defects in a case series of patients who developed TA-TMA after HCT.[34] The authors found that of the six patients with TA-TMA, 83% had heterozygous deletions in the complement factor H related protein (CFHR) genes, CFHR3 and CFHR1. This is much higher than the reported prevalence in general population of ~25%. Half of these patients also had presence of CFH autoantibodies compared with the control population who did not develop TA-TMA. Many genetic variants in complement genes have been identified that are thought to increase the risk of developing TA-TMA in patients after HCT. This was demonstrated in a recently published study that examined seven complement regulatory genes in a cohort of patients with TA-TMA. In this study, 65% of patients with TMA post-HCT had variants in these genes compared with only 9% in the patients without TA-TMA. This supports the concept that the presence of complement gene variants predisposes patients to develop TA-TMA.[68] Taken together, these findings demonstrate the important role of complement dysregulation in the pathogenesis of TA-TMA.

Clinical Presentation

Kidney

Kidney injury is the most common clinical manifestation of TA-TMA and includes proteinuria, HTN, and decreased GFR evidenced by elevated SCr levels. Kidney biopsy demonstrates a constellation of findings, including loss of endothelial cells, with subendothelial expansion and occlusion by schistocytes with fibrin deposits and mesangiolysis. C4d deposition, a marker of complement activation, is seen in glomerular capillaries in some patients with TA-TMA. Inflammatory infiltrates with CD8+ T-cells have been shown in tubules, glomeruli, and the interstitium.[32,69] These findings on kidney biopsy correlate with proteinuria, typically nephrotic range, and severe HTN. A worsening of preexisting HTN in HCT patients with need for more than one antihypertensive agent, in combination with increased proteinuria detected on random urine specimens, may be early markers for kidney involvement in TA-TMA.

Gastrointestinal Tract

The GI system is especially prone to complications from infection or GVHD. Because these can occur simultaneously with TA-TMA, it can be challenging to differentiate between these entities. Increased abdominal pain, diarrhea, and rectal bleeding that remain unresponsive to increased immunosuppression should raise clinical suspicion for TA-TMA. Histologic findings that support intestinal TMA include endothelial injury, which is seen as cell separation from the vessel wall with presence of microthrombi, denudation of intestinal mucosa, mucosal hemorrhages, crypt loss, and presence of schistocytes in the lumen of the small vessels.[70] Tissue analysis can prove crucial in establishing a diagnosis of TA-TMA in the gut, especially because this can coexist with GVHD. In fact, a recent study showed that in more than 90% of patients diagnosed clinically with gut GVHD, there was histologic evidence of TA-TMA.[71] Careful determination of presence of concurrent GVHD and TMA is valuable in the management of these patients. Although withdrawal of CNI has been reported to be helpful in treating intestinal TA-TMA, there could be a role for ongoing immunosuppression to reduce the risk of GVHD.

Lung

Lung involvement in TA-TMA includes significant pulmonary HTN that results from pulmonary arteriolar microangiopathy related to injured endothelium, microthrombi, and schistocytes in the interstitial tissue. It is important to recognize pulmonary involvement early because left untreated, the presence of pulmonary TA-TMA is associated with high fatality and is correlated with poor survival at 1 year post-HCT.[72]

Central Nervous System

TA-TMA in the central nervous system (CNS) can manifest with symptoms, such as altered mental status, seizures, headaches, and hallucinations. Although the mechanisms leading to CNS involvement are not fully understood, metabolic disturbances related to renal dysfunction or severe HTN are thought to play a role.[72] Patients are at risk for developing posterior reversible encephalopathy syndrome from uncontrolled severe HTN. This may reflect underlying endothelial injury in the brain in addition to resulting from severe HTN. Radiologic findings include presence of edema in parieto-occipital regions. In general, these findings are reversible with treatment of elevated blood pressures. In some instances, however, it can predispose to further CNS injury, including hemorrhagic stroke, leading to increased morbidity and mortality.[73]

Diagnosis

TA-TMA is a disease process that typically involves multiple organ systems owing to systemic endothelial injury and requires a high index of clinical suspicion. Several features of TA-TMA may be related to the HCT process itself rather than a distinct disease entity. Tissue diagnosis remains the gold standard but obtaining tissue specimens from HCT patients who are critically ill and at high risk of bleeding is often not feasible. As mentioned previously, kidney biopsies show the presence of thrombotic microangiopathy, including glomerular injury with thickened capillary loops, thrombotic lesions in small vessels, presence of endothelial injury, and fragmented RBC within mesangial matrix. Other organs, such as the GI tract and lung, have demonstrated similar TMA-related changes within tissue specimens. Published diagnostic criteria to assess risk of TMA are based on at least four different consensus criteria that have the common features of an elevated LDH, schistocytes on peripheral smear, in addition to anemia or thrombocytopenia.[74–76] More recently, new diagnostic criteria for TA-TMA have been proposed that include either a tissue diagnosis of TMA in the affected organ or a combination of proteinuria, HTN, de novo anemia, de novo thrombocytopenia, LDH, evidence of microangiopathy, such as schistocytes, or terminal complement activation.[77] The various published diagnostic criteria are outlined in Table 11.1. It is noteworthy that, although monitoring SCr is valuable, it is a late marker of kidney injury, especially in children and

Table 11.1   Diagnostic Criteria for Hematopoietic Cell Transplant Associated Thrombotic Microangiopathy

Category	LeukemiaNet International Working Group	Blood and Marrow Transplant Clinical Trials Network	Probable TMA Defined by Validation Study (Cho et al.)	Criteria by Jodele et al.
LDH	Increased	Increased	Increased	Increased
Schistocytes	> 4%	> 2 per hpf	> 2 per hpf	Microangiopathy (schistocytes or tissue biopsy)
Thrombocytopenia[a]	present	N/A	present	present
Hemoglobin	Decreased or increased pRBC transfusion	N/A	Decreased	Decreased or increased pRBC transfusion
Coombs test	N/A	Negative	Negative	N/A
Haptoglobin	Decreased	N/A	Decreased	N/A
Coagulation tests	Normal	Normal	Normal	N/A
Renal dysfunction[b] and/or neurologic dysfunction	N/A	N/A	N/A	Proteinuria > 30 mg/dL or HTN
Terminal complement activation	N/A	N/A	N/A	Elevate plasma level of sC5b-9

[a]Thrombocytopenia defined as platelets <50,000 or a >50% decrease from prior baseline.
[b]Renal dysfunction defined as doubling of serum creatinine or 50% decrease in creatinine clearance compared with baseline.
hpf, high power field; *HTN*, hypertension; *LDH*, lactate dehydrogenase; *N/A*, not applicable; *pRBC*, packed red blood cell; *TMA*, Thrombotic Microangiopathy.

those with low muscle mass at baseline. Cystatin C measurement can help determine GFR more accurately and can be used in combination with creatinine in GFR estimation equations to monitor renal function.[14] However, the utility of cystatin C can be limited by factors, such as steroid use, inflammation, and thyroid disease.

Studies have reported use of echocardiography as a tool to assess presence of pericardial effusion and/or pulmonary HTN. Both of these findings have been associated with TA-TMA in studies of HCT patients.[78,79] Once a diagnosis of TA-TMA is established, consideration of genetic testing for complement dysregulation should be considered. In HCT recipients, DNA specimens should come from a stored blood sample before transplant or from a tissue site other than blood.

Management

The approach to the management of TA-TMA includes both supportive and targeted therapy aimed at specific disease-causing mechanisms. Supportive care includes management of complications related to kidney injury, such as HTN, and early initiation of renal replacement therapies. Withdrawal of possible triggering agents, such as CNI or sirolimus, is an important strategy as well. However, in this population at risk for GVHD, stopping agents, such as CNI, requires careful consideration of risks and benefits. Early detection and treatment of viral infections, when possible, can also help. Limiting use of nephrotoxic medications, including iodinated contrast, can prove valuable in limiting further kidney injury as well.

Among targeted therapies, the most promising is eculizumab, an anti-C5 monoclonal antibody, which works by blocking the terminal complement pathway, and thereby prevents complement mediated endothelial injury. There are a small number of studies that have demonstrated efficacy in TA-TMA patients.[72,80]

Patient selection for therapy is important. Those with high-grade proteinuria, elevated serum levels of soluble MAC, and multiorgan dysfunction are thought to be appropriate candidates for a formal trial with eculizumab. Note that with some diseases, such as aHUS, this therapy is continued indefinitely. Conversely, in the HCT setting, it is typically discontinued after resolution of TA-TMA. In addition, the dosing of eculizumab in this population is different from the standard prescribed dosing. Patients tend to have variable clearance and may require individualized dosing regimens based on pharmacokinetic studies.[81] Typically, the initial dose is based on weight; however, subsequent doses may need to be adjusted and administered more frequently than weekly, especially in critically ill patients and/or those with significant GI bleeding. Using normal levels of terminal complement sC5b-9 (activated terminal complement complex) as a marker of efficacy can help determine dose and duration of treatment. Measuring total complement levels, CH50, can also be helpful unless there is coexisting hypocomplementemia for other reasons.

Another therapeutic option that has been considered is therapeutic plasma exchange (TPE). Recent studies between 2003 and 2011 demonstrated up to a 59% efficacy for TPE in uncontrolled studies of small populations.[69] Initiate TPE early in the course of TA-TMA because studies have demonstrated better efficacy when instituted early.[82] TPE has been performed daily for up to 5 days initially with goal of at least a one times plasma volume exchange per treatment. Treatments are then tapered gradually based on response of markers of TA-TMA. TPE also has a role in patients who have circulating antibodies, such as factor H autoantibody.[72]

Another agent that has been used in TA-TMA is rituximab, an anti-CD20 monoclonal antibody. There is a small number of patients who have been reported in the literature to have improvement with its use. Specifically, patients with autoantibodies to complement factor H have responded to rituximab, because it blocks production of antibody by B cells.[83,84]

Defibrotide is a drug that acts to inhibit TNF-α–mediated endothelial damage and has thrombolytic, antithrombotic, and antiinflammatory effects. It has been used in treatment of sinusoidal obstruction syndrome (SOS), with 30% to 60% efficacy reported by some European centers.[85] Currently, it is only approved in the United States for use in SOS and further studies are needed to determine efficacy for TA-TMA.

As with other complications following HCT, treatment of symptoms is a core component of the treatment plan for TA-TMA. As noted, the HTN seen in association with TMA is often severe and can result in negative consequences, including CNS symptoms. Given this, aggressive treatment of HTN in the setting of TMA is prudent. Similar to GVHD, and other kidney disorders that result in HTN and proteinuria, ACE-I or ARB therapy can be used to decrease blood pressure and degree of proteinuria.[38] More specifically related to TA-TMA, use of ACE-I in animal models of HUS has demonstrated a renoprotective effect.[86] Finally, as alluded to earlier, ACE-I/ARB can decrease the rate of progression to CKD by reducing inflammation and fibrosis in the kidney.[87] Of note, the use of ACE-I/ARB in the setting of significant AKI and volume depletion should be avoided to prevent further decline in kidney function.

Platelet transfusion in the setting of TA-TMA should be limited to patients with active bleeding and those undergoing invasive procedures because of the potential for worsening of the underlying pathophysiology of TMA. A similar approach should be taken when considering RBC transfusion. Decreased erythropoietin levels have been seen in patients with TA-TMA, and would suggest that the use of recombinant erythropoietin could be a beneficial treatment.[88] However, erythropoietin stimulating agents must be used with caution in patients with cancer, because an increase in mortality risk has been seen.[89]

Prognosis

TA-TMA has been reported to have significant morbidity and mortality, with centers reporting survival as low as 25% within 3 months of diagnosis. Factors such as proteinuria and elevated sC5b-C9 are associated with a worse prognosis, as reported by Jodele et al., with more than 80% mortality in patients with these findings at 1 year post-SCT.[72] Other reported prognostic factors include pulmonary HTN.[90] The absence of kidney dysfunction has been shown to correlate with better survival.[91]

Conclusion

TA-TMA is a frequent complication of HCT and is associated with poor outcomes. It is typically characterized by multiorgan involvement and requires a high index of suspicion for diagnosis. Multiple mechanisms are thought to play a role in the endothelial injury associated with TA-TMA, including complement dysregulation. In addition to supportive care, there is evidence to support the use of complement blockade therapy in patients with evidence of complement activation.

Key Points

- Graft-versus-host disease (GVHD) and transplant-associated thrombotic microangiopathy (TA-TMA) occur frequently and are associated with increased morbidity and mortality after HCT.
- Clinicians should have high index of suspicion for kidney involvement in GVHD and TA-TMA. Monitoring of markers of kidney injury, including proteinuria, hematuria, hypertension, and decline in kidney function, should be routinely conducted at regular intervals post-hematopoietic cell transplantation (post-HCT). Kidney biopsy should also be considered.
- Endothelial damage is a common pathway linking several complications following HCT, including GVHD and TA-TMA.
- Complement dysregulation is a major contributor to the pathophysiology of TA-TMA and therapies exist that specifically target this pathway. Genetic testing can help establish diagnosis of underlying risk of complement dysregulation and TA-TMA.
- Continuation of GVHD prophylaxis should be considered when signs of kidney injury related to GVHD are suspected.
- Kidney complications after HCT require a multidisciplinary approach targeting both symptoms and underlying pathologic processes within the context of patients' primary disease.

References

1. Hingorani S. Renal complications of hematopoietic-cell transplantation. *N Engl J Med.* 2016;374:2256-2267.
2. Mori J, Ohashi, K, Yamaguchi, T, et al. Risk assessment for acute kidney injury after allogeneic hematopoietic stem cell transplantation based on Acute Kidney Injury Network criteria. *Intern Med.* 2012;51:2105-2110.
3. Cruz DN, Perazella MA, Mahnensmith RL. Bone marrow transplant nephropathy: a case report and review of the literature. *J Am Soc Nephrol.* 1997;8:166-173.
7. Schmid PM, Bouazzaoui A, Schmid K, et al. Acute renal graft-versus-host disease in a murine model of allogeneic bone marrow transplantation. *Cell Transplant.* 2017;26:1428-1440.
8. Higo S, Shimizu A, Masuda Y. Acute graft-versus-host disease of the kidney in allogeneic rat bone marrow transplantation. *PloS One.* 2014;9:e115399.
12. Sadeghi B, Al-Chaqmaqchi H, Al-Hashmi S, et al. Early-phase GVHD gene expression profile in target versus non-target tissues: kidney, a possible target? *Bone Marrow Transplant.* 2013;48:284.
14. Hingorani S, Pao E, Schoch G, Gooley T, Schwartz GJ. Estimating GFR in adult patients with hematopoietic cell transplant: comparison of estimating equations with an iohexol reference standard. *Clin J Am Soc Nephrol.* 2015;10:601-610.
15. Mii A, Shimizu A, Kaneko T, et al. Renal thrombotic microangiopathy associated with chronic graft-versus-host disease after allogeneic hematopoietic stem cell transplantation. *Pathol Int.* 2011;61:518-527.
16. Sakellari I, Barbouti A, Bamichas G, et al. GVHD-associated chronic kidney disease after allogeneic haematopoietic cell transplantation. *Bone Marrow Transplant.* 2013;48:1329.
20. Laskin BL, Maisel J, Goebel J, et al. Renal arteriolar C4d deposition: a novel characteristic of hematopoietic stem cell transplantation–associated thrombotic microangiopathy. *Transplantation.* 2013;96:217.
23. Pilar F, Vazquez L, Caballero D, et al. Chronic graft-versus-host disease of the kidney in patients with allogenic hematopoietic stem cell transplant. *Eur J Haematol.* 2013;91:129-134.
24. Troxell ML, Higgins JP, Kambham N. Renal pathology associated with hematopoietic stem cell transplantation. *Adv Anat Pathol.* 2014;21:330-340.
27. Brukamp K, Doyle AM, Bloom RD, Bunin N, Tomaszewski JE, Cizman B. Nephrotic syndrome after hematopoietic cell transplantation: do glomerular lesions represent renal graft-versus-host disease? *Clin J Am Soc Nephrol.* 2006;1:685-694.
28. Numata A, Morishita Y, Mori M, et al. De novo postallogeneic hematopoietic stem cell transplant membranous nephropathy. *Exp Clin Transplant.* 2013;11:75-78.
31. Jodele S, Davies SM, Lane A, et al. Diagnostic and risk criteria for HSCT-associated thrombotic microangiopathy: a study in children and young adults. *Blood.* 2014;124:645-653.
32. Changsirikulchai S, Myerson D, Guthrie KA, McDonald GB, Alpers CE, Hingorani SR. Renal thrombotic microangiopathy after hematopoietic cell transplant: role of GVHD in pathogenesis. *Clin J Am Soc Nephrol.* 2009;4:345-353.
33. Tichelli A, Gratwohl A. Vascular endothelium as 'novel' target of graft-versus-host disease. *Best Pract Res Clin Haematol.* 2008;21:139-148.
35. Laskin BL, Nehus E, Goebel J, Khoury JC, Davies SM, Jodele S. Cystatin C-estimated glomerular filtration rate in pediatric autologous hematopoietic stem cell transplantation. *Biol Blood Marrow Transplant.* 2012;18:1745-1752.
37. Pulsipher MA, Skinner R, McDonald GB, et al. National Cancer Institute, National Heart, Lung and Blood Institute/Pediatric Blood and Marrow Transplantation Consortium First International Consensus Conference on late effects after pediatric hematopoietic cell transplantation: the need for pediatric-specific long-term follow-up guidelines. *Biol Blood Marrow Transplant.* 2012;18:334-347.
38. Hingorani SR, Seidel K, Lindner A, Aneja T, Schoch G, McDonald G. Albuminuria in hematopoietic cell transplantation patients: prevalence, clinical associations, and impact on survival. *Biol Blood Marrow Transplant.* 2008;14:1365-1372.
40. Hoffmeister PA, Hingorani SR, Storer BE, Baker KS, Sanders JE. Hypertension in long-term survivors of pediatric hematopoietic cell transplantation. *Biol Blood Marrow Transplant.* 2010;16:515-524.
51. Khosla J, Yeh AC, Spitzer TR, Dey BR. Hematopoietic stem cell transplant-associated thrombotic microangiopathy: current paradigm and novel therapies. *Bone Marrow Transplant.* 2018;53:129.
53. Seaby EG, Gilbert RD. Thrombotic microangiopathy following haematopoietic stem cell transplant. *Pediatr Nephrol.* 2017;33:1489-1500.
54. Shayani S, Palmer J, Stiller T, et al. Thrombotic microangiopathy associated with sirolimus level after allogeneic hematopoietic cell transplantation with tacrolimus/sirolimus-based graft-versus-host disease prophylaxis. *Biol Blood Marrow Transplant.* 2013;19:298-304.
55. Rosenthal J, Pawlowska A, Bolotin E, et al. Transplant-associated thrombotic microangiopathy in pediatric patients treated with sirolimus and tacrolimus. *Pediatr Blood Cancer.* 2011;57:142-146.
56. Goldberg RJ, Nakagawa T, Johnson RJ, Thurman JM. The role of endothelial cell injury in thrombotic microangiopathy. *Am J Kidney Dis.* 2010;56:1168-1174.
59. Robson M, Côte I, Abbs I, Koffman G, Goldsmith D. Thrombotic microangiopathy with sirolimus-based immunosuppression: potentiation of calcineurin-inhibitor-induced endothelial damage? *Am J Transplant.* 2003;3:324-327.
60. Willems E, Baron F, Seidel L, Frère P, Fillet G, Beguin Y. Comparison of thrombotic microangiopathy after allogeneic hematopoietic cell transplantation with high-dose or nonmyeloablative conditioning. *Bone Marrow Transplant.* 2010;45:689.
61. Chang A, Hingorani S, Kowalewska J, et al. Spectrum of renal pathology in hematopoietic cell transplantation: a series of 20 patients and review of the literature. *Clin J Am Soc Nephrol.* 2007;2:1014-1023.
65. Tang S, Zhang Y, Yin SW, et al. Neutrophil extracellular trap formation is associated with autophagy-related signalling in ANCA-associated vasculitis. *Clin Exp Immunol.* 2015;180:408-418.
66. Fuchs TA, Kremer Hovinga JA, Schatzberg D, Wagner DD, Lämmle B. Circulating DNA and myeloperoxidase indicate disease activity in

patients with thrombotic microangiopathies. *Blood.* 2012;120:1157-1164.

67. Gloude NJ, Khandelwal P, Luebbering N, et al. Circulating dsDNA, endothelial injury, and complement activation in thrombotic microangiopathy and GVHD. *Blood.* 130:2017;1259-1266.

68. Jodele S, Zhang K, Zou F, et al. The genetic fingerprint of susceptibility for transplant-associated thrombotic microangiopathy. *Blood.* 2016; 127:989-996.

69. Laskin BL, Goebel J, Davies SM, Jodele S. Small vessels, big trouble in the kidneys and beyond: hematopoietic stem cell transplantation–associated thrombotic microangiopathy. *Blood.* 2011;118:1452-1462.

71. Inamoto Y, Ito M, Suzuki R, et al. Clinicopathological manifestations and treatment of intestinal transplant-associated microangiopathy. *Bone Marrow Transplant.* 2009;44:43.

76. Cho B-S, Yahng SA, Lee SE, et al. Validation of recently proposed consensus criteria for thrombotic microangiopathy after allogeneic hematopoietic stem-cell transplantation. *Transplantation.* 2010;90: 918-926.

77. Jodele S, Dandoy CE, Myers KC, et al. New approaches in the diagnosis, pathophysiology, and treatment of pediatric hematopoietic stem cell transplantation-associated thrombotic microangiopathy. *Transfus Apher Sci.* 2016;54:181-190.

78. Dandoy CE, Hirsch R, Chima R, Davies SM, Jodele S. Pulmonary hypertension after hematopoietic stem cell transplantation. *Biol Blood Marrow Transplant.* 2013;19:1546-1556.

79. Lerner D, Dandoy C, Hirsch R, Laskin B, Davies SM, Jodele S. Pericardial effusion in pediatric SCT recipients with thrombotic microangiopathy. *Bone Marrow Transplant.* 2014;49:862.

80. Dhakal P, Giri S, Pathak R, Bhatt VR. Eculizumab in transplant-associated thrombotic microangiopathy. *Clin Appl Thromb Hemost.* 2017;23: 175-180.

83. Au WY, Ma ES, Lee TL, et al. Successful treatment of thrombotic microangiopathy after haematopoietic stem cell transplantation with rituximab. *Br J Haematol.* 2007;137:475-478.

84. Carella A, D'Arena G, Greco MM, Nobile M, Cascavilla N. Rituximab for allo-SCT-associated thrombotic thrombocytopenic purpura. *Bone Marrow Transplant.* 2008;41:1063.

85. Corti P, Uderzo C, Tagliabue A, et al. Defibrotide as a promising treatment for thrombotic thrombocytopenic purpura in patients undergoing bone marrow transplantation. *Bone Marrow Transplant.* 2002; 29:542.

86. Hingorani S. Chronic kidney disease after pediatric hematopoietic cell transplant. *Bone Marrow Transplant.* 2008;14:84-87.

90. Uderzo C, Jodele S, Missiry M, et al. Transplant-associated thrombotic microangiopathy (TA-TMA) and consensus based diagnostic and therapeutic recommendations: which TA-TMA patients to treat and when? *J Bone Marrow Res.* 2014;2:152.

A full list of references is available at Expertconsult.com

12 *Sinusoidal Obstruction Syndrome*

BRENDAN M. WEISS AND DEIRDRE SAWINSKI

Introduction

Sinusoidal obstruction syndrome (SOS) is a well-described complication of the high-dose conditioning regimens used in hematopoietic stem cell transplantation (HSCT), as well as certain hepatotoxic chemotherapies or radiation therapy used in other settings, and is a well-recognized cause of HSCT patient mortality. It was previously known as *hepatic veno-occlusive disease* based on the pathologic features, but the term was changed to SOS when it became clear that the initial injury is caused by changes in the hepatic sinusoidal cells.[1,2] The epidemiology of SOS is difficult to define because of differences in definitions and patient populations, and the clinical presentation ranges from mild, self-limited disease to severe SOS with multiorgan failure and mortality rates in excess of 80%.[2] In recent years, there has been improvement in the understanding of the pathogenesis of SOS and new strategies for both prevention and treatment.

Epidemiology

INCIDENCE

The incidence of SOS varies greatly in the literature, because of controversies in diagnosis, variable diagnostic criteria, and confounding factors, such as the patient population being studied. The published rates of SOS in all populations range from 0% to 60% of HSCT patients, but the mean incidence in a recent systematic review[2] was 13.7%. The incidence of SOS clearly varies by type of transplant; rates in fully myeloablative allogeneic transplants are 10% to 60%, whereas in reduced-intensity conditioning regimens and autologous transplants, the incidence is much lower, ranging from 5% to 30%.[2]

ADULTS

The average incidence of SOS in adults is 8% to 14% depending on the series and in a few studies is as high as 40%;[2] this is much lower than observed in children. The incidence of SOS has steadied now that there is a greater emphasis on use of reduced intensity conditioning regimens.

PEDIATRICS

In contrast to adults, SOS is a common complication of HSCT in children, occurring in approximately 20% to 30%

of patients overall[3] and as many as two-thirds of those at high risk for this complication.[4] One of the challenges of making this diagnosis in the pediatric population is the fact that one-third of children with SOS do not have hyperbilirubinemia;[5,6] therefore dependence on strict fulfillment of the Baltimore or modified Seattle criteria may miss the diagnosis, and children are more likely to present with late-onset SOS (20%).[4,7,8] Pediatric patients who do develop hyperbilirubinemia usually do so late in their disease progression or as a manifestation of more severe SOS. An early diagnostic clue in the pediatric population is thrombocytopenia that is refractory to platelet transfusion;[9] this usually precedes the diagnosis by 1 week. Children also can have more severe disease, with 30% to 60% developing multiorgan dysfunction.[4,10]

Risk Factors (Table 12.1)

PATIENT RELATED

Extremes of age increase the risk of SOS in both adults and children,[11,12] as does poor Karnofsky performance status ($< 90\%$)[13,14] or dependence on parenteral nutrition before transplant.[15] Advanced malignant disease, and the etiology of the underlying malignancy, are well-recognized risk factors.[11,16] In children, a diagnosis of osteopetrosis,[17] familial hemophagocytic lymphohistiocytosis,[15] juvenile myelomonocytic leukemia,[15] thalassemia major,[11] sickle cell disease,[18] neuroblastoma,[19] Wilms tumor,[20] or rhabdomyosarcoma[21] have all been associated with a higher risk of SOS. Laboratory abnormalities indicative of liver injury or inflammation, such as elevated transaminases, ferritin, or bilirubin, also are associated with a higher SOS risk.[15] Several genetic mutations predisposing to the condition have been identified, including GSTM1-null,[22] C282Y allele,[23] and the MTHFR 677CC/1298CC haplotype.[24] Patients with preexisting liver disease caused by viral hepatitis or iron overload are also at elevated risk for this complication.[15] Although it had been suggested in the past that there may be a gender difference in SOS, the increased risk for SOS development seems to be limited to women maintained on norethisterone to prevent gynecologic bleeding.[25]

PRETRANSPLANT TREATMENT RELATED

There are several pretransplant treatment characteristics associated with an elevated risk of SOS, including prior abdominal or liver radiation and baseline abnormalities in transaminases or bilirubin.[15,26,27] Certain salvage chemotherapies

Table 12.1   Risk factors for Development of Sinusoidal Obstruction Syndrome

Pretransplant	Transplant
Age < 1 year	Allogeneic > autologous
Increased transaminases	Haploidentical

Preexisting liver disease
    Viral hepatitis
    CMV positivity
	Conditioning regimen
	    Busulfan
	    Busulfan + cyclophosphamide (Cy)
	    Fludarabine
	    Carmustine (BCNU) + Cy +
	        etoposide

Underlying disease
    MDS
    Inborn errors of metabolism
    Leukemia
    CML
    Immunodeficiency
    Thalassemia
	Total body irradiation > 12 Gy + Cy

Interval between diagnosis
    and HCT > 12 months
	GVHD prophylaxis
	    Sirolimus + methotrexate _
	        tacrolimus
	    Methotrexate + cyclosporine
	    Cyclosporine

Deteriorating health
    pretransplant
    Diarrhea
    Fever
    Parenteral nutrition
	Non-T cell depleted grafts

Prior transplant	Peripheral blood > bone marrow
Prior abdominal radiation therapy	Acute hepatic or gut GVHD
Prior -ozogamicin agents	
Prior norethisterone	
Karnofsky index < 90%	
GSTM1 null phenotype	
Impaired pulmonary function	

Infections/antimicrobials
    Sepsis
    Vancomycin
    Acyclovir	

Ferritin > 1000 ng/mL	
Bilirubin > 26 μmol/L	

CML, chronic myeloid leukemia; *CMV*, cytomegalovirus; *GSTM1*, glutathione transferase mu- 1; *GVHD*, graft-versus-host disease; *Gy*, units of gray; *HCT*, hematopoietic cell transplantation, *MDS* , myelodysplastic syndrome.

used in leukemia to control disease and allow patients to proceed to HSCT deserve special mention. There are two antibody-drug conjugates that contain the same toxin, ozogamicin, that have been associated with SOS. Gemtuzumab ozogamicin (anti-CD33) was previously used in acute myeloma leukemia patients and was associated with SOS.[28,29] In patients exposed to gemtuzumab ozogamicin before HSCT, the risk of SOS was increased and fatalities resulting from SOS noted.[30] However, the use of the lower dose regimen may be associated with an acceptable SOS risk of around 8%.[31] This agent was taken off the market because of lack of use and toxicity concerns, but has recently been reapproved at a new dose.[32] Inotuzumab (anti-CD22)

ozogamicin has been approved for the salvage treatment of acute lymphoblastic leukemia and is associated with a 17% risk of SOS after HSCT.[33]

TRANSPLANTATION RELATED

In general, more intensive consolidating regimens and less well-matched transplants increase the risk of SOS. SOS is more common in fully myeloablative regimens than in reduced-intensity regimens,[34] but has been described as a complication of autologous transplants.[2] Use of fludarabine, cyclophosphamide, high-dose melphalan, and busulfan for consolidation have all been associated with SOS;[15] intravenous administration of busulfan may decrease the risk because of improved pharmacokinetic profiling of the dose.[35] High-dose or unfractionated total body irradiation increase SOS risk.[36] Second HSCT transplant recipients are also at increased risk for SOS because of their larger cumulative chemotherapeutic and radiation burden.[16]

Although SOS can occur in autologous SCT, it is much more common in allogeneic transplants. Unrelated donors, donors with a greater degree of human leukocyte antigen (HLA) mismatch, non-T cell depleted grafts, and peripheral blood stem cell transplants are all associated with an increased risk for development of SOS.[37,38] Posttransplant factors, such as choice of graft-versus-host disease (GVHD) prophylaxis, can also have an effect, with patients maintained on a calcineurin inhibitor, especially if given in combination with sirolimus and methotrexate, being at higher risk.[39]

Clinical Presentation

Patients present with volume overload, with ascites, and weight gain greater than 5% of baseline. They often have jaundice and painful hepatomegaly. Acute kidney injury is frequently a component and mimics the hepatorenal syndrome with hypotension, hyponatremia, and a low fractional excretion of sodium. Although most patients with SOS present with symptoms within the first 30 days of transplant, a subset of patients will develop late-onset disease.[7,8]

Diagnostic Criteria

There are two established clinical criteria for the diagnosis of SOS, the Baltimore[40] and modified Seattle[41] criteria (Table 12.2). Recently, the European Society for Blood and Marrow Transplantation (EBMT) proposed updated criteria[42] for adults and pediatrics to address the limitations of the Baltimore and modified Seattle criteria (Table 12.3). The rationale for this update was multiple—there are now effective therapies for SOS, making prompt diagnosis critical, and advances in our understanding of risk factors and imaging techniques to aid in diagnosis. In addition, there is a growing recognition that "late" SOS is a more common presentation than previously thought and that pediatric manifestations of the disease differ significantly from those seen in adults.

The modified Seattle criteria[41] specify that within the first 20 days after transplant, a patient must have two or more

Table 12.2 Clinical Diagnostic Criteria for Sinusoidal Obstruction Syndrome

Modified Seattle criteria	Baltimore criteria
In the first 20 days after HCT, ≥ 2 of the following:	In the first 21 days after HCT, bilirubin ≥ 2 mg/dL plus ≥ 2 of the following
Bilirubin > 2 mg/dL	Painful hepatomegaly
Hepatomegaly or pain in right upper quadrant	Ascites
Weight gain (> 2% basal weight)	Weight gain

HCT, Hematopoietic cell transplantation.

Table 12.3 Summary of British Committee for Standards in Haematology and British Society for Blood and Marrow Transplantation for the Diagnosis and Management of Sinusoidal Obstruction Syndrome

Diagnosis	Should be based on clinical criteria (modified Seattle or Baltimore) Ultrasound may be helpful Liver biopsy only in patients where SOS diagnosis unclear If performed, liver biopsy should be transjugular
Risk factors	Patients should be assessed pretransplant for risk factors, and managed when possible
Prophylaxis	Defibrotide is recommended in children with risk factors Defibrotide is suggested in adults with risk factors Prostaglandin E1, pentoxifylline, heparin, and antithrombin are not recommended Ursodeoxycholic acid is suggested
Treatment	Defibrotide is recommended in children and adults TPA and N-acetylcysteine are not recommended Methylprednisone may be considered with caveat for infectious risk Careful fluid management Early involvement of critical care specialists

SOS, Sinusoidal obstruction syndrome; *TPA*, tissue plasminogen activator.

of the following: bilirubin greater than 2 mg/dL, hepatomegaly or right upper quadrant pain, and weight gain (> 2% of baseline weight). The Baltimore criteria[40] specify that within the first 21 days after transplant, a patient must have a bilirubin greater than 2 mg/dL plus two or more of the following: painful hepatomegaly, ascites, or weight gain (> 5% of baseline weight).

The new EBMT criteria[42] for diagnosis of SOS in adults recognize two clinical entities: "classic" SOS and "late onset" SOS. Classic SOS by EBMT criteria presents within the first 21 days after transplant. Patients must have an elevated bilirubin level (≥ 2 mg/dL) and two of the following: painful hepatomegaly, weight gain more than 5% of baseline, or ascites. Late onset SOS is any patient with the classic presentation beyond day +21 or those with biopsy proven SOS; alternatively, any patient beyond day 21 after transplant with two or more of the following: bilirubin of

2 mg/dL or more, painful hepatomegaly, weight gain more than 5% of baseline, ascites, and hemodynamic or ultrasound findings suggestive of SOS (decrease in velocity or reversal of portal venous flow). Thrombocytopenia, although common in patients with SOS, is not an official part of the new diagnostic criteria.

The EMBT has also established new diagnostic criteria for children.[43] In these criteria, there is no longer a time limitation for the onset of symptoms. Patients require any two or more of the following: unexplained and transfusion refractory thrombocytopenia, unexplained weight gain for 3 days despite diuretics or weight gain more than 5% of baseline, hepatomegaly, ascites, and rising bilirubin for 3 consecutive days or an absolute bilirubin of 2 mg/dL or more.

Differential Diagnosis

The differential diagnosis of SOS includes hyperacute hepatic GVHD, autoimmune hepatitis, cholestasis of sepsis, biliary obstruction, infection including abscess or acute viral hepatitis, cholestasis caused by cyclosporine or tacrolimus, drug toxicity, iron overload, and right heart failure.[44,45]

Diagnostic Tests

LABORATORY TESTS

Adult patients with SOS often have elevated transaminases, hyperbilirubinemia, prolonged prothrombin time, elevated international normalized ratio, and low serum albumin. Approximately one-third of pediatric patients with SOS do not have hyperbilirubinemia.[46]

BIOMARKERS

Although the diagnosis of SOS remains a purely clinical one, there have been attempts to identify noninvasive biomarkers for the disease. Plasminogen activator inhibitor-1, an inhibitor of the fibrinolytic system, was one of the first biomarkers identified; levels increase in SOS patients concurrent with the rise in serum bilirubin.[47] Levels of thrombomodulin, von Willebrand factor (vWF), and soluble intercellular adhesion molecule-1 have all been shown to be elevated early in patients with SOS maintained on sirolimus for GVHD prophylaxis.[48] In one study,[48] levels of vWF 1400 IU/mL or greater and thrombomodulin 100 ng/dL or greater on day +7 were 100% sensitive and specific for the diagnosis of SOS. Using quantitative mass spectrometry based proteomics, Akil et al.[49] developed a diagnostic biomarker panel for SOS; suppression of tumorigenicity-2, angiopoietin-2, L-ficolin, hyaluronic acid, and vascular cell adhesion molecule-1 (VCAM-1) levels together were diagnostic of SOS with an area under the curve (AUC) of more than 0.81. These markers were able to identify patients at risk for SOS as early as the day of stem cell transplantation. In addition, L-ficolin, hyaluronic acid, and VCAM-1 levels predicted the severity of SOS disease with greater than 80% accuracy, when combined with clinical data.

LIVER BIOPSY

Transjugular liver biopsy with portal pressure measurement can be used to make a definitive diagnosis of SOS. Classic biopsy findings include acinar zone 3 necrosis and a wedged hepatic venous pressure gradient more than 10 mmHg is highly suggestive of the diagnosis.[50] However, liver biopsy is an invasive procedure with significant risks of bleeding and the possibility of misdiagnosis because of sampling error; therefore this approach is not commonly used.

TRANSIENT ELASTOGRAPHY

In much of general hepatology practice, liver biopsy has been supplanted by noninvasive measures of liver fibrosis, including transient elastography, which uses ultrasound waves to measure liver stiffness; this test is highly congruent with biopsy results, especially for patients with advanced fibrosis.[51,52] At least two studies have investigated the utility of transient elastography in the diagnosis of SOS in pediatric HSCT patients. In one study[53] of 25 patients, five developed SOS. Elastography measurements preconditioning did not differ between the groups, but as early as day +5, there was a significant increase in measured liver stiffness in the patients who eventually developed SOS; SOS was diagnosed at day +14 to 19 among these patients on the basis of modified Seattle criteria. The authors report that a velocity increase of 0.26 m/s over the baseline reading on day +5 was 60% sensitive and 90% specific for SOS. A second pediatric study[54] with 22 patients (four of whom developed SOS) noted similar findings; there was again no difference in baseline elastography among patients but those who developed SOS had an increase in liver stiffness 3 to 6 days before their clinical diagnosis. In the adult population,[55] a pretransplant liver stiffness of greater than 8 kPa was associated with significant hyperbilirubinemia posttransplant and posttransplant liver dysfunction, suggesting a role for transient elastography in identifying patients at risk for SOS in whom prophylactic defibrotide could be considered.

ULTRASOUND

Although ultrasound findings are not part of the official diagnostic criteria, they can assist in making the diagnosis and are useful for ruling out other etiologies in the differential diagnosis. On ultrasound,[56] patients can have ascites, hepatomegaly, gall bladder wall thickening, small portal vein diameter, elevated hepatic artery resistive index (> 0.75), or reversal of hepatic venous flow.

DISEASE SEVERITY GRADING

SOS can be classified as mild, moderate, or severe (Table 12.4). Patients with mild SOS can be managed with supportive care and their disease is usually self-limiting; in one series,[27] 9% of patients with mild SOS died of their disease. Those with moderate disease will benefit from analgesics, diuretics to manage fluid balance, and supportive measures; mortality in this group is around 25%.[27] Patients with severe SOS often have renal dysfunction and/or multiorgan system failure, with attendant mortality rates upwards of 80%.[2]

Table 12.4 A Proposed Grading System for Sinusoidal Obstruction Syndrome Severity

	Grade		
	Mild[a]	Moderate[a]	Severe[a]
Bilirubin (mg/dL)	2.0–3.0	3.1–5.0	> 5.0
Liver function	< 3× normal	3–5× normal	> 5× normal
Weight above baseline, %	2	2.1–5	> 5
Renal function	Normal	< 2× normal	≥ 2× normal
Rate of change, days	Slow (6–7)	Moderate (4–5)	Rapid (2–3)[b]

[a] Two or more of following, [b] Or creatinine clearance ≤ 50%.

The EMBT, in addition to updating the diagnostic criteria for SOS, have also proposed an updated grading system[42] for establishing the severity of disease in adults, which is modeled after the Common Terminology Criteria for Adverse Events reporting structure, ranging from grade 1 (mild) to grade 5 (death). This new system not only considers absolute laboratory values in grading disease severity, but considers the kinetics of laboratory and symptoms development; it also upgrades patients who are in between categories to a more serious classification of disease. The rationale for these changes was to prompt clinicians to institute therapy sooner, as earlier treatment with defibrotide has been associated with improved survival in SOS. Patients with mild disease have had a slow onset of symptoms, with bilirubin between 2 and 3 mg/dL, transaminases that are less than twice the upper limit of normal, weight gain less than 5%, and creatinine that is less than 20% above their baseline. Moderate disease has a quicker onset (5–7 days), with a bilirubin between 3 and 5 mg/dL, transaminases 2 to 5 times the upper limit of normal, weight gain between 5% and 10%, and no more than a 50% increase in serum creatinine. Patients with severe disease have a rapid onset, less than 4 days, with bilirubin in the 5 to 8 mg/dL range, with doubling in the past 48 hours, along with transaminases 5 to 8 times normal, weight gain less than10%, and creatinine may have doubled. Very severe disease is characterized by the presence of organ failure/dysfunction, with bilirubin greater than 8 mg/dL, transaminases eightfold above normal, more than 10% weight gain, and the need for renal replacement therapy.

There is also an updated EBMT severity grading scale for SOS in children,[43] with disease states categorized as mild, moderate, severe, and very severe/multiorgan failure. In mild disease, liver function tests (LFTs; aspartate transaminase, alanine transaminase, and glutamate dehydrogenase) are ≤ 2 times the upper limit of normal, thrombocytopenia has been present for less than 3 days, there is minimal ascites, glomerular filtration rate (GFR) is 89 to 60 mL/min, and there is minimal to no oxygen requirement. In moderate disease, LFTs are 2 to 5 times normal, thrombocytopenia has been present for 3 to 7 days, there is moderate ascites, GFR is 59 to 30 mL/min, and supplemental oxygen is required. Severe disease presents with LFTs greater than 5 times normal, more than 7 days of resistant thrombocytopenia, bilirubin 2 mg/dL or more, ascites requiring paracentesis, coagulopathy, GFR 29 to 15 mL/min, and ventilatory support is required. Very severe disease is similar with doubling of bilirubin in 48 hours, replacement of coagulation factors, renal replacement therapy, and cognitive impairment.

Prognosis

The prognosis of SOS depends on the severity of disease. In patients with mild disease, it is often self-limiting and they will improve with minimal clinical intervention. Those with moderate disease often require supportive care to manage their fluid balance and clinical symptoms. Severe disease, especially if accompanied by renal or pulmonary failure, is often fatal with mortality rates in excess of 80%.[2]

Pathophysiology

Ionizing radiation and the high-dose chemotherapy of the consolidation regimens are toxic to endothelial cells throughout the body; this injury manifests as thrombotic microangiopathy in the kidney, diffuse alveolar hemorrhage in the lung, and SOS in the liver.[57] Hepatic sinusoidal endothelial cells are particularly sensitive to this type of injury. Injured and activated endothelial cells detach and create gaps in the sinusoidal barrier. Erythrocytes, leukocytes, and platelets enter the space of Disse, furthering the endothelial injury. Detached endothelial cells obstruct the small intrahepatic venules, leading to local thrombosis. Cytokine release and activation of the fibrinolytic pathway magnifies this injury, leading to sinusoidal congestion, obstruction, and hepatic necrosis in acinar zone 3.

Management

Historically, the management of SOS was mainly supportive measures. Management focused on minimizing extracellular volume without compromising renal function. Anticoagulants and antifibrinolytics were selectively used with limited efficacy and substantial toxicity. Patients with severe SOS and multiorgan failure were transferred to intensive care settings with maximal support, including hemodialysis provided, but patient prognosis was poor. There are limited pharmacologic therapies for SOS and the best studied agent is defibrotide.

Prevention

Given the morbidity and mortality associated with severe SOS, there has been great interest in pharmacologic agents for the prevention of this disease. Different drugs have been trialed based on our pathophysiologic understanding of the disease and in extrapolation of treatments from other domains in medicine. Attempts have also been made to modify patient or transplant-related risk factors, such as use of reduced-intensity conditioning regimens, avoidance of busulfan, and selection of maximally HLA-compatible donors, whenever possible.

URSODIOL

Ursodiol is a hydrophilic bile acid that has been used to treat liver disease in other clinical settings. In one trial[58] of 67 patients undergoing allogeneic HSCT, patients were randomized to ursodiol prophylaxis (300 mg twice a day) or placebo; only 15% of the ursodiol patients developed SOS, whereas 40% of placebo treated patients did (p=.03). A metaanalysis[59] of six studies (four randomized control trials [RCTs] and two historically controlled trials), using ursodiol as prophylaxis, found a relative risk 0.34 (95% confidence interval [CI], 0.17–0.66) for SOS in patients receiving ursodiol. Congruent with the reduction in SOS, transplant-related mortality was as improved with use of ursodiol. A prospective, randomized, multicenter study of 132 patients comparing ursodiol with placebo demonstrated a lower rate of SOS in ursodiol treated patients (3%) versus 18.5% in placebo treated patients (p=.004). The British Committee for Standard in Haematology and the British Society for Blood and Marrow Transplantation guidelines[60] suggest the use of ursodiol for the prevention of SOS.

HEPARIN

Heparin, including low-molecular-weight heparin, has had mixed success when used as prophylaxis for SOS. One study[61] of 81 patients reported significantly lower rates of SOS in heparin treated patients (2.5% vs. 13.7%) with only minor bleeding complications. Although some cohort studies were positive,[62] a metaanalysis[63] of 12 studies failed to find a significant protective effect (relative risk 0.90; 95% CI, 0.62–1.29). Because of concerns of excess bleeding associated with the use of heparin as SOS prophylaxis, this is not currently recommended.

OTHER AGENTS

Smaller trials have explored alternative treatments, such as prostaglandin E1,[64] pentoxifylline,[65] and antithrombin;[66] these have either been shown to be ineffective, as in the case of pentoxifylline and antithrombin, or else have unacceptably high levels of side effects and toxicity[67] (prostaglandin E1).

Treatment

Traditionally, the mainstay of SOS treatment has been symptom management and supportive care; although these measures are still important, the emergence of defibrotide as an approved therapy for SOS in the United States has had a positive impact on patient survival.

DEFIBROTIDE

Defibrotide is a sodium salt of oligodeoxyribonucleotides derived from porcine mucosa. Its mechanism of action is incompletely understood, but it is thought to have antiinflammatory and antithrombotic properties.[68] In vitro data suggest that defibrotide binds to endothelial cells and restores nitric oxide synthase levels in treated endothelia, protecting them from reactive oxygen species.[68,69] It was approved for the treatment of SOS in 2013 in Europe and in 2016 in the United States.

Defibrotide is administered as 25 mg/kg/day in divided doses (four per day, every 6 hours). This dosing was determined in Phase II studies[70] that demonstrated 25 mg/kg/day had equivalent clinical efficacy with a higher dose (40 mg/kg/day) but less hypotension. It does not interact with the cytochrome P450 system and does not have systemic anticoagulant activity.[71] The main side effects of defibrotide therapy reported in clinical trials are hypotension and bleeding (pulmonary and/or gastrointestinal hemorrhage); however, these side effects were also very commonly encountered in control patients in the trials, leading to defibrotide approval. As renal dysfunction or failure can be a common complication of SOS, it is important to note that defibrotide does not require dose adjustment for reduced glomerular filtration rate or dialysis; dialysis does not affect defibrotide clearance and defibrotide does not accumulate in patients with advanced renal disease.[72]

Several studies have investigated the efficacy of defibrotide as treatment for SOS. The open-label, single arm Treatment IND study[73] (T-IND, NCT00628498) enrolled 642 patients across 78 centers in the United States, 89.3% of who had undergone an HSCT, and the vast majority of these were allogeneic transplants (87.8%). Investigators used the Baltimore and modified Seattle criteria to diagnose SOS and the main study outcome was patient survival at day 100+ after treatment with defibrotide. Overall 50.3% of HSCT patients enrolled met the study endpoint, with 45.3% survival in those with multiorgan dysfunction (MOD) and 58.1% survival in those without MOD. Better 100-day survival was also observed in the pediatric subgroup treated with defibrotide in the trial. Survival rates were noted to be higher in patients treated sooner after diagnosis with defibrotide. A subsequent study[74] compared outcomes for patients who were treated with defibrotide (25 mg/kg/day) with matched historical controls; in this study, 102 patients were enrolled and the main outcome was again day 100 survival. Survival rates were significantly higher in the defibrotide treated patients (38.2% vs. 25%, p=.0109) and the rates of adverse events were similar in both groups.

A secondary, posthoc analysis[75] from the T-IND study examined the impact of the timing of defibrotide therapy initiation on outcomes. Patients had better survival the earlier therapy was started; as little as 1-day delay in the initiation of therapy translated into an 8.8% increase in patient death. An open-label, RCT[4] from Europe has specifically investigated the use of defibrotide for SOS prevention; this study conducted at 28 centers in Europe enrolled 356 patients (adult and pediatric) with at least one SOS risk factor. Their intention to treat analysis demonstrated a lower rate of SOS in patients treated with defibrotide prophylaxis (12% vs. 20%, p=.0488), suggesting that this should be considered in high-risk patients. However, defibrotide is not yet approved for this indication in the United States, but there is an ongoing international clinical trial enrolling patients for this indication (NCT02851407).

ALTERNATIVE THERAPIES

A variety of alternative therapies for the treatment of SOS have been reported in the literature, all with a less robust clinical response than defibrotide. Methylprednisolone[76] has been trialed with some response, but there is concern because of the increased risk of infection associated with augmented immunosuppression in HSCT patients. N-acetylcysteine has been used as treatment, because of its antioxidant properties, but has not been found to be effective for this purpose.[77] Fibrinolytic therapies, such as tissue plasminogen activator or heparin, have been used; although a modest clinical response has been reported in some studies,[78] there were significant bleeding complications associated with both agents.[79]

SUPPORTIVE CARE

The administration of intravenous fluids and maintenance of appropriate fluid balance is vital for the care of patients with SOS. The endothelial damage caused by conditioning regimens leads to cytokine release and capillary leak syndrome, with third spacing of intravascular fluid. HSCT patients have large obligate fluid intakes with intravenous medications, blood product transfusions, and nutrition. Unaddressed volume overload increases patient mortality,[80] especially in those with acute kidney injury. Patients require strict monitoring of daily fluid intake and output, with prompt institution of diuretic therapy for those with volume overload. Care should be taken to avoid medications that are known to be nephrotoxic or hepatotoxic.

Summary

SOS remains an important complication of HSCT with evolving criteria for diagnosis and staging. Our understanding of the risk factors for this condition has improved and new therapeutic options for its prevention and treatment exist. These advances should translate into better outcomes for patients with SOS.

Key Points

- Sinusoidal obstruction syndrome is a well-described complication of the high-dose conditioning regimens used in hematopoietic stem cell transplantation and is a well-recognized cause of patient mortality.
- Patients present with volume overload, with ascites, and weight gain more than 5% of baseline. They often have jaundice and painful hepatomegaly. Acute kidney injury is frequent and mimics the hepatorenal syndrome with hypotension, hyponatremia, and a low fractional excretion of sodium.
- The differential diagnosis of sinusoidal obstruction syndrome includes hyperacute hepatic graft-versus-host disease, autoimmune hepatitis, cholestasis of sepsis, biliary obstruction, infection including abscess or acute viral hepatitis, cholestasis caused by cyclosporine or tacrolimus, drug toxicity, iron overload, and right heart failure.
- Ionizing radiation and the high-dose chemotherapy of the consolidation regimens are toxic to endothelial cells throughout the body; this injury manifests as thrombotic microangiopathy in the kidney, diffuse alveolar

hemorrhage in the lung, and sinusoidal obstruction syndrome in the liver.

- Traditionally, the mainstay of sinusoidal obstruction syndrome treatment has been symptom management and supportive care; although these measures are still important, the emergence of defibrotide as an approved therapy for sinusoidal obstruction syndrome in the United States has had a positive impact on patient survival.

References

1. DeLeve LD, Wang X, Kuhlenkamp JF, Kaplowitz N. Toxicity of azathioprine and monocrotaline in murine sinusoidal endothelial cells and hepatocytes: the role of glutathione and relevance to hepatic venoocclusive disease. *Hepatology.* 1996;23:589-599.
2. Coppell JA, Richardson PG, Soiffer R, et al. Hepatic veno-occlusive disease following stem cell transplantation: incidence, clinical course, and outcome. *Biol Blood Marrow Transplant.* 2010;16:157-168.
3. Bajwa RPS, Mahadeo KM, Taragin BH, et al. Consensus report by Pediatric Acute Lung Injury and Sepsis Investigators and Pediatric Blood and Marrow Transplantation Consortium Working Committees: supportive care guidelines for management of veno-occlusive disease in children and adolescents, Part 1: focus on investigations, prophylaxis and specific treatment. *Biol Blood Marrow Transplant.* 2017;23: 1817-1825.
4. Corbacioglu S, Cesaro S, Faraci M, et al. Defibrotide for prophylaxis of hepatic veno-occlusive disease in paediatric haemopoietic stem cell transplantation: an open-label, phase 3, randomized controlled trial. *Lancet.* 2012;379:1301-1309.
5. Myers KC, Dandoy C, El-Bieta J, Davies SM, Jodele S. Veno-occlusive disease of the liver in the absence of elevation in bilirubin in pediatric patients after hematopoietic stem cell transplantation. *Biol Blood Marrow Transplant.* 2015;21:379-381.
8. Carreras E, Rosiñol L, Terol MJ, et al. Veno-occlusive disease of the liver after high dose cytoreductive therapy with busulfan and melphalan for autologous blood stem cell transplantation in multiple myeloma patients. *Biol Blood Marrow Transplant.* 2007;13:1448-1454.
9. Rio B, Andreu G, Nicod A, et al. Thrombocytopenia in venocclusive disease after bone marrow transplantation or chemotherapy. *Blood.* 1986;67:1773-1776.
10. Richardson PG, Riches ML, Kernan NA, et al. Phase 3 trial of defibrotide for the treatment of severe veno-occlusive disease and multiorgan failure. *Blood.* 2016;127:1656-1665.
11. Cheuk DK, Wang P, Lee TL, et al. Risk factors and mortality predictors of hepatic veno-occlusive disease after pediatric hematopoietic stem cell transplantation. *Bone Marrow Transplant.* 2007;40:935-944.
12. Cesaro S, Pillon M, Talenti E, et al. A prospective survey on incidence, risk factors and therapy of hepatic veno-occlusive disease in children after hematopoietic stem cell transplantation. *Haematologica.* 2005;90: 1396-1404.
13. Carreras E, Bertz H, Arcese W, et al. Incidence and outcome of hepatic veno-occlusive disease after blood or marrow transplantation: a prospective cohort study of the European Group for Blood and Marrow Transplantation. European Group for Blood and Marrow Transplantation Chronic Leukemia Working Party. *Blood.* 1998;92: 3599-3604.
15. Dalle JH, Giralt SA. Hepatic veno-occlusive disease after hematopoietic stem cell transplantation: risk factors and stratification, prophylaxis, and treatment. *Biol Blood Marrow Transplant.* 2016;22: 400-409.
17. Corbacioglu S, Hönig M, Lahr G, et al. Stem cell transplantation in children with infantile osteopetrosis is associated with a high incidence of VOD, which could be prevented with defibrotide. *Bone Marrow Transplant.* 2006;38:547-553.
18. Corbacioglu S, Carreras E, Ansari M, et al. Diagnosis and severity criteria for sinusoidal obstruction syndrome/veno-occlusive disease in pediatric patients: a new classification from the European Society for Blood and Marrow Transplantation. *Bone Marrow Transplant.* 2018; 53:138-145.
19. Horn B, Reiss U, Matthay K, McMillan A, Cowan M. Veno-occlusive disease of the liver in children with solid tumors undergoing autologous hematopoietic progenitor cell transplantation: a high incidence in patients with neuroblastoma. *Bone Marrow Transplant.* 2002;29: 409-415.
22. Srivastava A, Poonkuzhali B, Shaji RV, et al. Glutathione S-transferase M1 polymorphism: a risk factor for hepatic venoocclusive disease in bone marrow transplantation. *Blood.* 2004;104:1574-1577.
25. Helmy A. Review article: updates in the pathogenesis and therapy of hepatic sinusoidal obstruction syndrome. *Aliment Pharmacol Ther.* 2006;23:11-25.
26. Carreras E, Diaz-Beyá M, Rosiñol L, Martínez C, Fernández-Avilés F, Rovira M. The incidence of venoocclusive disease following allogeneic hematopoietic stem cell transplantation has diminished and the outcome improved over the last decade. *Biol Blood Marrow Transplant.* 2011;17:1713-1720.
30. Wadleigh M, Richardson PG, Zahrieh D, et al. Prior gemtuzumab ozogamicin exposure significantly increases the risk of veno-occlusive disease in patients who undergo myeloablative allogeneic stem cell transplantation. *Blood.* 2003;102:1578-1582.
31. Battipaglia G, Labopin M, Candoni A, et al. Risk of sinusoidal obstruction syndrome in allogeneic stem cell transplantation after prior gemtuzumab ozogamicin treatment: a retrospective study from the Acute Leukemia Working Party of the EBMT. *Bone Marrow Transplant.* 2017;52:592-599.
34. Carreras E, Bertz H, Arcese W, et al. Incidence and outcome of hepatic veno-occlusive disease after blood or marrow transplantation: a prospective cohort study of the European Group for Blood and Marrow Transplantation. European Group for Blood and Marrow Transplantation Chronic Leukemia Working Party. *Blood.* 1998;92:3599-3604.
35. Kashyap A, Wingard J, Cagnoni P, et al. Intravenous versus oral busulfan as part of a busulfan/cyclophosphamide preparative regimen for allogeneic hematopoietic stem cell transplantation: decreased incidence of hepatic venoocclusive disease (HVOD), HVOD-related mortality, and overall 100-day mortality. *Biol Blood Marrow Transplant.* 2002;8:493-500.
36. Carreras E. Hepatic veno-occlusive disease following haematopoietic cell transplantation: pathogenesis, diagnosis, risk factors, prophylaxis and treatment VOD following cell transplantation. *Hematology.* 2013; 3:109-113.
37. Moscardó F, Urbano-Ispizua A, Sanz GF, et al. Positive selection for CD34+ reduces the incidence and severity of veno-occlusive disease of the liver after HLA-identical sibling allogeneic peripheral blood stem cell transplantation. *Exp Hematolo.* 2003;31:545-550.
39. Cutler C, Stevenson K, Kim HT, et al. Sirolimus is associated with veno-occlusive disease of the liver after myeloablative allogeneic stem cell transplantation. *Blood.* 2008;112:4425-4431.
40. Jones RJ, Lee KS, Beschorner WE, et al. Venoocclusive disease of the liver following bone marrow transplantation. *Transplantation.* 1987; 44:778-783.
42. Mohty M, Malard F, Abecassis M, et al. Revised diagnosis and severity criteria for sinusoidal obstruction syndrome/veno-occlusive disease in adult patients: a new classification from the European Society for Blood and Marrow Transplantation. *Bone Marrow Transplant.* 2016; 51:906-912.
43. Corbacioglu S, Carreras E, Ansari M, et al. Diagnosis and severity criteria for sinusoidal obstruction syndrome/veno-occlusive disease in pediatric patients: a new classification from the European Society for Blood and Marrow Transplantation. *Bone Marrow Transplant.* 2018;53: 138-145.
44. Carreras E. How I manage sinusoidal obstruction syndrome after haematopoietic cell transplantation. *Br J Haematol.* 2015;168: 481-491.
46. Myers KC, Dandoy C, El-Bietar J, Davies SM, Jodele S. Veno-occlusive disease of the liver in the absence of elevation in bilirubin in pediatric patients after hematopoietic stem cell transplantation. *Biol Blood Marrow Transplant.* 2015;21:379-381.
47. Salat C, Holler E, Kolb HJ, et al. Plasminogen activator inhibitor-1 confirms the diagnosis of hepatic veno-occlusive disease in patients with hyperbilirubinemia after bone marrow transplantation. *Blood.* 1997;89:2184-2188.
48. Cutler C, Kim HT, Ayanian S, et al. Prediction of veno-occlusive disease using biomarkers of endothelial injury. *Biol Blood Marrow Transplant.* 2010;16:1180-1185.
49. Akil A, Zhang Q, Mumaw CL, et al. Biomarkers for diagnosis and prognosis of sinusoidal obstruction syndrome after hematopoietic cell transplantation. *Biol Blood Marrow Transplant.* 2015;21:1739-1745.
50. Carreras EM, Grañena A, Navasa M, et al. Transjugular liver biopsy in BMT. *Bone Marrow Transplant.* 1993;11:21-26.

52. Talwalkar JA, Kurtz DM, Schoenleber SJ, West CP, Montori VM. Ultrasound-based transient elastography for the detection of hepatic fibrosis: systematic review and meta-analysis. *Clin Gastroenterol Hepatol.* 2007;5:1214-1220.

53. Reddivalla N, Robinson AL, Reid KJ, et al. Using liver elastography to diagnose sinusoidal obstruction syndrome in pediatric patients undergoing hematopoetic stem cell transplant. *Bone Marrow Transplant.* 2018. [Epub ahead of print].

54. Colecchia A, Marasco G, Ravaioli F, et al. Usefulness of liver stiffness measurement in predicting hepatic veno-occlusive disease development in patients who undergo HSCT. *Bone Marrow Transplant.* 2017;52: 494-497.

56. Lassau N, Leclère J, Auperin A, et al. Hepatic veno-occlusive disease after myeloablative treatment and bone marrow transplantation: value of gray-scale and Doppler US in 100 patients. *Radiology.* 1997; 204:545-552.

57. Carreras E, Diaz-Ricart M. The role of the endothelium in the short-term complications of hematopoietic SCT. *Bone Marrow Transplant.* 2011;46:1495-1502.

59. Tay J, Tinmouth A, Fergusson D, Huebsch L, Allan DS. Systematic review of controlled clinical trials on the use of ursodeoxycholic acid for the prevention of hepatic veno-occlusive disease in hematopoietic stem cell transplantation. *Biol Blood Marrow Transplant.* 2007;13:206-217.

60. Dignan FL, Wynn RF, Hadzic N, et al. BCSH/BSBMT guideline: diagnosis and management of veno-occlusive disease (sinusoidal obstruction syndrome) following haematopoietic stem cell transplantation. *Br J Haematol.* 2013;163:444-457.

63. Imran H, Tleyjeh IM, Zirakzadeh A, Rodriguez V, Khan SP. Use of prophylactic anticoagulation and the risk of hepatic veno-occlusive disease in patients undergoing hematopoietic stem cell transplantation: a systematic review and meta-analysis. *Bone Marrow Transplant.* 2006;37:677-686.

65. Attal M, Huguet F, Rubie H, et al. Prevention of regimen related toxicities after bone marrow transplantation by pentoxifylline: a prospective randomized trial. *Blood.* 1993;82:732-736.

67. Bearman SI, Shen DD, Hinds MS, Hill HA, McDonald GB. A phase I/II study of prostaglandin E1 for the prevention of hepatic venocclusive disease after bone marrow transplantation. *Br J Haematol.* 1993;84: 724-730.

68. Richardson PG, Triplett BM, Ho VT, et al. Defibrotide sodium for the treatment of hepatic veno-occlusive disease/sinusoidal obstruction syndrome. *Expert Rev Clin Pharmacol.* 2018;11:113-124.

70. Richardson PG, Soiffer RJ, Antin JH, et al. Defibrotide for the treatment of severe hepatic veno-occlusive disease and multiorgan failure after stem cell transplantation: a multicenter, randomized, dose-finding trial. *Biol Blood Marrow Transplant.* 2010;16:1005-1017.

72. Tocchetti P, Tudone E, Marier JF, Marbury TC, Zomorodi K, Eller M. Pharmacokinetic profile of defibrotide in patients with renal impairment. *Drug Des Devel Ther.* 2016;10:2631-2641.

A full list of references is available at Expertconsult.com

Thrombotic Microangiopathy

KEVIN W. FINKEL AND JAYA KALA

Introduction

Hematopoietic stem cell transplantation (HSCT) is a potentially curative therapy for patients with hematologic malignancies, bone marrow failure syndromes, immunodeficiency states, and metabolic disorders.[1] Thrombotic microangiopathy (TMA) is a well-recognized potentially lethal complication of HSCT. It is characterized by microangiopathic hemolytic anemia, thrombocytopenia, and multiple organ dysfunction.[2] The etiologies of this syndrome are diverse, and it requires a high degree of clinical suspicion for diagnosis. The incidence ranges between 0.5% and 63.6%.[3] This wide disparity in incidence rates is caused by the inability to obtain tissue biopsy in most circumstances and therefore diagnosis relies solely on clinical parameters. The etiology of posttransplant TMA is multifactorial, and its risk factors include high-dose chemotherapy, radiation therapy, unrelated bone marrow donor status, human leukocyte antigen (HLA) mismatch, exposure to calcineurin inhibitors (with or without concomitant exposure to mammalian target of rapamycin inhibitors, graft-versus-host disease [GVHD], and infections).[4] Genetic abnormalities in the complement system also contribute in a subset of patients.[5] Management of posttransplant TMA remains a therapeutic challenge mainly because of the diverse pathogenic mechanisms involved in this disorder and the limited treatment options.

Thrombotic Microangiopathy— General Background

TMA is a clinical syndrome of relative or absolute thrombocytopenia and microangiopathic hemolytic anemia. It leads to dysfunction of multiple organs, including the kidneys, resulting in acute kidney injury (AKI). In the past, the combination of TMA with severe AKI was simply referred to as *hemolytic uremic syndrome* (*HUS*). However, this classification scheme has been modified based on the understanding of the various pathogenic mechanisms underlying the development of TMA.

The primary site of injury in TMA is the endothelium, leading to microvascular thrombosis with fibrin and platelet-rich thrombi. Microthombi formation and fibrin stranding induce flow disturbances, leading to microangiopathic hemolytic anemia and thrombocytopenia. Kidney biopsy under light microscopy reveals arteriolar and/or intracapillary thrombosis with fragmented erythrocytes in the capillary lumens. On electron microscopy, there is separation of endothelium from the basement membrane with the accumulation of an electron-lucent material in the expanded subendothelial space. A newly formed thin basement membrane often follows the outline of the endothelial cells, leading to a "double contour" appearance (Fig. 13.1).

The clinical syndrome of TMA can be broadly categorized into four major entities based on pathogenesis (Table 13.1). All four types require the presence of absolute or relative (< 25% decrease from baseline) thrombocytopenia and microangiopathic hemolytic anemia (schistocytes on peripheral blood smear, elevated lactate dehydrogenase [LDH] levels, and decreased haptoglobin values). It is known that most types of TMA have a waxing and waning course, so that the absence of schistocytes on a single peripheral blood smear is not conclusive evidence that TMA is not present. Likewise, an elevated LDH level is not specific for hemolysis because it is increased in several other disorders, and, because haptoglobin is an acute-phase reactant, levels may not be reduced below normal values in the face of ongoing hemolysis. Dysfunction of numerous organs can develop with TMA, although the kidneys are typically the most severely affected.

Pathogenic mechanisms define the type of TMA and inform therapy. In patients who acquire an inhibitory autoantibody to the metalloproteinase enzyme ADAMTS-13 (a disintegrin and metalloproteinase with a thrombospondin type 1 motif, member 13) (or rarely have a genetic mutation in the protein), the inability to cleave large von-Willebrand factor leads to TMA. This disorder is referred to as *thrombotic thrombocytopenic purpura* (*TTP*) and is treated with therapeutic plasma exchange (TPE). The major benefit to TPE is the ability to infuse large volumes of fresh plasma to provide sufficient quantities of enzyme to overcome the autoantibody; removal of autoantibody with TPE plays a less significant role. It is impossible to differentiate TTP from other forms of TMA on clinical grounds alone, so it is mandatory that an ADAMTS-13 activity assay be tested before initiation of TPE. Patients with normal activity assays do not have TTP and will not benefit from plasma exchange. In fact, patients treated with TPE for TMA who have normal ADAMTS-13 activity, may show an improvement in both platelet counts and LDH levels, yet still experience a high rate of death and end-stage kidney disease.[6]

Patients can develop TMA associated with bloody diarrhea and severe AKI. The etiology is classically associated with infection with a shiga-toxin producing bacteria (typically *Escherichia coli* H-O157:H7). This syndrome is referred

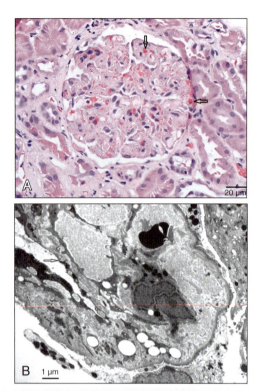

Fig. 13.1 Kidney biopsy from 49-year-old man with acute kidney injury receiving cyclosporine A, 98 days after allogeneic stem cell transplant for acute myelogenous leukemia. **A.** Kidney light microscopy (40X) of thrombotic microangiopathy. *Open arrows*: intracapillary thrombosis. *Closed arrow*: fragmented red blood cells (schistocytes). **B.** Kidney electronic microscopy of thrombotic microangiopathy. *Open arrow*: double contour of basement membrane. (Images courtesy William Glass, MD. Department of Pathology, UTHealth Science Center at Houston-McGovern Medical School.)

to as *shiga-toxin E. coli hemolytic uremic syndrome* (STEC-HUS). The infection is associated with eating uncooked meat, although the most recent outbreak occurred after ingestion of contaminated bean sprouts with *E. coli* serotype O104:H4. The disease is usually self-limited and only supportive care is necessary; antibiotics prolong shedding of the toxin. Direct injury of the endothelium by toxin leads to TMA and therefore there is no indication for TPE.

The most common form of TMA is HUS secondary to numerous medications (including chemotherapy), infections (including pneumonia and diarrhea [non-STEC HUS]), systemic diseases, various cancers (particularly adenocarcinomas), pregnancy, malignant hypertension, and transplantation (especially kidney and bone marrow) (Box 13.1). In most of these cases, the TMA is the result of direct endothelial injury or self-limited activation of the complement system and resolves with treatment of the underlying disorder or discontinuation of the triggering medication. Failure to improve after these measures may indicate that patients have an abnormality in the regulation of complement activation and actually have atypical HUS (aHUS) (vide infra). TPE does not address the pathogenic mechanism in cases of secondary HUS and is not indicated in these circumstances.

The final type of TMA is caused by continuous complement activation in patients with dysfunctional regulatory proteins, referred to as *aHUS*. Because of an inability to inhibit activated complement, unabated production of the membrane attack complex (C5b-9) directly injures the endothelium, leading to TMA. Untreated, 80% of patients either require permanent dialysis or have died at 3 years. TPE has no effect on clinical outcomes, although it can improve LDH levels and platelet counts in 60% to 70% of patients. Therefore hematologic response to TPE does not portend a good prognosis in such patients. Rather, treatment is directed at decreasing terminal complement activation with the anti-C5 monoclonal antibody, eculizumab. Because of the variable penetrance of the genetic abnormalities in the complement system, most patients with aHUS only present after a complement amplifying condition. Similar to the "two-hit" hypothesis, patients may have mild abnormalities in complement regulation and are disease free, but when complement is strongly stimulated, they are no longer able to stop activation and develop TMA. Key is the fact that most of the complement amplifying conditions that "unmask" aHUS can also cause secondary HUS. The clinical challenge in these scenarios is to determine whether the TMA is secondary to the underlying disease or medication, for example, a calcineurin inhibitor, or due to aHUS that has been unmasked by administration of the drug. There are no diagnostic tests to differentiate between the two. C3 levels are normal in 80% of aHUS cases; genetic testing takes too long and is negative in 30% of cases of aHUS. Therefore in such patients, treatment is directed toward the disease or drug associated with TMA. If TMA does not

Table 13.1   General Types of Thrombotic Microangiopathy

	TTP	STEC-HUS	Secondary HUS	Atypical HUS
ADAMTS-13 activity	< 10%	> 10%	> 10%	> 10%
Pathogenesis	Acquired autoantibody	Toxin induced endothelial injury	Direct endothelial injury	Dysregulated complement system
C3 level	Normal	Normal	Usually normal	Decreased in 20%
Response to TPE	+++	−	−	+/−
Treatment	TPE	Supportive care	Stop offending agent/treat underlying condition	Eculizumab

ADAMST-13, A disintegrin and metalloproteinase with a thrombospondin type 1 motif, member 13; *HUS*, hemolytic-uremic syndrome; *STEC*, shiga toxin producing *E. coli*; *TPE*, therapeutic plasma exchange; *TTP*, thrombotic thrombocytopenic purpura.

improve with appropriate therapy, aHUS should be suspected.

Pathogenesis of Post Bone Marrow Transplant Thrombotic Microangiopathy

Several factors have been implicated in the development of posttransplant TMA. These include conditioning regimens with high-dose chemotherapy, total body irradiation, infections, such as cytomegalovirus/human herpesvirus-6, use of calcineurin inhibitors, and GVHD.[7] The exact pathogenesis of TMA after HSCT remains incompletely understood, which limits the identification of patients at highest risk and appropriate selection of therapy. Although most cases of posttransplant TMA are a form of secondary HUS, some patients have been shown to have dysregulation of the complement system consistent with aHUS. In these patients, the histopathologic findings of the kidneys are identical to those reported in other cases of aHUS, including deposition of complement component C5b-9. Several investigators have demonstrated a genetic predisposition for the development of aHUS in patients with abnormalities in complement inhibitory factor H (CFH). Jodele et al. identified a high prevalence of deletions in CFH-related genes 3 and 1 and CFH autoantibodies in patients with posttransplant TMA.[5]

Risk Factors

The risk factors for development of posttransplant TMA include female gender, African American ethnicity, older age, prior medical history of severe hepatic dysfunction, and advanced primary disease. Treatment associated risk factors included unrelated donor transplant, HLA-mismatched donors, fludarabine based nonmyeloablative conditioning regimen, and busulfan with total body irradiation myeloablative conditioning. The use of calcineurin inhibitors, as well as infections and GVHD, also increases the risk of developing posttransplant TMA.

Pathologic and Clinical Features

Posttransplant TMA may be associated with long-term morbidity and chronic organ injury. It can manifest as a multisystem disease occurring as a result of various triggers of small vessel endothelial injury.[8] This leads to damage to tissues in different organs, most commonly the kidneys. The diagnosis is made when HSCT patients present with microangiopathic hemolytic anemia, de novo anemia, unexplained thrombocytopenia, elevated LDH, and schistocytes on peripheral blood smear. The diagnosis requires high index of suspicion because many of these findings are easily mistaken for common posttransplant complications, such as medication related hypertension, infections, or GVHD. Because of several comorbidities in HSCT patients, it is difficult to obtain tissue confirmation of TMA. It is therefore important to rely on clinical judgement to make a timely diagnosis of posttransplant TMA.

KIDNEYS

The kidneys are the most commonly affected organs in posttransplant TMA. The renal manifestations include AKI, proteinuria, and hypertension. The diagnosis of AKI requires high degree of clinical suspicion, because changes in serum creatinine levels may be an insensitive marker of alterations in glomerular filtration rate. One clue to the diagnosis is if a patient is requiring high doses of more than two antihypertensive medications for blood pressure control while receiving steroids or calcineurin inhibitors for GVHD treatment or prophylaxis.[9] Given the multiple etiologies that could result in this constellation of findings, including exposure to nephrotoxic agents, prohypertensive medications, and infections such as BK virus, the most reliable modality to diagnose posttransplant TMA in the kidney is histologic. However, kidney biopsy in posttransplant patients carries high risk of bleeding caused by thrombocytopenia and hypertension.

LUNGS

In the lungs, endothelial injury in the pulmonary arterioles results in microthrombosis and schistocyte extravasation into the lung interstitium. In a retrospective analysis by Dandoy et al., 40 patients with posttransplant TMA had an overall mortality rate of 55% (22/40); 86% (19/22) of the deaths were attributed to pulmonary hypertension.[10] Patients with pulmonary posttransplant TMA often succumb to severe acute pulmonary hypertension after presenting with unexplained hypoxemia. Although the differential diagnosis of respiratory symptoms after HSCT is broad, patients with unexplained hypoxemia or respiratory distress after transplantation should be evaluated for posttransplant TMA associated pulmonary involvement.

GASTROINTESTINAL TRACT

There is evidence that posttransplant TMA affects the small vessels of the gastrointestinal tract, leading to symptoms such as diarrhea, vomiting, bleeding, and abdominal pain. These symptoms are attributed to ischemic damage caused by microangiopathy. If untreated, it leads to significant morbidity and mortality.[11] The clinical diagnosis is difficult because similar symptoms are also seen with acute intestinal GVHD or infectious colitis. The histologic diagnosis is often crucial to help differentiate between GVHD and intestinal TMA. Tissue examination shows small vessel endothelial swelling, noninflammatory crypt degeneration, detachment or apoptosis of endothelial cells, and interstitial edema with hemorrhage or fragmented red blood cells. Inamoto et al. reported that 92% (80/87) of patients who underwent colonoscopic biopsy for a clinical diagnosis of acute intestinal GVHD had evidence of TMA.[12] Only 30% of the patients had histologic evidence of GVHD itself. Differentiation of intestinal TMA from GVHD is crucial because continuation of calcineurin inhibitors can significantly worsen symptoms of TMA.

CENTRAL NERVOUS SYSTEM

Manifestations of central nervous system (CNS) involvement of TMA include confusion, headaches, hallucinations, and seizures. The most common posttransplant TMA related CNS injury is caused by acute uncontrolled TMA associated hypertension, leading to posterior reversible encephalopathy (PRES) and intracranial hemorrhage.[8] This potential complication emphasizes the importance of aggressive blood pressure control in HSCT recipients and need to maintain normal hemostasis. Although the goal is usually to limit platelet transfusions with active microangiopathic hemolytic anemia, it may be necessary to prevent bleeding complications in PRES.

POLYSEROSITIS

It is common to find polyserositis with posttransplant TMA caused by the generalized vascular injury. Laskin et al., in their series of 20 patients evaluated for early clinical indicators of posttransplant TMA, found three of the six patients with confirmed posttransplant TMA had polyserositis.[2] Polyserositis often presents with refractory pericardial effusions, pleural effusions, and ascites without generalized edema. Lener et al. found the incidence of pericardial effusions to be 45% in patients with posttransplant TMA.[13] In a prospective study of 100 HSCT patients, Dandoy et al. found the incidence of pericardial effusions to be 52% using echocardiographic screening.[14] The pathogenesis is not well understood. Patients that have undergone HSCT who develop chest pain, tachycardia, cardiomegaly on chest x-ray, or have unexplained hypoxemia need to be evaluated for pericardial effusions.

Diagnostic Criteria

The general diagnostic workup for TMA was previously outlined in Fig. 13.1. However, in terms of post-HSCT TMA, the diagnostic criteria for posttransplant TMA have been published by several societies and are summarized in Table 13.2. The International Working Group requires five criteria for diagnosis whereas the Bone and Marrow Transplant Clinical Trials Network requires four criteria. Because haptoglobin is an acute-phase reactant, it may be elevated in many posttransplant patients because of an inflammatory response, thus reducing its specificity for detecting microangiopathic hemolytic anemia.[15] Identifying patients who are at highest risk of severe disease is challenging. In a study done by Jodele, 100 consecutive HSCT recipients were evaluated to determine the incidence of moderate and severe TMA and factors associated with poor overall outcomes.[16] Subjects with TMA had a significantly higher mortality unrelated to relapse at 1 year post-HSCT compared with those without TMA. Elevated LDH, proteinuria, and hypertension were early markers of TMA. In patients with TMA, proteinuria (> 30 mg/dL) and elevated serum C5b-9 levels at the time of diagnosis were associated with poor survival. Histologic analysis of tissue samples improves the diagnostic accuracy in TMA; however, the high risk of bleeding complications in these patients usually deters clinicians from obtaining a biopsy.

Table 13.2 Definition of Post Bone Marrow Transplant Thrombotic Microangiopathy

Parameter	Leukemia Net International Working Group	Blood and Marrow Transplant Clinical Trials Network	City of Hope (COH)	Overall Thrombotic Micro-Angiopathy (O-TMA) Grouping
LDH	increased	increased	> 2 × the upper limit of normal	increased
Platelet count	< 50 × 10⁹/L or < 50% of normal baseline	–	< 50 × 10⁹/L or ≥ 50% decrease from previous counts	< 50 × 10⁹/L or < 50% of normal baseline
Schistocytes	> 4%	>2/HPF	Presence of schistocytes, persistent nucleated RBCs	–
Creatinine	–	2 × baseline	> 1.5 × baseline	–
Haptoglobin	decreased	–	–	decreased
Transfusion	increased	–	–	–
Direct Coombs test	–	negative	–	negative

HPF, High power field; *LDH*, lactate dehydrogenase; *RBCs*, red blood cells.
Modified from Obut F, Kasinath V, Abdi R. Post-bone marrow transplant thrombotic microangiopathy. *Bone Marrow Transplant.* 2016;51:891–897.

Outcome and Prognosis

AKI and chronic kidney disease (CKD) are well-known consequences of posttransplant TMA. Other complications include hypertension, proteinuria, congestive heart failure, pulmonary hypertension, gastrointestinal and intracranial hemorrhage, and death.[9] In a prospective study of children and young adults receiving allogeneic HSCT, acute dialysis was required in 8.9% of patients within the first year after transplant.[8] The risk was higher in patients developing posttransplant TMA (12.8%) as compared with those without TMA (5.9%). Those subjects who developed posttransplant TMA were more likely to need antihypertensive medications, require intensive care unit admission, and developed significantly more gastrointestinal bleeding and respiratory failure.

In a retrospective study done in 100 patients who underwent T-cell depleted stem cell transplantation at Memorial Sloan-Kettering Cancer Center, 11 patients developed TMA.[9] The 2-year cumulative incidence of CKD was 30% in those patients who did not receive total body irradiation and was near 50% in those who did. The only significant predictor of severe CKD was TMA (hazard ratio 4.3; $p <. 0001$). The development of TMA was also associated with the development of hypertension. Because hypertension and CKD significantly affect cardiovascular morbidity and mortality, it is imperative to recognize the impact of TMA on long-term mortality of patients undergoing HSCT.

Finally, in a study done by Arai et al., 90 patients were retrospectively analyzed posttransplantation.[17] The 1-year overall survival was found to be significantly lower and nonrelapse mortality was significantly higher in the TMA group as compared with the non-TMA group. In patients with posttransplant TMA and multiple organ dysfunction, mortality reaches more than 90%. Patients with pulmonary involvement often die from progressive pulmonary hypertension.

Treatment

SUPPORTIVE CARE

Primary treatment for posttransplant TMA involves withdrawal of any offending agents, such as calcineurin inhibitors. Treatment of coexisting conditions, such as infections and GVHD, is also necessary because these disorders can trigger TMA either directly or by activating complement. Hypertension should be aggressively managed. All adjunctive therapies in patients with TMA post-HSCT should be evaluated on a case-by-case basis and the risks and benefits carefully considered for each patient. Modification of GVHD prophylaxis management should be done with caution to avoid any flares of GVHD because this can worsen TMA.

THERAPEUTIC PLASMA EXCHANGE

In the past, TPE had been used as a main treatment of TMA because of its ability to remove mutated complement, antibodies against complement, other triggering factors for endothelial dysfunction, and allow for administration of large quantities of fresh plasma. However, TPE is usually ineffective in treating posttransplant TMA, because the pathogenesis is rarely caused by an acquired autoantibody against ADAMTS-13 (TTP). Rather, most cases of posttransplant TMA are as a result of either secondary HUS or aHUS. Nevertheless, TPE is often started until the results of the ADAMTS-13 activity level are known. It should be pointed out that, in general, TTP tends to result in more profound thrombocytopenia and less severe AKI compared with other forms of TMA. In fact, in patients with a platelet count greater than 20 K/mm^3 and a serum creatinine greater than 2.5 mg/dL, HUS is 20-fold more likely than TTP.[18,19] This observation should be remembered, because indiscriminant use of TPE exposes patients to potential complications, such as hemorrhage, thrombosis, infection, and serum sickness.[20] In addition, randomized controlled studies demonstrating the benefit of TPE in posttransplant TMA are lacking. Some reports have shown response rates of less than 50% and mortality rates as high as more than 80%. The Blood and Marrow Transplant Clinical Trials Network toxicity committee concluded that the use of TPE for posttransplant TMA cannot be considered standard of care.[21] Despite the high risk of complications of TPE in patients with posttransplant TMA, it can be considered for use in those with documented evidence of Factor H autoantibodies or decreased ADAMTS-13 activity level. Of course, the decision to start TPE should be made after risk-benefit assessment.

DEFIBROTIDE

This is a polydeoxyribonucleotide salt with potent antithrombotic, antiischemic, antiinflammatory, and thrombolytic properties, without systemic anticoagulant effects. Defibrotide therapy improves outcomes in some patients who develop hepatic sinusoidal obstruction syndrome (SOS) after HSCT. Because the pathophysiology of SOS and posttransplant TMA is similar, Corti et al. administered oral defibrotide to 12 patients affected with posttransplant TMA. In this trial, three patients achieved partial remission and five achieved complete remission.[22] Larger trials are necessary to confirm the benefits of defibrotide.

RITUXIMAB

Little data on the use of the B-cell depleting agent rituximab in posttransplant TMA are available. In a study by Au et al., five patients with posttransplant TMA refractory to treatment with TPE and steroids were given with rituximab 375 mg/m^2/weekly for four doses.[23] Four patients attained complete remission. Because this is a case series, it makes it hard to recommend rituximab as therapy for posttransplant TMA.

COMPLEMENT BLOCKADE THERAPY

Dysregulation of the complement system may be involved in the pathogenesis of posttransplant TMA. In these circumstances, HSCT may be the complement amplifying condition that unmasks the presence of aHUS and suggests that complement inhibitors may be a reasonable therapeutic option for posttransplant TMA. Eculizumab is a monoclonal antibody against complement factor C5 that prevents the generation of the membrane attack complex, C5b-9. It is a proven effective therapy for paroxysmal nocturnal hemoglobinuria and aHUS, and is a promising agent for posttransplant TMA. However, the drug is expensive and is associated with increased susceptibility to encapsulated bacterial infections, particularly meningococcal disease. In a study of pediatric patients, Jodele et al. treated six patients with severe posttransplant TMA using eculizumab.[24] Posttransplant TMA resolved over time in four of the six patients. To achieve therapeutic drug levels and a clinical response, the children required higher doses or more frequent infusions than what is recommended for children with aHUS. Successful treatment with eculizumab has been published in several case reports and small studies.[25] Compared with aHUS, eculizumab for posttransplant TMA appears to require a longer induction time, with at least 4 to 6 weeks of therapy.[26] Although these results are encouraging, given the current information, it is unclear in whom eculizumab should be used, at what dose and frequency, and the duration of therapy. Given the high cost and risk of infection, treatment should be individualized, and randomized controlled trials should be encouraged.

Summary

TMA is a clinical syndrome of thrombocytopenia and microangiopathic hemolytic anemia often associated with multiple organ dysfunction, particularly the kidneys. TMA is a well-recognized complication following HSCT associated with significant morbidity and mortality. Risk factors for development of posttransplant TMA include female gender, African American ethnicity, older age, presence of severe liver disease, and advanced malignancy. Transplant-related risk factors are unrelated donor status, HLA mismatch, intensive conditioning regimens, GVHD, calcineurin inhibitor use, and various infections. Pathogenesis of posttransplant TMA is incompletely understood, but in many cases direct endothelial injury causing secondary HUS is implicated. On the other hand, HSCT may unmask an underlying disorder in complement regulation, resulting in aHUS. No specific treatment for posttransplant TMA is currently available. TPE rarely affects outcomes despite sometimes improving hematologic parameters (LDH levels and platelet counts) because it does not address the pathogenic mechanism in the majority of patients. Use of anticomplement therapy is promising although, at this time, given the difficulty in identifying patients with complement dysregulation and the cost and infection risks associated with such therapy, routine use cannot be recommended. For now, supportive care, treating underlying associated conditions, and discontinuation of offending medications are key. Any other adjuvant therapies should be individualized and based on risks and benefits, and ideally, randomized controlled trials.

Key Points

- Thrombotic microangiopathy is a well-recognized, potentially lethal complication of hematopoietic stem cell transplantation.

- Risk factors for hematopoietic stem cell associated thrombotic microangiopathy include high-dose chemoradiation, graft-versus-host disease, HLA mismatch, infection, use of calcineurin inhibitors, and dysregulation of the complement system.
- Hematopoietic stem cell associated thrombotic microangiopathy injures multiple organs although the kidneys are the most severely affected.
- Treatment is directed at supportive care and stopping/treating any contributing factors (infection, calcineurin inhibitors). Therapeutic plasma exchange is usually ineffective.
- Inhibition of complement factor C5 with a monoclonal antibody (eculizumab) can reverse thrombotic microangiopathy in a subset of patients with inherent complement dysregulation.

References

1. Thomas, ED. Karnofsky Memorial Lecture. Marrow transplantation for malignant diseases. *J Clin Oncol*. 1983;1:517-531.
2. Laskin BL, Goebel J, Davies SM, Jodele S. Small vessels, big trouble in the kidneys and beyond: hematopoietic stem cell transplantation-associated thrombotic microangiopathy. *Blood*. 2011;118:1452-1462.
3. George JN, Li X, McMinn JR, Terrell DR, Vesely SK, Selby GB. Thrombotic thrombocytopenic purpura-hemolytic uremic syndrome following allogeneic HPC transplantation: a diagnostic dilemma. *Transfusion*. 2004;44:294-304.
4. Rosenthal J. Hematopoietic cell transplantation-associated thrombotic microangiopathy: a review of pathophysiology, diagnosis, and treatment. *J Blood Med*. 2016;7:181-186.
5. Jodele S, Licht C, Goebel J, et al. Abnormalities in the alternative pathway of complement in children with hematopoietic stem cell transplant-associated thrombotic microangiopathy. *Blood*. 2013;122:2003-2007.
6. Laurence J, Haller H, Mannucci PM, Nangaku M, Praga M, Rodriguez de Cordoba S. Atypical hemolytic uremic syndrome (aHUS): essential aspects of an accurate diagnosis. *Clin Adv Hematol Oncol*. 2016;14:2-15.
7. Stavrou E, Lazarus HM. Thrombotic microangiopathy in haematopoietic cell transplantation: an update. *Mediterr J Hematol Infect Dis*. 2010;2:e2010033.
8. Jodele S, Laskin BL, Dandoy CE, et al. A new paradigm: diagnosis and management of HSCT-associated thrombotic microangiopathy as multi-system endothelial injury. *Blood Rev*. 2015;29:191-204.
9. Glezerman IG, Jhaveri KD, Watson TH, et al. Chronic kidney disease, thrombotic microangiopathy, and hypertension following T cell-depleted hematopoietic stem cell transplantation. *Biol Blood Marrow Transplant*. 2010;16:976-984.
10. Dandoy CE, Hirsch R, Chima R, Davies SM, Jodele S. Pulmonary hypertension after hematopoietic stem cell transplantation. *Biol Blood Marrow Transplant*. 2013;19:1546-1556.
11. Hewamana S, Austen B, Murray J, Johnson S, Wilson K. Intestinal perforation secondary to haematopoietic stem cell transplant associated thrombotic microangiopathy. *Eur J Haematol*. 2009;83:277.
12. Inamoto Y, Ito M, Suzuki R, et al. Clinicopathological manifestations and treatment of intestinal transplant-associated microangiopathy. *Bone Marrow Transplant*. 2009;44:43-49.
13. Lerner D, Dandoy C, Hirsch R, Laskin B, Davies SM, Jodele S. Pericardial effusion in pediatric SCT recipients with thrombotic microangiopathy. *Bone Marrow Transplant*. 2014;49:862-863.
14. Dandoy CE, Davies SM, Hirsch R, et al. Abnormal echocardiography 7 days after stem cell transplantation may be an early indicator of thrombotic microangiopathy. *Biol Blood Marrow Transplant*. 2015;21:113-118.
15. Obut F, Kasinath V, Abdi R. Post-bone marrow transplant thrombotic microangiopathy. *Bone Marrow Transplant*. 2016;51:891-897.
16. Jodele S, Davies SM, Lane A, et al. Diagnostic and risk criteria for HSCT-associated thrombotic microangiopathy: a study in children and young adults. *Blood*. 2014;124:645-653.

17. Arai Y, Yamashita K, Mizugishi K, et al. Serum neutrophil extracellular trap levels predict thrombotic microangiopathy after allogeneic stem cell transplantation. *Biol Blood Marrow Transplant*. 2013;19: 1683-1689.

18. Coppo P, Schwarzinger M, Buffet M, et al. Predictive features of severe acquired ADAMTS13 deficiency in idiopathic thrombotic microangiopathies: the French TMA reference center experience. *PLoS One*. 2010;5:e10208.

19. Zuber J, Fakhouri F, Roumenina LT, Loirat C, Frémeaux-Bacchi V, French Study Group for a HUS/C3G. Use of eculizumab for atypical haemolytic uraemic syndrome and C3 glomerulopathies. *Nat Rev Nephrol*. 2012;8:643-657.

20. Rizvi MA, Vesely SK, George JN, et al. Complications of plasma exchange in 71 consecutive patients treated for clinically suspected thrombotic thrombocytopenic purpura-hemolytic-uremic syndrome. *Transfusion*. 2000;40:896-901.

21. Ho VT, Cutler C, Carter S, et al. Blood and Marrow Transplant clinical trials network toxicity committee consensus summary: thrombotic microangiopathy after hematopoietic stem cell transplantation. *Biol Blood Marrow Transplant*. 2005;11:571-575.

22. Corti P, Uderzo C, Tagliabue A, et al. Defibrotide as a promising treatment for thrombotic thrombocytopenic purpura in patients undergoing bone marrow transplantation. *Bone Marrow Transplant*. 2002;29: 542-543.

23. Au WY, Ma ES, Lee TL, et al. Successful treatment of thrombotic microangiopathy after haematopoietic stem cell transplantation with rituximab. *Br J Haematol*. 2007;137:475-478.

24. Jodele S, Fukuda T, Vinks A, et al. Eculizumab therapy in children with severe hematopoietic stem cell transplantation-associated thrombotic microangiopathy. *Biol Blood Marrow Transplant*. 2014;20:518-525.

25. Dhakal P, Giri S, Pathak R, Bhatt VR. Eculizumab in transplant-associated thrombotic microangiopathy. *Clin Appl Thromb Hemost*. 2017;23:175-180.

26. Jodele S, Fukuda T, Mizuno K, et al. Variable eculizumab clearance requires pharmacodynamic monitoring to optimize therapy for thrombotic microangiopathy after hematopoietic stem cell transplantation. *Biol Blood Marrow Transplant*. 2016;22:307-315.

14 *Graft-Versus-Host Disease*

STEFAN KEMMNER AND UWE HEEMANN

Introduction

Since 1957, when the first bone marrow transplantation was performed by Thomas et al., hematopoietic stem cell transplantation (HSCT) has been used for the treatment of several hematologic and autoimmune disorders.[1] With the discovery of the human leukocyte antigen (HLA) system in 1958 and the subsequent better understanding of histocompatibility, allogeneic and autologous stem cell transplantations became standard practice.[2] In the 1970s the number of bone marrow transplantations was low and the 1-year patient survival was less than 50%.[3] Currently, nearly 20,000 HSCTs are performed in the United States and 5-year survival approaches 50% (https://bloodcell.transplant.hrsa.gov). Thus long-term complications of HSCT were almost unknown in early 1970s but today, with an increase in life expectancy of patients, they are significant.

Although the use of HSCT in hematologic practice has led to meaningful improvements in outcomes, the preparative regimens, procedures, posttransplant complications, infections, and drugs that have to be used either for the procedure or its complications may limit patient survival. Therefore the management of these issues is essential for a higher survival rate. HSCT related complications can be mainly classified into four categories: infections, early noninfectious complications, late noninfectious complications, and graft-versus-host disease (GVHD). In this chapter, we focus on GVHD-associated kidney diseases.

Acute Kidney Injury After Homologous Stem Cell Transplantation

Acute kidney injury (AKI) is one of the most severe complications of HSCT and is especially common after myeloablative allogeneic HSCT, because this procedure requires intense immunosuppression that may cause severe sepsis or liver failure. In addition, use of calcineurin inhibitors (CNIs) is routine for the first 100 days after myeloablative allogeneic HSCT.[4] It should not be forgotten that candidates for HSCT often have low muscle mass and low creatinine production, when compared with a healthy population. Hence a mildly elevated serum creatinine concentration may be an important marker of a severe kidney damage. In all of these settings, use of a confirmatory test, such as cystatin C, or measurement of clearance of an exogenous filtration marker, such as inulin, iohexol, or iothalamate, will provide a more accurate assessment of glomerular filtration rate (GFR) than creatinine-based formulas.

During the first days and weeks of HSCT, recipients are at a high risk of many forms of AKI. Prerenal syndromes and hypovolemia induced by vomiting or diarrhea are one of the most common causes. Mucositis secondary to chemotherapy can result in poor oral fluid intake and may trigger hypovolemia as well. Acute tubular necrosis (ATN) can develop from hypoperfusion injury or as a result of medications such as cytarabine, busulfan, and fludarabine. Amphotericin B and aminoglycosides are also well-known causes of ATN.[5]

HSCT patients are prone to develop sepsis caused by high immunosuppressive potential of chemotherapeutic agents. Sepsis can result in decreased effective circulating volume and hypotension and is thus a major risk factor for AKI (Box 14.1). On the other hand, sepsis may induce inflammation, which leads to increased capillary permeability and intravascular fluid leak, resulting in total body volume overload, while depleting effective circulating volume and end-organ perfusion.[6]

The most frequently investigated and published complication of HSCT is GVHD. Although skin, gut, liver, and other organ involvements and manifestations associated with GVHD are widely defined, the effects on the kidney still remain unclear.

Graft-Versus-Host Disease–Associated Kidney Disease

Despite the multiple etiologies of posttransplant renal dysfunction, GVHD has rarely been linked to the kidney, and it was believed that the kidney was not involved in acute GVHD. However, several reports suggest that both acute and chronic GVHD may cause kidney disease.[7]

Formerly, any manifestation of GVHD that manifested within the first 100 days after HSCT was defined as acute and beyond that as chronic. However, this classification led to some confusion if pathologic signs of acute or chronic GVHD occurred outside of these periods.

This situation led to development of a classification scheme based on clinical findings to differentiate between acute and chronic GVHD. The widely accepted National Institutes of Health consensus criteria for the diagnosis of GVHD classifies manifestations of GVHD as diagnostic or distinctive for chronic GVHD, or as common to both acute and chronic GVHD. In the 2014 version, it is accepted that in the absence of features fulfilling criteria for the diagnosis of chronic GVHD, the persistence, recurrence, or new onset of characteristic skin, gastrointestinal tract, or liver abnormalities should be classified as acute GVHD regardless of the time after transplantation.[8,9]

Both acute and chronic GVHD are almost completely different pathologic processes. In acute GVHD, patients mostly present with rash, diarrhea, and liver function test abnormalities, and can be treated with the addition of another immunosuppressive agent, such as steroids, antithymocyte globulin, antitumor necrosis factor α, and photopheresis.[10] Thirty to sixty percent of patients with acute GVHD progress to chronic GVHD, which mostly requires a lifelong immunosuppression with a CNI, a potential risk for chronic kidney disease (CKD).[11]

THE PATHOPHYSIOLOGY OF GRAFT-VERSUS-HOST DISEASE

Although GVHD is observed after HSCT, the process itself begins before the infusion of stem cells. Because of several factors, such as the underlying disease and its treatment, infections, or chemoradiotherapy, host tissues may secrete inflammatory cytokines, including tumor necrosis factor α and interleukin (IL)-1, which may result in endothelial apoptosis.[12] This hypothesis explains the increased risk of GVHD associated with intensive preparative regimens. After infusion of stem cells to the host, donor T-cell stimulation occurs, resulting in activation of host antigen presenting cells and the development of GVHD. Activation of CD8+ and CD4+ T-cells by major histocompatibility complex (MHC) Class I and Class II antigens leads to the activation of intracellular pathways that cause the release of cytokines, such as IL-2, interferon-γ, IL-4, IL-5, IL-10, and IL-13. The activation of Th1 cells enhances T-cell proliferation and activates monocytes and macrophages. This in turn induces the migration of macrophages and their successive binding to the endothelium and subsequent extravasation from the vessels.[13–15] Finally, macrophages can produce high amounts of nitric oxide (NO) as a result of activation and NO contributes to the deleterious effects of GVHD on target tissues, inhibits repair mechanisms especially in the gut and skin, and enhances GVHD-induced immunosuppression.[16,17]

CLINICAL FEATURES OF GRAFT-VERSUS-HOST DISEASE

In acute GVHD, skin, liver, and gastrointestinal tract are primarily affected. Skin rash with blisters, abdominal pain,

nausea and vomiting, and the elevation of liver enzymes are typical symptoms. Acute GVHD is staged according to number and extent of organs involved into four grades (I-IV).[18] Acute GVHD is an important risk factor for the development of AKI.[19] The contribution of GVHD to AKI can be attributed to cytokine-induced inflammation affecting renal structures, the use of potential nephrotoxic drugs, and the increased risk of infections.[20] The pathology of the kidney in acute GVHD has been studied in some animal models. In these studies, infiltration of mononuclear cells in the renal tubule-interstitium, mainly around small arteries and veins, is typically identified, as well as acute glomerulonephritis and acute endarteritis.[7] Whereas acute GVHD has strong inflammatory components, chronic GVHD displays more autoimmune and fibrotic features. Fibrotic injury in chronic GVHD is characterized by accumulation of collagen. Fibroblasts take up the place of parenchymal cells and disrupt normal tissue function.[21,22]

Although kidneys are not traditionally considered to be the target organ for GVHD after HSCT, GVHD has been implicated as the cause of glomerular injuries. In acute GVHD, kidney dysfunction is predominantly related to causes, such as hypovolemia, nephrotoxic drugs, infections, and sepsis. Although these factors could contribute to chronic GVHD as well, an association of glomerular disease with chronic GVHD was reported in several cases and the cumulative incidence of nephrotic syndrome was given as 8% to 27.7%.[23–25] Membranous glomerulonephritis is the most frequent glomerular manifestation of chronic GVHD. Other reported forms of glomerulonephritis include minimal change disease, focal segmental glomerulosclerosis, membranoproliferative glomerulonephritis, antineutrophil cytoplasmic antibodies–associated glomerulonephritis, proliferative glomerulonephritis, and immunoglobulin A nephropathy.[26]

All of these renal disorders typically occur within 8 to 14 months after HSCT, especially after the cessation or dose reduction of CNIs.[27,28] Treatment for GVHD associated nephrotic syndrome is similar to that in other settings, and it includes steroids and the resumption of CNIs[28,29] and angiotensin-converting enzyme inhibitors or angiotensin receptor blockers. As in other forms of kidney diseases, albuminuria is an important indicator of the progression and risk of death.[30]

Another important disorder associated with GVHD and HSCT is thrombotic microangiopathy (TMA). Although it is more closely associated with chronic GVHD, TMA was present in 20% of kidneys at autopsy in patients after HSCT. The risk of TMA is increased fourfold in patients with acute GVHD. The incidence of TMA syndromes in the setting of HSCT ranges between 2% and 21%.[31] TMA is defined by hemolytic anemia with erythrocyte fragmentation, thrombocytopenia, and renal failure. Thickening of glomerular and arteriolar vessels caused by endothelial damage are caused by the fragmentation of erythrocytes and thrombosis, which are typical findings of TMA.[32,33] The progression of TMA is usually slow and results in CKD. However, acute flares may cause AKI. Risk factors for the development of TMA after HSCT include use of CNIs, total body irradiation, and GVHD.[34] In the treatment of TMA, therapeutic plasma exchange is usually ineffective and is not routinely recommended. Some patients are found to have dysregulation of their complement system and benefit from administration of the anti-C5 monoclonal antibody, eculizumab.[33] Because CNIs are considered to be one of the risk factors for TMA, alternative agents for prophylaxis or treatment of GVHD, such as mycophenolate mofetil, corticosteroids, or IL-2 receptor antagonists, should be considered.[35,36]

Summary

Although the use of HSCT in hematologic practice has led to meaningful improvements in outcomes, the preparative regimens, procedures, posttransplant complications, infections, and drugs that have to be used either for the procedure or its complications may limit patient survival. Therefore the management of these issues is essential for a higher survival rate. Despite the multiple etiologies of posttransplant renal dysfunction, GVHD has rarely been linked to the kidney, and it was believed that the kidney is not involved in acute GVHD. However, several reports suggest that both acute and chronic GVHD may cause kidney disease. Kidney disease in acute GVDH typically results from volume depletion, drug toxicity, or infection associated with development or treatment of GVHD. However, there is increasing evidence that acute GVHD can also induce AKI by directly stimulating an inflammatory response in the kidneys. In chronic GVHD, the kidneys display more autoimmune and fibrotic features, leading to CKD. In addition, chronic GVHD has been associated with development of the nephrotic syndrome, with varied pathologic findings.

Key Points

- Both acute and chronic graft-versus-host disease (GVHD) can cause kidney disease.
- Acute kidney injury associated with acute GVHD can be attributed to cytokine induced inflammation.
- Chronic GVHD promotes fibrogenesis and can result in progressive chronic kidney disease.
- Chronic GVHD is associated with glomerular injury, resulting in nephrotic syndrome most commonly caused by membranous nephropathy.
- GVHD is also associated with the development of thrombotic microangiopathy.

References

1. Thomas ED, Lochte HL Jr, Lu WC, Ferrebee JW. Intravenous infusion of bone marrow in patients receiving radiation and chemotherapy. *N Engl J Med*. 1957;257:491-496.
2. Dausset J. Iso-leuco-anticorps. *Acta Haematol*. 1958;20:156-166.
3. Thomas E, Storb R, Clift RA, et al. Bone-marrow transplantation (first of two parts). *N Engl J Med*. 1975;292:832-843.
4. Magee C. Kidney disease in liver, cardiac, lung, and hematopoietic cell transplantation. In: Johnson J, Feehally J, Floege J (eds) *Comprehensive clinical nephrology*. 5th ed. 2014, 1262-1264. Elsevier Saunders, Aachen, Germany.
5. Kersting S, Koomans HA, Hené RJ, Verdonck LF. Acute renal failure after allogeneic myeloablative stem cell transplantation: retrospective analysis of incidence, risk factors and survival. *Bone Marrow Transplant*. 2007;39:359-365.
6. Wan L, Bagshaw SM, Langenberg C, Saotome T, May C, Bellomo R. Pathophysiology of septic acute kidney injury: what do we really know? *Crit Care Med*. 2008;36:S198-S203.
7. Higo S, Shimizu A, Masuda Y, et al. Acute graft-versus-host disease of the kidney in allogeneic rat bone marrow transplantation. *PLoS One*. 2014;9:e115399.
8. Filipovich AH, Weisdorf D, Pavletic S, et al. National Institutes of Health consensus development project on criteria for clinical trials in chronic graft-versus-host disease: I. Diagnosis and staging working group report. *Biol Blood Marrow Transplant*. 2005;11:945-956.
9. Jagasia MH, Greinix HT, Arora M, et al. National Institutes of Health Consensus Development Project on criteria for clinical trials in chronic graft-versus-host disease: I. The 2014 Diagnosis and Staging Working Group report. *Biol Blood Marrow Transplant*. 2015;21:389-401.
10. Reddy P. Pathophysiology of acute graft-versus-host disease. *Hematol Oncol*. 2003;21:149-161.
11. Sawinski D. The kidney effects of hematopoietic stem cell transplantation. *Adv Chronic Kidney Dis*. 2014;21:96-105.
12. Ferrara JL, Cooke KR, Teshima T. The pathophysiology of acute graft-versus-host disease. *Int J Hematol*. 2003;78:181-187.
13. Xun CQ, Thompson JS, Jennings CD, Brown SA, Widmer MB. Effect of total body irradiation, busulfan-cyclophosphamide, or cyclophosphamide conditioning on inflammatory cytokine release and development of acute and chronic graft-versus-host disease in H-2-incompatible transplanted SCID mice. *Blood*. 1994;83:2360-2367.
14. Hill GR, Crawford JM, Cooke KJ, Brinson YS, Pan L, Ferrara JL. Total body irradiation and acute graft versus host disease. The role of gastrointestinal damage and inflammatory cytokincs. *Blood*. 1997;90:3204-3213.
15. Shlomchik WD, Couzens MS, Tang CB, et al. Prevention of graft versus host disease by inactivation of host antigen-presenting cells. *Science*. 1999;285:412-415.
16. Falzarano G, Krenger W, Snyder KM, Delmonte J, Karandikar M, Ferrara JL. Suppression of B cell proliferation to lipopolysaccharide is mediated through induction of the nitric oxide pathway by tumor necrosis factor-a in mice with acute graft-versus-host disease. *Blood*. 1996;87:2853-2860.
17. Krenger W, Falzarano G, Delmonte J, Snyder KM, Byon JC, Ferrara JL. Interferon-suppresses T-cell proliferation to mitogen via the nitric oxide pathway during experimental acute graft versus-host disease. *Blood*. 1996;88:1113-1121.
18. Jacobsohn DA, Vogelsang GB. Acute graft versus host disease. *Orphanet J Rare Dis*. 2007;2:35.
19. Lopes JA, Jorge S. Acute kidney injury following HCT: incidence, risk factors and outcome. *Bone Marrow Transplant*. 2011;46:1399-1408.
20. Krishnappa V, Gupta M, Manu G, Kwatra S, Owusu OT, Raina R. Acute kidney injury in hematopoietic stem cell transplantation: a review. *Int J Nephrol*. 2016;2016:5163789.
21. Duffield JS, Forbes SJ, Constandinou CM, et al. Selective depletion of macrophages reveals distinct, opposing roles during liver injury and repair. *J Clin Invest*. 2005;115:56-65.
22. Gangadharan B, Hoeve MA, Allen JE, et al. Murine gammaherpesvirus-induced fibrosis is associated with the development of alternatively activated macrophages. *J Leukoc Biol*. 2008;84:50-58.
23. Hu SL. The role of graft-versus-host disease in haematopoietic cell transplantation-associated glomerular disease. *Nephrol Dial Transplant*. 2011;26:2025-2031.
24. Colombo AA, Rusconi C, Esposito C, et al. Nephrotic syndrome after allogeneic hematopoietic stem cell transplantation as a late complication of chronic graft-versus-host disease. *Transplantation*. 2006;81:1087-1092.
25. Sakellari I, Barbouti A, Bamichas G, et al. GVHD-associated chronic kidney disease after allogeneic haematopoietic cell transplantation. *Bone Marrow Transplant*. 2013;48:1329-1334.
26. Barbouch S, Gaied H, Abdelghani KB, et al. Chronic graft versus host disease and nephrotic syndrome. *Saudi J Kidney Dis Transpl*. 2014;25:1062-1064.
27. Brukamp K, Doyle AM, Bloom RD, Bunin N, Tomaszewski JE, Cizman B. Nephrotic syndrome after hematopoietic cell transplantation: do glomerular lesions represent renal graft-versus-host disease? *Clin J Am Soc Nephrol*. 2006;1:685-694.
28. Abboud I, Peraldi MN, Hingorani S. Chronic kidney diseases in long-term survivors after allogeneic hematopoietic stem cell transplantation: monitoring and management guidelines. *Semin Hematol*. 2012;49:73-82.
29. Niscola P, Tendas A, Luo XD, et al. The management of membranous glomerulopathy in allogeneic stem cells transplantation: Updated literature. *Cardiovasc Hematol Agents Med Chem*. 2013;11:67-76.

30. Hingorani S. Renal complications of hematopoietic-cell transplantation. *N Engl J Med.* 2016;374:2256-2267.
31. Changsirikulchai S, Myerson D, Guthrie KA, McDonald GB, Alpers CE, Hingorani SR. Renal thrombotic microangiopathy after hematopoietic cell transplant: role of GVHD in pathogenesis. *Clin J Am Soc Nephrol.* 2009;4:345-353.
32. Batts ED, Lazarus HM. Diagnosis and treatment of transplantation-associated thrombotic microangiopathy: real progress or are we still waiting? *Bone Marrow Transplant.* 2007;40:709-719.
33. Khosla J, Yeh AC, Spitzer TR, Dey BR. Hematopoietic stem cell transplant-associated thrombotic microangiopathy: current paradigm and novel therapies. *Bone Marrow Transplant.* 2018;53:129-137.
34. Hingorani S, Angelo JR. Hematopoietic stem cell transplant–related kidney disease. In: *Onco-Nephrology Curriculum.* American Society of Nephrology; 2016. Available at available here: https://www.asn-online.org/education/distancelearning/curricula/onco/.
35. Choi CM, Schmaier AH, Snell MR, Lazarus HM. Thrombotic microangiopathy in haematopoietic stem cell transplantation: diagnosis and treatment. *Drugs.* 2009;69:183-198.
36. Wolff D, Wilhelm S, Hahn J, et al. Replacement of calcineurin inhibitors with daclizumab in patients with transplantation-associated microangiopathy or renal insufficiency associated with graft-versus-host disease. *Bone Marrow Transplant.* 2006;38:445-451.

15 Chronic Kidney Disease, End-Stage Renal Disease, and Bone Marrow Transplant

CLAUDE BASSIL

Introduction

Hematopoietic stem cell transplantation (HSCT) is commonly used as a treatment for malignant and nonmalignant diseases. Over the past decade, there has been more focus on the chronic complications post-HSCT, in particular chronic kidney disease (CKD), which is associated with high mortality in this population, especially in patients who progress to end-stage renal disease (ESRD) requiring dialysis. Although the HSCT may be curative of the underlying malignancy, it trades one set of problems with many chronic conditions associated with CKD.

The incidence of CKD post-HSCT is variable and ranges from 13% to 66%.[1-4] It develops from 6 months to 10 years[5,6] post-HSCT. The etiologies of CKD post-HSCT are not well identified; however, the occurrence of CKD has been associated with many risk factors.

Hingorani and her colleagues[4] have shown in a cohort study that the presence of acute renal failure (ARF) and graft-versus-host disease (GVHD), but not total body irradiation (TBI), were associated with the occurrence of CKD. Similar findings were duplicated in other clinical studies.[7-9] The variability in incidence rates of CKD, in adult and pediatric populations, likely reflects a lack of a standard definition of post-HSCT CKD. Differences are further compounded by the different HSCT modalities (autologous vs. allogeneic) and differences in the variable periods of follow-up.

Albuminuria and Chronic Kidney Disease After Hematopoietic Stem Cell Transplantation

Albuminuria, defined as a urine albumin:urine creatinine ratio (ACR) of 30 to 300 mg/g, is commonly used as a surrogate marker of systemic endothelial dysfunction and inflammation, affecting many organs, including the kidney. Albuminuria occurs frequently after HSCT and it correlates with acute GVHD (aGVHD), bacteremia, hypertension (HTN), and progression of renal disease.[10] Albuminuria at day 100 post-HSCT was associated with CKD at 1 year,[10] as defined by a glomerular filtration rate (GFR) below 60 mL/min/1.73 m^2, using the abbreviated modification of diet in renal disease equation, after adjusting for chronic GVHD (c-GVHD), HTN, diabetes, and age. In addition, Hingorani

and colleagues proposed a possible intrarenal inflammation after HSCT, by identifying elevated urinary levels of proinflammatory cytokines (interleukin [IL]-6, IL-15, and elafin), which were associated with the development of albuminuria and proteinuria (Table 15.1 and Fig. 15.1). Urinary elafin is an endogenous serine protease inhibitor, produced by epithelial cells and macrophages in response to tissue inflammation.[11] An elevated urinary elafin level is associated with both acute kidney injury and CKD.[11] Furthermore, albuminuria and proteinuria within the first 100 days post-HSCT are associated with decreased overall survival.[12]

Relationship Between Graft-Versus-Host Disease and Chronic Kidney Disease

A formal pathologic criterion of proper renal GVHD (r-GVHD) does not exist yet. However, a probable relationship between GVHD and kidney injury may be demonstrated. In a mouse model of GVHD, many changes were described, highlighting an immune-mediated renal injury. There was an upregulation of antigen presenting pathways in the kidney, adaptive and innate immune responses. In addition, infiltration of the kidney by CD3+ T cells, and expression of vascular adhesion molecules were seen, which favor an underlying endothelial injury.[13] Furthermore, Mii and colleagues[14] described the kidney as a potential target of c-GVHD by identifying renal tubulitis, peritubular capillaritis, and glomerulitis. In addition to the T-cell infiltration, the kidney may be the target of chronic inflammatory state of GVHD, which may lead to renal injury. Several proinflammatory cytokines were seen in the urine of these patients.[15,16]

In the majority of cases of CKD post-HSCT, the cause is either idiopathic or multifactorial. However, several clinical syndromes of CKD in long-term survivors of HSCT have been proposed and that include:

- Transplant associated thrombotic microangiopathy (TA-TMA) also known as *bone marrow transplant nephropathy*.
- Nephrotic syndrome.
- Viral infections and renal diseases.
- Idiopathic: includes "progression of old acute injury," and "multifactorial" CKD category.

Table 15.1 Association Between Different Urinary Cytokines, Albuminuria, and Acute Kidney Disease/Chronic Kidney Disease[11,12]

Cytokines	Association
*IL-6 and IL-15	Microalbuminuria and persistent macroalbuminuria
Elafin	Development of micro- and macroalbuminuria, AKI, and CKD
MCP-1	Development of CKD at 1 year post-HSCT

AKI, Acute kidney injury; *CKD*, chronic kidney disease; *HSCT*, hematopoietic stem cell transplantation; *IL*, interleukin; *MCP-1*, monocyte chemoattractant protein-1.

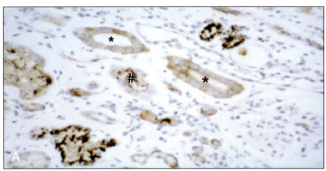
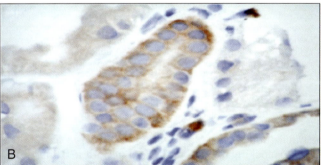

Fig. 15.1 Elafin staining in hematopoietic cell transplantation and control kidney samples. **A.** Intermediate-power image shows positive staining in a subset of tubules and negative glomerulus (*arrowhead*). This case demonstrated several patterns, including diffuse finely (*) and coarsely (upper right and lower left) granular, as well as coarse luminal granules (#) (3,3'-diaminobenzidine; original magnification, ×200). **B.** Finely granular cytoplasmic staining was most commonly diffusely distributed within the cytoplasm. (From Hingorani SFL, Pao E, Lawler R, Schoch G, McDonald GB, Najafian B, et al. Urinary elafin and kidney injury in hematopoietic cell transplant recipients. *Clin J Am Soc Nephrol.* 2015;10: 12–20.)

TA-TMA Category

TA-TMA is a serious complication, associated with higher morbidity and mortality compared with other complications occurring post-HSCT. Patients who survive the TA-TMA course end up with long-term morbidity and chronic organ injury, including CKDs or ESRDs.

Although the exact pathogenic mechanism resulting in TA-TMA is not well identified, significant advances have been made. The complement activation plays a significant role in the pathogenesis, and TA-TMA may coincide and be an endothelial variant of GVHD. The incidence of TA-TMA

varies widely, ranging from 0.5% to 63%.[17] This wide variation can be explained by the diagnostic uncertainty of TA-TMA criteria among many cancer centers. Jodele and her colleagues[18] reported an incidence of 39% in their prospective study, but the incidence of TA-TMA in many other retrospective studies ranges around 15% to 18%.[19,20] Many reported risks factors have been associated with the development of TA-TMA after allogeneic HSCT, in particular aGVHD (especially grade 2–4) and unrelated donor type,[21–28] in addition to other important risk factors including: older age; female sex; advanced primary cancer disease; unrelated donor transplants; conditioning regimen (high-dose busulfan—16 mg/kg), human leukocyte antigen mismatch, nonmyeloablative transplants (NMAT), TBI, cyclosporine or tacrolimus use, rapamycin inhibitor use, aGVHD, and other infections.

CLINICAL PRESENTATION AND DIAGNOSIS

Many proposed definitions of TA-TMA have been used, but the most relevant criteria used to diagnose TA-TMA[18,29–31] are Blood and Marrow Transplant Clinical Trials Network (BMT-CTN) and International Working Group (IWG) criteria (Table 15.2). TA-TMA should be diagnosed in patients who present with hemolytic anemia, excessive transfusion requirements, thrombocytopenia, elevated lactate dehydrogenase (LDH), and presence of schistocytes on the peripheral smear. If TA-TMA is described on a kidney biopsy, no further criteria need to be met. However, if there is elevated LDH, proteinuria (random urinalysis protein concentration of $\geq$ 30 mg/dL), and HTN, closer monitoring is required. Although biochemical parameters are important in early diagnosis, the earliest sign of TA-TMA is HTN. Therefore a high degree of suspicion is needed in an HSCT recipient who requires more than two antihypertensive medications until proven otherwise.[32] Renal manifestations of TA-TMA include: impaired GFR; proteinuria; and HTN.[33,34]

The definitive diagnosis of renal associated thrombotic microangiopathy requires a tissue biopsy, because many kidney diseases share clinical similarities with TA-TMA.

Table 15.2 Diagnosis of Hematopoietic Stem Cell Transplantation-Associated Thrombotic Microangiopathy: Blood and Marrow Transplant Clinical Trials Network and International Working Group Criteria

Test	BMT-CTN Criteria[29]	IWG Criteria
Schistocytes	$\geq$ 2 per high power field	> 4%
Elevated LDH	+	+
Thrombocytopenia	–	+
Decreased hemoglobin or need for transfusion	–	+
Negative Coombs test	+	+
Decreased haptoglobin	–	+
Renal dysfunction	+	–
Neurologic dysfunction	+	–

HSCT, Hematopoietic stem cell transplantation; *LDH*, lactate dehydrogenase; *TMA*, thrombotic microangiopathy.

However, because of the increased risk of bleeding in HSCT patients, kidney biopsies are rarely done.

For the pathologic findings associated with TA-TMA see Table 15.3 and Fig. 15.2.

Various definitions for the diagnosis of transplant-associated thrombotic microangiopathy are employed.

Per BMT-CTN, IWG, all criteria are needed under each group of guidelines to make the diagnosis of TA-TMA. "+" refers to included in the guidelines and "−" refers to not included.

TREATMENT

A systematic approach to monitor and diagnose a patient with TA-TMA is needed (Fig. 15.3). All patients with HSCT should be monitored closely every 2 to 4 weeks by checking their blood pressure, renal function, urinalysis, proteinuria, and LDH. If the patients are considered suspicious of having TA-TMA, their blood pressure and other biomarkers including hemoglobin, platelets, LDH, serum creatinine, and proteinuria should be monitored closely. Once the diagnosis of TA-TMA is certain, a kidney biopsy will be needed if no absolute contraindications exist, such as severe thrombocytopenia, hemodynamic instability, etc. However, if TA-TMA is unlikely, alternate causes of renal dysfunction, proteinuria, and HTN should be examined. If the diagnosis of TA-TMA is highly probable, supportive measures are needed, such as removal of precipitating factors, including calcineurin inhibitor (CNI), and/or sirolimus, and replacing them with other appropriate GVHD treatment/prophylaxis.

Because of the probable relationship between TA-TMA and GVHD, and the lack of conclusive data, stopping CNI may be harmful in a patient with life-threatening GVHD, but it may be acceptable in a mild TA-TMA case. Other supportive measures include: platelet and red blood cell transfusion, tight blood pressure control with renin-angiotensin pathway inhibitors, and renal support with various modalities of renal replacement therapy. In terms of immunomodulatory agents, data are limited and most of the treatment options include: plasmapheresis, with a variable response rate between 59% and 65%. The mechanism includes removal of potential inhibitor/antibody of the alternative complement cascade.[32,37,38] However many reported serious side effects were associated with this therapy, including bleeding, infections, and hypotension.

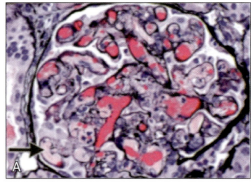

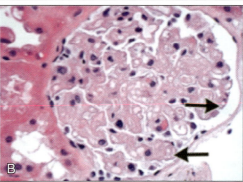

Fig. 15.2 Pathologic changes in the kidney caused by acute and chronic thrombotic microangiopathy. **A.** The glomerulus has capillary congestion with focal mesangial lysis and extensive fibrin thrombi (*arrow*). Membrane duplication is visible only in rare segments (Jones's methenamine silver stain, high magnification). **B.** The normocellular glomerulus has diffuse membrane duplication (*arrows*) and narrowed capillary lumens (hematoxylin and eosin, high magnification). (From Hingorani S. Renal Complications of Hematopoietic-Cell Transplantation. *N Engl J Med.* 2016;374: 2256–2226.)

Daclizumab[39] was reported in few cases as alternative to CNI, by blocking the IL-2 pathway, but skin rash, infections, and autoimmune diseases were reported as potential side effects of this therapy. Moreover, rituximab has been used successfully in 15 patients with an 80% response rate without major side effects, except infusion reactions and infections.[38,40,41] However, eculizumab is the only drug with promising results, because of the relevant role of complement activation mechanism in the pathogenesis of TA-TMA. Eculizumab was used in a total of 25 patients[33,42–44] with a 67% response rate and two reported side effects,

Table 15.3 Pathologic Findings from Kidney Biopsies in Patients With Transplant-Associated Thrombotic Microangiopathy (see Fig. 15.1A)

	TA-TMA
Light microscopy	• Glomerular endothelial swelling • Basement membrane (BM) duplication • Mesangiolysis with diffuse arteriolonecrosis[35] • Occluded vascular lumens • Tubular injury with interstitial fibrosis[36] • Formation of inner glomerular BM leading to the classic double contour appearance
Immunofluorescence	• Negative for any immune complexes, although nonspecific staining may be seen with fibrin
Electron microscopy	• Arteriolar and/or glomerular thrombi with subendothelial space widening[36] • Extensive or focal podocyte foot effacement[36]

TA-TMA, Transplant-associated thrombotic microangiopathy.

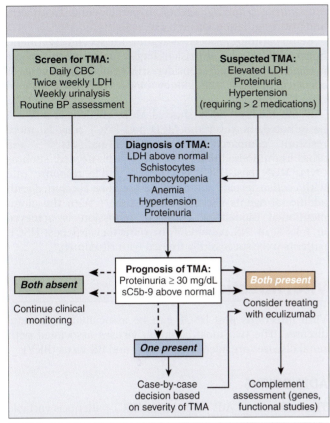

Fig. 15.3 Algorithm for the evaluation of thrombotic microangiopathy (TMA) after hematopoietic stem cell transplantation (HSCT). Screening for TMA includes monitoring lactate dehydrogenase (LDH), complete blood count (CBC), and routine urinalyses. TMA should be suspected in HSCT recipients with an acute elevation of LDH, proteinuria greater than 30 mg/dL, and hypertension more severe than expected with calcineurin or steroid therapy, usually requiring more than 2 antihypertensive medications. Clinical interventions should be considered for patients with both proteinuria > 30 mg/dL and elevated sC5b-9. *BP*, Blood pressure. (From Jodele S, Davies SM, Lane A, Khoury J, Dandoy C, Goebel J, et al. Diagnostic and risk criteria for HSCT-associated thrombotic microangiopathy: a study in children and young adults. *Blood*. 2014; 124: 645–653.)

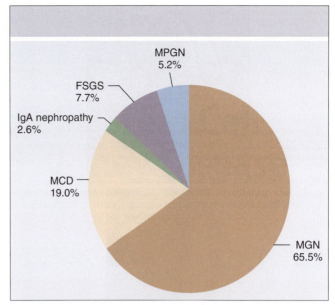

Fig. 15.4 Renal pathology observed in nephrotic syndrome after hematopoietic stem cell transplantation. MPGN indicates membranoproliferative glomerulonephritis. *FSGS, IgA,* immunoglobulin A; *MCD,* minimal change disease; *MGN,* membranous nephropathy. (From Beyar-Katz O, Davila E, Zuckerman T, Fineman R, Haddad N, Okasha D, et al. FSGS: focal and segmental glomerulosclerosis. Adult nephrotic syndrome after hematopoietic stem cell transplantation: renal pathology is the best predictor of response to therapy. *Biol Blood Marrow Transplant. 2016;* 22: 975–981.)

including infections and bleeding. Furthermore, the patients with high risk TA-TMA, defined as patients with proteinuria and activated terminal complement pathway and multiorgan involvement, who received eculizumab, had a better survival than untreated patients (62% vs. 9%) at 1 year from TMA diagnosis (*p*=.007).[43]

Nephrotic Syndrome

c-GVHD is well described in many organs, but the effect on the kidney is not well recognized. A review of the literature supports the existence of r-GVHD, associated clinically with nephrotic syndrome (NS). Most of the case reports found temporal associations of glomerular alterations with GVHD and tapering of immunosuppressive agents, used for GVHD prophylaxis.[45] The common pathologic lesions found on kidney biopsies in these patients were membranous nephropathy (MGN) in two-thirds of the cases followed by minimal change disease (MCD)[45–47] (Fig. 15.4). c-GVHD is a

well-described entity occurring postallogeneic HSCT, but its pathophysiology is poorly understood. Experimental models of c-GVHD showed that autoantibody formation plays a prominent role in the pathophysiology of the disease. But despite the murine models of c-GVHD, where renal involvement was described, the same findings may not be clearly identified in humans. However, most patients with c-GVHD have evidence of autoantibodies to several cell surface, intracellular antigens,[48,49] and against minor histocompatibility antigens, which may play a major role in the pathogenesis of c-GVHD in humans.[50–52]

EPIDEMIOLOGY

NS post-HSCT is extremely rare, with an incidence around 1%;[46–54] however, NMAT HSCT is associated with a higher incidence of NS at 6%.[55] Colombo et al. found a NS incidence of 8% in patients with c-GVHD, with a markedly higher probability in patients who received peripheral blood stem cells compared with bone marrow cells.[56]

PATHOLOGY

The development of NS usually happens in the late posttransplant period more than 6 months post-HSCT.[57] The two most common renal pathologies for NS post-HSCT are MGN (Fig. 15.5) in two-thirds of the cases followed by MCD.

PATHOPHYSIOLOGY

In general, NS develops after the cessation or tapering of immunosuppressive therapy, which suggests that NS could be a

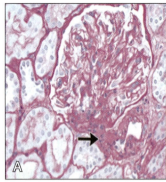

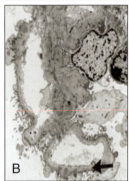

Fig. 15.5 A. A normocellular glomerulus with slightly thickened basement membranes and barely visible membrane spikes. The beadlike hyalinosis (*arrow*) of the artery may be a result of treatment with calcineurin inhibitors (periodic acid-Schiff, medium magnification). **B.** An electron micrograph of the same kidney-biopsy specimen shows scattered epimembranous and intramembranous electron-dense deposits (*arrow*) and effacement of the foot process focally (uranyl acetate). (From Hingorani S. Renal Complications of Hematopoietic-Cell Transplantation. *N Engl J Med.* 2016;374: 2256–2226.)

manifestation of c-GVHD. Many hypotheses were proposed to explain the pathophysiology of NS post-HSCT (Table 15.4).

TREATMENT

It is unclear whether the same management used in idiopathic NS works for NS post-HSCT. In general, nonspecific therapy is adopted by initiating the angiotensin-converting enzyme inhibitors or angiotensin receptor blockers as

proteinuria reducing agents, hyperlipidemia treatment, and anticoagulation for high-risk patients.

Renal pathology is needed to guide the specific treatment; however, because of the risk of biopsy in thrombocytopenic patients, one should consider the empiric treatment of corticosteroids, if the kidney biopsy is contraindicated (Fig. 15.6).

If the kidney biopsy showed MCD, corticosteroids will be initiated, however the MCD post-HSCT may be more resistant, compared with non-HSCT patients,[66,67] and other immunomodulatory agents will be needed, such as CNIs. MGN post-HSCT has less favorable response rate with corticosteroids alone and it should be combined with additional agents like idiopathic MGN.[39] With the aforementioned modalities, complete remission is achieved in 63.5% of NS patients.[68] In refractory NS post-HSCT, patients were successfully treated with rituximab.[47,50]

Viral Infections

Viral infections post-HSCT can be associated with renal diseases. The two most common viruses associated with renal diseases are adenovirus (AdV) and BK virus (BKV).

ADENOVIRUS

The incidence of AdV infection in HSCT patients is variable between 9% and 31.3%.[69–72] Early diagnosis and effective treatment are essential in treating systemic adenovirus infection, to avoid severe complications. Furthermore, the diagnosis of AdV disease requires the presence of prodromal symptoms, including hemorrhagic cystitis, fever, urodynia, and hematuria, in addition to the AdV isolation and/or frequent detection of the AdV genome by polymerase chain reaction in urine/sera. Primary infections, transmission with a transplant organ, or reactivation of a latent infection are the different modes of transmission of AdV. AdV nephritis can be complicated by renal failure in 90% of infected patients.[42] Pathologic features of AdV nephritis include: interstitial nephritis, with the presence of viral inclusions in tubular cells; presence of granulomas around the tubules; and in severe cases, it can present as necrotizing

Table 15.4 Pathophysiology of Nephrotic Syndrome Posthematopoietic Stem Cell Transplantation

Theory	Mechanism	Role for T/B Cells or Cytokines
Murine models	▪ Membranous changes in the recipient kidney after donor lymphocyte infusion[58]	▪ Dysregulation of B and T cells[59] ▪ Dysregulation of cytokines[59]
T cells	▪ Alloreactive donor T cells (ADT) targets host major and/or minor histocompatibility antigens[60] ▪ ADT targets the kidney and induce podocyte expression of CD80, mainly in MCD[61]	▪ Role for alloreactive T cells ▪ Levels of regulatory T cells are lower in NS HSCT patients compared with non-NS[62]
B cells	▪ Role of B cells in c-GVHD: dysregulation of B cells with high prevalence of autoantibodies[63] ▪ Improvement of MGN post-rituximab[64]	▪ Dysregulation of B cells in c-GVHD
Cytokines	▪ Association between TNF-α (from allogeneic T cells) and NS[62] ▪ TNF-α and IFN-γ higher level in NS[65]	▪ Role of TNF-α and IFN-γ in NS

c-GVHD, Chronic graft-versus-host disease; *HSCT,* hematopoietic stem cell transplantation; *INF-γ,* interferon γ; *MCD,* minimal change disease; *MGN,* membranous nephropathy; *NS,* nephrotic syndrome; *TNF-α,* tumor necrosis factor α.

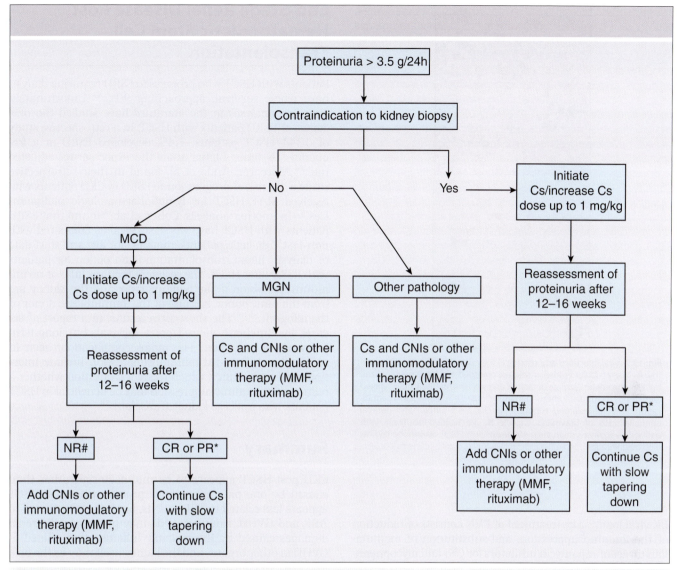

Fig. 15.6 Management of nephrotic syndrome after hematopoietic stem cell transplantation. *CR or PR**, Complete response defined as a reduction in proteinuria levels greater than 5 g/day, and partial response defined as a reduction in proteinuria greater than 50% relative to baseline values; *Cs*, corticosteroid; *CNIs*, calcineurin inhibitors; *MMF*, mycophenolate mofetil; *NR#*, no reduction in proteinuria level. (From Beyar-Katz O, Davila E, Zuckerman T, Fineman R, Haddad N, Okasha D, et al. Adult nephrotic syndrome after hematopoietic stem cell transplantation: renal pathology is the best predictor of response to therapy. *Biol Blood Marrow Transplant.* 2016; 22: 975–981.)

tubulointerstitial nephritis.[73] Moreover, adenovirus nephritis can lead to ureteral obstruction and hydronephrosis.[73,74] Cidofovir is commonly used to treat life-threatening AdV infections, with similar pharmacokinetics between pediatric patients and adults.[75]

BK NEPHRITIS AND HEMORRHAGIC CYSTITIS (Fig. 15.7)

Polyomavirus nephropathy (PVN) has been more reported as a cause of renal failure in native kidneys post-HSCT. It is often underdiagnosed, because CKD post-HSCT is usually attributed to other etiologies. Moreover, patients with BKV infection do not have any prodromal symptoms, and high degree of suspicion is needed. After a primary infection in early childhood, BKV appears to establish latency in the genitourinary tract.[76] After immunosuppression, asymptomatic viral replication occurs, as manifested by a viruria, and some patients will progress to invasive infection of the kidney, termed *PVN*. BKV infection causes several clinical manifestations in addition to nephropathy and hemorrhagic cystitis.[77] For the diagnosis of PVN (polyomavirus), high BK viral loads in the urine and the blood, and the presence of decoy cells, will help as a potential diagnostic surrogate; however the final diagnosis of PVN is confirmed by a kidney biopsy. Renal histopathologic changes of PVN include: tubulointerstitial nephritis,[78,79] with interstitial inflammation; tubular injury; and tubulitis. SV40 stains positively in the tubulointerstitium, showing viral inclusions. Moreover, BKV can cause hemorrhagic cystitis, urethritis, and urinary tract obstruction. The severity of renal damage has been shown to be dependent on the

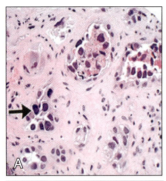

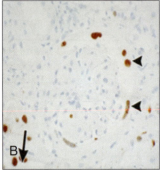

Fig. 15.7 Viral infections and chronic kidney disease. BK virus nephropathy. **A.** Many tubular epithelial cells are enlarged and have marginalized nuclear chromatin (*arrow*); detached and necrotic epithelial cells mixed with debris fill tubular lumens (hematoxylin and eosin, medium magnification). Several enlarged tubular epithelial cells (*arrow*) and parietal epithelial cells of Bowman's capsule **B.** are stained positively with antibodies against simian virus 40 (*arrowheads*) (3,3'-diaminobenzidine, high magnification). (From Hingorani S. Renal Complications of Hematopoietic-Cell Transplantation. *N Engl J Med*. 2016;374: 2256–2226.)

BK viral load.[80] The treatment of PVN consists of reduction of the immunosuppression, and substitution of mammalian target of rapamycin inhibitors for CNI and mycophenolate. Cidofovir can be tried in some patients with severe hemorrhagic cystitis.[81] Because of the nephrotoxicity of cidofovir, its use is limited in the management of PKN despite the hydration and the use of probenecid to decrease its nephrotoxicity.[82]

Idiopathic Chronic Kidney Disease

If the patients with CKD post-HSCT do not meet the criteria for TMA or NS, and they do not have BKV or AdV infections, their CKD will be considered as idiopathic. The incidence of idiopathic CKD post-TMA is around 17.5%,[3] and up to 66% in NMAT.[2] Major risk factors associated with idiopathic CKD post-MAT include acute and chronic GVHD and ARF,[2,3] but for NMAT, other risk factors were described: CKD; old autologous transplant; and CNI use.[2,3] The associations between GVHD and idiopathic CKD may be explained by the T cell-mediated renal damage, or via the inflammatory and cytokine cascade.[83,84] CNI nephrotoxicity may be exacerbated in the presence of chronic inflammatory process. CKD post-HSCT appears more as multifactorial in origin, related to GVHD, chronic inflammatory process, and exacerbated by nephrotoxic medications.

End-Stage Renal Disease Post-Hematopoietic Stem Cell Transplantation

Patients with HSCT who progress to ESRD requiring dialysis have worse survival, approaching 90%.[85] Unfortunately, only few analyses in the literature have studied the outcomes of ESRD patients with HSCT. In a retrospective study of 1341 HSCT patients, 1.4% developed ESRD at a frequency 16 times higher than the expected age-adjusted rate.[86] Moreover, Ando et al. found in their retrospective study a 4% risk of progression to ESRD in CKD patients who received MAT HSCT for lymphohaematologic malignancies.[87] In another analysis, Cohen et al.[85] found that ESRD patients with HSCT have worse survival as compared with non-HSCT diabetic patients, matched for age and start date of dialysis. Renal transplantation is an option for patients with ESRD after HSCT. The recipient requires little or no immunosuppression if the bone marrow and the kidney are from the same donor, because of the immunologic donor of the allograft.[88,89] The short-term results, in a report of six cases by Butcher,[3] showed good survival, but long-term follow-up is unknown. The major complications seen in recipients who needed immunosuppression include infections and malignancy, which raises the question whether a reduction in immunosuppression may be beneficial in HSCT patients who undergo kidney transplant.[88]

Summary

CKD post-HSCT appears to be multifactorial rather than caused by one pathophysiologic process. CKD post-HSCT appears less related to TBI or CNIs, but it is more related to ARF and GVHD. However, CNIs may potentiate the renal damages caused by the systemic inflammation related to GVHD in other organs, and the kidney itself may be the host in GVHD. In conclusion, it is essential for us to understand the pathogenic mechanisms of CKD post-HSCT, so that we can design targeted therapies, and therefore improve the prognosis of CKD post-HSCT.

Key Points

- Chronic kidney disease post-hematopoietic stem cell transplantation (HSCT) appears as multifactorial in origin, related to graft-versus-host disease, chronic inflammatory process, and exacerbated by nephrotoxic medications.
- Intrarenal inflammation after HSCT is identified by an elevated urinary level of proinflammatory cytokines (interleukin [IL]-6, IL-15, and elafin), which are associated with the development of albuminuria and proteinuria.
- Hypertension is the earliest sign of TA-TMA.
- Rituximab may have a role in refractory nephropathic syndrome post-HSCT.
- Renal transplantation is an option for patients with end-stage renal disease following HSCT, and the recipient requires little or no immunosuppression if the bone marrow and the kidney are from the same donor.

References

1. Cohen EP. Radiation nephropathy after bone marrow transplantation. *Kidney Int*. 2000;58:903-918.
2. Weiss AS, Sandmaier BM, Storer B, Storb R, McSweeney PA, Parikh CR. Chronic kidney disease following non-myeloablative hematopoietic cell transplantation. *Am J Transplant*. 2006;6:89-94.
3. Hingorani S. Risk factors for chronic kidney disease after hematopoietic cell transplant. *Biol Blood Marrow Transplant*. 2005;11:72-73.
4. Hingorani S, Guthrie KA, Schoch G, Weiss NS, McDonald GB. Chronic kidney disease in long-term survivors of hematopoietic cell transplant. *Bone Marrow Transplant*. 2007;39:223-229.
5. Ileri T, Ertem M, Ozcakar ZB, et al. Prospective evaluation of acute and chronic renal function in children following matched related donor hematopoietic stem cell transplantation. *Pediatr Transplant*. 2010; 14:138-144.
6. Abboud I, Porcher R, Robin M, et al. Chronic kidney dysfunction in patients alive without relapse 2 years after allogeneic hematopoietic stem cell transplantation. *Biol Blood Marrow Transplant*. 2009; 15:1251-1257.
11. Hingorani S, Finn LS, Pao E, et al. Urinary elafin and kidney injury in hematopoietic cell transplant recipients. *Clin J Am Soc Nephrol*. 2015;10:12-20.
12. Hingorani S, Gooley T, Pao E, Sandmaier B, McDonald G. Urinary cytokines after HCT: evidence for renal inflammation in the pathogenesis of proteinuria and kidney disease. *Bone Marrow Transplant*. 2014;49: 403-409.
13. Sadeghi B, Al-Chaqmaqchi H, Al-Hashmi S, et al. Early-phase GVHD gene expression profile in target versus non-target tissues: kidney, a possible target? *Bone Marrow Transplant*. 2013;48:284-293.
14. Mii A, Shimizu A, Kaneko T, et al. Renal thrombotic microangiopathy associated with chronic graft-versus-host disease after allogeneic hematopoietic stem cell transplantation. *Pathol Int*. 2011;61:518-527.
17. George JN, Li X, McMinn JR, Terrell DR, Vesely SK, Selby GB. Thrombotic thrombocytopenic purpura-hemolytic uremic syndrome following allogeneic HPC transplantation: a diagnostic dilemma. *Transfusion*. 2004; 44:294-304.
18. Jodele S, Davies SM, Lane A, et al. Diagnostic and risk criteria for HSCT-associated thrombotic microangiopathy: a study in children and young adults. *Blood*. 2014;124:645-653.
19. Willems E, Baron F, Seidel L, Frère P, Fillet G, Beguin Y. Comparison of thrombotic microangiopathy after allogeneic hematopoietic cell transplantation with high-dose or nonmyeloablative conditioning. *Bone Marrow Transplant*. 2010;45:689-693.
21. Ye Y, Zheng W, Wang J, et al. Risk and prognostic factors of transplantation associated thrombotic microangiopathy in allogenic hematopoietic stem cell transplantation: a nested case control study. *Hematol Oncol*. 2017;35:821-827.
22. Uderzo C, Bonanomi S, Busca A, et al. Risk factors and severe outcome in thrombotic microangiopathy after allogeneic hematopoietic stem cell transplantation. *Transplantation*. 2006;82:638-644.
23. Daly AS, Hasegawa WS, Lipton JH, Messner HA, Kiss TL. Transplantation-associated thrombotic microangiopathy is associated with transplantation from unrelated donors, acute graft-versus-host disease and venoocclusive disease of the liver. *Transfus Apher Sci*. 2002;27:3-12.
29. Ho VT, Cutler C, Carter S, et al. Blood and Marrow Transplant Clinical Trials Network Toxicity Committee Consensus Summary: thrombotic microangiopathy after hematopoietic stem cell transplantation. *Biol Blood Marrow Transplant*. 2005;11:571-575.
30. Ruutu T, Barosi G, Benjamin RJ, et al. Diagnostic criteria for hematopoietic stem cell transplant-associated microangiopathy: results of a consensus process by an international working group. *Hematologica*. 2007;92:95-100.
31. Cho BS, Yahng SA, Lee SE, et al. Validation of recently proposed consensus criteria for thrombotic microangiopathy after allogeneic hematopoietic stem cell transplantation. *Transplantation*. 2010;90: 918-926.
32. Laskin BL, Goebel J, Davies SM, Jodele S. Small vessels, big trouble in the kidneys and beyond: hematopoietic stem cell transplantation-associated thrombotic microangiopathy. *Blood*. 2011;118:1452-1462.
33. Jodele S, Laskin BL, Dandoy CE, et al. A new paradigm: diagnosis and management of HSCT-associated thrombotic microangiopathy as multi-system endothelial injury. *Blood Rev*. 2015;29:191-204.
34. Hoffmeister PA, Hingorani SR, Storer BE, Baker KS, Sanders JE. Hypertension in long-term survivors of pediatric hematopoietic cell transplantation. *Biol Blood Marrow Transplant*. 2010;16:515-524.
35. Antignac C, Gubler MC, Leverger G, Broyer M, Habib R. Delayed renal failure with extensive mesangiolysis following bone marrow transplantation. *Kidney Int*. 1989;35:1336-1344.
36. Chang A, Hingorani S, Kowalewska J, et al. Spectrum of renal pathology in hematopoietic cell transplantation: a series of 20 patients and review of the literature. *Clin J Am Soc Nephrol*. 2007;2:1014-1023.
37. Jodele S, Laskin B, Goebel J, et al. Does early initiation of therapeutic plasma exchange improve outcome in pediatric stem cell transplant-associated thrombotic microangiopathy? *Transfusion*. 2013;53:661-667.
40. Au WY, Ma ES, Lee TL, et al. Successful treatment of thrombotic microangiopathy after haematopoietic stem cell transplantation with rituximab. *Br J Haematol*. 2007;137:475-478.
42. Jodele S, Fukuda T, Vinks A, et al. Eculizumab therapy in children with severe hematopoetic stem cell transplantation associated thrombotic microangiopathy. *Biol Blood Marrow Transplant*. 2013;20:518-525.
45. Brukamp K, Doyle AM, Bloom RD, Bunin N, Tomaszewski JE, Cizman B. Nephrotic syndrome after hematopoietic cell transplantation: do glomerular lesions represent renal graft-versus-host disease? *Clin J Am Soc Nephrol*. 2006;1:685-694.
46. Reddy P, Johnson K, Uberti JP, et al. Nephrotic syndrome associated with chronic graft-versus-host disease after allogeneic hematopoietic stem cell transplantation. *Bone Marrow Transplant*. 2006;38: 351-357.
48. Graze PR, Gale RP. Chronic graft versus host disease: a syndrome of disordered immunity. *Am J Med*. 1979;66:611-620.
50. Ratanatharathorn V, Ayash L, Reynolds C, et al. Treatment of chronic graft-versus-host disease with anti-CD20 chimeric monoclonal antibody. *Biol Blood Marrow Transplant*. 2003;9:505-511.
55. Srinivasan R, Balow JE, Sabnis S, et al. Nephrotic syndrome: an underrecognised immune-mediated complication of non-myeloablative allogeneic haematopoietic cell transplantation. *Br J Haematol*. 2005; 131:74-79.
57. Rao PS. Nephrotic syndrome in patients with peripheral blood stem cell transplant. *Am J Kidney Dis*. 2005;45:780-785.
58. Bruijn JA, van Elven EH, Hogendoorn PC, Corver WE, Hoedemaeker PJ, Fleuren GJ. Murine chronic graft-versus-host disease as a model for lupus nephritis. *Am J Pathol*. 1988;130:639-641.
59. Otani M, Aoki I, Miyagi Y, et al. Glomerulonephritis induced by murine chronic graft-versus-host reaction. *Acta Pathol Jpn*. 1992; 42:325-332.
60. Lee SJ, Vogelsang G, Flowers ME. Chronic graft-versus-host disease. *Biol Blood Marrow Transplant*. 2003;9:215-233.
62. Luo XD, Liu QF, Zhang Y, et al. Nephrotic syndrome after allogeneic hematopoietic stem cell transplantation: etiology and pathogenesis. *Blood Cells Mol Dis*. 2011;46:182-187.
63. Morris SC, Cheek RL, Cohen PL, Eisenberg RA. Autoantibodies in chronic graft versus host result from cognate T-B interactions. *J Exp Med*. 1990;171:503-517.
66. Mak SK, Short CD, Mallick NP. Long-term outcome of adult-onset minimal-change nephropathy. *Nephrol Dial Transplant*. 1996;11: 2192-2201.
68. Beyar-Katz O, Davila EK, Zuckerman T, et al. Adult nephrotic syndrome after hematopoietic stem cell transplantation: renal pathology is the best predictor of response to therapy. *Biol Blood Marrow Transplant*. 2016;22:975-981.
69. Flomenberg P, Babbitt J, Drobyski WR, et al. Increasing incidence of adenovirus disease in bone marrow transplant recipients. *J Infect Dis*. 1994;169:775-781.
73. Bruno, B, Zager RA, Boeckh MJ, et al. Adenovirus nephritis in hematopoietic stem-cell transplantation. *Transplantation*. 2004;77:1049-1057.
76. Chesters PM, Heritage J, McCance DJ. Persistence of DNA sequences of BK virus and JC virus in normal human tissues and in diseased tissues. *J Infect Dis*. 1983;147:676-684.
80. Haines HL, Laskin BL, Goebel J, et al. Blood, and not urine, BK viral load predicts renal outcome in children with hemorrhagic cystitis following hematopoietic stem cell transplantation. *Biol Blood Marrow Transplant*. 2011;17:1512-1519.
83. Ferrara J. Pathogenesis of acute graft-versus-host disease: cytokines and cellular effectors. *J Hematother Stem Cell Res*. 2000;9:299-306.
85. Cohen EP, Piering WF, Kabler-Babbitt C, Moulder JE. End stage renal disease (ESRD) after bone marrow transplantation: poor survival compared to other causes of ESRD. *Nephron*. 1998;79:408-412.

A full list of references is available at Expertconsult.com

Chemotherapy and Radiation Related Kidney Diseases

16 *Conventional Chemotherapy*

BEN SPRANGERS, LAURA COSMAI, AND CAMILLO PORTA

Introduction

Several conventional chemotherapeutics have been associated with renal side effects including kidney function deterioration, electrolyte disorders, tubular injury, glomerular lesions, tubulointerstitial nephritis, and the development of thrombotic microangiopathy (TMA) (Tables 16.1–16.3).[1-5] Multiple risk factors for chemotherapy-induced nephrotoxicity have been identified (Box 16.1). The quality of data available regarding these kidney side effects is low, because subtle kidney damage goes frequently unrecognized and therefore the true incidence of nephrotoxicity is difficult to determine. Most episodes of medication-induced acute kidney injury (AKI) are reversible, but chronic kidney disease (CKD) can develop because of glomerular scarring or tubulointerstitial inflammation.

AKI is a common condition in cancer patients and is associated with higher cost, longer length of hospital stay, increased morbidity, and mortality. A Danish population study reported an 18% incidence of AKI in the first year after cancer diagnosis.[6] A study from the MD Anderson Cancer Center demonstrated that the rate of AKI in hospitalized cancer patients is significantly higher than in noncancer patients, and AKI occurrence correlated significantly with the administration of chemotherapy.[7] AKI developed in many patients during admission and was associated with longer hospital stay, increased costs, and increased mortality.[7] Even small increases in serum creatinine in cancer patients are associated with a prolonged stay at the intensive care unit (ICU) and increased mortality.[8] In cancer patients admitted to an ICU, 32% required dialysis and hospital, and 6-month mortality rates were 64% and 73%, respectively.[9] In survivors, kidney function recovered completely in 82% and partially in 12%, whereas 6% required chronic dialysis therapy.[9]

Recently, CKD has been reported as a long-term complication in cancer survivors and has been associated with decreased survival.[10,11] Chronic nephrotoxicity in cancer patients may have multiple causes, including chemotherapy, radiotherapy exposure of the kidneys, kidney surgery, supportive care drugs, iodine-containing contrast agents, and tumor-related factors. A particularly vulnerable group of patients to develop chronic renal side effects are pediatric patients.[12-21] Long-term childhood cancer survivors are at increased risk to develop elevated blood pressure[12] and decreased kidney function.[14,15] Unilateral nephrectomy, abdominal radiotherapy, treatment with cisplatin and ifosfamide, higher cisplatin dose, and cumulative carboplatin dose have all been associated with an increased risk of persistent nephrotoxicity.[13-15] Chronic glomerular and tubular nephrotoxicity developed in 20% to 50% and 60% to 80% of children treated with ifosfamide and cisplatin, respectively, and after nephrectomy, 20% of children displayed evidence of chronic glomerular damage.[18] Overall, childhood cancer survivors have a ninefold higher risk of developing kidney failure compared with their siblings.[18] Each drug has its own pattern of injury and in this chapter, we attempt to provide a detailed overview of specific chemotherapeutic drug-associated kidney side effects.

Furthermore, the kidneys are a major excretion pathway for a number of antineoplastic drugs and their metabolites. Thus kidney impairment often results in delayed and/or decreased drug excretion and metabolism of cytotoxic chemotherapeutics, possibly leading to increased toxicity. Therefore many antineoplastic agents require dose adjustment when administered in the setting of acute kidney disease or CKD (Table 16.4). Unfortunately, because severe renal impairment is usually an exclusion criterion in clinical trials, we do lack information on the excretion and metabolism of anticancer agents in this setting, though specific studies in these patients have been advocated; consequently, in patients with end-stage renal disease (ESRD) undergoing dialysis, the situation is even more complex, because antineoplastic agents' excretion and metabolism are not fully known.[22] Recommendations on dose adjustments of chemotherapeutics in patients with kidney dysfunction are based on our own experience and inspired by different published guidelines (see Table 16.4).[23-26]

Estimation of Kidney Function

There are two main pathways for drug excretion by the kidney: glomerular filtration and tubular secretion. For those drugs that are excreted by the kidneys, dose adjustments are often required when kidney function is impaired, which is common in cancer patients.[10] Because it is practically impossible to evaluate serum drug concentrations in every cancer patient, the most precise evaluation of kidney function possible is mandatory. Different methods can be used, although each method is in some way flawed and there is no consensus on an ideal tool to be used, especially in oncologic patients.[27,28] A creatinine clearance (CrCl) calculation, based upon a 24-hour collection of urine, is cumbersome and subject to error, mainly because of the need for urine collection, which is often troublesome for the patient, especially in the outpatient setting. Estimation equations, such as the Cockcroft-Gault (CG), the Modification of Diet in Renal Disease (MDRD), and the Chronic Kidney Disease Epidemiology Collaboration (CKD-EPI) are presently the most common methods used in routine clinical practice. Most of

Table 16.1   Conventional Chemotherapeutics, Mechanism of Action, Cancer Types Treated

Drug Class	Drug	Anti-Cancer MoA	Types of Cancers Treated
Platinum-based chemotherapeutics	Carboplatin	Inhibition of DNA replication	Head/neck, lung, ovarian, breast, and testicular
	Cisplatin		Testicular, germ cell, ovarian, cervical, breast, bladder, head/neck, esophageal, lung, mesothelioma
	Oxaliplatin		Colorectal, gastrointestinal
Alkylating agents	Busulfan	Cross-linking of DNA strands	Bone marrow transplantation conditioning, leukemia, lymphoma, myeloproliferative disorders
	Cyclophosphamide	Inhibition of RNA production	Lymphoma, multiple myeloma, leukemia, ovarian, breast, small cell lung, neuroblastoma, sarcoma
	Diaziquone		Primary brain
	Ifosfamide		Hodgkin and non-Hodgkin lymphoma, soft tissue sarcomas, osteosarcoma, testicular, breast, ovarian, cervical
	Melphalan		Multiple myeloma
	Procarbazine		Hodgkin lymphoma, brain
	Temozolomide		Brain, melanoma
	Trabectedin		Soft tissue sarcoma, ovarian
Antimetabolites	Azacitidine	Inhibition of DNA production by incorporation of chemically altered nucleotides or by depletion of nucleotides	Myelodysplastic syndrome, acute myeloid leukemia
	Capecitabine		Metastatic breast and colorectal, esophageal, gastric, prostate, ovarian, pancreas
	Cladribine		Hairy cell leukemia, chronic lymphocytic leukemia
	Clofarabine		Relapsed or refractory acute myeloid leukemia, lymphoblastic leukemia
	Cytarabine		Acute myeloid leukemia, acute lymphocytic leukemia, chronic myelogenous leukemia, Hodgkin and non-Hodgkin lymphoma
	Deoxycofomycin		Hairy cell leukemia, chronic lymphocytic leukemia, adult T-cell leukemia/lymphoma
	Fludarabine		Acute myeloid/lymphocytic leukemia, chronic lymphocytic leukemia, non-Hodgkin lymphoma
	5-Fluorouracil		Colorectal, esophageal, gastric, pancreatic, breast, cervical
	Gemcitabine		Breast, ovarian, non-small cell lung, pancreatic, bladder, cholangiobiliary
	Mercaptopurine		Acute leukemia, chronic leukemia
	Methotrexate		Breast, lung, head/neck, bladder, leukemia, lymphoma, osteosarcoma
	Pemetrexed		Non-small lung cancer, mesothelioma
	Thioguanine		Acute leukemia, chronic myeloid leukemia
Antitumor antibiotics	Anthracyclines	DNA intercalation resulting in blocking of DNA/RNA synthesis	Acute myeloid leukemia, acute lymphoid leukemia, chronic myelogenous leukemia, neuroblastoma, Kaposi sarcoma, breast, non-Hodgkin lymphoma
	Bleomycin		Hodgkin and non-Hodgkin lymphoma, testicular, ovarian, cervical
	Mitomycin C		Bladder, esophageal, anal, breast
Chloroethylnitrosourea		Interstrand cross-linking of DNA	Brain, multiple myeloma, Hodgkin and non-Hodgkin lymphoma, beta cell, chronic lymphocytic leukemia, prostate
Microtubule inhibitors	Taxanes	Inhibition of microtubules assembly/function	Breast, head/neck, gastric, prostate, non-small cell lung, ovarian, Kaposi sarcoma, cervical, pancreatic, urothelial
	Vinca alkaloids		Acute leukemia, Hodgkin lymphoma, lung, bladder, breast, small cell lung, sarcoma
Topoisomerase inhibitors	Etoposide	Single-DNA strand breaks	Lung, lymphoma, testicular
	Irinotecan		Colon, small cell lung
	Topotecan		Ovarian, small cell lung
Others	Tamoxifen	Degradation of PML-RARα	Acute promyelocytic leukemia
		Binding of estrogen-receptor	Breast

DNA, Deoxyribonucleic acid; *PML-RARα*, promyelocytic leukemia retinoic acid receptor; *RNA*, ribonucleic acid.

the available data suggest that all these formulae provide similar levels of concordance in the measurement of glomerular filtration rate (GFR) in cancer patients, and are thus adequate enough for the purpose of dosing cancer drugs excreted by the kidneys.[29] However, a recent report suggested that the CG equation underestimates GFR compared with the MDRD and CKD-EPI formulas, at least in Asian patients.[30] More recently, the most accurate and least biased method to estimate GFR was described;[31] this method applied a new multivariable linear model for GFR calculation using statistic regression analysis.[31] Chromium-51 labeled ethylenediamine tetraacetic acid (^{51}Cr-EDTA) GFR was compared with the estimated GFR (eGFR) from seven published models and the new model proposed; the new model improved the eGFR accuracy compared with all published models. Importantly, the new model reduced the fraction of

Table 16.2 Conventional Chemotherapeutics and Clinical Renal Syndromes

Drug Class	Drug	Clinical Renal Syndromes
Platinum-based chemotherapeutics	Carboplatin	AKI, CKD, hypomagnesemia, hypokalemia, hyponatremia, TMA
	Cisplatin	AKI, CKD, hypomagnesemia, Fanconi syndrome, distal RTA, polyuria, TMA, salt-wasting syndrome, SIADH
	Oxaliplatin	AKI, ATN, hypokalemia, TMA
Alkylating agents	Busulfan	AKI
	Cyclophosphamide	SIADH, hyponatremia, hemorrhagic cystitis
	Diaziquone	AKI
	Ifosfamide	AKI, CKD, ATN, Fanconi syndrome, distal and proximal RTA, nephrogenic diabetes insipidus, hypokalemia, interstitial nephritis, glomerular disease, hemorrhagic cystitis, SIADH
	Melphalan	AKI, nephrotic syndrome, SIADH
	Procarbazine	AKI
	Temozolomide	AKI
	Trabectedin	AKI
Antimetabolites	Azacitidine	AKI, Fanconi syndrome, RTA, polyuria, nephrogenic diabetes insipidus
	Capecitabine	AKI
	Cladribine	AKI
	Clofarabine	AKI, proteinuria, collapsing glomerulopathy
	Cytarabine	AKI, TMA
	Deoxycoformycin	AKI, hematuria, dysuria, TMA
	Fludarabine	AKI
	5-Fluorouracil	AKI, hyponatremia, hypokalemia
	Gemcitabine	AKI, proteinuria, hematuria, TMA
	Mercaptopurine	AKI, Fanconi syndrome
	Methotrexate	Crystalline nephropathy, ATN, AKI
	Pemetrexed	ATN, interstitial edema, distal RTA, nephrogenic diabetes insipidus, CKD
	Thioguanine	AKI
Antitumor antibiotics	Anthracyclines	Nephrotic syndrome, glomerular diseases (MCD, FSGS), TMA, CKD
	Bleomycin	TMA
	Mitomycin C	TMA
Chloroethylnitrosourea		AKI, chronic interstitial nephritis, CKD, uric acid nephrolithiasis, nephrogenic diabetes insipidus, Fanconi syndrome, proximal RTA, TMA
Microtubule inhibitors	Taxanes	Hyponatremia, TMA, (ATN), hypokalemia
	Vinca alkaloids	(AKI), SIADH
Topoisomerase inhibitors	Etoposide	None
	Irinotecan	AKI
	Topotecan	AKI
Others	Arsenic trioxide	Acute tubulointerstitial injury
	Tamoxifen	Nephrotic syndrome

AKI, Acute kidney injury; *ATN*, acute tubular necrosis; *CKD*, chronic kidney disease; *FSGS*, focal segmental glomerulosclerosis, *MCD*, minimal change disease, *RTA*, renal tubular acidosis; *SIADH*, syndrome of inappropriate antidiuretic hormone secretion; *TMA*, thrombotic microangiopathy.

Table 16.3 Causes of the Most Common Clinical Renal Syndromes Associated With Conventional Chemotherapeutics

Clinical Renal Syndrome	Conventional Chemotherapeutic
AKI/ATN	Carboplatin, cisplatin, oxaliplatin, (busulfan), diaziquone, ifosfamide, melphalan, procarbazine, temozolomide, trabectedin, azacitidine, (capecitabine), cladaribine, clofarabine, cytarabine, deoxycofymycin, fludarabine, 5-fluorouracil, gemcitabine, mercaptopurine, methotrexate, pemetrexed, thioguanine, chloroethylnitrosourea, (taxanes, vinca alkaloids), irinotecan, (topotecan)
CKD	Carboplatin, cisplatin, ifosfamide, pemetrexed, anthracyclines, chloroethylnitrosourea
Crystalline nephropathy	Methotrexate
Distal RTA	Cisplatin, ifosfamide, pemetrexed
Dysuria	Deoxycofomycin
Fanconi syndrome	Cisplatin, ifosfamide, mercaptopurine, chloroethylnitrosourea
Glomerular disease	Ifosfamide, clofarbine, anthracyclines
Hematuria	Deoxycoformycin, gemcitabine
Hemorrhagic cystitis	Cyclophosphamide, ifosfamide

Table 16.3 Causes of the Most Common Clinical Renal Syndromes Associated With Conventional Chemotherapeutics—cont'd

Clinical Renal Syndrome	Conventional Chemotherapeutic
Hypokalemia	Platinum derivatives, ifosfamide, 5-fluorouracil, taxanes
Hypomagnesemia	Carboplatin, cisplatin
Hyponatremia	Platinum derivatives, cyclophosphamide, 5-fluorouracil, taxanes
Interstitial nephritis/injury	Ifosfamide, pemetrexed, chloroethylnitrosourea, arsenic trioxide
Nephrogenic diabetes insipidus	Ifosfamide, azacitidine, pemetrexed, chloroethylnitrosourea
Nephrotic syndrome	Melphalan, methotrexate, anthracyclines, tamoxifen
Proteinuria	Clofarabine, gemcitabine
Proximal RTA	Ifosfamide, azacitidine, chloroethylnitrosourea
SIADH	Cyclophosphamide, ifosfamide, melphalan, vinca alkaloids, cisplatin
TMA	Carboplatin, cisplatin, oxaliplatin, cytarabine, deoxycofomycin, gemcitabine, anthracyclines, bleomycin, mitomycin C, chloroethylnitrosourea, taxanes
Uric acid nephrolithiasis	Chloroethylnitrosourea

AKI, Acute kidney injury; *ATN*, acute tubular necrosis; *CKD*, chronic kidney disease; *RTA*, renal tubular acidosis; *SIADH*, syndrome of inappropriate antidiuretic hormone secretion; *TMA*, thrombotic microangiopathy.

Box 16.1   Risk Factors for Chemotherapy-Induced Nephrotoxicity

Patient Factors

- Older age
- Acute or chronic renal dysfunction
- Genetic factors: gene mutations in hepatic/renal CYP450 enzyme systems and transport proteins

Intrinsic Chemotherapeutic Nephrotoxicity

- Cumulative drug dose
- Crystal formation by drug or metabolites
- Direct nephrotoxic effects
- Combination with other nephrotoxins (e.g., NSAID, iodine-containing contrast agent, nephrotoxic antibiotics)

Tumor-Related Risk Factors

- Volume depletion (diarrhea, vomiting, malignant ascites or pleuritis, sepsis)
- Tumor lysis syndrome
- Hyperuricemia, hypercalcemia
- Renal infiltration
- Urinary obstruction caused by tumor or radiation therapy-induced fibrosis
- Paraprotein-related kidney disease
- Paraneoplastic glomerulonephritis

Renal Drug Handling

- Accumulation and high metabolic rate in renal tubular cells
- Hypoxic renal environment
- Concentration of drug/toxin in the interstitium and medulla

NSAID, Nonsteroidal anti-inflammatory drug.
Adapted from Perazella MA. Onco-nephrology: renal toxicities of chemo-therapeutic agents. *Clin J Am Soc Nephrol.* 2012; 7:1713-1721.

---

patients with a carboplatin dose absolute percentage error greater than 20% to 14.17%, in contrast to 18.62% for the body surface area (BSA)-adjusted CKD-EPI, and 25.51% for the CG formula. Notably enough, this new model has been externally validated, and should now be considered a new "gold standard."[31]

Platinum-Based Chemotherapeutics

CARBOPLATIN

Carboplatin is a second-generation platinum-based chemotherapeutic (including cisplatin, heptaplatin, lobaplatin, nedaplatin, oxaliplatin) and is used to treat a variety of cancers, such as head/neck cancer, lung cancer, ovarian cancer, brain cancer, and testicular cancer. Compared with cisplatin, carboplatin is better tolerated but less potent.

Mechanism of Action

The mechanism of cytotoxicity of carboplatin is similar to that of cisplatin (discussed in detail in the cisplatin section), because it also interferes with deoxyribonucleic acid (DNA) duplication.

Pharmacokinetics

Carboplatin or cis-diammine (1,1-cyclobutane dicarboxylate) platinum(II) is administered intravenously. In general, the dosage of carboplatin is four times the dosage of cisplatin.[32] More than 50% of the administered dosage is excreted unchanged in the urine within 24 hours.[31] The importance of renal clearance to the metabolism and excretion of carboplatin is highlighted by its usual dosing schema, which is based upon an eGFR, along with the desired level of drug exposure, according to the area under the concentration-time curve (AUC, mg/mL × min), rather than the more common dosing calculation based upon the BSA (mg/m^2). Using the desired target AUC (which typically varies between 5 and 7 mg/mL/min) and the eGFR, the dose of carboplatin is then calculated using the Calvert formula: dose (mg) = AUC (mg/mL × min) × [GFR (mL/min) + 25 (mL/min)].[33] This dose calculation using the Calvert formula has to be repeated before each course of carboplatin to take into account possible changes in weight or renal function. A possible issue related to the use of this formula is the appropriate weight to use when calculating the eGFR. The original CG formula to estimate GFR used actual body

Table 16.4   Dose Adjustment of Chemotherapeutic Drugs in Patients With Renal Dysfunction

Chemotherapeutic agent	>90	90–80	80–70	70–60	60–50	50–40	40–30	30–20	20–10	10–0	HD	PD
Carboplatin	No DR (Calvert Formula)						250 mg/m² max dose		CI			
Cisplatin		no DR		DR 25%		DR 50% (consider carboplatin)					DR 50–75%	DR 50%
Oxaliplatin				no DR				consider DR			?	?
Busulfan							no DR					
Cyclophosphamide				no DR					DR25%	DR50%		DR 25%
Diaziquone							no DR					
Ifosfamide		no DR		DR 25%		DR50%			CI		DR 50%	DR 50%
Melphalan			no DR				DR25%			DR 50%	DR 50%	?
Temozolomide					no DR						LD	LD
Trabectedin				no DR			CI				CI	CI
Cytarabine		no DR		DR 40%		DR 50%		CI for high dose			LD	LD
Deoxycofomycin		no DR		DR 25%		DR 50%		CI				
Fludarabine	no DR			DR 20–50%				CI			LD	DR 50%
5-Fluorouracil					no DR			consider DR			LD	LD
Gemcitabine					no DR			DR			no DR	LD
Mercaptopurine	no DR	increase dose interval 24–36h					increase dose interval 48hr					
Methotrexate		no DR		avoid high dose			DR 50%		CI		DR 50–75%	CI
Pemetrexed			no DR				CI					
Thioguanine		no DR					consider DR					
Bleomycin			no DR				DR 25%		DR 50%			
Mitomycin C					no DR				DR 25%		DR 25%?	
Streptozocin			no DR				DR 25%		stop	LD		
Iomustine			no DR				DR 25%		DR 50%		DR 50%–75%	
Bendamustine			no DR					CI				
Carmustine		no DR		DR 20%			DR25%				no DR	
Estramustine						no DR						
Lomustine		no DR		DR 25%		DR 50%	CI					
Taxanes						no DR					no DR	
Vincristine						no DR						
Vinblastine						no Dr						
Vinorelbine						no DR						
Eribulin			no DR				consider DR		CI			
Etoposide			no DR				DR 25%			DR 50%	DR 50%	DR 50%
Topotecan			no DR				DR 50%			DR 75%	CI	

CI, contraindicated; DR dose reduction; HD, hemodialysis; LD, limited data available; PD, peritoneal dialysis.

weight, but none of the patients considered were obese. Most clinicians use actual body weight in the CG formula for nonobese patients. However, the use of actual body weight in the CG calculation can overestimate the GFR resulting in higher carboplatin dose in obese individuals.[34] The Gynecological Oncology Group (GOG) recommends that actual weight be used to determine eGFR when using the CG equation as long as patients have a body mass index (BMI) of less than 25.[35] For other patients, the use of an adjusted weight is suggested (adjusted weight [kg] = [{actual weight − ideal weight} × 0.40] + ideal weight). Another issue is that the Calvert formula was developed measuring GFR using Cr-EDTA, whereas in clinical practice CrCl or eGFR (using the MDRD or CKD-EPI formula) are used. It is not clear at this point how accurate it is to calculate the carboplatin dosage using these estimates. Carboplatin should not be administered to patients with CrCl lower than 20 mL/min and a maximum carboplatin dose of 250 mg/m^2 has been suggested in patients with CrCl=20 to 39 mL/min.

As far as carboplatin administration in patients undergoing dialysis concerns, polychemotherapy regimens incorporating carboplatin have been successfully used in patients undergoing hemodialysis (HD) and peritoneal dialysis (PD) without evidence of increased toxicity or reduced efficacy.[36–41] Few cases of HD patients treated with carboplatin, either alone or in combination, are reported in the literature. The Calvert formula has been initially used in HD patients by assuming that GFR is zero. This is applicable to patients who receive HD within 12 to 18 hours after carboplatin infusion. After the first 24 hours, the majority of carboplatin, which is bound to serum proteins, is not easily dialyzable and remains in the blood stream despite repeated sessions of HD. Guddati et al. have proposed a correction factor to calculate the resultant AUC in HD patients; the AUC can increase by eightfold in patients who received the adjusted dose, but whose HD was delayed beyond 24 hours after infusion. The correction factor proposed can also be used to calculate the dose adjustment required, a priori, in patients who may receive delayed HD.[42] The same authors have also developed a formula to adjust carboplatin dosage in PD patients; this formula takes into account the frequency of dialysis sessions and the time delay between carboplatin infusion and the initiation of dialysis, and predicts an approximately similar dosage of carboplatin as that of the Calvert formula in patients undergoing PD 4 times per day, if dialysis is initiated 12 hours after infusion.[43] In another patient, HD was performed for 3.5 hours starting 90 minutes after completion of carboplatin, and pharmacokinetic assessments were performed at 1, 2, 4, and 12 hours after its infusion. Total carboplatin concentrations in plasma and platinum ultrafiltrate were measured. The plasma concentration of free platinum at the end of the infusion was 31,000 ng/mL and the AUC was 2.9 minutes times mg/mL. No significant carboplatin-related toxicities were reported. This case report clearly indicates that carboplatin can be safely administered in HD patients.[44]

Toxicity

In general, platinum-based chemotherapeutics are associated with numerous and potentially severe side effects. Most common side effects include nausea, bone marrow suppression, and electrolyte disturbances.

Kidney Toxicity

Although carboplatin is a nephrotoxic drug,[45–51] its nephrotoxicity is much lower compared with cisplatin. Carboplatin is significantly less nephrotoxic than carboplatin because of its enhanced stability; this is mainly related to the fact that carboplatin has carboxylate and cyclobutane moieties in the cis position, rather than chloride. In a study involving patients treated with carboplatin

in combination with vincristine, a 19% decrease in CrCl was observed as early as from the second course.[51] In contrast, in another study comparing patients treated with carboplatin alone or in combination with etoposide and bleomycin, no significant change in kidney function before and after (1 month, < 3 months, and > 3 months) treatment with carboplatin was noted.[52] AKI has been anecdotally reported in patients who have been treated with intraperitoneal carboplatin,[47] in association with high dose carboplatin (1500–2000 mg/m^2)[49,50] or in combination with ifosfamide and etoposide.[50] In this setting, AKI occurs within days after carboplatin administration and is often only partially reversible.

In a single center study including 50 children with Wilms tumors, treated between 2002 and 2012 and followed for 2 years, it was reported that patients treated with cyclophosphamide and carboplatin were at higher risk of kidney function deterioration.[53] Skinner et al. evaluated the long-term nephrotoxicity of platinum-based chemotherapy in 63 childhood cancer survivors (27 cisplatin, 24 carboplatin, and 12 both cisplatin and carboplatin).[15] There was no significant overall change in kidney function over time in any treatment group except for a slight reduced median GFR (84 mL/min/1.73 m^2) and serum magnesium level (0.68 mmol/L) in the cisplatin-treated group. At 10 years, reduced GFR (< 60 mL/min/1.73 m^2) and need for magnesium supplements were present in 11% and 7% of cisplatin-treated patients, respectively.[15] In the patients treated with carboplatin, older age was associated with lower GFR during follow-up, higher cumulative carboplatin dose associated with lower serum magnesium levels at 1 year, and increased nephrotoxicity at 1 and 10 years.[15] Hypomagnesemia is a frequent complication in childhood cancer survivors (7%–29%).[21] Both cisplatin and carboplatin are associated with the development of Fanconi syndrome.[54] The occurrence of hypomagnesemia after carboplatin administration has been widely reported.[55–58] In one study, 6 months following carboplatin therapy, hypomagnesemia was observed in 15.6% of the children treated for solid tumors.[55] In combination with the antiepidermal growth factor receptor monoclonal antibody, cetuximab (which also causes hypomagnesemia[59]), grade 3 to 4 hypomagnesemia occurred in 3% to 7.5% in lung cancer patients.[57,58] Also in combination with proton pump inhibitors, carboplatin is associated with the development of severe hypomagnesemia.[60] Hypokalemia and hyponatremia may also rarely occur after carboplatin administration.[58,61,62] Carboplatin has only rarely been associated with the development of TMA[63] and most often in combination with other chemotherapeutics (gemcitabine, cyclophosphamide and thiotepa, docotaxel and trastumab).[64–66] Finally, there are case reports concerning obstructive AKI caused by bladder obstruction by blood clots in two patients with ovarian cancer treated with carboplatin, in combination with paclitaxel.[67,68]

Prevention of nephrotoxicity of platinum-based chemotherapeutics through sufficient hydration is essential. In patients with preexisting kidney impairment secondary to cisplatin, the effectiveness of hydration was shown in patients treated with carboplatin (800 mg/m^2) with or without hydration (250 mL/h of isotonic saline 3 hours before and after carboplatin infusion).[49] Without hydration, a decrease in CrCl of 36% to 61% was noted versus no reduction in patients receiving hydration.[49]

CISPLATIN

Cisplatin, the best known of the platinums, is widely used to treat testicular cancer, germ cell cancer, ovarian cancer, cervical cancer, breast cancer, bladder cancer, head/neck cancer, esophageal cancer, lung cancer, mesothelioma, brain tumors, and neuroblastoma. All platinum-based chemotherapeutics have been associated with early nephrotoxicity. Although carboplatinum and oxaliplatin have fewer side effects compared with cisplatin, cisplatin is still used extensively, because it is more potent in some cancers, resulting in better survival rates.[69,70]

Pharmacokinetics

Cisplatin is nonenzymatically transformed into multiple metabolites after its administration. Cisplatin and its metabolites are removed from the body through the kidney (20%–80% within 24 hours) and the dose has to be reduced in patients with a decreased CrCl. In clinical trials, it is commonly required that patients receiving cisplatin have a serum creatinine of less than 2.0 mg/dL or a CrCl of 60 mL/min or higher. We suggest a 25% dose reduction for CrCl 46 to 60 mL/min and a 50% dose reduction for CrCl 30 to 45 mL/min. Cisplatin has been administered to patients undergoing HD[23,71,72] and 50% to 75% and 50% dose reductions are suggested for patients undergoing HD and PD, respectively.[23,73,74] HD should be performed within 3 hours after administration of cisplatin. Furthermore, it has been suggested to consider carboplatin instead of cisplatin in patients with CrCl less than 45 mL/min.

Mechanism of Action

The main mechanism of action of cisplatin is the binding of DNA and inhibition of DNA replication (Fig. 16.1). Inhibition of DNA replication mainly affects rapidly proliferating cells. After administration, cisplatin undergoes

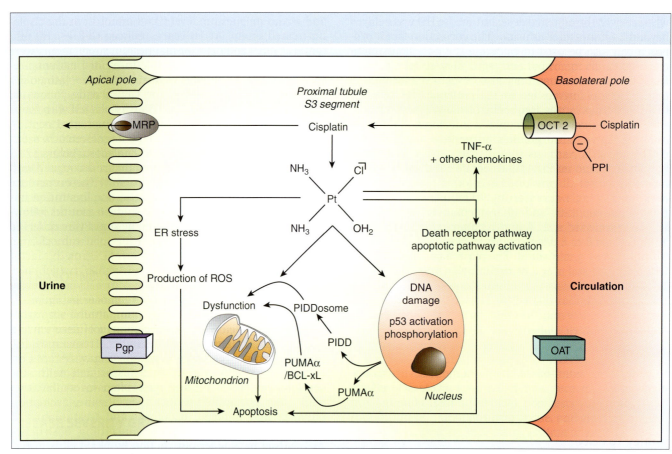

Fig. 16.1 Cisplatin nephrotoxicity. Cisplatin enters the proximal tubular cells through organic cation transporter-2 (OCT2) and accumulates in the cell cytoplasm. Cisplatin-mediated cellular injury involves several mechanisms. Cisplatin induces endoplasmic reticular stress (ER stress) and production of reactive-oxygen species (ROS), resulting in apoptosis. Moreover, cisplatin induces mitochondrial dysfunction, which is also associated with caspase-independent and caspase-dependent apoptosis. Moreover, cisplatin induces deoxyribonucleic acid (DNA) damage with phosphorylation and activation of p53. p53 subsequently induces transcription of apoptic genes such as *PUMA*-α and *PIDD*. PIDD forms the PIDDosome and activation of caspase 2 and caspase-independent apoptosis. PUMA-α neutralizes Bcl-XL, resulting in mitochondrial dysfunction and caspase-dependent apoptosis. Finally, cisplatin activates the death receptor pathway apoptosis pathway. Cisplatin also induces inflammation through the production of tumor necrosis factor (TNF)α and other chemokines. *MRP*, Multidrug-resistant protein; *OAT*, organic anion transporter; *OCT*, organic cation transporter; *Pgp, P* glycoprotein.

aquation intracellularly, in which one of the two chloride ligands is replaced by H_2O. This aqua ligand is thereafter displaced by a DNA base, preferentially guanine. Cross-linking of DNA interferes with mitosis and results in apoptosis.

Toxicity

The most commonly reported side effects associated with cisplatin include nephrotoxicity, nausea/vomiting, bone marrow suppression and hemolytic anemia, ototoxicity, and neurotoxicity.

Kidney Toxicity

As far as the clinical manifestations of cisplatin kidney injury, AKI has been reportedly observed in approximately 20% to 30% of patients, but the more common one is hypomagnesemia, observed between 40% and 100% of the cases.[75] Other rarer, but not less challenging, manifestations include Fanconi-like syndrome, distal renal tubular acidosis (RTA), renal concentrating defect, and TMA. Cisplatin-induced nephrotoxicity mostly affects the corticomedullary S3 segment of the proximal tubule and to a lesser degree the loop of Henle and distal tubular segments. In proximal tubular cells in the S3 segment, cisplatin accumulates to a great degree, resulting in a cisplatin concentration 5 times higher than the serum concentration.[76] After cisplatin enters the tubular cell, it appears to undergo a complex series of reactions that results in the formation of more potent (toxic) metabolites. However, it is unclear if all cisplatin-induced cytotoxic effects are mediated via its activated metabolites. Once within the tubular cell, cisplatin exerts many different biological effects, which culminate in cell apoptosis/necrosis (see Fig. 16.1). Although cisplatin targets nuclear DNA, it has been reported that only 1% of the cytosolic cisplatin is present within the nucleus.[77] Multiple cellular targets have been identified for cisplatin toxicity, including: (1) DNA damage; (2) cytoplasmic organelle dysfunction, with endoplasmic reticulum stress and mitochondrial dysfunction; (3) apoptotic pathways both caspase-dependent and death receptor-mediated; (4) oxidative stress with formation of reactive oxygen species; and (5) inflammation mediated via tumor necrosis factor and other chemokines.[78] In addition, there also appears to be an immune component to cisplatin-induced nephrotoxicity.[79,80] Several nonmodifiable factors have been identified to increase the risk for cisplatin-induced nephrotoxicity, such as genetic factors, race, gender, age, cardiac disease, malnutrition, dehydration, comorbidities such as diabetes or cirrhosis (hypoalbuminemia is associated with a higher unbound fraction of cisplatin, resulting in greater peak plasma concentrations), concomitant use of other nephrotoxic agents, or preexisting kidney diseases.[81-85]

It is well known that cisplatin-induced kidney injury is dose-, duration-, and frequency-dependent.[86,87] Higher peak plasma concentrations result in greater injury.[20] Furthermore, a higher cumulative dose has also been shown to increase the risk for future kidney injury.[88] Early trials with cisplatin reported that greater than 70% of patients developed dose-related AKI. In more recent trials, at high cisplatin doses, 42% of treated patients had nephrotoxic injury. A recent study reported cisplatin-induced nephrotoxicity to occur in more than one-third of patients after the fourth cycle of chemotherapy and preventive strategies were ineffective.[89] In a meta-analysis of randomized phase 2 and 3 clinical trials comparing first-line platinum-based chemotherapy with the same regimen without platinum, platinum was associated with a significant increase in nephrotoxicity (18 trials; 4384 patients; odds ratio, 3.09; 95% confidence interval, 1.88–5.06; $p <$ .0001).[90] With improved survival in cancer patients, it has become evident that cytotoxic chemotherapeutics can also result in CKD. In childhood cancer, loss of GFR occurs, especially in older children treated with ifosfamide and higher doses of cisplatin.[13,15] The long-term effect of cisplatin on kidney function in 859 adult patients treated with cisplatin who had survived 5 years or more after initial dose showed most patients experienced small but permanent declines in eGFR, although none progressed to ESRD requiring HD.[91]

Cisplatin is associated with the development of TMA[92] either as monotherapy[93,94] or in combination with other chemotherapeutics (with bleomycin and vincristine/vinblastine,[95,96] with bleomycin and epirubicin,[97,98] with bleomycin and methotrexate,[99] with gemcitabine,[100] with 5-fluorouracil [5-FU],[101] with cyclophosphamide and adriamycin[102]). TMA can develop up to 4 months after the last administration of cisplatin. There is no established treatment for cisplatin-induced TMA as variable efficacies have been described for plasma exchange and infusion of fresh frozen plasma, aspirin, and dipyridamole.

Clinical practice guidelines have been published on the prevention of cisplatin-induced kidney injury.[27,103,104] Different preventive strategies have been tested to reduce cisplatin-induced nephrotoxicity. A recent systematic review concluded that: (1) hydration is essential for all patients; (2) short-duration, low-volume, outpatient hydration regimens appear to be safe and feasible, even in patients receiving intermediate- to high-dose cisplatin; (3) magnesium supplementation (8–16 mEq) may limit cisplatin-induced nephrotoxicity; and (4) mannitol might be considered for high-dose cisplatin regimens and/or for patients with preexisting hypertension. These findings have broad implications for clinical practice and represent best practice principles for the prevention of cisplatin-induced nephrotoxicity.[105] In animal models, amifostine (a free radical scavenger) ameliorates cisplatin-mediated nephrotoxicity. However, cisplatin-induced nephrotoxicity cannot be completely prevented with current available measures and several aspects regarding optimal management are still controversial, such as duration of hydration, use of magnesium, and use of diuretics.[103,106-110] Diuretics should probably be avoided in patients receiving platinum-based chemotherapy, because they are potentially harmful.[106] Cisplatin is transported into the tubular cell by the basolateral organic cation transporter 2 (OCT2) channel; therefore blockers of the OCT2 channel have potential to prevent/reduce nephrotoxicity. A recent trial demonstrated that proton pump inhibitors (which are known blockers of the OCT2 channel) are associated with reduced cisplatin-mediated nephrotoxicity.[111]

OXALIPLATIN

Oxaliplatin is a member of platinum-based chemotherapeutics. Oxaliplatin is used to treat colorectal cancer (and other gastrointestinal cancers) and is often combined with 5-FU and leucovorin.

Mechanism of Action

As other platinum-based chemotherapeutics, its action is through the blockade of DNA production. Oxaliplatin forms both inter- and intrastrand cross-links in DNA, causing cell death. However, recently it was reported that oxaliplatin does not only kill cells through DNA damage response, but also by inducing ribosome biogenesis stress.[112] This might explain the distinct clinical implementation of oxaliplatin compared with other platinum-based chemotherapeutics.

Pharmacokinetics

Oxaliplatin undergoes extensive nonenzymatic biotransformation and platinum is mainly excreted by the kidneys. Approximately half of the total dose is recovered in the urine by day 5. Dose reduction is recommended in patients with a CrCl less than 20 mL/min. Doses up to 130 mg/m^2 every 3 weeks proved to be well tolerated in patients with CrCl greater than 20 mL/min and do not require dose reduction.[113] Some experts recommend oxaliplatin dose reduction in patients with ESRD undergoing HD.[23] Although others suggest this is not necessary if HD is performed shortly after drug administration, and the dosing interval is extended to 3 weeks.[114]

Toxicity

Common side effects include neurotoxicity (peripheral neuropathy), fatigue, nausea and vomiting, neutropenia, nephrotoxicity, and ototoxicity (less than cisplatin and carboplatin). Other serious side effects include allergic reactions and rhabdomyolysis.

Kidney Toxicity

Oxaliplatin is less nephrotoxic than cisplatin and carboplatin,[115–118] but all platinum-based chemotherapeutics cause proximal tubular cell damage.[119] There are few cases of AKI associated with oxaliplatin-induced immune-mediated intravascular hemolysis[120–123] and the occurrence of acute tubular necrosis (ATN).[121,122] In these reported cases, the evolution was favorable with recovery of kidney function. Another well-known side effect of oxaliplatin is the development of hypokalemia during treatment.[115,116] In a prospective study of 772 patients treated with oxaliplatin, seven patients developed hypokalemia rapidly after oxaliplatin administration.[124] It is suggested that oxaliplatin shifts potassium into cells. Oxaliplatin has also been associated with the development of TMA.[125–131] Data from the Oklahoma thrombotic thrombocytopenic purpura-hemolytic uremic syndrome (TTP-HUS) registry and BloodCenter of Wisconsin concluded that there was a definite association between oxaliplatin and the occurrence of TMA.[131] It has been suggested that TMA associated with oxaliplatin is immune mediated.[132–134] Prevention of platinum-based chemotherapeutic-related nephrotoxicity is based on intravenous (IV) administration of isotonic saline fluids and treatment of nausea and vomiting.[135]

Alkylating Agents

Alkylating agents were among the earliest anticancer drugs, dating back to the 1940s. Alkylating agents react with electron-rich atoms to form covalent bonds. The common alkane transferred by classical alkylating agents is a single-carbon methyl group that also includes longer hydrocarbons. The most important reactions with regard to the agents' antitumor activities are reactions with DNA bases; indeed, some alkylating agents are monofunctional and react with only one strand of DNA, whereas others are bifunctional and react with an atom on both strands of DNA, producing a cross-link that covalently links the two strands of the DNA double helix. Unless repaired, this lesion will prevent the cell from replicating effectively.

BUSULFAN

Busulfan is part of the conditioning regimen for bone marrow transplantation in patients with leukemia, lymphoma, and myeloproliferative disorders.

Mechanism of Action

Busulfan is an alkylating chemotherapeutic.

Pharmacokinetics

Busulfan is extensively metabolized in the liver and these metabolites are predominantly excreted as inactive metabolites by renal excretion. No dose reductions are recommended in patients with renal dysfunction.

Toxicity

Busulfan-associated side effects include interstitial pulmonary fibrosis, seizures, hepatic veno-occlusive disease, and wasting syndrome.

Kidney Toxicity

The nephrotoxicity of busulfan seems to be limited.[136] In a phase I study, only one of 15 refractory acute leukemia patients received busulfan and clofarabine, as preparation for allogeneic hematopoietic stem cell transplantation, developed AKI (attributed to clofarabine).[137]

CYCLOPHOSPHAMIDE

Cyclophosphamide is used to treat lymphoma, multiple myeloma, leukemia, ovarian cancer, breast cancer, small cell lung cancer, neuroblastoma, and sarcoma.

Mechanism of Action

Cyclophosphamide is an alkylating agent and a member of the nitrogen mustard family. It acts through interfering with DNA replication and ribonucleic acid (RNA) production. The active metabolite of cyclophosphamide is phosphoramide mustard. This metabolite is only formed in cells that have low levels of aldehyde dehydrogenase activity. Phosphoramide mustard forms DNA inter- and intrastrand cross-links, which leads to cell apoptosis.

Pharmacokinetics

When administered orally, cyclophosphamide is rapidly absorbed and converted to its active metabolites in the liver. Several metabolites are produced: 4-hydroxycyclophosphamide, aldophosphamide, carboxycyclophosphamide (Fig. 16.2). A fraction of aldophosphamide diffuses into cells and is there metabolized into phosphoramide mustard (the active metabolite of cyclophosphamide) and acrolein. Aldophosphamide is

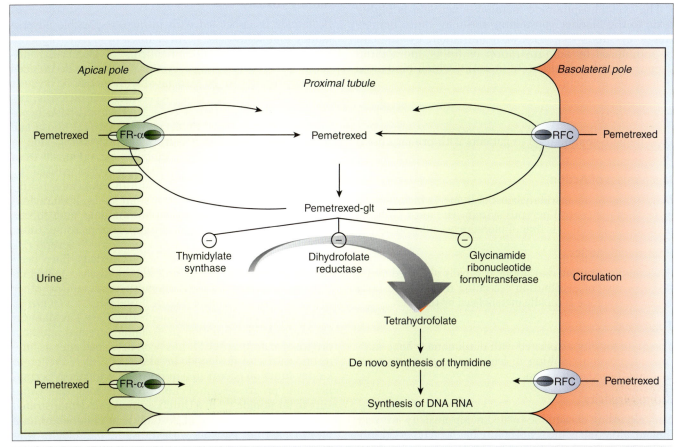

Fig. 16.2 Ifosfamide nephrotoxicity. Ifosfamide is transported in the proximal tubular cells through organic cation transporter-2 (OCT2). Ifosfamide undergoes substantial metabolization with the production of acrolein (responsible for bladder irritation and hemorrhagic cystitis) and chloroacetaldehyde (responsible for development of proximal tubulopathy). In this figure, the metabolism of ifosfamide is represented in the renal tubular cells, while this happens mainly in liver cells. *FR-α*, folate receptor-alpha; *RFC*, reduced folate carrier.

oxidized to carboxycyclophosphamide by the enzyme aldehyde dehydrogenase, and the formation of phosphoramide mustard only occurs in cells with low aldehyde dehydrogenase activity. Similarly, it has been demonstrated that high aldehyde dehydrogenase activity results in cyclophosphamide resistance in certain leukemia cell lines.[138] Conversion of aldophosphamide to carboxycyclophosphamide by aldehyde dehydrogenase prevents toxicity as carboxycyclophosphamide does not result in nitrogen mustard formation and alkylation.

Some 30% of the cyclophosphamide dose is excreted in unchanged form in the urine, whereas highly protein-bound metabolites are primarily excreted through the kidney. Cyclophosphamide pharmacokinetics are clearly altered in patients with renal insufficiency.[139] However, there is no consensus whether cyclophosphamide dose adjustments are needed in patients with reduced kidney function, because studies are unable to demonstrate an association between kidney function and cyclophosphamide clearance or hematologic toxicity.[140,141] We recommend no dose reduction, a 25% dose reduction, and a 50% dose reduction in patients with a CrCl greater than 20 mL/min, 10 to 20 mL/min, and less than 10 mL/min, respectively. Cyclophosphamide is moderately hemodialyzable and should always be administered after HD and HD held until 12 hours later.[23,142] In PD patients, a 25% dose reduction has been suggested.[23,142]

Toxicity

Common adverse effects include low white blood cell counts, nausea/vomiting, hair loss, and hemorrhagic cystitis. Other severe adverse effects include increased future risk of cancer, infertility, allergic reactions, and pulmonary fibrosis. Cardiotoxicity occurs mainly with high cumulative doses of cyclophosphamide. Infertility has been reported in both females and males, and the risk for infertility increases with both cumulative dose of cyclophosphamide and patient age.

Kidney Toxicity

Cyclophosphamide nephrotoxicity includes syndrome of inappropriate antidiuretic hormone secretion (SIADH) with hyponatremia, and hemorrhagic cystitis. Cyclophosphamide might either directly induce SIADH[143–145] or stimulate ADH through cyclophosphamide-induced nausea.[146,147] Hyponatremia typically occurs with high dose IV cyclophosphamide but has also been reported after oral cyclophosphamide or low-dose IV cyclophosphamide. Hyponatremia often resolves after drug discontinuation, but high-dose IV cyclophosphamide and concomitant IV fluids to prevent hemorrhagic cystitis, the combination of SIADH, and enhanced water administration can lead to severe, occasionally fatal hyponatremia.[145] Therefore it is recommended to administer isotonic saline rather than hypotonic solutions.

The cyclophosphamide metabolite acrolein is highly toxic to the bladder epithelium and may cause hemorrhagic cystitis.[148] The risk of hemorrhagic cystitis can be minimized by administration of fluids and sodium 2-mercaptoethane sulfonate (mesna), which binds and inactivates acrolein.[149,150]

DIAZIQUONE

Diaziquone is mainly used in patients with primary brain tumors.

Mechanism of Action

Diaziquone is an aziridinylbenzoquinone, which rapidly penetrates the central nervous system. The most probable mechanism of action is that of bioreductive alkylation.

Pharmacokinetics

After administration, diaziquone is rapidly absorbed and it has a volume of distribution exceeding that of total body water. Diaziquone is rapidly metabolized by the liver.

Toxicity

The main toxicity associated with diaziquone is bone marrow suppression resulting in leukopenia, granulocytopenia, and thrombocytopenia.

Kidney Toxicity

Data regarding diaziquone-related nephrotoxicity are very limited, although acute renal failure has been reported subsequent to treatment with diaziquone.[151]

IFOSFAMIDE

Ifosfamide is used in the treatment of Hodgkin and non-Hodgkin lymphoma, soft tissue and osteosarcoma, lung cancer, testicular cancer, breast cancer, ovarian cancer, and cervical cancer.

Mechanism of Action

Ifosfamide is an alkylating agent and a member of the nitrogen mustard family. It is believed to act through interfering with DNA replication and RNA production.

Pharmacokinetics

Ifosfamide is primarily excreted in the urine (80% to the total dose as unchanged ifosfamide). Guidelines vary substantially in regard to dosing in patients with kidney failure. We recommend a 25% dose reduction in patients with a CrCL 40 to 60 mL/min, a 50% dose reduction for patients with a CrCl 10 to 40 mL/min, and drug discontinuation in patients with CrCl lower than 10 mL/min. Ifosfamide is dialyzable, and it should be administered after HD with a dose reduction of 50%.[152] The same dose reduction is recommended for PD patients. No dialysis should be performed for 12 hours after ifosfamide administration.

Toxicity

Common side effects include hair loss, vomiting, nephrotoxicity, neurotoxicity (encephalopathy and peripheral neuropathy), and bone marrow suppression.

Kidney Toxicity

Ifosfamide is associated with numerous possible adverse kidney manifestations;[153] AKI caused by ATN,[154] Fanconi syndrome,[54,154] interstitial nephritis,[155] glomerular disease,[156] and hemorrhagic cystitis.[157] Ifosfamide-induced tubular toxicity can be associated with metabolic acidosis with a normal anion gap (hyperchloremic acidosis) because of type 1 (distal) or type 2 (proximal) RTA; hypophosphatemia induced by decreased proximal phosphate reabsorption; renal glucosuria, aminoaciduria, and a marked increase in β_2-microglobulin excretion, all from generalized proximal dysfunction; polyuria caused by nephrogenic diabetes insipidus; and hypokalemia, resulting from increased urinary potassium losses. Ifosfamide is more nephrotoxic than cyclophosphamide and this is caused by selective uptake of ifosfamide in proximal tubular cells through the OCT2 (see Fig. 16.2).[158] Several risk factors for ifosfamide-induced nephrotoxicity have been identified including preexisting kidney disease, combination with platinum-based chemotherapy and/or other nephrotoxins, cumulative dose of ifosfamide (> 119 g/m^2), and renal irradiation.[17] Although there are few data on long-term kidney function in ifosfamide-treated adults, a progressive decline in GFR has been described after as little as one course of ifosfamide in adults.[159] This reduction in kidney function occurs in a minority of patients, is permanent and progressive, and can also occur long after exposure to ifosfamide.[160] In a Dutch study, it was demonstrated that patients who received ifosfamide in childhood had a lower GFR than patients with the same pathologies who did not receive this treatment.[14] The main risk factors for nephrotoxicity in children are a cumulative dose greater than 45 mg/m^2, young age (< 3 years), previous or concurrent cisplatin treatment, Wilms tumor, and unilateral nephrectomy.[161] Hemorrhagic cystitis can occur even when mesna is used.[157]

Tubular involvement is generally very prolonged, potentially progressive and may lead to advanced CKD.[19,162] Ifosfamide-induced proximal tubular toxicity is characterized by aminoaciduria (28%), glucosuria (90%), low molecular weight proteinuria, Fanconi syndrome (1%–7%), hypophosphatemia, proximal RTA, hypokalemia, phosphaturia, and more rarely, calciuria, magnesiuria, and natriuria.[161] Distal tubular toxicity has also been reported with type 1 RTA, a defect in urine concentration, and nephrogenic diabetes insipidus. Ifosfamide can induce SIADH characterized by hyponatremia, plasma hypoosmolality, and inadequate urinary osmolality.[163,164]

Mesna and hydration are the main measures to minimize the urogenital and nephrologic involvement of ifosfamide, but N-acetylcysteine is recommended by some.[165,166] Patients who received ifosfamide should be followed long-term to detect CKD early.

MELPHALAN

Melphalan is an alkylating agent and is used in the treatment of multiple myeloma.

Mechanism of Action

Melphalan is a member of the nitrogen mustard alkylating agent family. Melphalan alkylates guanine, which results in inter- and intrastrand links of DNA. This results in the inhibition of DNA and RNA synthesis and cytotoxicity.

Pharmacokinetics

Melphalan is metabolized primarily in the liver, and 10% to 30% is eliminated by the kidneys. Melphalan is both secreted and reabsorbed in the renal tubules.[140] In patients with decreased kidney function, elimination of melphalan is reduced and systemic exposure is increased, which may result in bone marrow suppression.[167] Recommendations regarding dose reduction for decreased kidney function differ substantially. We recommend a 25% dose reduction in patients with CrCl between 10 and 50 mL/min and a 50% dose reduction with CrCl less than 10 mL/min. Melphalan is removed during dialysis and should be administered at 50% of the dose after HD.

Toxicity

The most common side effects are nausea, vomiting, and bone marrow suppression.

Kidney Toxicity

Nearly 19% of 80 consecutive patients with AL amyloidosis treated with high-dose melphalan followed by peripheral blood stem cell transplantation developed AKI.[168] Patients who developed AKI had a worse 1-year survival ($p=.03$).[168] A few case reports note nephrotic syndrome after melphalan administration.[169,170] During 1-year follow-up, kidney function improved with disappearance of the nephrotic syndrome.[170] Finally, melphalan has been associated with the development of SIADH.[171,172]

PROCARBAZINE

Procarbazine is used, in combination with other chemotherapeutics, to treat Hodgkin lymphoma and brain cancers, such as glioblastoma multiforme.

Mechanism of Action

Procarbazine is an alkylating agent. Its mechanism of action is incompletely understood but involves inducing breaks in DNA strands.

Pharmacokinetics

Oral procarbazine is rapidly metabolized in the liver. After 24 hours, up to 70% of the dose is recovered in the urine. The use of procarbazine is not recommended in patients with severe kidney impairment, and a 50% dose reduction is recommended with a serum creatinine greater than 2.0 mg/dL.

Toxicity

Common side effects include: bone marrow suppression, nausea, vomiting, peripheral neuropathy, and fatigue. In combination with ethanol, procarbazine may cause a disulfiram-like reaction.

Kidney Toxicity

Procarbazine monotherapy is not nephrotoxic. However, renal insufficiency after administration of procarbazine and high doses of methotrexate has been reported.[173] The authors suggested procarbazine augmented the nephrotoxicity of methotrexate.[173]

TEMOZOLOMIDE

Temozolomide is an alkylating agent used in the treatment of brain tumors (astrocytoma and glioblastoma multiforme) and melanomas, at least before the area of targeted agents and immunotherapy.

Mechanism of Action

Temozolomide is an alkylating agent that alkylates/methylates guanine residues, resulting in DNA damage and cell death.

Pharmacokinetics

Temozolomide is administered orally and the kidney is the major route of elimination (5%–10% as unchanged temozolomide and 90–95% as metabolites). However, studies in patients with mild to moderate kidney dysfunction showed unaltered pharmacokinetics, suggesting no dose adjustment is required.[174] Experience with temozolomide in HD patients is very limited.[175]

Toxicity

The main toxicity associated with the use of temozolomide is bone marrow suppression.[176]

Kidney Toxicity

Temozolomide nephrotoxicity appears to be very limited.[176–179] Few AKI cases were described with temozolomide treatment.[180–182] Only one of 42 patients treated with temozolomide and irinotecan died after developing AKI.[180]

TRABECTEDIN

Trabectedin is an alkylating agent used to treat soft tissue sarcoma and ovarian cancer.

Mechanism of Action

Trabectedin is an alkylating agent that binds DNA at the N2 position of guanine promoting degradation of RNA polymerase and generating DNA double-strand breaks. Furthermore, trabectedin blocks DNA binding of the transcription factor FUS-CHOP and reverses the oncogenic phenotype of liposarcoma cells.[183]

Pharmacokinetics

Dose adjustments are not recommended in patients with CrCl greater than 30 mL/min and no data are available in patients with more severe kidney disease. Therefore the drug, which is not dialyzable, should not be used in patients with CrCl lower than 30 mL/min.[184,185]

Toxicity

Adverse effects associated with trabectedin include bone marrow suppression, hepatotoxicity, nausea, vomiting, and fatigue.

Kidney Toxicity

Cases of AKI (occasionally fatal) have been reported, some of which are attributable to rhabdomyolysis.[186–191] Furthermore, elevations in serum creatinine grade 3 or 4 were observed in 4.2% of patients treated with trabectedin for liposarcoma or leiomyosarcoma. Nephrotoxicity complicated by hepatic failure and death was reported in a

79-year-old patient with sarcoma after a second course of trabectedin.[186]

Antimetabolites

Antimetabolites interfere with DNA production and cell division by impairing DNA replication machinery, either by incorporation of chemically altered nucleotides, or by depleting the supply of deoxynucleotides needed for DNA replication and cell proliferation. Antimetabolite drugs are used to treat a variety of solid, and hematologic, malignancies.

AZACITIDINE

Azacitidine and its derivative, decitabine or 5-aza-2'deoxycytidine, are used to treat patients with myelodysplastic syndrome[192] and acute myeloid leukemia.[193] Recently, an oral form of azacitidine (CC-486) was developed,[194–196] which is currently being evaluated in phase III studies in myelodysplastic syndrome and acute myeloid leukemia.[197]

Mechanism of Action

Azacitidine is a chemical analog of cytidine and is incorporated in DNA and RNA, resulting in cytotoxic effects on hematopoietic cells in the bone marrow at high doses. Azacitidine is incorporated in RNA more than in DNA, and incorporation of azacitidine into RNA results in disaggregation of polyribosomes, accumulation of 80S ribosomes, decreased transfer RNA acceptor activity, and inhibition of protein synthesis.[198–201] At low doses, azacitidine inhibits DNA methyltransferase by formation of covalent bonds between DNA-cytosine methyltransferase and DNA containing 5-azacytosine, resulting in DNA hypomethylation.[202–205] Decitabine is a deoxyribonucleoside that can only be incorporated in DNA.

Pharmacokinetics

Azacitidine and its metabolites are primarily excreted by the kidneys, thereby requiring close monitoring in patients with kidney disease. Although the initial dose does not require adjustment, a 50% reduction is recommended when an unexplained elevation in serum creatinine occurs. The next azacitidine cycle should be postponed until kidney function normalizes.

Toxicity

The most common toxicity associated with azacitidine is hematologic toxicity: anemia, neutropenia, and thrombocytopenia. Hepatotoxicity has also been reported, especially in patients with underlying liver abnormalities. Therefore azacitidine is contraindicated in patients with advanced hepatic tumors. Other reported toxicities include gastrointestinal adverse effects (nausea, diarrhea, constipation, anorexia, vomiting), fever, arthralgia, headache, and dizziness.

Kidney Toxicity

Adverse kidney effects are variable and range from increased serum creatinine levels to AKI.[206] Risk of AKI is increased in patients receiving IV azacitidine in combination with other chemotherapeutics, and possibly in patients with preexisting kidney disease.[207] Fanconi syndrome has been reported with azacitidine use in combination with etoposide for the treatment of chronic myelogenous leukemia. RTA, polyuria, aminoaciduria, phosphaturia, and glucosuria have also been observed. Two patients with very severe hypophosphatemia and associated muscle cramps have been reported (serum phosphate levels 0.6–1 mg/dL).[208] Nine of 22 patients with acute leukemia treated with azacitidine at a dose of 200 mg/m^2/day developed glucosuria, whereas seven had polyuria.[209] In addition, nephrogenic diabetes insipidus has been reported with azacitidine. Treatment of azacitidine-associated nephrotoxicity is drug discontinuation.

CAPECITABINE

Capecitabine is used to treat metastatic breast and colorectal cancer, esophageal cancer, gastric cancer, prostate cancer, renal cell cancer, ovarian cancer, and pancreatic cancer.

Mechanism of Action

Capecitabine is an oral fluoropyrimidine (besides 5-FU and tegafur) with approximately 100% bioavailability and is converted to 5-FU by thymidylate phosphorylase. 5-FU inhibits thymidylate synthase, resulting in the inhibition of thymidine monophosphate production necessary for de novo DNA synthesis. High levels of thymidylate phosphorylase are found in several tumor cells and hepatocytes, rendering these cells more susceptible to toxicity.

Pharmacokinetics

Capecitabine is primarily removed from the body by the kidneys (up to 96% of the dose is recovered in the urine) and therefore dose reduction is required for kidney dysfunction. A 25% dose reduction in patients with CrCl between 30 to 50 mL/min and no administration of capecitabine with CrCl less than 30 mL/min are recommended.[210] Some experts have suggested that capecitabine can be administered to patients with CrCl less than 30mL/min with close monitoring and dose adjustments. To this point, 12 patients with a CrCl less than 30 mL/min (including HD patients) were treated with capecitabine in reduced dose (up to 50%) and the drug was well tolerated. It is recommended that capecitabine is administered after HD.[211]

Toxicity

The most common dose-limiting adverse effects associated with capecitabine monotherapy are hyperbilirubinemia, diarrhea, and hand-foot syndrome. Other adverse effects include abdominal pain, vomiting, weakness, fatigue, and myelosuppression. Bolus capecitabine is associated with more frequent hand-foot syndrome but less stomatitis, alopecia, neutropenia, diarrhea, and nausea.[212]

Kidney Toxicity

Because capecitabine is usually given in combination with other cytotoxics and/or targeted agents, it is difficult to appreciate the relative role of each agent within a given combination causing nephrotoxicity. Kidney function, along with BSA and age, are factors associated with risk of early-onset nephrotoxicity with capecitabine-based anti-cancer regimens.[213] However, exclusion of capecitabine-based treatments in patients with kidney disease, but otherwise good performance status, may not be justified with appropriate dosing modifications.[214] In fact, good renal tolerance of capecitabine was reported with no delayed toxicity greater than grade 2.[215] Also, in the elderly, capecitabine is not associated with deterioration of kidney function.[216] An incidence of hypokalemia of 20%, which was reversible in 91% of cases, occurred with capecitabine but did not require treatment discontinuation.[217]

CLADRIBINE

Cladribine is used in the treatment of hairy cell leukemia and chronic lymphocytic leukemia.

Mechanism of Action

Cladribine is a prodrug, which undergoes intracellular phosphorylation only in lymphocytes. Phosphorylated cladribine is a purine analog and is similar to adenosine. It inhibits the enzyme adenosine deaminase, which results in inhibition of DNA production.

Pharmacokinetics

Approximately 20% of the administered dose is recovered in the urine. There are insufficient data available to make recommendations regarding dose reduction in patients with kidney disease.

Toxicity

The most important adverse effect of cladribine is bone marrow suppression and increased susceptibility for infections.

Kidney Toxicity

Nephrotoxicity of cladribine is limited and there is only one case available in the literature reporting AKI after high doses of cladribine, in combination with other chemotherapeutics and irradiation.[218] In animal studies, renal proximal tubule injury was reported with cladribine.[219]

CLOFARABINE

Clofarabine is used for the treatment of relapsed or refractory acute myeloid and lymphoblastic leukemia.

Mechanism of Action

Clofarabine is a purine analog and inhibits DNA synthesis and the enzyme ribonucleotide reductase.

Pharmacokinetics

As clofarabine is partially removed from the body through renal excretion (60% of the dose is excreted unchanged in the urine after 24 hours), underlying kidney disease increases drug exposure, which might worsen treatment-related toxicity.[220,221] Therefore 50% dose reduction is advised with a CrCl between 30 and 60 mL/min. No recommendation can be made for patients with CrCl lower than 30 mL/min: we consider this a contraindication for clofarabine administration. It has been suggested that clofarabine is not dialyzable.[222] When kidney function deterioration develops during clofarabine treatment, the drug should be discontinued and restarted at 75% of the original dose after kidney function recovery.

Toxicity

Clofarabine-associated adverse effects include bone marrow suppression, hepatotoxicity, gastrointestinal complaints, and fatigue.

Kidney Toxicity

Two case reports have been reported on nephrotoxicity after clofarabine administration.[223,224] AKI and need for renal replacement therapy were described in a 48-year-old man with refractory acute myeloid leukemia treated with clofarabine.[223] The second case demonstrated AKI and proteinuria in a 65-year-old man treated with clofarabine for relapsed acute myeloid leukemia.[224] Twenty-nine cases of adverse kidney events were described in the Food and Drug Administration Adverse Event Reporting System.[223] Collapsing glomerulopathy, severe tubular injury, or a combination of both may be the mechanism of clofarabine-induced AKI. Unfortunately, biopsy data are lacking. In clinical trials involving clofarabine in adults with acute myeloid leukemia, nephrotoxicity was reported in 10% to 42% of patients, and severe kidney injury in 6% to 19% of treated patients.[225–229] In patients undergoing hematopoietic stem cell transplantation, the incidence of AKI was 55% and age and clofarabine AUC were notable risk factors.[230]

CYTARABINE

Cytosine arabinoside or cytarabine is used to treat acute myeloid leukemia, acute lymphocytic leukemia, chronic myelogenous leukemia, and non-Hodgkin lymphoma. Cytarabine is administered intravenously or intrathecal for the treatment/prophylaxis of meningeal leukemia.

Mechanism of Action

Cytarabine is an antimetabolic agent and blocks the function of DNA polymerase. After cellular uptake, cytarabine is converted to cytarabine-5′-triphosphate, which is the active metabolite incorporated into DNA during DNA synthesis. This results in a cell cycle arrest in the S phase. In cohorts of both pediatric and adult patients with acute myeloid leukemia, the response to cytosine arabinoside-containing therapy was inversely correlated with sterile α motif and HD domain-containing protein 1 or SAMHD1 (this protein has deoxynucleoside triphosphate triphosphohydrolase activity) expression levels.[231,232]

Pharmacokinetics

Cytarabine is concentrated in the liver, where a major portion is inactivated by the enzyme cytidine deaminase. After 24 hours, 80% of the drug is eliminated either unchanged or as inactive metabolite in the urine. There are no data available on the use of cytarabine in HD patients. Dose reductions are recommended for high-dose cytarabine (1–3 g/m^2): a 40% dose reduction and a 50% dose reduction in patients with a CrCl of 46 to 60 mL/min and 31 to 45 mL/min, respectively. High-dose cytarabine should not be administered in patients with a CrCl less than 30 mL/min.

Toxicity

The side effects of cytarabine include bone marrow suppression (leukopenia, thrombocytopenia, anemia), stomatitis, conjunctivitis, pneumonitis, and dermatologic side effects.

Kidney Toxicity

Cytarabine may be potentially nephrotoxic, although there are very few data available in the literature reporting its nephrotoxicity. AKI is probably the most common renal side effect.[233–235] In a study by Slavin et al., 85% of patients experienced a doubling of serum creatinine or a decrease in CrCl greater than 50%.[233] Histologic examination showed interstitial edema and dilation of tubules with flattening, focal atypia, and occasional mitotic figures in tubular epithelium.[233] Besides AKI, hypokalemia and hypocalcemia have been reported in patients treated with cytarabine, especially in patients experiencing diarrhea.[233] TMA has also been described although all patients were also receiving other agents associated with the development of TMA.[236–239]

DEOXYCOFOMYCIN

Deoxycofomycin or pentostatin is used in the treatment of hairy cell leukemia, chronic lymphocytic leukemia, and adult T-cell leukemia/lymphoma.

Mechanism of Action

Deoxycofomycin is a purine analog and antimetabolite, which inhibits adenosine deaminase and DNA replication.

Pharmacokinetics

Deoxycofomycin is administered intravenously and is primarily excreted unchanged in the urine (30%–90%) within 24 hours. To prevent deoxycofomycin-induced nephrotoxicity, 250 to 600 mL/m^2 of 5% dextrose solution or 0.45% sodium chloride should be administered before each injection of pentostatin and 300 mL/m^2 after each administration. Dose reduction is required in patients with decreased CrCl: 25% and 50% dose reduction are recommended in patients with a CrCl of 40 to 59 mL/min and 35 to 39 mL/min, respectively. Deoxycofomycin should not be administered with CrCl less than 35 mL/min.

Toxicity

Deoxycofomycin is a well-tolerated chemotherapeutic, whose main toxicities are nausea/vomiting, neurologic toxicity, opportunistic infections, and nephrologic toxicity. The toxicity seen with pentostatin is dose-dependent and therefore the dose of deoxycofomycin should never exceed 4 mg/m^2.

Kidney Toxicity

Deoxycofomycin possesses dose-dependent nephrotoxicity.[151] The risk for AKI is increased with doses of deoxycofomycin greater than 4 g/m^2/week.[240] In addition, hematuria and dysuria develop with deoxycofomycin use,[241] whereas TMA has also been associated with deoxycofomycin.[131,242–245] Data from the Oklahoma TTP-HUS registry and BloodCenter of Wisconsin concluded that there was a definite association between deoxycofomycin and the occurrence of TMA.[131]

FLUDARABINE

Fludarabine is used in the treatment of acute leukemia (myeloid and lymphocytic), chronic lymphocytic leukemia, and non-Hodgkin lymphoma.

Mechanism of Action

Fludarabine is a purine analog and inhibits DNA duplication.

Pharmacokinetics

Approximately 50% to 60% of the fludarabine dose is excreted by the kidneys within 24 hours, making dose adjustments necessary in patients with kidney disease.[246] A 20% to 50% dose reduction is advised for patients with a CrCl of 30 to 70 mL/min and fludarabine should not be given to patients with CrCl less than 30 mL/min. In HD patients, no recommendations can be made. A 50% dose reduction has been suggested for PD patients.

Toxicity

The most common adverse effects are nausea, diarrhea, fever, rash, and dyspnea. Cardiac and hematologic toxicity also occur with fludarabine.[246,247]

Kidney Toxicity

Fludarabine is not considered to be significantly nephrotoxic.[246,247] However, in a retrospective study of 241 patients receiving allogeneic bone marrow transplantation, fludarabine and older age were risk factors for the development of posttransplant AKI.[248]

5-FLUOROURACIL

5-FU is used in the treatment of colon cancer, esophageal cancer, gastric cancer, pancreatic cancer, breast cancer, and cervical cancer.

Mechanism of Action

5-FU is a pyrimidine analog and an inhibitor of thymidylate synthase, which blocks production of DNA. Thymidylate synthase converts deoxyuridine monophosphate to thymidine monophosphate. 5-FU administration reduces deoxythymidine monophosphate, blocks DNA synthesis, and causes cell death. Calcium folinate stabilizes the complex between 5-FU and thymidylate synthase and thus augments 5-FU cytotoxicity.

Pharmacokinetics

5-FU is a prodrug that requires intracellular activation to exert its effects: more than 80% of the administered 5-FU dose is eliminated by catabolism through dihydropyrimidine dehydrogenase, which is highest in the liver. The metabolism of 5-FU is significantly reduced by older age, high serum alkaline phosphatase, length of drug infusion, and low peripheral blood mononuclear cell dihydropyrimidine dehydrogenase activity. Dose reduction of 5-FU should only be considered in patients with severe kidney failure.

Toxicity

Common adverse effects include stomatitis, bone marrow suppression, hair loss, and nausea.

Kidney Toxicity

5-FU alone is not nephrotoxic. However, in combination with folinic acid in high doses,[249] mitomycin,[250–252] and cisplatin,[253] 5-FU may be nephrotoxic. Folinic acid augments 5-FU cytotoxicity, and treatment with this drug combination decreased CrCl by 50% in three patients with normal baseline kidney function.[249] Tubular damage was observed in all patients. Also in combination with cisplatin, 5-FU may be associated with hyponatremia. Hyponatremia occurred in all patients with gastric cancer; 20% of patients had a serum sodium less than 125 mmol/L.[254] In patients with cervical cancer, severe hyponatremia (grade 3–4) was found in 11.1% of patients treated with cisplatin and 5-FU.[255] The combination of cisplatin and 5-FU may also cause hypokalemia.[256] Finally, 5-FU may be associated with TMA.[257,258]

GEMCITABINE

Gemcitabine is used in the treatment of various cancers including breast cancer, ovarian cancer, non-small cell lung cancer, pancreatic cancer, bladder cancer, and cholangiobiliary carcinomas.

Mechanism of Action

Gemcitabine is a cell cycle-specific pyrimidine antagonist and blocks the production of DNA resulting in cell death.

Pharmacokinetics

Gemcitabine is rapidly metabolized by cytidine deaminase. Active metabolites have not been detected in plasma or urine. However, greater than expected toxicity (mainly hematologic toxicity) has been reported in patients with reduced kidney function,[259] requiring dose reduction in patients with CrCl less than 30 mL/min. HD patients have been treated with gemcitabine,[260] with retrospective reports suggesting that gemcitabine treatment in ESRD with intermittent standard HD treatment is safe and well tolerated. Pharmacokinetic data suggest that dose adjustment of gemcitabine should be avoided to ensure its full cytotoxic activity, and that HD treatment should be initiated 6 to 12 hours after its administration to minimize the potential side effects of its noncytotoxic metabolite 2',2'-difluorodeoxyuridine.[260–265] There are no data available regarding gemcitabine administration in PD patients.

Toxicity

Common adverse effects include bone marrow suppression, hepatic toxicity, vomiting and nausea, fever, rash, dyspnea, and hair loss. Rare but potentially severe toxic effects include reversible posterior encephalopathy syndrome, capillary leak syndrome, and adult respiratory stress syndrome.

Kidney Toxicity

A meta-analysis of 979 patients treated with gemcitabine noted that AKI occurred in 0.7% of patients. However, proteinuria and hematuria developed in 36% and 31% of patients, respectively.[266] The most severe adverse kidney effect associated with gemcitabine is TMA.[131,267–276] The incidence of gemcitabine-induced TMA is estimated to range from 0.015% to 2.7%, and it usually develops within 1 to 2 months following gemcitabine therapy.[267,276,277] Data from the Oklahoma TTP-HUS registry and BloodCenter of Wisconsin concluded that there was a definite association between gemcitabine and the occurrence of TMA.[131] Prior treatment with mitomycin C or cisplatin, prolonged treatment with gemcitabine (> 18 courses), and a cumulative dose of gemcitabine (> 20 g/m^2) are risk factors for the development of gemcitabine-induced TMA.[268,269,278] The clinical picture consists of arterial hypertension, decreased renal function, nonnephrotic range proteinuria, and microscopic hemolytic anemia and thrombocytopenia.

Besides cessation of gemcitabine, different treatment modalities have been used to treat gemcitabine-induced TMA, but the best prevention and/or treatment strategy has not been established. Plasma exchange, infusion of fresh frozen plasma, HD, immunoadsorption, plasmapheresis, azathioprine, corticosteroids, vincristine, antiplatelet/anticoagulant therapies, and splenectomy have all been used. The role of plasma exchange in the management of gemcitabine-induced TMA is unclear. Although an improvement in hematologic parameters is often observed during plasma exchange, the beneficial effect on kidney function is less obvious.[267] In addition, doxycycline may be useful in the treatment of gemcitabine-induced TMA.[267,279] The C5 inhibitor eculizumab has been increasingly used for the treatment of gemcitabine-induced TMA.[280–286] Early diagnosis improves chances of renal function recovery, whereas delayed diagnosis is associated with development of CKD, progression to ESRD, and death. The overall outcome of gemcitabine-induced TMA is poor, with a reported mortality ranging from 40% to 90%.[287]

MERCAPTOPURINE

Mercaptopurine is used in the treatment of both acute and chronic leukemia.

Mechanism of Action

Mercaptopurine is an antimetabolite and member of the thiopurine family, which includes azathioprine, 6-mercaptopurine, and 6-thioguanine. As inactive prodrugs, the thiopurines require intracellular activation—catalyzed by multiple enzymes—to exert cytotoxicity. The cytotoxic effects of thiopurine drugs are achieved through different mechanisms: inhibition of de novo purine synthesis by methylmercaptopurine nucleotides, inhibition of Rac1 inducing apoptosis, incorporation of thio-deoxyguanosine triphosphate, and thioguanine triphosphate into DNA and RNA, respectively.

Pharmacokinetics

The clearance of mercaptopurine is mainly hepatic, and renal clearance is only important when high doses of mercaptopurine are administered. The dose interval should be increased in patients with decreased kidney function to 24 to 36 hours and to 48 hours in patients with a CrCl of 50 to 80 mL/min and 10 to 50 mL/min, respectively.

Toxicity

Common adverse effects include rash, flu-like symptoms, bone marrow suppression, hepatotoxicity, pancreatitis, nausea and vomiting, and bone marrow suppression. The toxicity of mercaptopurine can be linked to genetic polymorphisms in thiopurine S-methyltransferase, nudix hydrolase 15, and inosine triphosphate pyrophosphatase.

Kidney Toxicity

Mercaptopurine has only been associated with AKI when tumor lysis syndrome follows tumor therapy. Fanconi syndrome has also been associated with mercaptopurine.[288]

METHOTREXATE

Methotrexate is used in the treatment of breast cancer, lung cancer, head/neck cancer, bladder cancer, leukemia, lymphoma, and osteosarcoma.

Mechanism of Action

Methotrexate can be given orally or by injection. Methotrexate is an antimetabolite and is a competitive inhibitor of dihydrofolate reductase, an enzyme involved in tetrahydrofolate synthesis. Tetrahydrofolate is needed for de novo synthesis of the nucleoside thymidine. Methotrexate inhibits the production of DNA, RNA and proteins.

Pharmacokinetics

Methotrexate is predominantly (60%–90%) excreted by glomerular filtration and tubular secretion. Methotrexate is excreted by the kidneys both in the intact form and as its insoluble metabolite 7-hydroxymethotrexate. In acid urine (pH < 5.5) both compounds precipitate, whereas solubility is 10-fold greater at neutral pH. AKI is associated with higher incidence of bone marrow suppression and gastrointestinal toxicity. Guidelines regarding dose recommendations of methotrexate in patients with kidney disease vary.[140] We advise that high-dose methotrexate should be administered only when CrCl is greater than 60 mL/min before the start of treatment. A 50% dose reduction is advised in patients with CrCl between 10 to 50 mL/min and the drug should be avoided with CrCl lower than 10 mL/min.[73] Methotrexate is protein-bound and only partially removed by HD,[289,290] although HD using high-flux HD membranes can remove more methotrexate. For HD patients treated with low-dose oral methotrexate, a 50% to 75% dose reduction and administration after dialysis is advised (no dialysis for 12 hours after administration)[23] Methotrexate is contraindicated in PD patients. High-dose methotrexate should be avoided in ESRD patients.

Toxicity

The most common adverse effects include hepatotoxicity, stomatitis, bone marrow suppression, nausea, fatigue, pneumonitis, rarely pulmonary fibrosis, and neurotoxicity (including amnesia).

Kidney Toxicity

Doses of methotrexate lower than 0.5 to 1.0 g/m^2 are usually not associated with nephrotoxicity, unless underlying kidney disease is present. Methotrexate-induced crystalline nephropathy is caused by the precipitation of the drug and/or its metabolite in the renal tubule, causing tubular obstruction (promoted by urinary pH < 7) and ATN.[291–293] Direct tubular injury mediated by methotrexate has also been reported. The incidence of AKI associated with methotrexate varies widely, with reports from the 1970s and 1980s noting AKI in 30% to 50% of patients after high-dose methotrexate therapy with leucovorin rescue.[294–295] In contrast, only 1.8% of patients with osteosarcoma who were treated with high-dose methotrexate developed significant nephrotoxicity.[296] The variable incidence of high-dose methotrexate-induced AKI may be genetically determined. Anionic drugs such as methotrexate can be eliminated by multidrug resistance protein 2 (MRP2) transporter (encoded by the gene ABCC2), which is expressed at the luminal side of renal proximal tubular cells. A heterozygous mutation of MRP2 is associated with reduced methotrexate excretion and increased nephrotoxicity.[297] In addition, organic anion transporters also appear to play a role in crystalluria and tubular dysfunction.[298,299] Nephrotoxicity mainly occurs in patients who are volume-depleted and are treated with high doses of methotrexate.[300–302] In children, it was shown that nephrotoxicity is determined by the dose administered and not the cumulative dose.[303] Because of low solubility of methotrexate at low urinary pH, metabolic changes resulting in tubular acidification are an additional risk factor for AKI. Methotrexate administration is also associated with short-term transient decrease in GFR, with complete recovery within 8 hours of discontinuing the drug as a consequence of afferent arteriolar constriction or mesangial cell constriction.[304] In most cases, methotrexate-induced AKI is reversible and kidney function will usually recover in 1 to 3 weeks. However, even at low doses, methotrexate administration can be associated with a significant decrease in CrCl and progressive kidney dysfunction.[305] One of 19 psoriatic patients with normal kidney function receiving methotrexate for prolonged period of time experienced AKI, which showed interstitial fibrosis and focal calcifications of renal tubular cells.[306] Methotrexate has also been associated with the development of the SIADH and polyuria.[307]

Prevention of methotrexate nephrotoxicity includes adjusting the methotrexate dose for kidney function, assuring euvolemia of the patients along with intense hydration, urinary alkalization to obtain a urine pH greater than 7.5, co-administration of high-dose leucovorin, thymidine, and discontinuation of other potentially nephrotoxic drugs.[308–312] Several drugs have been associated with increased nephrotoxicity when coadministered with methotrexate because they compete with the renal tubular secretion of methotrexate, for example, probenecid, salicylates, sulfisoxazole, penicillins, and nonsteroidal antiinflammatory drugs (NSAIDs), and these drugs should be avoided.[313–316] Glucarpidase (carboxypeptidase-G_2), in combination with leucovorin, may be considered in cases of nephrotoxicity attributed to high-dose methotrexate administration or methotrexate intoxication. Administration of glucarpidase, which cleaves methotrexate to inactive metabolites, is associated with a rapid and near total reduction in methotrexate levels (plasma methotrexate concentrations decreased by 98.7% within 15 minutes after glucarpidase administration).[317] HD and continuous venovenous hemodiafiltration can also decrease methotrexate serum levels.[318,319]

PEMETREXED

Pemetrexed is a derivative of methotrexate that is approved for treatment of advanced non-small cell lung cancer and pleural mesothelioma.

Mechanism of Action

Pemetrexed is a novel multitargeted antifolate that inhibits three or more enzymes involved in folate metabolism and purine and pyrimidine synthesis (Fig. 16.3). These enzymes include thymidylate synthase, dihydrofolate reductase, and glycinamide ribonucleotide formyltransferase. Tetrahydrofolate is needed for de novo synthesis of the nucleoside thymidine, required for DNA synthesis. Similar to methotrexate, pemetrexed inhibits the production of DNA, RNA, and proteins.

Pharmacokinetics

The most important route of excretion of pemetrexed is the kidney (70%–90% of dose as unchanged pemetrexed). Pemetrexed should be avoided in patients with a CrCl less than 45 mL/min. In patients with a creatinine clearance CrCl of 45 mL/min or greater, no dose adjustment is needed but prior use of NSAID is contraindicated.[320] Data regarding the use of pemetrexed in dialysis-dependent patients are lacking.

Toxicity

Most common adverse effects associated with pemetrexed include fatigue, nausea, vomiting, diarrhea, stomatitis, bone marrow suppression, and skin irritation.

Kidney Toxicity

Pemetrexed has been associated with ATN, interstitial edema, distal RTA, and nephrogenic diabetes insipidus.[321–323] Pemetrexed is nephrotoxic as monotherapy or in combination with other cytotoxic agents. Risk factors for the development of pemetrexed-associated nephrotoxicity include dehydration, hypertension, baseline kidney disease, and pre-existing diabetes.[323,324] Nephrotoxicity of pemetrexed is correlated with renal reabsorption; pemetrexed, as it is similar to folic acid, is reabsorbed via folate renal receptors (see Fig. 16.3) and via brush border vesicles and tubular reabsorption is increased at acidic pH.[325]

The risk of pemetrexed-associated AKI is in general low (1%–5%), but a higher risk has been reported by others (up to 50%), mainly in patients with lung cancer treated with combination chemotherapy.[323,324] Moderate kidney dysfunction has been observed in patients in phase I and II studies.[326–328] A grade 1/2 increase in serum creatinine was observed in 20% of patients with colorectal or renal

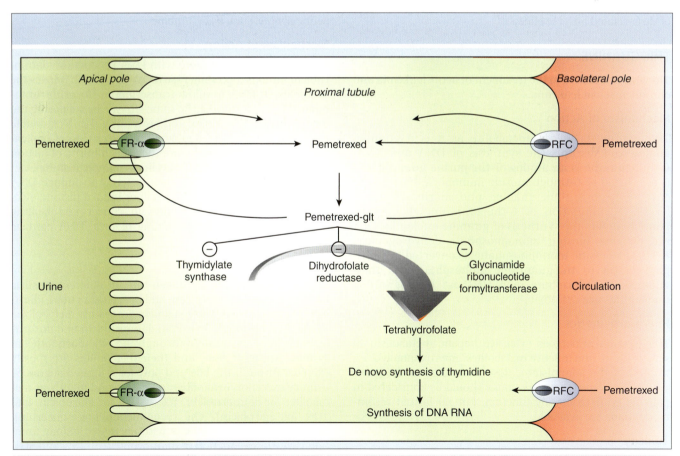

Fig. 16.3 Pemetrexed nephrotoxicity. Pemetrexed enters the proximal tubular cell through the apical folate receptor α (FR-α) and basolateral reduced folate carrier (RFC) transporter. Inside the cell, pemetrexed is polyglutamylated, which inhibits the transport of the drug out of the cells. Polyglutamylated pemetrexed inhibits enzymes involved in the tetrahydrofolate pathway, resulting in the depletion of tetrahydrofolate and inhibition of the de novo synthesis of thymidine, resulting in the inhibition of deoxyribonucleic acid (DNA) and ribonucleic acid (RNA) synthesis.

cancer receiving pemetrexed at a dose of 600 mg/m² every 21 days.[327] In a study of patients receiving pemetrexed in combination with gemcitabine, nephrotoxicity occurred in 13% of patients.[329] In patients receiving pemetrexed and bevacizumab for non-small cell lung cancer, 33% of patients discontinued dual treatment because of adverse events and in 54% of cases this adverse event was nephrotoxicity.[330] Pemetrexed-induced AKI may not always be reversible.[323,324] Interestingly, there is evidence that the combination of pemetrexed + cisplatin is less nephrotoxic than cisplatin alone.[329] Pemetrexed may also cause ATN with interstitial fibrosis.[321,325,331,332] This pathologic finding occurred between the second and sixth pemetrexed course. In addition, despite pemetrexed discontinuation, CKD developed.[325] Pemetrexed may be particularly nephrotoxic with prolonged exposure, by a mechanism of accumulation of pemeterexed polyglutamate derivatives within renal cells. In addition, pemetrexed may also be the cause of nephrogenic diabetes insipidus and RTA.[321,322]

To reduce the risk of pemetrexed toxicity, folic acid and vitamin B12 should be administered. To limit the reabsorption of pemetrexed, alkalization of the urine and hydration are recommended.[321] In addition, concomitant administration of potentially nephrotoxic medication should be avoided, especially NSAIDs, angiotensin-converting enzyme inhibitors and/or angiotensin-receptor antagonists, and statins, because these drugs may decrease the elimination of pemetrexed and therefore increase the occurrence of dose-related adverse effects.[333]

THIOGUANINE

Thioguanine is used in the treatment of acute leukemia and chronic myeloid leukemia.

Mechanism of Action

Thioguanine is an antimetabolite as it is a guanine analog and disrupts the synthesis of DNA and RNA. 6-Thioguanine is an analog of the purine guanine and is converted to 6-thioguanosine monophosphate by the enzyme hypoxanthine-guanine phosphoribosyl transferase. Accumulation of 6-thioguanosine monophosphate hampers the synthesis of guanine nucleotides via the enzyme inosine monophosphate dehydrogenase. 6-Thioguanosine monophosphate is converted by phosphorylation to thioguanosine diphosphate and thioguanosine triphosphate, and all these 6-thioguanine nucleotides are cytotoxic.

Pharmacokinetics

Thioguanine undergoes extensive hepatic metabolism to several active and inactive metabolites. Approximately 25% to 50% of the administered dose is excreted in the urine within 24 hours. Dose reductions should be considered in patients with kidney dysfunction, but no formal recommendations are available.

Toxicity

Common adverse effects include bone marrow suppression, hepatotoxicity, nausea and vomiting, and stomatitis. Those with a genetic deficiency in thiopurine S-methyltransferase are at higher risk of adverse effects.

Kidney Toxicity

The nephrotoxicity of thioguanine is limited and only cases of tumor lysis syndrome-induced AKI have been reported. In 37 patients with Burkitt lymphoma developing tumor lysis syndrome, 11 patients were treated with BACT (BCNU, cytosine arabinoside, cyclophosphamide, thioguanine).[334]

Antitumor Antibiotics

Antitumor antibiotics are a heterogeneous family of anticancer agents and they act mainly by DNA intercalation, causing a block in the synthesis of DNA and RNA, or through other different, more complex and at a certain extent still ill-defined, mechanisms (especially anthracyclines).

ANTHRACYCLINES

Daunorubicin, doxorubicin, epirubicin, mitoxantrone, and idarubicin are anthracyclines. Daunorubicin is mainly used in the treatment of hematologic malignancies, such as acute myeloid leukemia, acute lymphoid leukemia, chronic myelogenous leukemia, neuroblastoma, and Kaposi sarcoma. Epirubicin is mainly used in the treatment of patients with breast cancer, whereas mitoxantrone is also used in acute myeloid leukemia and non-Hodgkin lymphoma. Anthracyclines are usually combined with other chemotherapeutic agents, such as cytarabine.

Mechanism of Action

All anthracyclines interfere with DNA production: daunorubicin inhibits topoisomerase II enzyme, which relaxes the supercoils in DNA to allow transcription. Doxorubicin inhibits the progression of the same enzyme by stabilizing the topoisomerase II complex and preventing the DNA double helix from being resealed and halting the process of replication.[335,336] More recently, another mechanism of action was described for the anthracyclines, namely histone eviction.[337,338] Independent of their potency to induce DNA double strand breaks, anthracyclines induce histone eviction, deregulating transcription in cancer and healthy tissues. This results in dampening of local DNA damage responses.[337,338]

Pharmacokinetics

Daunorubicin is rapidly taken up in different tissues, including liver, kidney, spleen, and heart. Doxorubin, idarubicin, mitoxantrone, and epirubicin are mainly metabolized in the liver, although liposomal daunorubicin and doxorubicin are probably cleared through the reticuloendothelial system. Anthracyclines and their metabolites are mostly excreted through the bile and only for a limited degree by urinary excretion (estimated to be 25% and mainly as metabolites for daunorubicin, 5% to 16% for idarubicin, and 10% for epirubicin). The recommendations concerning dose adjustments in patients with decreased kidney function vary. Dose reduction of daunorubicin of 25% and 50% has been suggested in patients with a serum creatinine of 1.2 to 3 mg/dL and more than 3 mg/dL, respectively. For liposomal daunorubicin, a 50% dose reduction is recommended in patients with a serum creatinine greater than

3 mg/dL, whereas for liposomal doxorubicin and IV doxorubicin, no dose reduction is required with kidney dysfunction. For idarubicin, a dose reduction of 50% is suggested in patients with a serum creatinine of 1.13 to 1.98 mg/dL and in HD patients, a 50% dose reduction has been suggested. For epirubicin, dose reductions should be considered only in patients with CrCl lower than 10 mL/min. For mitoxantrone, no dose reduction is recommended in patients with kidney dysfunction. It has been recommended that no dose adjustments are needed for doxorubicin and epirubicin in HD patients and that administration should be done after HD.[23,73]

Toxicity

The most common adverse effects associated with anthracycline use are vomiting, hair loss, bone marrow suppression, and oral ulcers. Severe adverse effects include cardiomyopathy and tissue necrosis at the side of injection.[339]

Kidney Toxicity

Anthracyclines, especially when combined with the anti-HER2 monoclonal antibody trastuzumab, may cause significant cardiotoxicity, with possible secondary kidney damage.[340] However, anthracyclines, alone or combined with trastuzumab, at present are considered to have limited nephrotoxicity. When injected in rodents, doxorubicin induces glomerular injury similar to noncollapsing focal segmental glomerulosclerosis[341,342] and podocyte injury appears to be mediated by the receptor for advanced glycation end-products.[343] Anthracyclines have been reported to be associated with nephrotic syndrome and several glomerular diseases. There are a few case reports linking anthracyclines with minimal change disease.[344,345] Anthracyclines have also been associated with both collapsing and noncollapsing focal segmental glomerulosclerosis.[346–349] Few cases of proteinuria associated with the administration of epirubicin have been reported in a phase II study in patients with small cell lung cancer.[350] Three cases of TMA were diagnosed in patients treated with PEGylated liposomal doxorubicin.[347,351] One patient was also treated with bevacizumab and all patients had received high cumulative doses of PEGylated liposomal doxorubicin (880–1445 mg/m^2). All patients presented with hypertension, nonnephrotic range proteinuria, and decreased kidney function. Symptoms only improved partially after withdrawal of PEGylated liposomal doxorubicin. In addition, 23% of 56 patients treated with PEGylated liposomal doxorubicin (by itself or in combination with other chemotherapeutic agents) developed stage 3 to 4 CKD and hypertension.[351] PEGylated liposomal doxorubicin has also been associated with the development of nephrotic syndrome and AKI.[352] Nephrotoxicity occurs in 1% of patients treated with idarubicine and especially when combined with cytarabine.[353–356] Mitoxantrone has limited nephrotoxicity.[357] Renal tubular toxicity mediated by anthracyclines was described in a study including 66 pediatric cancer patients.[358]

BLEOMYCIN

Bleomycin is used in the treatment Hodgkin lymphoma, non-Hodgkin lymphoma, testicular cancer, ovarian cancer, and cervical cancer.

Mechanism of Action

Bleomycin is an antitumor antibiotic derived from *Streptomyces verticillus*.[359] It is believed to degrade DNA.[360] Bleomycin demonstrates sequence selective DNA binding and cleavage, resulting in DNA degradation.[360,361] In addition, bleomycin inhibits the incorporation of thymidine into DNA. In vitro, bleomycin-induced DNA degradation is dependent on oxygen and metal ions, such as iron. Bleomycin chelates iron, resulting in a pseudoenzyme generating hydroxide free radicals and superoxide that will subsequently cleave DNA.[362,363] Other mechanisms involved in bleomycin-induced cytotoxicity are lipid peroxidation, topoisomerase II enzyme inhibition, and oxidative RNA degradation.[364,365]

Pharmacokinetics

Bleomycin can be administered intravenously, intramuscularly, and subcutaneously. Inactivation of bleomycin occurs primarily in the liver. Two-thirds of the administered dose is excreted unchanged in the urine. Few patients with kidney impairment receiving bleomycin have been studied.[366,367] A 25% dose reduction is recommended in patients with CrCl 10 to 50 mL/min and 50% dose reduction is recommended in patients with CrCl lower than 10 mL/min.

Toxicity

The most common adverse effects associated with bleomycin include fever, weight loss, vomiting, rash, hyperpigmentation, alopecia, and Raynaud phenomena. Serious adverse effects include anaphylaxis and pulmonary fibrosis. The pathophysiology of bleomycin-induced pulmonary fibrosis has been hypothesized to be related to its oxygen toxicity and involves proinflammatory cytokines such as interleukin (IL)-18 and IL-1β.[368] Bleomycin is excreted by the kidney and kidney disease increases the risk for bleomycin-related toxicity.[369–371]

Kidney Toxicity

Bleomycin has been associated with TMA characterized by the combination of hemolytic microangiopathic anemia and AKI.[239,257,270,372,373] Bleomycin-associated TMA occurred with combination chemotherapy, including bleomycin.

MITOMYCIN C

Mitomycin C is used in the treatment of bladder cancer (also by bladder installation), esophageal carcinoma, anal cancers, and breast cancer.

Mechanism of Action

Mitomycin C is an alkylating chemotherapeutic. After administration, mitomycin C is converted to mitosene, which will alkylate guanine, causing cross-linking in the DNA.

Pharmacokinetics

Only 20% of the mitomycin C dose is excreted in the urine[140] and therefore mitomycin C can be administered to patients with kidney disease, without dose reductions. The percentage of the mitomycin C dose excreted in the urine increases with increasing doses. Some guidelines have recommended withholding mitomycin C in patients with a serum creatinine greater than 1.7 mg/dL, whereas others recommend a 25% dose reduction in patients with CrCl less than 10 mL/min.[73] There are no recommendations regarding the use of mitomycin C in HD patients, although the same dose reduction of 25% can be applied.

Toxicity

The most common toxicity is bone marrow suppression. It may result in pulmonary and renal toxicity.

Kidney Toxicity

Mitomycin C causes dose-dependent nephrotoxicity, which occurs at cumulative doses of greater than 30 mg/m^2 and above.[374] The main adverse kidney effect is TMA, which is often severe and has a variable time of onset (from immediately after treatment up to 9 months after treatment). However, this lesion is most likely to occur after at least 6 months of therapy, with an overall incidence related to cumulative dose.[257,375,376] As an example, in one series, kidney complications developed in 2%, 11%, and 28% of patients receiving cumulative doses of 50, 50 to 69, and more than 70 mg/m^2, respectively.[257,375,377–380] TMA is presumed to result from direct endothelial injury.[375] In experimental animals, direct renal artery infusion of mitomycin C into anesthetized rats produced classic microangiopathic lesions.[381] Recovery of the kidney function can occur, but usually kidney dysfunction is progressive and dialysis is required in nearly one-third of patients. Mitomycin C-induced TMA has a high case fatality rate (75%) and the median time to death is approximately 4 weeks.[375,380,382] Treatment of mitomycin C-induced TMA consists of prompt diagnosis, early discontinuation of the drug, and supportive treatment. Plasmapheresis appears to be ineffective. However, mitomycin C-induced TMA unresponsive to plasma exchanges experienced a dramatic improvement of hematologic parameters and kidney function after eculizumab infusion.[383]

Chloroethylnitrosourea Compounds Carmustine, Semustine, Streptozocin, Bendamustine, Estramustine, Lomustine

The chloroethylnitrosourea family includes carmustine, semustine, streptozocin, bendamustine, estramustine, and lomustine. Nitrosoureas are a group of cell cycle phase-nonspecific, lipid soluble, alkylating agents that are able to cross the blood-brain barrier; among them, streptozocin is an antibiotic that contains a nitrosourea group and differs somewhat in action from the other nitrosoureas. Carmustine is a nitrogen mustard β-chloro-nitrosourea compound used in the treatment of patients with different forms of brain cancer, multiple myeloma, and Hodgkin and non-Hodgkin lymphoma. Carmustine is often used in combination with alkyl guanine transferase inhibitors or fludarabine and melphalan (when used in preparation of hematopoietic stem cell transplantation). Semustine is another member of this family of chemotherapeutics and is structurally similar

to lomustine. Streptozocin is used in the treatment of metastatic cancer of the islets of Langerhans, which cannot be managed surgically. Streptozocin is highly toxic to β cells and is used in experimental models to induce diabetes mellitus. Bendamustine is used in the treatment of chronic lymphocytic leukemia and non-Hodgkin lymphoma. Estramustine is used in the treatment of prostate cancer and lomustine in the treatment of brain cancers.

Mechanism of Action

Chloroethylnitrosourea forms interstrand cross-links in DNA, which halts DNA replication and transcription. Streptozocin is a glucosamine-nitrosourea compound and causes DNA damage, as all other nitrosourea agents, and because streptozocin is structurally similar to glucose it is transported into the cells through the GLUT2 glucose-transporter. Because β cells express high levels of the GLUT2 transporter, these cells are particularly susceptible for streptozocin toxicity.

Pharmacokinetics

Carmustine is partially metabolized to active metabolites by hepatic microsomal enzymes. Some 60% to 70% of the total carmustine dose is excreted in the urine within 3 days. Estramustine is excreted partially in the urine and lomustine metabolites are primarily excreted by the kidneys. Little is known regarding dose adjustment of chloroethylnitrosoureas in patients with kidney impairment. In our opinion, streptozocin, because of its high intrinsic nephrotoxicity, should not be administered in patients with preexisting kidney disease. When kidney failure develops during therapy, the dose should be reduced with 25% in patients with CrCl between 10 to 50 mL/min and therapy should be stopped with CrCl lower than 10 mL/min. There are no data regarding streptozocin in HD patients. For lomustine, dose reductions of 25% and 50% are recommended for CrCl of 10 to 50 mL/min and less than 10 mL/min, respectively. For HD patients, the dose of lomustine should be reduced by 50% to 75%. In patients with CrCl of 40 to 80 mL/min,[384] the pharmacokinetics of bendamustine are unaltered. In patients with CrCl less than 40 mL/min, grade 3 or 4 side effects might be higher[385] and therefore bendamustine is contraindicated. Dose reduction of 20% and 25% is recommended for carmustine in patients with CrCl of 45 to 60 mL/min and 30 to 45 mL/min, respectively. No dose reduction is needed for HD patients. For estramustine, no adjustments are required in patients with kidney dysfunction. A 25% and 50% dose reduction are recommended in patients with CrCl of 45 to 60 mL/min and 30 to 45 mL/min, respectively. Lomustine should not be administered to patients with CrCl lower than 30 mL/min and in HD patients.

Toxicity

Pulmonary toxicity is the most notable side effect of the chloroethylnitrosourea compounds.

Kidney Toxicity

Chloroethylnitrosoureas can trigger systemic hypotension and renal hypoperfusion with prerenal azotemia. Treatment of hypotension consists of the administration of IV crystalloid fluids and reduced rate of chemotherapy infusion. Sometimes vasopressors are required. Antihypertensive treatment should be discontinued 24 hours before the administration of chloroethylnitrosoureas.

The metabolites of the chloroethylnitrosoureas are primarily considered nephrotoxic and they persist in the urine for up to 72 hours.[386] Irreversible chronic interstitial nephritis and CKD have been reported in patients treated with carmustine, iomustine, and streptozocin.[387,388,389] Tubular toxicity is thought to result from alkylation of tubular cell protein. Streptozocin is associated with nephrotoxicity in up to 75% of patients who chronically receive this drug. Streptozocin-induced nephrotoxicity is rarely seen in patients who received less than 15 g/m²/week.[390] Streptozocin has also been associated with uric acid nephrolithiasis, AKI, and diabetes insipidus.[391,392] Finally, Fanconi syndrome is rarely associated with the use of streptozocin. Treatment of this complication consists of immediate cessation of further chemotherapy, because irreversible renal damage will develop with continued administration.

Adverse kidney effects associated with streptozocin are mild proteinuria and an increase in plasma creatinine concentration. Thereafter, signs and symptoms of tubular dysfunction will occur including phosphaturia, glycosuria, aminoaciduria, uricosuria, and bicarbonaturia. In 52 patients treated with streptozocin for advanced islet cell carcinoma, 51% had proteinuria, 17% proximal RTA, 13% complete or partial Fanconi syndrome, and 26% decreased kidney function.[393] It was estimated that nephrotoxicity contributed to death in 11% of patients.[393]

Nephrotoxicity can be delayed several years after cessation of chloroethylnitrosoureas and therefore long-term follow-up is recommended. Several cases of lomustine-related nephrotoxicity have been reported.[387,388,394–396] In patients receiving nitrosourea treatment for more than 1 year, 17 of 18 patients who received at least six courses, and all nine patients who received more than 10 courses, developed impaired kidney function.[388] In addition, four patients subsequently developed ESRD.[388] Preexisting hypertension and kidney disease, prolonged treatment with nitrosourea, and high cumulative dose have been linked with increased risk for nephrotoxicity. Kidney biopsy demonstrated the presence of glomerulosclerosis, tubular atrophy, interstitial fibrosis, and inflammation.[387,388] Kidney impairment associated with lomustine tends to be progressive, despite discontinuation of nitrosourea treatment.[310]

Semustine is associated with kidney injury, as described in 35 patients with semustine-related nephrotoxicity.[397] High risk of nephrotoxicity occurs when the cumulative dose exceeds 1200 mg/m². Notably, the onset of kidney dysfunction might be considerably delayed.[397] Semustine has also been associated with the development of TMA.[398] Adverse kidney effects of bendamustine are limited and may be related to tumor lysis syndrome developing after drug therapy.[399,400] In patients with multiple myeloma, bendamustine has been administered to patients with preexisting renal insufficiency without negative effect on kidney function.[401,402] The recommended treatment of chloroethylnitrosourea-induced nephrotoxicity is interruption of treatment and preadministration forced diuresis.[403]

Microtubule Inhibitors

TAXANES

The taxane family includes docetaxel, paclitaxel, and cabazitaxel. Docetaxel is used in the treatment of breast cancer, head/neck cancer, gastric cancer, prostate cancer, and non-small cell lung cancer. Paclitaxel is used in the treatment of ovarian cancer, breast cancer, lung cancer, Kaposi sarcoma, cervical cancer, and pancreatic cancer. Cabazitaxel is used in the treatment of prostate cancer.

Mechanism of Action

Taxanes bind to microtubules, disrupting their normal function and halting cell division. Binding of docetaxel to microtubules prevents microtubule depolymerization/disassembly. This results in decreased levels of free tubulin, which is needed for microtubule formation. Docetaxel inhibits mitotic spindle assembly and paclitaxel stabilizes the microtubule polymer and protects it from disassembly.

Pharmacokinetics

Taxanes are mainly removed from the body in the bile (75% of the total dose), whereas kidney excretion (6% of the total dose) is limited. Therefore dose reduction is not necessary in patients with kidney disease,[73] even in HD patients.[404–407] Cabazitaxel is a novel taxane that has limited information about nephrotoxicity and dosing.

Toxicity

Adverse effects associated with docetaxel and paclitaxel include vomiting, hair loss, and muscle cramps. Serious adverse effects include cardiac and pulmonary problems.

Kidney Toxicity

Nephrotoxicity associated with docetaxel administration seems to be limited,[408] although occurrence of hyponatremia[409] and TMA[410] have been reported. Because urinary β2 microglobulin levels are increased after docetaxel administration, docetaxel may have some tubular toxicity.[411]

Although nephrotoxicity of paclitaxel monotherapy has been suggested,[412,413] there are no data from reported clinical trials available to corroborate this. Paclitaxel is known to potentiate platinum-based chemotherapeutic-associated nephrotoxicity. In patients with gynecologic cancers, treated with cisplatin or cisplatin in combination with paclitaxel, a higher incidence of nephrotoxicity in the combination group was noted.[414] In addition, hypokalemia and hyponatremia have been reported with paclitaxel.[57,61,415]

VINCA ALKALOIDS

The vinca alkaloid family includes vincristine, vinblastine, vinorelbine, and eribulin. Vincristine is used in the treatment of hematologic tumors (acute leukemia and Hodgkin lymphoma) and lung cancer. Vinblastine is used in the treatment of Hodgkin lymphoma, lung cancer, bladder cancer, and other types of cancer. Vinorelbine is used in the treatment of breast cancer and non-small cell lung cancer, and eribulin is used in the treatment of breast cancer and sarcoma.

Mechanism of Action

Vinca alkaloids bind to tubulin, resulting in the inhibition of the microtubules assembly and mitotic spindle formation. Eribulin binds predominantly at the plus ends of existing microtubules.

Pharmacokinetics

Vinca alkaloids are mainly eliminated from the body through the liver, with a minor contribution from the kidneys (33% of the vinblastine dose within 72 hours, 10% of the vincristine dose within 24 hours, 20% of the vinorelbine dose). For vincristine, vinblastine, and vinorelbine, no doses adjustments are recommended in patients with kidney dysfunction, except for HD patients for whom a lower starting dose of vinorelbine has been proposed.[23] For eribulin, a lower staring dose is recommended for CrCl between 30 and 49 mL/min and eribulin should be avoided for the time being with CrCl lower than 30 mL/min.[74] The only available data suggest that patients with moderate or severe kidney impairment can tolerate doses of 1.4 mg/m² without unexpected toxicity.

Toxicity

Toxicities associated with vinca alkaloids are numerous and include hair loss, gastrointestinal complaints, bone marrow suppression, dermatologic and neurologic toxicities.

Kidney Toxicity

To our knowledge, there are no data on possible nephrotoxicity associated with vincristine, vinblastine, vinorelbine, or eribulin in monotherapy.[416] In combination with eroltinib, vinorelbine has been associated with the development of diarrhea and hypokalemia.[417] In addition, there are several cases of SIADH after administration of vinca alkaloids, although the prevalence appears to be low (1.3/100,000). For example, vincristine combined with itraconazole and in combination with cyclophosphamide, doxorubicin, prednisone (CHOP protocol) has been associated with SIADH.[418,419] SIADH has never been reported for the newer compound of this family, vinflunine. The only reported adverse kidney effect of erlotinib is urinary tract infections, with a reported incidence of 10% among 503 patients with metastatic breast cancer.[420]

Topoisomerase Inhibitors

ETOPOSIDE

Etoposide is used in patients with lung cancer, lymphoma, testicular cancer, and other cancers.

Mechanism of Action

Etoposide is a semisynthetic podophyllotoxin derived from the root of *Podophyllum peltatum* (May apple or mandrake). It causes single-strand breaks in DNA and inhibits DNA topoisomerase II. Etoposide mainly exerts its cell cytotoxicity during the late S and G2 phase.

Pharmacokinetics

Etoposide has a bioavailability of approximately 50% and is metabolized in the liver via the cytochrome p450 system (CYP3A4). Some 50% to 60% of etoposide is excreted in unaltered form by the kidneys and 40% to 50% through biliary excretion.[421] Kidney disease is associated with increased (mainly hematologic) toxicity.[422,423] Dose reductions of 25% and 50% are recommended for CrCl of 15 to 50 mL/min and less than 15 mL/min, respectively. Etoposide has been administered to HD patients (50% dose reduction either before or after dialysis).[23,40,424,425] Also a dose reduction of 50% is suggested in PD patients.

Toxicity

The toxicity of etoposide is mainly manifested by hematologic toxicity. Other reported toxicities are hypersensitivity reactions, transient hypotension, stomatitis and phlebitis.

Kidney Toxicity

No particular nephrotoxicity has been reported in the literature.[412,426,427]

IRINOTECAN

Irinotecan is used in the treatment of colon cancer and small cell lung cancer, either alone or in combination with other chemotherapeutics, such as 5-FU and cisplatin.

Mechanism of Action

After administration, irinotecan is converted in vivo by carboxylesterase enzymes into SN-38, its active metabolite. SN-38 is a potent inhibitor of topoisomerase I and this inhibition results in inhibition of DNA replication and transcription.

Pharmacokinetics

Irinotecan is eliminated by the liver via glucuronidation and biliary excretion. SN-38 can be excreted intact, lactone-hydrolyzed and excreted, or glucuronidated. Urine excretion of SN-38 accounts for less than 20% of drug elimination.[428] The plasma concentration of SN-38 is significantly increased with CrCl less than 20 mL/min and in HD patients.[429] Despite the fact that the kidneys are responsible for only a small fraction of drug clearance (19.9% of irinotecan and 0.25% of SN-38),[430] ESRD patients treated with irinotecan experience increased toxicity and even single doses of greater than 125 mg/m² have been associated with severe adverse events.[431–433] Weekly doses of irinotecan, not exceeding 50 to 80 mg/m²,[432] are appropriate of HD patients (administered after HD).[23] Specific guidelines for irinotecan use in PD patients are lacking.

Toxicity

The most common side effects associated with the use of irinotecan are diarrhea, vomiting, bone marrow suppression, and fever. Other reported severe side effects are colitis, anaphylactic reaction, and thrombosis.

Kidney Toxicity

The intrinsic nephrotoxicity of irinotecan is limited. AKI in patients treated with irinotecan is caused by tumor lysis syndrome or diarrhea-induced dehydration.[434–436]

TOPOTECAN

Topotecan is primarily used in the treatment of ovarian cancer and lung cancer.

Mechanism of Action

Topotecan is a derivative of camptothecin and a topoisomerase inhibitor. Topotecan prevents topoisomerase from religating cleaved DNA strand and subsequently DNA damage occurs. Inactivation of topoisomerase results in apoptosis and cell death.

Pharmacokinetics

Topotecan and its open ring form are predominantly cleared by the kidneys, and increased toxicity is reported in patients with moderate kidney impairment.[73,437] Drug dosing in patients with kidney disease is controversial. A recent pharmacodynamic and pharmacokinetic study of oral topotecan, in patients with advanced solid tumors, concluded that dose adjustments are not required in patients with mildly impaired kidney function, whereas reduced doses are required for patients with moderate or severe kidney impairment.[438] However, from a previous phase I and pharmacokinetic study of topotecan, in patients with impaired kidney function, it was clear that dose adjustments are required in patients with moderate, but not mild, kidney impairment.[437] We recommend a 50% dose reduction for patients with CrCl of 10 to 50 mL/min, a 75% dose reduction for patients with CrCl less than 10 mL/min and avoidance in HD patients.[73]

Toxicity

Topotecan-related toxicity includes bone marrow suppression, gastrointestinal complaints (diarrhea, nausea, constipation), stomatitis, and fatigue.

Kidney Toxicity

Topotecan is not nephrotoxic to our knowledge.[412] In a study of 27 patients, decreased kidney function was noted in two patients, but deemed not related to topotecan.[439]

Others

ARSENIC TRIOXIDE

Arsenic trioxide is mainly used in patients with acute promyelocytic leukemia.

Mechanism of Action

The *promyelocytic leukemia retinoic acid receptor (PML-RARα)* gene is pathognomonic of acute promyelocytic leukemia, because it causes the arrest of myeloid cell development at the promyelocyte stage. Arsenic trioxide has been shown to cause degradation of *PML-RARα*, promoting differentiation.

Pharmacokinetics

Arsenic is stored mainly in liver, kidney, heart, lung, hair, and nails. The toxic metabolites of arsenic trioxide are eliminated from the body through renal excretion and therefore drug exposure is probably higher in patients with severe kidney impairment.[440] No clear recommendations are available regarding dose reduction in patients with CrCl less than 30 mL/min, although close monitoring for toxicity and consideration of dose reduction is advised. No data are available regarding use of this agent in HD patients.

Toxicity

Arsenic trioxide side effects include gastrointestinal complaints (nausea, vomiting, diarrhea and abdominal pain), and fatigue.

Kidney Toxicity

It is well established that exposure to arsenic results in rhabdomyolysis and acute tubulointerstitial disease;[114] however, exposure to low doses of arsenic trioxide is only rarely associated with adverse kidney effects.[441]

TAMOXIFEN

Tamoxifen is used in the prevention and treatment of breast cancer.

Pharmacokinetics and Mechanism of Action

Tamoxifen is a selective estrogen-receptor modulator. Tamoxifen is a prodrug that is metabolized in the liver into its active metabolites, 4-hydroxytamoxifen and N-desmethyl-4-hydroxytamoxifen, which are potent ligands of the estrogen receptor and blocks cell proliferation.

Toxicity

Adverse effects associated with tamoxifen include induction of menopause (irregular periods, hot flashes), limited increased risk of endometrial cancer, stroke, and thrombo-embolic events.

Kidney Toxicity

To our knowledge, only one case report noted nephrotic syndrome after treatment with tamoxifen in a 56-year-old woman.[442] No histology is reported in this case report. The nephrotic syndrome disappeared after cessation of tamoxifen and treatment of corticosteroids.[442]

Key Points

- Several conventional chemotherapeutics have been associated with renal side effects including kidney function deterioration, electrolyte disorders, tubular injury, glomerular lesions, tubulointerstitial nephritis and the development of thrombotic microangiopathy (TMA).
- AKI is a common condition in cancer patients and is associated with higher cost, longer length of hospital stay, increased morbidity and mortality.
- Chronic kidney disease (CKD) has been reported as a long-term complication in cancer survivors, and pediatric patients are a particularly vulnerable group.
- The kidneys are a major excretion pathway for many antineoplastic agents and thus require dose adjustment when administered in the setting of acute kidney disease or CKD.
- Additional studies are needed to determine the optimal dosage of chemotherapeutic agents in patients decreased kidney function and dialysis.

References

1. Perazella MA. Onco-nephrology: renal toxicities of chemotherapeutic agents. *Clin J Am Soc Nephrol.* 2012;7:1713-1721.

3. Airy M, Raghavan R, Truong LD, Eknoyan G. Tubulointerstitial nephritis and cancer chemotherapy: update on a neglected clinical entity. *Nephrol Dial Transplant.* 2013;28:2502-2509.

4. Garcia G, Atallah JP. Antineoplastic agents and thrombotic microangiopathy. *J Oncol Pharm Pract.* 2017;23:135-142.

5. Troxell ML, Higgins JP, Kambham N. Antineoplastic treatment and renal injury: an update on renal pathology due to cytotoxic and targeted therapies. *Adv Anat Pathol.* 2016;23:310-329.

6. Christiansen CF, Johansen MB, Langeberg WJ, Fryzek JP, Sørensen HT. Incidence of acute kidney injury in cancer patients: a Danish population-based cohort study. *Eur J Intern Med.* 2011;22:399-406.

7. Salahudeen AK, Doshi SM, Pawar T, Nowshad G, Lahoti A, Shah P. Incidence rate, clinical correlates, and outcomes of AKI in patients admitted to a comprehensive cancer center. *Clin J Am Soc Nephrol.* 2013;8:347-354.

8. Samuels J, Ng CS, Nates J, et al. Small increases in serum creatinine are associated with prolonged ICU stay and increased hospital mortality in critically ill patients with cancer. *Support Care Cancer.* 2011;19:1527-1532.

9. Soares M, Salluh JI, Carvalho MS, Darmon M, Rocco JR, Spector N. Prognosis of critically ill patients with cancer and acute renal dysfunction. *J Clin Oncol.* 2006;24:4003-4010.

10. Launay-Vacher V, Oudard S, Janus N, et al. Prevalence of renal insufficiency in cancer patients and implications for anticancer drug management: the renal insufficiency and anticancer medications (IRMA) study. *Cancer.* 2007;110:1376-1384.

11. Janus N, Launay-Vacher V, Byloos E, et al. Cancer and renal insufficiency results of the BIRMA study. *Br J Cancer.* 2010;103:1815-1821.

12. Knijnenburg SL, Jaspers MW, van der Pal HJ, et al. Renal dysfunction and elevated blood pressure in long-term childhood cancer survivors. *Clin J Am Soc Nephrol.* 2012;7:1416-1427.

13. Mulder RL, Knijnenburg SL, Geskus RB, et al. Glomerular function time trends in long-term survivors of childhood cancer: a longitudinal study. *Cancer Epidemiol Biomarkers Prev.* 2013;22:1736-1746.

14. Dekkers IA, Blijdorp K, Cransberg K, et al. Long-term nephrotoxicity in adult survivors of childhood cancer. *Clin J Am Soc Nephrol.* 2013;8:922-929.

16. Skinner R, Parry A, Price L, Cole M, Craft AW, Pearson AD. Glomerular toxicity persists 10 years after ifosfamide treatment in childhood and is not predictable by age or dose. *Pediatr Blood Cancer.* 2010;54:983-989.

23. Janus N, Thariat J, Boulanger H, Deray G, Launay-Vacher V. Proposal for dosage adjustment and timing of chemotherapy in hemodialyzed patients. *Ann Oncol.* 2010;21:1395-1403.

27. Launay-Vacher V, Chatelut E, Lichtman SM, Wildiers H, Steer C, Aapro M. Renal insufficiency in elderly cancer patients: International Society of Geriatric Oncology clinical practice recommendations. *Ann Oncol.* 2007;18:1314-1321.

29. Dooley MJ, Poole SG, Rischin D. Dosing of cytotoxic chemotherapy: impact of renal function estimates on dose. *Ann Oncol.* 2013;24:2746-2752.

30. Rhee J, Kwon JM, Han SH, et al. Cockcroft-Gault, Modification of Diet in Renal Disease, and Chronic Kidney Disease Epidemiology Collaboration equations for estimating glomerular filtration rates in cancer patients receiving cisplatin-based chemotherapy. *Kidney Res Clin Pract.* 2017;36:342-348.

31. Janowitz T, Williams EH, Marshall A, et al. New model for estimating glomerular filtration rate in patients with cancer. *J Clin Oncol.* 2017;35:2798-2805.

42. Guddati AK, Joy PS, Marak CP. Dose adjustment of carboplatin in patients on hemodialysis. *Med Oncol.* 2014;31:848.

54. Hall AM, Bass P, Unwin RJ. Drug-induced renal Fanconi syndrome. *QJM.* 2014;107:261-269.

69. Hotta K, Matsuo K, Ueoka H, Kiura K, Tabata M, Tanimoto M. Meta-analysis of randomized clinical trials comparing cisplatin to carboplatin in patients with advanced non-small-cell lung cancer. *J Clin Oncol.* 2004;22:3852-3859.

75. Schilsky RL, Anderson T. Hypomagnesemia and renal magnesium wasting in patients receiving cisplatin. *Ann Intern Med.* 1979;90:929-931.

78. Manohar S, Leung N. Cisplatin nephrotoxicity: a review of the literature. *J Nephrol.* 2018;31:15-25.

89. Prasaja Y, Sutandyo N, Andrajati R. Incidence of cisplatin-induced nephrotoxicity and associated factors among cancer patients in Indonesia. *Asian Pac J Cancer Prev.* 2015;16:1117-1122.

90. D'Addario G, Pintilie M, Leighl NB, Feld R, Cerny T, Shepherd FA. Platinum-based versus non-platinum-based chemotherapy in advanced non-small-cell lung cancer: a meta-analysis of the published literature. *J Clin Oncol.* 2005;23:2926-2936.

91. Latcha S, Jaimes EA, Patil S, Glezerman IG, Mehta S, Flombaum CD. Long-term renal outcomes after cisplatin treatment. *Clin J Am Soc Nephrol.* 2016;11:1173-1179.

111. Ikemura K, Oshima K, Enokiya T, et al. Co-administration of proton pump inhibitors ameliorates nephrotoxicity in patients receiving chemotherapy with cisplatin and fluorouracil: a retrospective cohort study. *Cancer Chemother Pharmacol.* 2017;79:943-949.

131. Reese JA, Bougie DW, Curtis BR, et al. Drug-induced thrombotic microangiopathy: experience of the Oklahoma Registry and the BloodCenter of Wisconsin. *Am J Hematol.* 2015;90:406-410.

150. Bryant BM, Jarman M, Ford HT, Smith IE. Prevention of isophosphamide-induced urothelial toxicity with 2-mercaptoethane sulphonate sodium (mesnum) in patients with advanced carcinoma. *Lancet.* 1980;2:657-659.

159. Farry JK, Flombaum CD, Latcha S. Long term renal toxicity of ifosfamide in adult patients–5 year data. *Eur J Cancer.* 2012;48:1326-1331.

160. Akilesh S, Juaire N, Duffield JS, Smith KD. Chronic ifosfamide toxicity: kidney pathology and pathophysiology. *Am J Kidney Dis.* 2014;63:843-850.

171. Sørensen JB, Andersen MK, Hansen HH. Syndrome of inappropriate secretion of antidiuretic hormone (SIADH) in malignant disease. *J Intern Med.* 1995;238:97-110.

213. Meulendijks D, van Hasselt JGC, Huitema ADR, et al. Renal function, body surface area, and age are associated with risk of early-onset fluoropyrimidine-associated toxicity in patients treated with capecitabine-based anticancer regimens in daily clinical care. *Eur J Cancer.* 2016;54:120-130.

214. Lichtman SM, Cirrincione CT, Hurria A, et al. Effect of pretreatment renal function on treatment and clinical outcomes in the adjuvant treatment of older women with breast cancer: Alliance A171201, an ancillary study of CALGB/CTSU 49907. *J Clin Oncol.* 2016;34:699-705.

256. Ajani JA, Rodriguez W, Bodoky G, et al. Multicenter phase III comparison of cisplatin/S-1 with cisplatin/infusional fluorouracil in advanced gastric or gastroesophageal adenocarcinoma study: the FLAGS trial. *J Clin Oncol.* 2010;28:1547-1553.

267. Izzedine H, Isnard-Bagnis C, Launay-Vacher V, et al. Gemcitabine-induced thrombotic microangiopathy: a systematic review. *Nephrol Dial Transplant.* 2006;21:3038-3045.

293. Garneau AP, Riopel J, Isenring P. Acute methotrexate-induced crystal nephropathy. *N Engl J Med.* 2015;373:2691-2693.

294. Von Hoff DD, Penta JS, Helman LJ, Slavik M. Incidence of drug-related deaths secondary to high-dose methotrexate and citrovorum factor administration. *Cancer Treat Rep.* 1977;61:745-748.

295. Abelson HT, Fosburg MT, Beardsley GP, et al. Methotrexate-induced renal impairment: clinical studies and rescue from systemic toxicity with high-dose leucovorin and thymidine. *J Clin Oncol.* 1983;1:208-216.

305. Seideman P, Müller-Suur R, Ekman E. Renal effects of low dose methotrexate in rheumatoid arthritis. *J Rheumatol.* 1993;20:1126-1128.

317. Widemann BC, Balis FM, Kim A, et al. Glucarpidase, leucovorin, and thymidine for high-dose methotrexate-induced renal dysfunction: clinical and pharmacologic factors affecting outcome. *J Clin Oncol.* 2010;28:3979-3986.

320. Mita AC, Sweeney CJ, Baker SD, et al. Phase I and pharmacokinetic study of pemetrexed administered every 3 weeks to advanced cancer patients with normal and impaired renal function. *J Clin Oncol.* 2006;24:552-562.

325. Chauvet S, Courbebaisse M, Ronco P, Plaisier E. Pemetrexed-induced acute kidney injury leading to chronic kidney disease. *Clin Nephrol.* 2014;82:402-406.

343. Guo J, Ananthakrishnan R, Qu W, et al. RAGE mediates podocyte injury in adriamycin-induced glomerulosclerosis. *J Am Soc Nephrol.* 2008;19:961-972.

346. Mohamed N, Goldstein J, Schiff J, John R. Collapsing glomerulopathy following anthracycline therapy. *Am J Kidney Dis*. 2013;61:778-781.

374. Verwey J, de Vries J, Pinedo HM. Mitomycin C-induced renal toxicity, a dose-dependent side effect? *Eur J Cancer Clin Oncol*. 1987;23:195-199.

383. Faguer S, Huart A, Frémeaux-Bacchi V, Ribes D, Chauveau D. Eculizumab and drug-induced haemolytic-uraemic syndrome. *Clin Kidney J*. 2013;6:484-485.

390. Sadoff L. Nephrotoxicity of streptozotocin (NSC-85998). *Cancer Chemother Rep*. 1970;54:457-459.

438. Devriese LA, Witteveen PE, Mergui-Roelvink M, et al. Pharmacodynamics and pharmacokinetics of oral topotecan in patients with advanced solid tumours and impaired renal function. *Br J Clin Pharmacol*. 2015;80:253-266.

A full list of references is available at Expertconsult.com

17 Targeted Cancer Therapies (Biologics)

VIDHI DESAI, JYOTSANA THAKKAR, RIMDA WANCHOO, AND KENAR D. JHAVERI

Introduction

In the past decade, advances in cell biology have led to the development of anticancer agents that target specific molecular pathways. The National Cancer Institute (NCI) defines targeted therapies as "drugs or substances that block the growth and spread of cancer by interfering with specific molecules involved in tumor growth and progression." Targeted therapies are now commonly used in cancer treatment and it is vital that their kidney toxicities be recognized and investigated. Early reports suggest that targeted therapies are associated with a range of toxicities from hypertension (HTN) to acute kidney injury (AKI). Table 17.1 and Fig. 17.1 summarize the renal effects of targeted therapies. Many of these drugs, however, have been associated with significant kidney complications, ranging from electrolyte disorders to AKI requiring dialysis.[1-3] This chapter will cover renal toxicities seen with several classes of molecularly targeted and biologic agents, including preventive strategies. Immune-mediated renal toxicity associated with checkpoint inhibitor immunotherapy (ipilimumab, pembrolizumab, nivolumab, duravalumab, atezolizumab) is discussed in Chapter 18.

VASCULAR ENDOTHELIAL GROWTH FACTOR INHIBITORS

Angiogenesis, the process by which new blood vessels form, plays an integral role in tumorigenesis and is mediated by vascular endothelial growth factors (VEGF).[4] Accordingly, drugs that inhibit this pathway have emerged as an effective anticancer therapy in various malignancies, such as lung, breast, colon, renal cell carcinoma, and ovarian cancer. VEGF inhibition works by several proposed mechanisms, including monoclonal antibodies against the VEGF molecule, small molecule tyrosine kinase inhibitors (TKIs) of the VEGF receptors, soluble decoy receptors, and ribozymes that target VEGF messenger ribonucleic acid.[5] Bevacizumab, ramucirumab, and aflibercept (a soluble decoy receptor of VEGF) are monoclonal antibodies that bind to the VEGF molecule, preventing it from binding to the receptor, thus inhibiting endothelial cell proliferation and vessel formation, whereas the small molecule TKIs (sunitinib, sorafenib, pazoponib, axinitib, cabozatinib, lenvatinib, regorafanib, and vendatinib) block the intracellular domain of VEGF.[2,6]

Proteinuria is a class effect of all VEGF inhibitors; however, the exact mechanism is unclear. VEGF plays an important role in the regulation of renal vascular endothelium and maintenance of normal kidney function. VEGF is found on both endothelial cells and podocytes (renal epithelial cells) among other cells, and the interaction between the glomerular endothelial cells and podocytes via the VEGF pathway is necessary to maintain glomerular filtration by preserving the integrity of the glomerular slit diaphragm. It has been theorized that VEGF inhibition can lead to podocyte injury and can therefore lead to proteinuria. Histologic findings in these patients can show renal limited thrombotic microangiopathy (TMA) (Fig. 17.2) and in some cases minimal change disease (MCD) or focal segmental glomerulosclerosis (FSGS)[7] (Fig. 17.3). Preexisting kidney disease and renal cell carcinoma may be predisposing factors. Treatment can be continued in those cases where proteinuria is not in the nephrotic range, and HTN and proteinuria can be aggressively managed with angiotensin-converting enzyme inhibitor (ACEI) or angiotensin receptor blocker (ARB) inhibition.[8] AKI, especially when caused by TMA, is an indication for drug discontinuation.

HTN frequently accompanies proteinuria. Several mechanisms have been proposed in the pathogenesis of HTN, including decreased nitrous oxide and microvasculature rarefaction leading to nitrous oxide dysregulation (Fig. 17.4). The adverse effects of both proteinuria and HTN were initially described with bevacizumab, the first anti-VEGF drug introduced to clinical practice. The HTN appears to be dose dependent, as observed in several studies, with one study reporting the relative risk of HTN of 3.0 in low-dose bevacizumab (3, 5 or 7.5 mg/kg) as compared with high-dose (10 or 15 mg/kg).[9] Another study by Yang et al. demonstrated that the rate of HTN was 3% in the low-dose bevacizumab group (3 mg/kg), compared with 36% in the high-dose cohort (10 mg/kg).[10] Similarly, the HTN reported with small molecule TKIs appears to be dose dependent as well. Interestingly, the development of HTN may portend a better response to therapy, and therefore should encourage physicians to continue treatment while managing the blood pressure.[11-13] The choice of antihypertensive agents should be individualized with ACEIs or ARBs as first-line options and calcium channel blockers as a reasonable second line.[2]

A small number of patients develop more severe kidney disease, manifested by nephrotic range proteinuria and AKI. Unfortunately, few undergo diagnostic kidney biopsy. Review of reported cases highlights that the most common histopathologic lesion, acute TMA, has been reported in patients with advanced cancers treated with bevacizumab and VEGF trap (aflibercept). Other anti-VEGF therapy induced kidney lesions included FSGS, mesangioproliferative

Table 17.1   Renal Side Effects of Selected Targeted Therapies

Name of Agent	Mechanism of Action of the Targeted Therapy	Reported Nephrotoxicities
Bevacizumab	VEGF inhibitor	HTN, proteinuria, nephrotic syndrome, preeclampsia-like syndrome, renal limited TMA
Aflibercept	VEGF inhibitor	HTN, proteinuria
Sunitinib	Multi-kinase TKI	HTN, proteinuria, MCD/FSGS, AIN, chronic interstitial nephritis
Pazopanib	Multi-kinase TKI	HTN, proteinuria
Axitinib	Multi-kinase TKI	HTN, proteinuria
Sorafenib	Multi-kinase TKI	HTN, proteinuria, MCD/FSGS, AIN, chronic interstitial nephritis, hypophosphatemia
Imatinib	Cellular TKI (BCR-ABL)	ATN, HTN, hypocalcemia, hypophosphatemia
Dasatinib	Multi-kinase TKI	Proteinuria
Nilotinib	Multi-kinase TKI	HTN
Ponatinib	Multi-kinase TKI	HTN
Cetuximab	EGFR inhibitor	Hypomagnesaemia, hypokalemia, AKI, hyponatremia, glomerulonephritis
Panitumumab	EGFR inhibitor	Hypomagnesaemia, AKI, hypokalemia
Erlotinib	EGFR inhibitor	AKI, hypomagnesaemia
Afatinib	EGFR inhibitor	AKI, hyponatremia
Gefitinib	EGFR inhibitor	AKI, hypokalemia, fluid retention, minimal change disease, proteinuria
Vemurafenib	B-RAF inhibitor	AIN, ATN, hypophosphatemia, Fanconi syndrome
Dabrafenib	B-RAF Inhibitor	AIN, ATN, hypophosphatemia, nephrotic syndrome (in combination with MEK inhibitor)
Crizotinib	ALK inhibitor	ATN, renal cysts
Ipilimumab	CTLA-4 inhibitor	AIN, MN, MCD, hyponatremia, TMA
Nivolumab	PD-1 Inhibitor	AIN, ATN, podocytopathies
Pembrolizumab	PD-1 Inhibitor	AIN, ATN, podocytopathies
Temsirolimus	mTOR inhibitor	ATN, FSGS
Carfilzomib	Proteasome inhibitor	Prerenal, ATN, TMA
Bortezomib	Proteasome inhibitor	TMA
Lenalidomide	Immunomodulator	Fanconi syndrome, AIN, MCD
Trametinib	MEK inhibitor	AKI, nephrotic syndrome (in combination with BRAF)

AIN, Acute interstitial nephritis; *AKI*, acute kidney injury; *ALK*, anaplastic lymphoma kinase; *ATN*, acute tubular necrosis; *BCR-ABL*, breakpoint cluster region–abelson; *CTLA*, cytotoxic T lymphocyte antigen−4; *EGFR*, epidermal growth factor receptor; *FSGS*, focal segmental glomerulosclerosis; *HTN*, hypertension; *MCD*, minimal change disease; *MEK*, mitogen-activated protein kinase; *MN*, membranous nephropathy; *PD*, programmed cell death; *TKI*, tyrosine kinase inhibitor; *TMA*, thrombotic microangiopathy; *VEGF*, vascular endothelial growth factor.

glomerulonephritis, cryoglobulinemic glomerulonephritis, immune complex glomerulonephritis, glomerular endotheliosis, and acute interstitial nephritis (AIN). All patients developed proteinuria, whereas half developed HTN or AKI. In most of the cases, kidney function normalized or stabilized, proteinuria resolved, and blood pressure control improved after discontinuation of the agent.[14,15] Fig. 17.5 summarizes the VEGF effects on blood pressure and proteinuria.

TYROSINE KINASE INHIBITORS

Protein kinases are important mediators of the signal transduction process and regulate cell proliferation, differentiation, migration, metabolism, and antiapoptotic signaling. The most important protein kinases are the serine/threonine and tyrosine kinases, which are characterized by their ability to catalyze the phosphorylation of serine/threonine or tyrosine residues in proteins, respectively.[16] There are two types of tyrosine kinases: receptor and cellular tyrosine kinases. Receptor tyrosine kinases consist of an extracellular ligand binding domain, a transmembrane domain, and an intracellular catalytic domain. They are activated by ligand binding to the extracellular domain. Cellular tyrosine kinases play a role in the downstream signal transduction pathway, in the cytoplasm or nucleus. Tyrosine kinases are involved in several steps of neoplastic development and progression; the signaling pathways normally prevent unregulated proliferation; however, these pathways are usually genetically altered in cancer cells, thus allowing for constitutive activity of the tyrosine kinases and unregulated cell

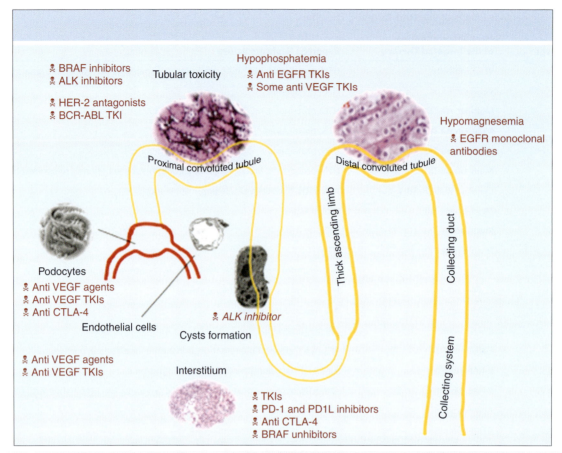

Fig. 17.1 Summary of renal adverse events noted with targeted therapies. *ALK*, Anaplastic lymphoma kinase; *BCR-ABL*, breakpoint cluster region–abelson; *BRAF*, v-RAF murine sarcoma viral oncogene homolog B; *CTLA*, cytotoxic T lymphocyte antigen−4; *EGFR*, epidermal growth factor receptor; *HER-2*, human epidermal growth factor−2; *PD*, programmed cell death; *TKI*, tyrosine kinase inhibitors; *VEGF*, vascular endothelial growth factor. Reproduced with permission from Jhaveri KD, Wanchoo R, Sakhiya V, Ross DW, Fishbane S. Adverse renal effects of novel molecular oncologic targeted therapies: a narrative review. *Kidney Int Rep.* 2016;2(1):108-123.

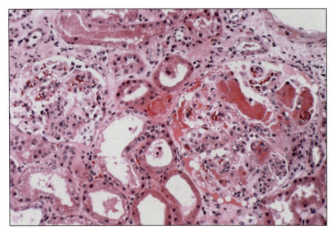

Fig. 17.2 A 56-year-old male with history of renal cell cancer receives bevacizumab presents with acute rise in creatinine, hypertension, and proteinuria. The kidney biopsy depicted shows acute thrombotic microangiopathy (light microscopy view).

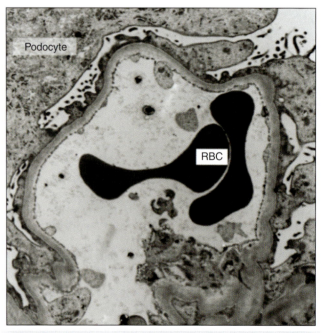

Fig. 17.3 A 78-year-old male with history of renal cell cancer receives sunitinib and presents with sudden onset nephrotic syndrome. The kidney biopsy depicted reveals minimal change nephropathy (electron microscopy view). *RBC*, Red blood cell.

growth and proliferation.[17] Thus TKIs are effective anti-cancer agents, because they interfere with this unregulated process. Receptor TKIs target the epidermal growth factor receptor (EGFR), platelet derived growth factor receptor (PDGFR), and vascular endothelial growth factor

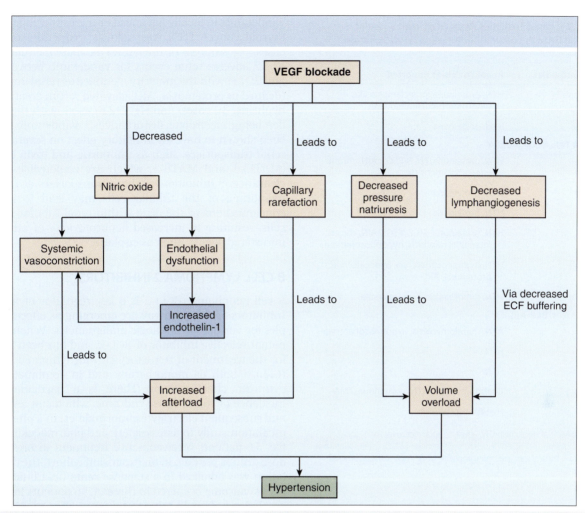

Fig. 17.4 Multiple mechanisms by which vascular endothelial growth factor (VEGF) blockade induces hypertension. VEGF signaling blockade inhibits nitrous oxide (NO) production, enhances endothelin-1 secretion, and causes capillary rarefaction. All of these effects cause increased afterload and consequent increased blood pressure. In addition, VEGF blockade shifts the pressure-natriuresis curve and decreases lymphangiogenesis, and both of these effects contribute to volume overload and hypertension. *ECF*, Extracellular fluid.

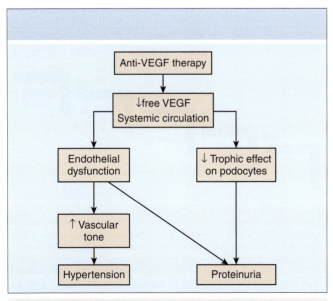

Fig. 17.5 Summary of the antivascular endothelial growth factor (anti-VEGF) therapy on blood pressure and podocytes.

receptor (VEGFR), whereas cellular TKIs can target breakpoint cluster region–abelson (BCR-ABL) (imatinib) and Bruton's kinase (ibrutinib). These agents could target single receptors, such as EGFR (geftinib), or could be multitargeted, such as sunitinib, which targets VEGFR, PDGFR, kit, Flt3, and RET. Some of the renal side effects of common TKIs, such as sunitinib and sorafenib, were discussed earlier with anti-VEGF therapy, as their effects are similar on the kidney.

Like anti-VEGF drugs, the small molecule TKIs of the VEGFR family (sunitinib, sorafenib, pazopanib, axitinib, cabozantinib, lenvatinib, and vandetanib) are also potent inhibitors of angiogenesis, and thus have a similar adverse effect profile. Sunitinib and sorafenib target multiple receptor kinases including VEGFR, PDGFR, c-kit among others. Sunitinib, sorafenib, pazopanib, and axitinib have known effects of HTN, proteinuria, TMA, and chronic and acute interstitial nephritis. Sorafenib is also known to cause hypophosphatemia and hypocalcemia, thought to be related to pancreatic dysfunction from the drug leading to vitamin D malabsorption and secondary hyperparathyroidism.[2] Table 17.2 summarizes reported renal toxicities specific to VEGF inhibitors.

Table 17.2 Renal Toxicities Associated With Vascular Endothelial Growth Factor Inhibitors and Tyrosine Kinase Inhibitors

VEGF/R Antibodies	Renal Toxicities Reported
Bevacizumab	HTN, proteinuria, preeclampsia-like syndrome, renal limited TMA
Aflibercept	HTN, proteinuria
RECEPTOR TKIs, VEGF FAMILY	
Sunitinib	HTN, proteinuria, MCD/FSGS, AIN, chronic interstitial nephritis
Pazopanib	HTN, proteinuria
Axitinib	HTN, proteinuria
Sorafenib	HTN, proteinuria, MCD/FSGS, AIN, chronic interstitial nephritis, hypophosphatemia
Regorafenib	HTN, hypophosphatemia, hypocalcemia, proteinuria, AKI
Vandetanib	HTN, hypokalemia, hypocalcemia
CELLULAR TKIs, BCR-ABL	
Imatinib	ATN, rhabdomyolysis, hypophosphatemia
Nilotinib	HTN
Ponatinib	HTN
Dasatinib	Rhabdomyolysis, ATN, proteinuria, TMA
Bosutinib	Hypophosphatemia

AIN, Acute interstitial nephritis; *ATN*, acute tubular necrosis; *FSGS*, focal segmental glomerular sclerosis; *HTN*, hypertension; *MCD*, minimal change disease; *TMA*, thrombotic microangiopathy; *VEGF*, vascular endothelial growth factor.

Lenvatinib also targets several tyrosine kinases including RET, KIT, VEGFR, and PDGFRA. No significant renal toxicities have been reported with this drug.[3] Regorafenib is associated with several electrolyte abnormalities, including hypophosphatemia, hypocalcemia, hyponatremia, and hypokalemia. However, these abnormalities are usually mild to moderate and do not require dose adjustments or interruptions in treatment. As with other VEGF inhibitors, there is a significant incidence of HTN. In the initial trial evaluating regorafenib as monotherapy for previously untreated metastatic colorectal cancer, the incidence of HTN was 28%, with 7% reported as grade 3. The incidence of proteinuria was lower at 7%, with 1% reported as grade 3.[18] Unlike bevacizumab, the HTN associated with regorafenib does not appear to be dose dependent. A systematic review by Wang et al. evaluated 1069 patients from five clinical trials. The incidence of all grade and high-grade HTN were 44.4% and 12.5%, respectively.[19] An analysis of the U.S. Food and Drug Administration (FDA) Adverse Event Reporting System (FAERS) database confirmed HTN as the most common adverse event (57 cases of 125 total cases of regorafenib-related toxicity), followed by AKI (40 cases) and hypophosphatemia (8 cases).[3]

Vandetanib targets VEGFR2, EGFR, and RET. This agent has also been associated with several electrolyte disturbances, such as hypocalcemia, hypokalemia, hyponatremia, and hypercalcemia. Similar to other VEGF inhibitors, there is also a significant incidence of HTN. In a phase 2 trial of vandetanib, in locally advanced or metastatic differentiated thyroid cancer, HTN was seen as frequently as 34% of cases.[20,21] Analysis of the FAERS database identified a total of 57 adverse renal events for vandetanib between 2011 and 2015, with the majority identified as renal impairment (defined as proteinuria, AKI, elevated serum creatinine +/- nephritis, 30 cases) and HTN (21 cases), with the remainder being electrolyte disturbances.[3] Vandetanib has also been shown to have an inhibitory effect on several human renal transporters, such as multidrug and toxin exclusion (MATE)-1 and MATE-2, which are responsible for drug clearance.[20] Inhibition of these transporters at the apical membrane of the tubular cells may lead to increased concentrations of the drug within renal tubular epithelial cells, resulting in increased nephrotoxicity of other coadministered agents, such as cisplatin.[20,21]

B CELL LYMPHOMA 2 INHIBITORS

B cell lymphoma (BCL)-2 is a key regulator of apoptosis. Inhibitors of this pathway are emerging as effective therapies for various hematologic malignancies. Venetoclax is a potent selective inhibitor of BCL-2, and has been approved for the treatment of refractory chronic lymphoid leukemia (CLL),[22] both as monotherapy and in combination with cytotoxic chemotherapy. There is a particularly high incidence of tumor lysis syndrome, which can lead to AKI and subsequent electrolyte abnormalities. In a phase 1 dose escalation study to assess safety and pharmacokinetic profile, 56 patients received active treatment in one of eight dose groups per day; in an expansion cohort, the dose escalation was adjusted to a stepwise ramp up. Clinical tumor lysis syndrome occurred in three of 56 patients in the dose escalation cohort but was not present after adjustments to the dose escalation schedule were made in the expansion cohort.[23] Thus a stepwise dose escalation strategy (Fig. 17.6), with close monitoring of renal function and electrolytes, is advised to reduce the risk of tumor lysis syndrome.[23]

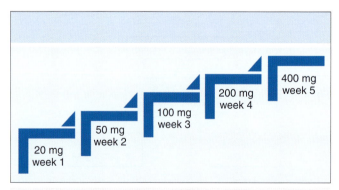

Fig. 17.6 Recommended once daily dosing schedule for venetoclax 5-week dose ramp up used in clinical trials for patients with chronic lymphocytic leukemia. There is high risk for tumor lysis syndrome with this agent, with any measurable lymph nodes with largest diameter greater than 10 cm OR absolute lymphocyte count greater than 25 × 10⁹/L AND any measurable lymph node with largest diameter greater than 5 cm, then the first doses of 20 mg and 50 mg should be inpatient dosing and laboratory monitoring done at 0, 4, 8, 12, and 24 hours. Hydration with 1 to 2 L/day of fluids with rasburicase recommended. Early nephrology consultation in certain very high-risk situations.

BCR-ABL AND KIT INHIBITORS

The *bcr-abl* oncogene, present in 95% of patients with chronic myelogenous leukemia (CML), codes for the constitutively activated tyrosine kinase that is implicated in the pathogenesis of this disease.[24] The introduction of BCR-ABL inhibitors have changed the landscape of CML, improving overall survival and inducing higher rates of complete cytogenetic response and major molecular response.[24] Several small molecule inhibitors of BCR-ABL exist, including imatinib, dasatinib, nilotinib, bosutinib, and ponatinib.

Imatinib is a first generation TKI that targets BCR-ABL, KIT, and PDGFR. Both AKI and chronic kidney injury have been reported in patients treated with imatinib. In one study of 105 CML patients, 7% of patients developed AKI and 12% patients developed chronic kidney disease (CKD). The mean decrease in estimated glomerular filtration rate (GFR) was 2.77 mL/min/1.73 m^2 per year.[25] Potential mechanisms of renal injury include tumor lysis syndrome and acute tubular injury; sometimes an isolated Fanconi syndrome develops.[26–29] Rhabdomyolysis has also been reported. The kidney injury does appear to be dose dependent, as seen with renal cell cancer treatment, with higher doses associated with a higher incidence of renal tubular damage.[30] Two common electrolyte abnormalities reported are hypocalcemia and hypophosphatemia. In one case series, the incidence of hypophosphatemia was close to 10% and associated with low calcium and 25-OH vitamin D levels. The underlying mechanism for hypophosphatemia is unclear, but may be related to the inhibition of tubular reabsorption of phosphorus.[31]

Dasatinib is a second generation TKI used in imatinib-resistant CML. It also has effects on PDGFR and KIT. There have been several cases of AKI reported with the use of this drug, including one patient who developed rhabomyolysis,[32] and another patient who developed thrombotic thrombocytopenic purpura.[33] In addition, there is a 5% incidence of proteinuria with this agent. Nephrotic syndrome has also been described.[34,35] Of the BCR-ABL TKIs, dasatinib is the only one associated with proteinuria. In all cases the proteinuria resolved upon discontinuation of the drug or switching to imatinib.

Nilotinib is also an inhibitor of BCR-ABL, c-KIT, and PDGFR. It has been associated with HTN. The effect of nilotinib on CKD was evaluated in animal models, where it has been shown to be nephroprotective. Interestingly, treatment with nilotinib significantly decreased renal cortical expression of profibrogenic genes (such as *IL-1B* and *monocyte chemotactic protein-1*), which correlated with tubulointerstitial damage; in addition, nilotinib significantly prolonged survival. These results suggest that nilotinib may limit the progression of CKD.[36]

Bosutinib is a dual TKI that targets the ABL and SRC pathways that is approved for the treatment of refractory CML. The only renal toxicities reported with this agent are hypophosphatemia and an apparently reversible decline in GFR.[37] Ponatinib is a multitargeted TKI, with VEGF being one of the molecular targets. As such, the renal toxicities that are a class effect of VEGF can be seen with this agent.

V-RAF MURINE SARCOMA VIRAL ONCOGENE HOMOLOG B INHIBITORS

Mutations that drive signaling pathways critical to tumor growth are attractive molecular targets for cancer therapy. The mitogen-activating protein kinase (MAPK) pathway is one such pathway, estimated to be dysregulated in about 50% of malignancies. RAF is a kinase along this pathway that, once activated, phosphorylates mitogen-activated protein kinases (MEK) and activates MAPK, which in turn stimulates cell growth.[38] Mutations in v-RAF murine sarcoma viral oncogene homolog B (BRAF), most commonly a valine-to-glutamic acid substitution at codon 600 (V600E), have been demonstrated in approximately 50% of patients with melanoma. Vemurafenib, an inhibitor of mutated BRAF, has shown significant improvements in survival when compared with standard therapy. The initial phase III study did not report significant renal toxicity. In 2016 Wanchoo et al.[39] did a comprehensive review of AKI with BRAF inhibitors; the most common findings were acute tubulointerstitial damage and decreased GFR in 1 month and some nonnephrotic range proteinuria. The mechanism of AKI is not clear; however, kidney biopsies, when done, showed acute tubulointerstitial damage and interstitial fibrosis (Fig. 17.7).[40] Multiple other publications have reported various renal toxicities. One series of eight cases from France demonstrated decrease in GFR,[41] whereas another case reported Fanconi syndrome with severe hypokalemia, which improved after interruption of therapy.[42] Another study showed that vemurafenib induces a dual mechanism of increase in plasma creatinine with both an inhibition of creatinine tubular secretion and slight impairment in kidney function. However, this adverse effect is mostly reversible when vemurafenib is discontinued and should not dissuade physicians from continuing treatment if effective.[43] Finally, an analysis of the FAERS database reported 132 cases of AKI, more commonly identified in older men. There were 13 reported cases of AKI with dabrafenib in the same review period. Eight cases of electrolyte disorders were reported (hypokalemia and hyponatremia); however, no cases of hypophosphatemia were found, contrary to prior reports.[44]

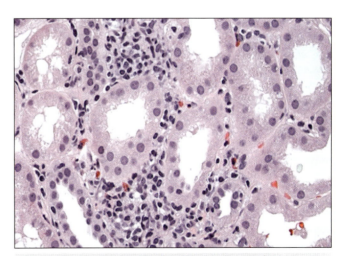

Fig. 17.7 A 78-year-old male with melanoma on vemurafenib presents with acute rise in serum creatinine, and the kidney biopsy depicted shows acute interstitial nephritis (light microscopy view).

MITOGEN-ACTIVATED PROTEIN KINASES INHIBITORS

MEK inhibitors have clinical activity in melanoma patients who harbor that V600 mutation and are mostly used in combination with BRAF inhibitors. Trametinib and cobimetinib are potent, highly specific inhibitors of MEK1/ MEK2. There have been no published cases of nephrotoxicity with trametinib. Monotherapy with this agent can lead to HTN.[45] Renal insufficiency, hyponatremia, and rare cases of glomerulonephritis have been described in patients treated with the combination of a BRAF and MEK inhibitor; however, this may reflect the additive effect of the BRAF inhibitor rather than a sole effect of the MEK inhibitor.[46] In the unique case of glomerulonephritis and granulomatous vasculitis of the kidney, kidney function recovered completely after withdrawal of the therapy.[47]

ANAPLASTIC LYMPHOMA KINASE TARGET INHIBITORS

Anaplastic lymphoma kinase (ALK) is a member of the insulin receptor tyrosine kinase family. *ALK* gene mutations are linked with many cancers, including non-small cell lung cancer (NSCLC), anaplastic large cell lymphoma, Hodgkin lymphoma, rhabdomyosarcoma, and neuroblastoma.[48-50]

Among the patients with NSCLC (most common lung cancer type), a small subgroup with mutation of echinoderm microtubule-associated protein-like 4 (EML4)-ALK are highly sensitive to ALK TKIs.[51] Crizotinib is the first FDA-approved ALK target inhibitor medication. It has been associated with several adverse renal effects. In a retrospective review done by Brosnan et al. at the University of Colorado, crizotinib therapy was associated with a mean reduction in GFR by 23.9% within first 12 weeks.[52] However, the mechanism for decline in GFR was unclear. Most patients recovered their estimated GFR (eGFR) after cessation of crizotinib therapy. Hence the authors hypothesized that the drop in GFR could be attributable to interference of tubular secretion of creatinine by crizotinib, given that it occurred rapidly and was largely reversible on stopping the drug. As a result, they postulate that crizotinib is not directly nephrotoxic. However, there has been a single case report of biopsy proven acute tubular necrosis (ATN) after crizotinib use by Gastaud et al.[53] There is an increased risk of new renal cysts (primarily complex cysts) formation and progression of preexisting cysts associated with the use of crizotinib.[54-56] Renal cyst changes were observed in 22% of patients in Taiwan, after crizotinib treatment, and spontaneously regressed after stopping the drug.[54] A single case of spontaneous regression of crizotinib associated complex renal cysts despite continuous crizotinib therapy has been reported.[54,55] Electrolyte disorders, such as hypokalemia and hyponatremia, have also been observed with crizotinib use in FDA Adverse Event Reporting System (FAERS) analysis.[3] A recent review on adverse renal effects of crizotinib have reported additional adverse effects, including peripheral edema.[57]

EPIDERMAL GROWTH FACTOR RECEPTOR 1 TARGET INHIBITORS

EGFR inhibitors are divided into two major classes. The first class includes monoclonal antibodies, namely cetuximab and panitumumab. The second class comprises three small molecule TKIs: erlotinib, geftinib, and afatinib. Major adverse renal effects of EGFR target inhibitors are electrolyte abnormalities.[58]

Cetuximab is used in the treatment of metastatic colorectal cancer and was approved by the FDA in February 2004.[59,60] Shortly after its approval for colorectal cancer, Schrang et al., at Memorial Sloan-Kettering Cancer Center, observed profound hypomagnesemia in a patient with metastatic colon cancer treated with cetuximab.[61] This prompted the investigators to review the laboratory profiles for 154 colorectal cancer patients treated with cetuximab over the first 6 months of its commercial availability at the institution. However, only 22% of patients had magnesium level checked as none of the practice guidelines required serum magnesium surveillance after its approval. Among these patients, 24% had severe hypomagnesemia.[61] Subsequently, several studies reported hypomagnesemia associated with cetuximab use. In 2006, Fakih et al. observed an incidence of grade 3 ($< 0.9–0.7$ mg/dL) and grade 4 (< 0.7 mg/dL) hypomagnesemia as 27%.[62] Although these earlier studies reported a high incidence of grade 3 to 4 hypomagnesemia, recent studies have reported an incidence of grade 3 to 4 hypomagnesemia as 5.6%, 2.9%, and 3.7% of patients, respectively.[63-65] Similarly, discrepancies are also seen in the incidence of overall hypomagnesemia, with two largest metaanalyses reporting between 25.8% to 36.7%.[63,64] Risk factors for development of hypomagnesemia are duration of treatment, age, and baseline magnesium level.[63] The mechanism of action for hypomagnesemia, is a reduction of transport of transient receptor potential melastatin (TRPM) 6/7 ion channels. Both EGFR and TRMP 6 are expressed in the distal convoluted tubule, which is the main active site of renal magnesium handling. EGFR activation is required for activity and movement of TRPM 6 ion channels into the apical membrane. Therefore blockage of EGFR by cetuximab impairs TRPM 6 ion channels activity, causing magnesium wasting in the distal convoluted tubule[58] (Fig. 17.8).

A review by Faikh et al. provides a detailed description about management of hypomagnesemia.[66] No magnesium replacement is necessary for grade 1 hypomagnesemia, because these patients are typically asymptomatic. Oral magnesium supplementation can be given for grade 2 (0.9–1 mg/dL) hypomagnesemia. An alternative therapy is weekly intravenous replacement of magnesium sulfate (4 g) in patients who are unable to tolerate oral magnesium. Patients with severe grade 3 and 4 hypomagnesemia are at increased risk of developing cardiac arrhythmias and require much higher doses of intravenous magnesium sulfate, ranging from 6 to 10 g daily. Hypokalemia and hypocalcemia may also develop from hypomagnesemia. Potassium wasting by the kidney occurs from loss of magnesium inhibitory effect on renal outer medullary potassium channels, whereas release and effect of parathyroid hormone is impaired with hypomagnesemia, promoting hypocalcemia. Monitoring of serum magnesium levels every other day is helpful to guide the frequency of replacement in these patients. An alternative approach for these patients is to stop cetuximab for 2 months and then restart. In addition, medications associated with development of hypomagnesemia, such as thiazide diuretics and proton

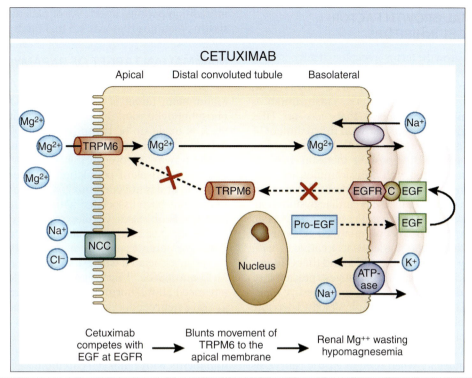

Fig. 17.8 Cetuximab (C) is an epidermal growth factor receptor (EGFR) antibody that causes kidney magnesium wasting by competing with EGF for its receptor. Normally, EGF binds its receptor (EGFR) and stimulates magnesium reabsorption in the distal convoluted cell. EGFR activation is associated with magnesium absorption through transient receptor potential M6 (TRPM6) in the apical membrane. *ATPase*, adenosine triphosphatase; *NCC*, sodium chloride cotransporter. Reproduced from Perazella MA. Onconephrology: renal toxicities of chemotherapeutic agents. *Clin J Am Soc Nephrol.* 2012;7:1713-1721.

pump inhibitors, should be stopped. As per FAERS review, cetuximab has the second highest number of events for any of the targeted therapies.[3] About 467 individuals had adverse renal events. Interestingly, out of these, 172 had AKI, although the most commonly reported side effect is hypomagnesemia on literature search.[61–69]

So far, only one clinical trial has reported kidney failure in about 2% of the patients.[67] Two cases of glomerular diseases have also been described with cetuximab use.[68,69] Given the very high number of cases associated with AKI in FAERS data, it certainly needs to be studied in the future. Other electrolyte abnormalities associated with its usage are hyponatremia and hypokalemia.[70,71]

Panitumumab is another monoclonal antibody EGF target inhibitor. The most commonly reported adverse renal effect with panitumumab therapy is hypomagnesemia. The incidence of hypomagnesemia was about 36% in a clinical trial where panitumumab was used for colorectal cancer.[72] In a recent randomized trial on patients with head and neck cancer performed in 26 countries, panitumumab therapy caused hypomagnesemia in approximately 12% and hypokalemia in 10% of the study population.[73] Therefore frequent monitoring and repletion of magnesium levels should be done for patients on monoclonal antibody EGFR target inhibitor chemotherapy.

Erlotinib, gefitinib, and afatinib are TKIs that act on EGFR. A phase I trial including sorafenib and erlotinib combination in patients with advanced solid tumors reported hypophosphatemia in about 76% of the patients.[74]

In this trial, it is unclear how much sorafenib contributed to hypophosphatemia, which is a known complication of this drug.[74–76] Broniscer et al. conducted a trial in which erlotinib was administered concurrently with radiotherapy, and noted a 30% incidence of hypophosphatemia.[77] A phase II trial with erlotinib for advanced NSCLC reported hypokalemia, elevation in serum creatinine, and hypomagnesemia in 5%, 4%, and 1% of the patients, respectively.[78] In 2009, a single case of crescentic glomerulonephritis with erlotinib use was described by Kurita et al.[79] In FAERS analysis, 63 cases of AKI and eight cases of hypomagnesemia have been reported.[3]

Gefitinib is used in the treatment of NSCLC. Its use has been associated with the development of nephrotic syndrome. Kidney biopsy in a patient from Japan who developed nephrotic syndrome with gefitinib therapy demonstrated MCD.[80] A recent case of MCD had remission of proteinuria after discontinuation of gefitinib therapy.[81] In addition to MCD, immunoglobulin A nephropathy, tubulointerstitial nephritis, and AKI have also been reported with gefitinib therapy.[82,83] On review of the FAERS database, 15 cases of adverse renal effects were seen and about a half of them were AKI.[3]

In a randomized control trial, afatinib therapy was associated with hypokalemia in approximately 34% of patients.[84] No other published data on nephrotoxicity with this agent are available. Twenty-six cases of AKI, six cases of hypokalemia, and five cases of hyponatremia were noted in FAERS review.[3]

HUMAN EPIDERMAL GROWTH FACTOR RECEPTOR 2 TARGET INHIBITORS

Human epidermal growth factor receptor (HER) 2 is a member of transmembrane EGFR with tyrosine kinase activity. Overexpression of this receptor is observed in approximately 20% of breast cancers. Trastuzumab is a humanized monoclonal antibody that acts on HER 2 receptor. Trastuzumab has a major role in the treatment of HER 2-positive metastatic breast cancer.[85] It is also used as an adjuvant therapy in HER 2-positive metastatic gastric cancer. It has been associated with anhydramnios and fetal nephrotoxicity in three separate case reports.[86–88] One of the major complications seen after its use is cardiac dysfunction, which requires regular cardiac screening with MUGA scan or echocardiography.[89,90] Russo et al. analyzed echocardiograms of 499 patients who underwent treatment with trastuzumab therapy for 12 months and found that GFR less than 78 mL/min/1.73 m^2 was the strongest predictor of cardiotoxicity.[91] Cardiac toxicity leading to congestive heart failure can cause AKI from cardiorenal physiology. Therefore routine monitoring of renal function should be considered in patients receiving this medication. In a randomized control trial, trastuzumab in combination with other chemotherapy caused more nephrotoxicity when used in gastric cancer, as compared with standard chemotherapy.[92] Approximately 124 cases of AKI associated with trastuzumab have been reported in the FAERS database.[3] Electrolyte disorders, such as hypokalemia, hyponatremia, and hypomagnesemia have also been reported. Tumor lysis syndrome from trastuzumab use was recently described.[93] Ado-trastuzumab emtansine is a conjugate of trastuzumab linked to cytotoxic agent emtansine (DM1). Hypokalemia is observed in about 10% of patients treated with this agent.[94,95]

Pertuzumab binds to the extracellular dimerization domain of HER 2 and is used primarily in combination with trastuzumab for treatment of HER 2-positive breast cancer. Analysis of FAERS data revealed approximately 100 cases of nephrotoxicity. Out of these, 46 cases had AKI.[3] However, there are no published data on nephrotoxicity with this agent in clinical trials or case reports.

Lapatinib is a dual TKI and blocks both EGFR (erbB1) and HER 2 (erbB2) pathways. The only published data available on adverse renal effects with this agent is hyponatremia.[96] There are 171 cases documented in the FAERS database. Most cases had hypokalemia and AKI, whereas a small number had HTN, hypomagnesemia, and hyponatremia.[3]

BURTON KINASE INHIBITOR

Ibrutinib is a burton kinase inhibitor used for treatment of CLL and mantle cell lymphoma. It is largely excreted in the feces (90%) and less than 10% is excreted in urine. As a result, there is no dose adjustment recommendation for patients with CKD. A multicenter study undertaken in patients with relapsed or refractory CLL, treated with ibrutinib, reported a 13% incidence of HTN and 21% incidence of peripheral edema.[97] In another study involving patients with mantle cell lymphoma, serum creatinine elevation was seen in approximately 35% of patients.[98] Out of these, approximately 5% had grade 3 kidney failure; however, preexisting HTN and dehydration were confounding factors in these cases. As per

medication package insert, 9% of patients had an increase in serum creatinine that was 1.5 to 3 times normal.[99]

MAMMALIAN TARGET OF RAPAMYCIN INHIBITORS

Mammalian target of rapamycin (mTOR) is a member of phosphatidylinositol-3-kinase-related kinases (PIKKs) family. It is made up of two protein complexes, mTORC1 and mTORC2, both of which are important in cellular regulation. Sirolimus was approved by the FDA in 1997. It has been used in organ transplant population for prevention of allograft rejection and is not currently used as an anticancer medication. It has been associated with proteinuria and podocytopathies. Four cases of biopsy proven ATN with mTOR inhibitors have been described in the literature.[100] Temsirolimus is a parenterally administered mTOR inhibitor, which has been associated with ATN and podocytopathies, such as MCD and FSGS.[101] Everolimus is used for the treatment of advanced HER2/hormone receptor breast cancer and progressive neuroendocrine tumors of pancreatic, gastrointestinal, and lung origin. It is also used as a second-line agent for renal cell carcinoma. In a retrospective analysis, there was a high incidence of everolimus-associated AKI (16.2%) in patients with renal cell carcinoma.[102] An increased incidence of AKI with decreasing eGFR was also observed with this drug. Recently, a case report of AKI from everolimus use in a breast cancer patient was reported.[103]

PROTEASOME INHIBITORS

The proteasome pathway is important for cell cycle, cell function, and survival, and it plays a crucial role in targeted destruction of cellular proteins, making proteasome inhibition an important target in cancer therapy. Bortezomib, a boronate peptide, is a reversible inhibitor of chymotrypsin-like activity of the 26S proteasome. It is the first-generation proteasome inhibitor approved in 2003 for the treatment of multiple myeloma. There have been five case reports of AKI and TMA associated with the use of bortezomib.[104–108] A possible mechanism for development of TMA includes inhibition of the ubiquitination of inhibitor of κB, thereby preventing nuclear factor κB from entering the nucleus, leading to decreased VEGF production.[109,110] There has also been one reported case of bortezomib associated AIN.[111]

Carfilzomib, a tetra peptide epoxyketone, is an irreversible inhibitor of chymotrypsin-like activity of 20S proteasome. It is approved for the treatment of relapsed or refractory multiple myeloma.[112] AKI was initially reported in 25% of 266 patients in the phase 2 study of this drug.[113] Multiple cases of AKI have been reported with this drug; likely mechanisms include prerenal causes, tumor lysis syndrome, and biopsy-proven TMA.[114–118] There are 12 reported cases of TMA associated with carfilzomib.[119,120] Yui et al. published the largest case series of 11 patients who developed proteasome inhibitor-induced TMA, eight from carfilzomib and three from bortezomib.[121] In the carFilzOmib for advanCed refractory mUltiple myeloma European Study (FOCUS) trial that compared carfilzomib to low-dose steroids in relapsed multiple myeloma, the investigators found that the incidence of grade 3 AKI was 8% in the carfilzomib group compared with 3% in the control group.[122] In this cohort, up to 24% of patients developed adverse renal events.[122]

DRUG DOSING IN CHRONIC KIDNEY DISEASE AND DIALYSIS PATIENTS

Because the majority of the targeted therapies are associated with potential systemic toxicity and nephrotoxicity, accurate dosing in CKD and patients on dialysis is of great importance. As noted in prior chemotherapy trials, most trials excluded patients on dialysis or with severe CKD (GFR < 30 ml/min). This limits our understanding of dosing in CKD and dialysis patients. In Table 17.3, we summarize the existing published literature on dosing of these agents in CKD and dialysis (wherever data are available).

Summary

The use of novel targeted anticancer therapies has led to a significant improvement in survival and overall prognosis with many malignancies. However, there is evolving knowledge on adverse renal events with these agents. Timely recognition of these toxicities can aid in the proper management of cancer patients. In this chapter, we recognized that there are multiple mechanisms by which targeted therapies can have an impact on kidney function. Box 17.1 summarizes the recommended monitoring strategy for patients receiving these agents. In addition, newer targeted agents are entering clinical trials and we must be alert to potential toxicity. However, because it is exceedingly difficult to keep up with all the new drugs and their associated nephrotoxicities, it is important that the medical community advocates for an international database registry for targeted therapies, to facilitate accurate data on the nephrotoxicity of this group of drugs.

Acknowledgements

We thank Dr. Vanesa Bijol, nephropathologist at Northwell Health, for Figs. 17.2, 17.3, and 17.7.

Table 17.3 Approved Hematology and Oncology Indications for Targeted Therapies Along With Dosing in Chronic Kidney Disease and End-Stage Renal Disease

Generic Name of Targeted Therapy (trade name)	Target	Cancer	Renal Excretion	Dose Adjustment for GFR 30–90 mL/min/1.73 m^2	Dialysis Dose Adjustment
Afatineb (Gilotrif)	EGFR TKI	Metastatic NSCLC	< 5%	No	No data
Axitinib (Inlyta)	Multi target TKI	Pancreatic cancer, RCC, CML	< 25%	No	No
Aflibercept (Eylea or Zaltrap)	VEGF	Colorectal cancer	No	No	No
Bevacizumab (Avastin)	VEGF	Colorectal cancer, NSCLC, RCC, breast cancer, epithelial ovarian cancer, GBM	No	No	No
Bosutinib (Bosulif)	BCR-ABL TKI	CML	No	Reduce dose to 300 mg once daily	No data
Cetuximab (Erbitux)	EGFR	Colorectal cancer, head and neck SCC	No	No	No
Crizotinib (Xalkori)	ALK	NSCLC	No	No	No
Dabrafenib (Tafinlar)	BRAF	Melanoma	< 25%	No	No data
Dasatinib (Sprycel)	BCR-ABL TKI	CML	< 5%	No	No data
Erlotinib (Tarceva)	EGFR TKI	NSCLC, pancreatic cancer	< 10%	No	No
Gefitinib (Iressa)	EGFR TKI	NSCLC	< 5%	No	No
Ibrutinib (Imbruvica)	Bruton kinase TKI	CLL, mantle cell lymphoma	No	No data	No data
Imatinib (Gleevec)	BCR-ABL TKI	Gastrointestinal stromal tumors, CML	< 15%	No	No
Ipilimumab (Yervoy)	CTLA4	Melanoma	No	No	No data
Lapatinib (Tykerb)	ERBB2	Breast cancer	< 5%	No	No
Nivolumab (Opdivo)	PD-1	Melanoma, NSCLC, Hodgkin lymphoma, RCC	No	No	No data
Nilotinib (Tasigna)	BCR-ABL TKI	CML	No	No	No data
Panitumumab (Vectibix)	EGFR	Colorectal cancer	No	No	No
Pazopanib (Votrient)	Multitarget TKI	RCC, soft tissue sarcoma	< 4%	No	No
Pembrolizumab (Keytruda)	PD-L1	Melanoma, NSCLC, Hodgkin lymphoma	No data	No	No

Continued

Table 17.3   Approved Hematology and Oncology Indications for Targeted Therapies Along With Dosing in Chronic Kidney Disease and End-Stage Renal Disease—cont'd

Generic Name of Targeted Therapy (trade name)	Target	Cancer	Renal Excretion	Dose Adjustment for GFR 30–90 mL/min/1.73 m²	Dialysis Dose Adjustment
Pertuzumab (Perjeta)	ERBB2	Breast cancer	No	No	No data
Ponatanib (Iclusig)	BCR-ABL TKI	CML, ALL	No	No	No data
Regorafenib (Stivarga)	Multitarget TKI	Colorectal cancer, gastrointestinal stromal tumors	< 20%	No	No
Sorafenib (Nexavar)	Multitarget TKI	RCC, hepatocellular carcinoma, thyroid carcinoma	< 20%	No	No
Sunitinib (Sutent)	Multitarget TKI	RCC, gastrointestinal stromal tumors, pancreatic neuroendocrine tumors	< 20%	No	No
Trametinib (Mekinist)	MEK	Melanoma	< 20%	No	No data
Trastuzumab (Herceptin)	ERBB2	Breast cancer	No	No	No
Vandetanib (Caprelsa)	Multitarget TKI	Medullary thyroid cancer	< 25%	No	No data
Vemurafenib (Zelboraf)	BRAF	Melanoma, thyroid cancer, colorectal cancer	< 5%	No	No data

ALK, Anaplastic lymphoma kinase; *ALL,* acute lymphocytic leukemia; *BCR-ABL,* breakpoint cluster region–abelson; *CLL,* chronic lymphocytic leukemia; *CML,* chronic myelogenous leukemia; *CTLA,* cytotoxic T lymphocyte antigen−4; *EGFR,* epidermal growth factor receptor; *GBM,* glioblastoma multiforme; *MEK,* mitogen-activated protein kinase; *NSCLC,* non-small cell lung cancer; *PD,* programmed cell death; *RCC,* renal cell carcinoma; *SCC,* squamous cell cancer; *TKI,* tyrosine kinase inhibitor; *VEGF,* vascular endothelial growth factor. Information obtained from package inserts of agents, clinical trials, and published case reports. No data available for most agents for dose adjustments for glomerular filtration rate < 30 mL/min/1.73 m² except vandetanib, which requires dose adjustment.

Box 17.1   Recommended Routine Physical Examination, Imaging, and Serum and Urine Monitoring With Various Targeted Therapies

Blood pressure monitoring[a]
Peripheral edema examination[b]
Serum creatinine
Serum electrolytes (K, Na, Cl, Phos)
Serum magnesium[c]
Complete blood count
Urinalysis and urine sediment evaluation
Urinary spot protein/creatinine ratio[a]
LDH[a]
Haptoglobin[a]
CK[d]
Renal sonogram evaluation for cysts[b]

[a]Antivascular endothelial growth factor (VEGF) agents, tyrosine kinase inhibitors
[b]Crizotinib.
[c]Epidermal growth factor (EGFR) inhibitors.
[d]BCR-ABL tyrosine kinase inhibitors.
CK, Creatinine kinase; *LDH,* lactate dehydrogenase.
Most targeted therapies require all the tests listed subsequently, and a few require extra tests that are labeled with the subsequent legend.

Key Points

- Novel targeted anticancer therapies have resulted in improvement in patient survival compared with standard chemotherapy. Renal toxicities of targeted agents are increasingly being recognized.
- The incidence, severity, and pattern of renal toxicities may vary according to the respective target of the drug.

- A number of adverse renal effects occur with several of the currently approved targeted cancer therapies targeting EGFR, HER2, BRAF, MEK, ALK, VEGF/R, and TK signaling.
- Electrolyte disorders, renal impairment, and hypertension are the most commonly reported events.
- The early diagnosis and prompt recognition of these renal adverse events are essential for the general nephrologist taking care of these patients.

References

1. Launay-Vacher V, Aapro M, De Castro G Jr, et al. Renal effects of molecular targeted therapies in oncology: a review by the Cancer and the Kidney International Network (C-KIN). *Ann Oncol.* 2015; 26(8):1677-1684.
2. Jhaveri KD, Wanchoo R, Sakhiya V, Ross DW, Fishbane S. Adverse renal effects of novel molecular oncologic targeted therapies: a narrative review. *Kidney Int Rep.* 2017;2(1):108.
3. Jhaveri KD, Sakhiya V, Wanchoo R, Ross D, Fishbane S. Renal effects of novel anticancer targeted therapies: a review of the Food and Drug Administration Adverse Event Reporting System. *Kidney Int.* 2016; 90(3):706-707.
4. Murukesh N, Dive C, Jayson GC. Biomarkers of angiogenesis and their role in the development of VEGF inhibitors. *Br J Cancer.* 2010;102: 8-18.
6. Merchan JR, Jhaveri KD. Chemotherapy nephrotoxicity and dose modification in patients with renal insufficiency: molecularly targeted agents. In: Savarese D, ed. UpToDate. October 31, 2017. Available at: http://www.uptodate.com/contents/chemotherapy-nephrotoxicity-and-dose-modification-in-patients-with-renal-insufficiency-molecularly-targeted-agents.
8. Hayman SR, Grande JP, Garovic VD. VEGF inhibition, hypertension, and renal toxicity. *Curr Oncol Rep.* 2012;14(4):285-294.
11. Perazella MA. Onco-nephrology: renal toxicities of chemotherapeutic agents. *Clin J Am Soc Nephrol.* 2012;7(10):1713-1721.

12. Yang JC, Haworth L, Sherry RM, et al. A randomized trial of bevacizumab, an anti-vascular endothelial growth factor antibody, for metastatic renal cancer. *N Engl J Med.* 2003;349:427-434.

15. Izzedine H, Rixe O, Billemont B, Baumelou A, Deray G. Angiogenesis inhibitor therapies: focus on kidney toxicity and hypertension. *Am J Kidney Dis.* 2007;50:203-218.

18. Grothey A, Custem EV, Sobrero A, et al. Regorafenib monotherapy for previously treated metastatic colorectal cancer (CORRECT): an international, multicenter, randomized, placebo-controlled, phase 3 trial. *Lancet.* 2013;381(9863):303-312.

19. Wang Z, Xu J, Nie W, Huang G, Tang J, Guan X. Risk of hypertension with regorafenib in cancer patients: a systematic review and meta-analysis. *Eur J Clin Pharmacol.* 2014;70:225-231.

20. Shen H, Yang Z, Zhao W, Zhang Y, Rodrigues AD. Assessment of vandetanib as an inhibitor of various human renal transporters: inhibition of multidrug and toxin extrusion as a possible mechanism leading to decreased cisplatin and creatinine clearance. *Drug Metab Dispos.* 2013;41:2095-2103.

23. Druker BJ, Talpaz M, Resta DJ, et al. Efficacy and safety of a specific inhibitor of the BCR-ABL tyrosine kinase in chronic myeloid leukemia. *N Engl J Med.* 2001;344:1031-1037.

25. Marcolino MS, Boersma E, Clementino NC, et al. Imatinib treatment duration is related to decreased estimated glomerular filtration rate in chronic myeloid leukemia patients. *Ann Oncol.* 2011;22(9):2073-2079.

30. Barta VS, Uppal NN, Pullman JM, et al. Acute tubular injury associated with imatinib (Gleevec): a case report and review of the literature. *J Onco-Nephrol.* 2017;1(1):57-61.

31. Berman E, Nicolaides M, Maki RG, et al. Altered bone and mineral metabolism in patients receiving imatinib mesylate. *N Engl J Med.* 2006;354(19):2006-2013.

35. Hirano T, Hashimoto M, Korogi Y, et al. Dasatinib-induced nephrotic syndrome. *Leuk Lymphoma.* 2016;57(3):726-727.

36. Iyoda M, Shibata T, Hirai Y, Kuno Y, Akizawa T. Nilotinib attenuates renal injury and prolongs survival in chronic kidney disease. *J Am Soc Nephrol.* 2011;22(8):1486-1496.

37. Cortes JE, Gambacorti-Passerini C, et al. Effects of bosutinib treatment on renal function in patients with Philadelphia chromosome-positive leukemias. *Clin Lymphoma Myeloma Leuk.* 2017;17(10):684-695.

39. Wanchoo R, Jhaveri KD, Deray G, Launay-Vacher V. Renal effects of BRAF inhibitors: a systematic review by the Cancer and the Kidney International Network. *Clin Kidney J.* 2016;9(2):245-251.

43. Launay-Vacher V, Zimner-Rapuch S, Poulalhon N, et al. Acute renal failure associated with the new BRAF inhibitor vemurafenib: a case series of 8 patients. *Cancer.* 2014;120:2158-2163.

44. Jhaveri, K, Fishbane S, Fishbane S. Nephrotoxicity of the BRAF inhibitors vemurafenib and dabrafenib. *JAMA Oncol.* 2015;1(8):1133-1134.

45. Abdel-Rahman O, ElHalwani H, Ahmed H. Risk of selected cardiovascular toxicities in patients with cancer treated with MEK inhibitors: a comparative systematic review and meta-analysis. *J Glob Oncol.* 2015;1(2):73-82.

52. Brosnan EM, Weickhardt AJ, Lu X, et al. Drug-induced reduction in estimated glomerular filtration rate in patients with ALK-positive non-small cell lung cancer treated with the ALK inhibitor crizotinib. *Cancer.* 2014;120:664-674.

54. Lin YT, Wang YF, Yang JC, et al. Development of renal cysts after crizotinib treatment in advanced ALK-positive non-small cell lung cancer. *J Thorac Oncol.* 2014;9:1720-1725.

57. Izzedine H, El-fekih RK, Perazella MA. The renal effects of ALK inhibitors. *Invest New Drugs.* 2016;34:643-649.

61. Schrag D, Chung KY, Flombaum CD, Saltz L. Cetuximab therapy and symptomatic hypomagnesemia. *J Natl Cancer Inst.* 2005;97:1221-1224.

63. Cao Y, Liao C, Tan A, Liu L, Gao F. Meta-analysis of incidence and risk of hypomagnesemia with cetuximab for advanced cancer. *Chemotherapy.* 2010;56:459-465.

64. Chen P, Wang L, Li H, Liu B, Zou Z. Incidence and risk of hypomagnesemia in advanced cancer patients treated with cetuximab: a meta-analysis. *Oncol Lett.* 2013;5:1915-1920.

66. Fakih M. Management of anti-EGFR-targeting monoclonal antibody-induced hypomagnesemia. *Oncology (Williston Park).* 2008;22:74-76.

72. Van Cutsem E, Peeters M, Siena S, et al. Open-label phase III trial of panitumumab plus best supportive care compared with best supportive care alone in patients with chemotherapy-refractory metastatic colorectal cancer. *J Clin Oncol.* 2007;25:1658-1664.

73. Vermorken JB, Stohlmacher-Williams J, Davidenko I, et al. Cisplatin and fluorouracil with or without panitumumab in patients with recurrent or metastatic squamous-cell carcinoma of the head and neck (SPECTRUM): an open label phase 3 randomized trial. *Lancet Oncol.* 2013;14:697-710.

74. Duran I, Hotté SJ, Hirte H, et al. Phase I targeted combination trial of sorafenib and erlotinib in patients with advanced solid tumors. *Clin Cancer Res.* 2007;13:4849-4857.

77. Broniscer A, Baker SJ, Stewart CF, et al. Phase I and pharmacokinetic studies of erlotinib administered concurrently with radiotherapy for children, adolescents, and young adults with high-grade glioma. *Clin Cancer Res.* 2009;15:701-707.

78. Jackman DM, Yeap BY, Lindeman NI, et al. Phase II clinical trial of chemotherapy-naive patients > or = 70 years of age treated with erlotinib for advanced non-small-cell lung cancer. *J Clin Oncol.* 2007;25:760-766.

81. Maruyama K, Chinda J, Kuroshima T, et al. Minimal change nephrotic syndrome associated with gefitinib and a successful switch to erlotinib. *Intern Med.* 2015;54:823-826.

84. Miller VA, Hirsh V, Cadranel J, et al. Afatinib versus placebo for patients with advanced, metastatic non-small-cell lung cancer after failure of erlotinib, gefitinib, or both, and one or two lines of chemotherapy (LUX-Lung 1): a phase 2b/3 randomized trial. *Lancet Oncol.* 2012;13:528-538.

88. Gotschalk I, Berg C, Harbeck N, Stressig R, Kozlowski P. Fetal renal insufficiency following trastuzumab treatment for breast cancer in pregnancy: case report and review of the current literature. *Breast Care (Basel).* 2011;6(6):475-478.

91. Russo G, Cioffi G, Di Lenarda A, et al. Role of renal function on the development of cardiotoxicity associated with trastuzumab-based adjuvant chemotherapy for early breast cancer. *Intern Emerg Med.* 2012;7:439-446.

92. Bang YJ, Van Cutsem E, Feyereislova A, et al. Trastuzumab in combination with chemotherapy versus chemotherapy alone for treatment of HER2-positive advanced gastric or gastro-oesophageal junction cancer (ToGA): a phase 3, open-label, randomised controlled trial. *Lancet.* 2010;376:687-697.

97. Byrd JC, Furman RR, Coutre SE, et al. Targeting BTK with ibrutinib in relapsed chronic lymphocytic leukemia. *N Engl J Med.* 2013;369:32-42.

98. Wang ML, Blum KA, Martin P, et al. Long-term follow-up of MCL patients treated with single-agent ibrutinib: updated safety and efficacy results. *Blood.* 2015;126:739-745.

100. Izzedine H, Escudier B, Rouvier P, et al. Acute tubular necrosis associated with mTOR inhibitor therapy: a real entity biopsy-proven. *Ann Oncol.* 2013;24(9):2421-2425.

102. Ha SH, Park JH, Jang HR, et al. Increased risk of everolimus-associated acute kidney injury in cancer patients with impaired kidney function. *BMC Cancer.* 2014;14:906.

104. Mehta N, Saxena A, Niesvizky R. Bortezomib-induced thrombotic thrombocytopaenic purpura. *BMJ Case Rep.* 2012;pii:2012006461.

111. Cheungpasitporn W, Leung N, Rajkumar SV, et al. Bortezomib-induced acute interstitial nephritis. *Nephrol Dial Transplant.* 2015;30:1225-1229.

113. Siegel DS, Martin T, Wang M, et al. A phase 2 study of single-agent carfilzomib (PX-171-003-A1) in patients with relapsed and refractory multiple myeloma. *Blood.* 2012;120:2817-2825.

114. Jhaveri KD, Chidella S, Varghese J, Mailloux L, Devoe C. Carfilzomib-related acute kidney injury. *Clin Adv Hematol Oncol.* 2013;11:604-605.

119. Hobeika L, Self SE, Velez JC. Renal thrombotic microangiopathy and podocytopathy associated with the use of carfilzomib in a patient with multiple myeloma. *BMC Nephrol.* 2014;15:156.

121. Yui JC, Van Keer J, Weiss BM, et al. Proteasome inhibitor associated thrombotic microangiopathy. *Am J Hematol.* 2016;91:E348-E352.

122. Hájek R, Masszi T, Petrucci MT, et al. A randomized phase III study of carfilzomib vs low-dose corticosteroids with optional cyclophosphamide in relapsed and refractory multiple myeloma (FOCUS). *Leukemia.* 2017;31:107-114.

A full list of references is available at Expertconsult.com

18 Adverse Kidney Effects of Immunotherapies

DANIELLE L. SALY AND MARK A. PERAZELLA

Introduction

The scope of oncology has changed greatly over the past decade as therapies for cancer have moved toward creating or intensifying an immune response against it.[1] The ever-growing number of therapies uses a multitude of different mechanisms, including blockade of specific immune checkpoints, manipulation of T-cells, or direct stimulation of the immune system to enhance killing of tumor cells. Many of the newly available cancer immunotherapies leverage knowledge that the anticancer effects of the immune system (recognizing tumor antigen) are typically balanced by checkpoints that guard against autoimmunity (recognizing self-antigen). These immune checkpoints participate in cancer surveillance and tumor eradication, allowing tumor killing; however, different cancers are able to co-opt these checkpoints to evade surveillance and allow unchecked tumor cell proliferation and metastasis. This immune evasion, which is one of the hallmarks of cancer, leaves the immune system unable to mount an effective antitumor response.[2] The modern immunotherapies work to create robust, antitumor responses by manipulation of the immune system through a variety of mechanisms.

Understanding the basics of the immune system's role in cancer cell surveillance is critical to recognizing the utility of various immunotherapies. In general, the acquired immune response involves antigen presentation to naïve T-cells, which leads to their subsequent activation and proliferation. T-cell activation requires three signals, which include the T-cell receptor interacting with antigen-bound major histocompatibility complex (MHC) on an antigen-presenting cell (APC). This interaction initiates a second intracellular signaling cascade that is modulated by a second signal from a costimulatory or coinhibitory molecule on the T-cell surface. Lastly, signals produced by cytokines and other molecules further refine the immune response.[3,4]

Enhancing or suppressing T-cell activation via costimulatory or coinhibitory molecules modifies the effector T-cell response and provides a "checkpoint" for immune regulation. Several different receptors on the T-cell surface participate in this process. The constitutively expressed T-cell membrane receptor, CD28, is stimulated and interacts with the CD80 or CD86 receptor on the APC surface when the T-cell receptor engages with MHC/antigen complex. The costimulatory signal promotes recruitment and activation of phosphatidylinositol-3-kinase, which causes intracellular accumulation of 3-phosphorylated lipids that are able to bind and activate pleckstrin-homology-containing proteins.[5–8] Activation of these intracellular signaling proteins increases cellular metabolism, expression of survival factors, and cell progression through the cell cycle. This T-cell activation cascade can be inhibited at various steps, known as *checkpoints* (Fig. 18.1). Two receptors that play an important role in regulating T-cell activation and continued function via these intracellular signaling pathways are programmed cell death 1 (PD-1) and cytotoxic lymphocyte-associated antigen 4 (CTLA-4).

PD-1 receptor is a transmembrane protein that is expressed on activated effector and regulatory T-cells, B-cells, and APCs that binds the ligands (PD-L1 and PD-L2), which are expressed on tumor cells, APCs, and other cells.[3] Upon ligand binding, the PD-1 receptor cytoplasmic domain is phosphorylated at two different sites following ligand binding, which recruits two tyrosine phosphatases,[9,10] which dephosphorylate signaling intermediates and reduce downstream effects, thereby blunting T-cell activation. CTLA-4 receptor is expressed on the T-cell surface when there is significant T-cell receptor stimulation and competes with CD28 to bind CD80/CD86, thereby reducing the magnitude of the CD28 costimulatory response.[11,12] CTLA-4 receptor binding can also inhibit T-cell activation in the absence of CD28 by directly antagonizing T-cell receptor-driven signaling pathways.[13] Ultimately, CTLA-4 receptor activation disrupts effective T-cell signal transmission and T-cell proliferation and inhibits cell cycle progression.[14,15] This pathway also suppresses effector T-cells and promotes the development of regulatory T-cells.[16–19]

Ligand binding to PD-1 and CTLA-4 receptors modifies the immune system response to antigens by inhibiting T-cell activation and allows immunologic self-tolerance. Experimental blockade of PD-1 and CTLA-4 receptors provides insight into the importance of these checkpoints in preventing autoimmunity. PD-1 receptor blockade in both wild type and CD28 deficient mice resulted in an accelerated and severe form of autoimmune encephalomyelitis, marked by increased antigen-specific T-cell expansion and cytokine production.[20] In addition, PD-1 receptor deficient mice had increased B-cell proliferation and reduced expression of CD5 (negative regulator of B-cell activation) compared with control animals.[21] CTLA-4 receptor blockade mice enhanced antitumor immunity, but also elicited autoimmune responses.[22,23] Enhanced autoimmunity in a variety of end organs was also noted in six of 14 patients with metastatic melanoma patients, whereas three patients had significant antitumor effects.[24]

Novel immunotherapies include immune checkpoint inhibitors (ICIs), which are monoclonal antibodies aimed at

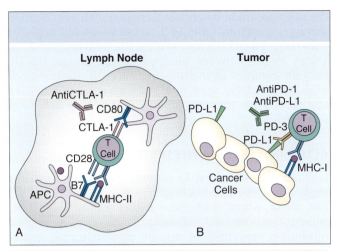

Fig. 18.1 Immune checkpoint inhibitor target sites. A, At the level of the lymph node, cytotoxic lymphocyte-associated antigen 4 (CTLA-4) receptor is expressed on T-cells and competes with CD28 to bind to CD80. This competitive binding reduces the magnitude of the CD28 costimulatory response, thus inhibiting the potency of T-cell activation. CTLA-4 receptor blockade leads to T-cells activation and antitumor effects. B, In the tumor microenvironment, programmed cell death 1 (PD-1) receptor is a protein expressed on T-cells that binds to ligands on tumor cells, PD-L1 and PD-L2. When PD-1 binds to these ligands, T-cell activation is blunted. Anti PD-1 and anti–PD-L1 receptor blockade leads to further T-cell activation (or blocks deactivation of T-cells) and antitumor effects. *APC*, Antigen presenting cell; *CD80, MHC*, major histocompatibility complex.

targeting specific immune checkpoints via their ligand-receptor interactions. CTLA-4 is a receptor that, when activated, limits T-cell activation.[1] PD-1 receptor is expressed primarily on the surface of activated T-cells, and is a negative costimulatory receptor.[25,26] When PD-1 receptor binds to one of its ligands, such as programmed death ligand 1 (PD-L1) or programmed death ligand 2 (PD-L2), an otherwise cytotoxic T-cell response is inhibited (see Fig. 18.1).[27,28] As noted, various cancers use this pathway to evade T-cell induced antitumor activity.[29] At present, ICIs available for clinical use include ipilimumab, a CTLA-4 receptor antagonist approved for advanced melanoma, and nivolumab and pembrolizumab, PD-1 receptor antagonists approved for advanced melanoma and non-small cell lung cancer. Other drug trials are underway examining the utility of these monoclonal antibodies for various malignancies.

Another novel modality of harnessing the immune system for its antitumor effects includes chimeric antigen receptor (CAR) T-cell therapy. CAR T-cells are modified using a single-chain variable fragment from an antibody along with a costimulatory domain to target an extracellular antigen. This T-cell manipulation evokes an immune response targeted at specific antigens alone. Clinical trials have focused on targeting CD19, which is expressed ubiquitously on B-cells, thus CD19 targeted CAR T-cells have been used to treat B-cell malignancies.[29] In October 2017, axicabtagene ciloleucel, a CAR T-cell therapy, was approved to treat adult patients with some types of large B-cell lymphoma that have relapsed, or have not responded, to two types of therapy thus far.[30] Given the novelty of the field, the potential targets for CAR T-cell therapy, and the malignancies it may be used in, have not yet been fully discovered.

Interferon alpha (IFN-α) is an older immunologic therapy that has been used in the treatment of chronic myeloid leukemia since 1981. Its use has since been expanded to include metastatic melanoma and hairy cell leukemia (HCL). IFN-α was initially described to have antiviral activity and later realized to have antitumor activity.[31] IFN-α activates the immune system by promoting effector T-cell mediated responses (such as interleukin [IL]-12 secretion) via several signaling events. This robust immune response leads to successful antitumor activity.[32]

IL-2 is a cytokine with both activating and regulatory immune functions. IL-2 mediates the immune system by binding to several different receptors. These receptors are found on activated T-cells, T regulatory cells, memory T-cells, and natural killer cells.[33] Administration of high doses of IL-2 thus leads to a robust immune response, which has been used in the treatment of patients with metastatic renal cell carcinoma since 1991, and with metastatic melanoma since 1998, with improvement in survival.[33]

With the advent of immunotherapy, starting with IFN-α, followed by IL-2 and more recently with ICIs and CAR T-cell therapy, survival for many different cancers has been extended. Most notably, the landscape for metastatic melanoma, non-small cell lung cancer, metastatic renal cell carcinoma, HCL, and B-cell lymphomas has markedly improved. However, these immunotherapies have the potential to result in many different types of nephrotoxicity. In this chapter, we outline each class of immunotherapy, the types of cancer they are approved to treat, and the resultant potential mechanisms of nephrotoxicity.

Immune Checkpoint Inhibitors

The scope of malignancies that can be treated with ICIs continues to grow, as more clinical trials show promising results. Ipilimumab, the CTLA-4 receptor antagonist, is currently approved for patients with advanced melanoma.[34] Pembrolizumab, a PD-1 receptor antagonist, is currently approved for use in subsets of patients with advanced non-small cell lung cancer, advanced melanoma, advanced urothelial bladder cancer, advanced head and neck squamous cell cancer, classic Hodgkin lymphoma, and microsatellite instability-high tumors.[35,36] Nivolumab, another PD-1 receptor antagonist, is approved for a subset of patients with advanced non-small cell lung cancer, advanced melanoma, advanced urothelial bladder cancer, advanced head and neck squamous cell cancer, classic Hodgkin lymphoma, but can also be used in select patients with hepatocellular carcinoma, advanced renal cell cancer, and mismatch repair deficient or microsatellite instability-high metastatic colorectal cancer.[37]

Although these ICIs bring much promise to the treatment of many advanced malignancies, the robust immune response that they generate lends itself to a myriad of different side effects. Almost all organs can be affected by ICI therapy; the most highlighted side effects in the literature are dermatitis, colitis, hypophysitis, pneumonitis, and endocrinopathies. Organs known to be affected by immune-related toxicities include the skin, the endocrine glands, the lungs, the gastrointestinal tract, the central nervous system, the kidneys, the hematologic cells, the

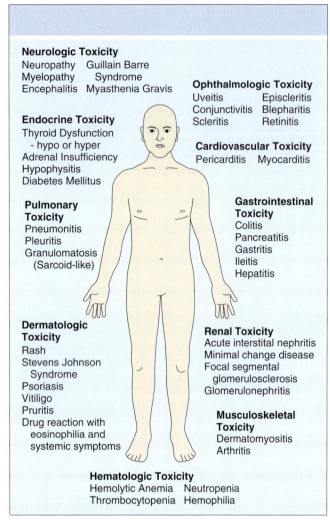

Neurologic Toxicity
Neuropathy   Guillain Barre
Myelopathy   Syndrome
Encephalitis   Myasthenia Gravis

Endocrine Toxicity
Thyroid Dysfunction
- hypo or hyper
Adrenal Insufficiency
Hypophysitis
Diabetes Mellitus

**Pulmonary
Toxicity**
Pneumonitis
Pleuritis
Granulomatosis
  (Sarcoid-like)

**Dermatologic
Toxicity**
Rash
Stevens Johnson
  Syndrome
Psoriasis
Vitiligo
Pruritis
Drug reaction with
  eosinophilia and
  systemic symptoms

Ophthalmologic Toxicity
Uveitis   Episcleritis
Conjunctivitis   Blepharitis
Scleritis   Retinitis

Cardiovascular Toxicity
Pericarditis   Myocarditis

**Gastrointestinal
Toxicity**
Colitis
Pancreatitis
Gastritis
Ileitis
Hepatitis

Renal Toxicity
Acute interstital nephritis
Minimal change disease
Focal segmental
  glomerulosclerosis
Glomerulonephritis

**Musculoskeletal
Toxicity**
Dermatomyositis
Arthritis

Hematologic Toxicity
Hemolytic Anemia   Neutropenia
Thrombocytopenia   Hemophilia

Fig. 18.2 Adverse effect profile of immune checkpoint inhibitor therapy by organ system. Various organs can be involved in the setting of immune checkpoint inhibitor therapy. Modified from Champiat S, Lambotte O, Barreau E, et al. Management of immune checkpoint blockade dysimmune toxicities: a collaborative position paper. *Ann Oncol.* 2016;27: 559-574.

musculoskeletal system, the cardiovascular system, and the eyes (Fig. 18.2).[38] The scope and mechanisms of the nephrotoxicities caused by ICI therapy are outlined subsequently.

The best estimate of the incidence of nephrotoxicity cause by ICI therapy comes from Cortazar et al. They analyzed data from phase II and III clinical trials with the goal of estimating the overall incidence of acute kidney injury (AKI), while on ICI therapy. From a total of 3695 patients, they found that the overall incidence of AKI was 2.2%. The incidence of grade III or IV AKI (increase in serum creatinine greater than threefold above baseline, an increase in serum creatinine greater than 4.0 mg/dL, or the need for renal replacement therapy) was 0.6%. When stratified, AKI occurred more frequently with combination therapy with ipilimumab and nivolumab (4.9%), than in patients on monotherapy with ipilumab (2%), nivolumab (1.9%), or pembrolizumab (1.4%).[39] These data suggest that although the incidence of ICI-induced AKI is generally low,

the risk appears to be greatly increased with combination therapy. As seen in Table 18.1, acute interstitial nephritis (AIN) (Fig. 18.3) is by far the most common drug-induced kidney lesion; however, minimal change disease (MCD), immune-complex glomerulonephritis (GN), membranous nephropathy, focal segmental glomerulosclerosis (FSGS), and thrombotic microangiopathy (TMA) have also been described.[37,39-45]

ACUTE INTERSTITIAL NEPHRITIS

Cortazar et al. described 13 patients, from seven academic medical centers, with AKI occurring in the setting of ICI use, all of whom underwent kidney biopsy.[39] Of these patients, six were on ipilimumab monotherapy, one on nivolumab monotherapy, one on pembrolizumab monotherapy, and four were on combination therapy with ipilimumab and nivolumab. Seven of these patients had a documented immune related adverse event (IRAE) before AKI and one patient had a concurrent IRAE with AKI. The most common extrarenal IRAEs were colitis and hypophysitis. The timing of AKI from initiation of ICI therapy ranged from 21 to 245 days, and the timing of AKI compared with the last dose of ICI ranged from 7 to 63 days. Of these patients, eight had pyuria, three had hematuria, and one had eosinophilia. Mean peak serum creatinine was 4.5 mg/dL and the majority of patients had subnephrotic proteinuria. AIN was found in 12 of the 13 patients; one patient had acute TMA. AIN was predominantly lymphocytic with some plasma cells and eosinophils whereas three out of the 12 AIN cases had granulomatous features. One patient with AIN also had evidence of subepithelial and intramembranous deposits; however, an antinuclear antibody titer was negative, the patient had no evidence of infection, and ultimately no explanation was found for these deposits.

ICI therapy was discontinued in 12 of 13 patients because of AKI and other IRAEs. Of the patients with AIN, 10 out of the 12 received treatment with glucocorticoids as did the patient with TMA. Glucocorticoid therapy in AIN patients on glucocorticoids was associated with partial recovery of kidney function in seven and complete recovery in two. The patient with TMA did not recover kidney function and was dialysis dependent. Two patients with AIN who were not treated with glucocorticoids did not recover kidney function, and one became dialysis dependent. Two patients with AIN required transient hemodialysis before recovering. Two patients who recovered after glucocorticoid treatment were rechallenged with ICI therapy and neither developed AKI.[39]

Shirali et al. reported six cases of AKI caused by biopsy-proven AIN in patients with non-small cell lung cancer following treatment with the PD-1 inhibitors, nivolumab and pembrolizumab.[7] In one of the cases, nivolumab was combined with ipilimumab. AKI developed after 3 to 16 months of drug exposure with a median time of 10.5 months. Four of the patients were on other medications, five on proton-pump inhibitors for greater than 3 months and one on ibuprofen for greater than 12 months. In these patients, serum creatinine ranged from 1.8 to 10.6 mg/dL with a mean serum creatinine of 4.1 mg/dL. None of the patients had clinical evidence of an allergic drug reaction except for

Table 18.1   Kidney Lesions Associated With Immune Checkpoint Inhibitor Therapy

Reference	Immune Checkpoint Inhibitor Therapy	Onset of AKI After Initiation of ICI	Kidney Presentation	Urinalysis/Urine Sediment	Kidney Biopsy	Treatment	Outcome
Cortazar et al.[39]							
	Ipilimumab	54 days	AKI	5–10 WBCs, 2 RBCS	AIN with granuloma	Drug DC, prednisone	PR
	Ipilimumab + Nivolumab	91 days	AKI	2–3 WBCS, 3–5 RBCS	AIN with granuloma	Drug DC, prednisone	CR
	Ipilimumab + Nivolumab	69 days	AKI	5–10 WBCS, 0 RBCS	AIN with granuloma	Drug DC, prednisone	PR
	Ipilimumab	70 days	AKI	0–2 WBC casts, 16–34 WBCS	AIN	Drug DC only	NR
	Ipilimumab + Nivolumab	245 days	AKI	5 WBCS, 1 RBC	AIN	Drug DC, MP, then prednisone	PR
	Ipilimumab	183 days	AKI	0 WBC, 0 RBC	AIN	Drug DC, MP, then prednisone	NR
	Nivolumab	224 days	AKI	0 WBC, 0 RBC	AIN	Drug DC, prednisone	PR
	Ipilimumab	154 days	AKI	6–9 WBCs, 0–3 RBCs	TMA	Drug DC, prednisone	NR
	Ipilimumab + Nivolumab	42 days	AKI	9 WBCs, 8 RBCs	AIN	Drug DC, MP, prednisone, MMF	PR
	Ipilimumab	120 days	AKI	3 WBCs/RBCs, WBC casts	AIN and IC deposits	Drug continued	NR
	Ipilimumab	60 days	AKI	50–100 WBCs, 0–2 RBCs	AIN	Drug DC, prednisone	PR
	Pembrolizumab	21 days	AKI	20–50 WBCs, 0–2 RBCs	AIN	Drug DC, MP, then prednisone	PR
	Pembrolizumab	231 days	AKI	11–20 WBCs, 0 RBCs	AIN	Drug DC, MP, then prednisone	CR
Shirali et al.[41]							
	Nivolumab	11 months	AKI	Bland	AIN	Drug continued initially then held	CR 6 months after drug DC
	Nivolumab	16 months	AKI	2 WBC casts/HPF	AIN	Drug DC, prednisone	CR
	Nivolumab + bevacizumab	10 months	AKI	2–5 WBCs/LPF	AIN	Drug continued, MP, then prednisone	CR
	Pembrolizumab	3 months	AKI	Numerous WBCs/HPF	AIN	Drug DC, prednisone x 2 courses	CR after 2nd steroid course
	Nivolumab + Ipilimumab	8 months	AKI	1 WBC cast/LPF	AIN	Drug DC, recurrent AKI with retrial treated with MP and prednisone	CR, recurrent AKI with retrial, PR after steroids

Continued

Table 18.1   Kidney Lesions Associated With Immune Checkpoint Inhibitor Therapy—cont'd

Reference	Immune Checkpoint Inhibitor Therapy	Onset of AKI After Initiation of ICI	Kidney Presentation	Urinalysis/Urine Sediment	Kidney Biopsy	Treatment	Outcome
Izzedine et al.[46]	Pembrolizumab	365 days	AKI	15–30 WBCs/HPF	AIN	Drug DC, prednisone	CR
	Ipilimumab	42 days	AKI	35 WBCs/HPF, 70 RBCs/HPF	AIN	Drug DC, prednisone	CR
	Ipilimumab	42 days	AKI	N/A	AIN with granuloma	Drug DC, prednisone	CR
Belliere et al.[82]	Nivolumab	48 days	AKI	Bland	AIN with granuloma	Drug DC, steroids	PR
	Pembrolizumab	137 days	AKI	Bland	AIN	Drug DC, steroids	PR
	Ipilimumab	130 days	AKI	Bland	AIN	Drug DC, steroids	CR
Murakami et al.[17]	Nivolumab + Ipilimumab	21 days	AKI	9 WBCs/HPF, 8 RBCs/HPF, WBC and granular casts	AIN	Drug DC, MP and prednisone, MMF after failure	NR, fatal septic shock
Kitchlu et al.[43]	Pembrolizumab	1 month	NS, AKI	N/A	MCD, mild ATI	Drug DC, prednisone, dexamethasone	PR
	Ipilimumab	18 months	NS	N/A	MCD	Drug DC, prednisone	CR, relapse of NS with retrial, CR with DC
Fadel et al.[49]	Ipilimumab	21 days	NS	25 RBCs/cubic mm	Lupus nephritis	Drug DC, prednisone	CR
Jung et al.[50]	Nivolumab	10 months	AKI	Numerous RBCs, 3–5 WBCs, 1–3 granular casts	IgA dominant GN	Drug DC, MP followed by prednisone	HD dependent for 6 months, CR off HD
Daanen et al.[44]	Nivolumab	1.5 months	NS, AKI	Many hyaline casts, few WBCs/RBCs	FSGS	Drug DC, MP, then prednisone	PR
Lin et al.[83]	Nivolumab	2 months	NS	Bland	Membranous nephropathy	Drug DC, prednisone	PR
Kidd et al.[37]	Ipilimumab	N/A	NS, AKI	N/A	MCD	Drug DC, prednisone	CR (NS), PR (AKI)
Ray et al.[45]	Nivolumab	14 days	AKI	N/A	Collapsing FSGS	Drug DC, steroids	NR, HD dependent

AKI, Acute kidney injury; *AIN,* acute interstitial nephritis; *ATI,* acute tubular injury; *CR,* complete remission; *DC,* discontinuation; *FSGS,* focal segmental glomerulosclerosis; *GN,* glomerulonephritis; *HD,* hemodialysis; *HPF,* high power field; *Ig* immunoglobulin; *LPF,* low power field; *MCD,* minimal change disease; *MP,* methylprednisolone; *MMF,* mycophenolate mofetil; *NR,* no remission; *NS,* nephrotic syndrome; *PR,* partial remission; *RBC,* red blood cells; *TMA,* thrombotic microangiopathy; *WBC,* white blood cells.

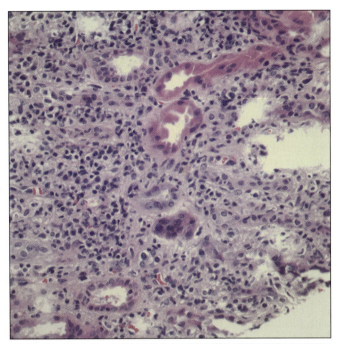

Fig. 18.3 Acute interstitial nephritis complicating immune checkpoint inhibitor therapy. Treatment with immune checkpoint inhibitors can cause acute interstitial nephritis, which is the most common kidney lesion seen. In this image, a diffuse interstitial infiltrate composed of inflammatory cells (lymphocytes, plasma cells, eosinophils) is observed (hematoxylin and eosin stain).

two patients with a mild serum eosinophilia (6% and 7 %, respectively). Urine studies were suggestive of an inflammatory kidney lesion in four of six patients who had sterile pyuria ($n = 3$) or white blood cell casts ($n = 2$). One patient had completely bland urine sediment. Following discontinuation of the ICIs (and other culprit drugs) and corticosteroid therapy in all but one patient, five patients had complete recovery of kidney function. One patient had partial recovery with serum creatinine remaining slightly above baseline. No patient required transient or permanent dialysis.

In 2014 Izzedine and colleagues reported the association of the anti–CTLA-4 antibody ipilimumab with two cases of granulomatous AIN.[46] In addition to these two cases, literature review revealed several cases of AIN (clinical and biopsy diagnosis) and one case of an immune-complex GN from this CTLA-4 antagonist. Murakami et al. also described biopsy-proven AIN following exposure ICI therapy.[14] A 75-year-old male treated with combination therapy of ipilimumab and nivolumab developed AKI after his second cycle of treatment. Kidney biopsy revealed diffuse extensive interstitial inflammation without granuloma. Treatment with glucocorticoids was initially associated with improvement in kidney function; however, a week later AKI redeveloped. The patient was treated again with pulse dose steroids and mycophenolate mofetil. Unfortunately, the patient suffered from septic shock and died. This case contrasts the other reported cases, where glucocorticoid treatment resulted in some kidney recovery.

Review of the aforementioned publications highlights the clear link between the ICIs and AIN presenting clinically as AKI. In addition, there appears to be a lack of consistent concomitant allergic symptoms and signs in patients developing ICI-mediated AIN. In reviewing the 13 cases compiled by Cortazar et al., seven patients had developed an IRAE before occurrence of AKI. Only two of Shirali's six cases had mild eosinophilia at the time of AKI. Urine studies were suggestive of an inflammatory kidney lesion (sterile pyuria, white blood cell [WBC] casts) in some but not all patients with biopsy-proven AIN, making laboratory studies unreliable. In our opinion, a kidney biopsy should be pursued for most patients who develop AKI in the setting of ICI therapy, as our personal experience supports that a significant number of patients with AKI in this setting have another kidney lesion (acute tubular injury [ATI]/acute tubular necrosis [ATN]). As such, a reasonable diagnostic clinical approach is the following: clinicians must be watchful for AKI when patients are on ICI therapy, particularly once an initial IRAE occurs. There is no expected timeline for when AKI develops, which contrasts IRAEs affecting other organs that have more expected time courses. For example, dermatologic side effects typically occur within the first few weeks of ICI initiation, gastrointestinal IRAEs tend to occur within 5 to 10 weeks of initiation, and endocrinopathies and hepatic side effects occur after approximately 6 weeks.[47] In addition, the timeline for ICI-mediated AIN is more variable than seen with traditional drug-induced AIN. ICI-mediated AIN has the potential to develop long after the first and last dose of drug. Laboratory findings in the setting of ICI-induced AIN are generally not helpful, with classic allergic findings, such as rash, fever, and eosinophilia, not present. Sterile pyuria and WBC casts seen on urine sediment examination may provide a clue to the presence of drug-induced AIN, which is largely insensitive and quite often nonspecific (seen in other kidney lesions).

Collectively, the data suggest that complete or partial recovery of kidney function may be achieved with some combination of drug discontinuation and glucocorticoid treatment. However, a small number may require long-term dialysis. Although initial drug discontinuation is prudent in the setting of AKI (and biopsy-proven AIN), the feasibility of restarting ICI versus permanent discontinuation is unknown. At present, experts recommend permanent cessation of ICI therapy if a patient develops grade III or IV nephrotoxicity, which is defined as tripling of serum creatinine concentration or need for renal replacement therapy.[48] However, patients who improved on glucocorticoid therapy and were retrialed on ICI therapy did not develop recurrent AKI/AIN.[5] However, one patient developed a recurrence of AKI, when rechallenged with ICI therapy.[41] Thus ICI rechallenge may be feasible in some but not all patients—close monitoring is warranted. With regards to the role of glucocorticoid treatment in ICI-mediated AIN, nine out of 10 patients with AIN (Cortazar's study) who received glucocorticoids had some degree of kidney recovery as compared with the two untreated patient who did not recover.[5,6] In the report by Shirali and coworkers, five of the six patients received glucocorticoid therapy and recovered kidney function to or near baseline, supporting use of this treatment in patients with biopsy-proven AIN.[7] Although these represent case reports, the literature thus far leads the clinician to believe that there is a clearer role for glucocorticoid use in ICI-mediated AIN.

The mechanism underlying kidney injury with ICI therapy has not been clearly worked out. It is possible that ICI-induced AIN may be the result of reprogramming of the host's immune system, which subsequently leads to loss of tolerance against endogenous kidney antigens not normally targeted. This contrasts the delayed-type hypersensitivity reaction typically seen in AIN from other medications.[39] This mechanism may ultimately explain the long latency period from drug exposure to kidney injury that has been observed in the cases previously reported.[5–7] In addition, it is possible that ICI therapy with activation of T-cells lowers normal host tolerance to concomitantly prescribed medications linked to AIN (nonsteroidal antiinflammatory drugs [NSAIDs] and proton-pump inhibitors), thereby precipitating drug-induced AIN.[41]

OTHER KIDNEY LESIONS

Although AIN is by far the most common nephrotoxicity of ICI therapy, immune-complex GN has also been reported. Fadel et al. described a patient with metastatic melanoma who received ipilimumab intravenously every 3 weeks. After two rounds of treatment, the patient was found to have a serum creatinine of 1.01 mg/dL with a urinary protein excretion rate of 7.5 g/day. Antinuclear antibody was mildly positive at 1:100 and antidouble stranded deoxyribonucleic acid (DNA) antibodies were positive. On kidney biopsy, a mildly proliferative glomerular lesion with thick capillary loops was seen on light microscopy with extramembranous and mesangial desposits of immunoglobulin (Ig)G, IgM, C3, and C1q on immunofluorescence. Granular, electron-dense extramembranous deposits were seen on electron microscopy. The findings were indicative of lupus nephritis and ipilimumab was discontinued. With cessation of ICI therapy, the antidouble stranded DNA antibodies became negative; however, 6 months later the patient continued to have nephrotic range proteinuria and developed a venous thrombotic event. He was subsequently started on prednisone therapy and his proteinuria improved to nonnephrotic range at 12 months postdiagnosis. Given the normalization of the antidouble stranded DNA with withdrawal of the ICI therapy, ipilimumab was thought to be the potential cause of this lupus nephritis-like glomerulopathy.[49]

Jung et al. described a patient with metastatic renal cell cancer on nivolumab treatment, every 2 weeks, who developed an AKI 10 months into treatment. Serum creatinine rose to 10.08 mg/dL from a value of 1.67 mg/dL the month prior. Antinuclear antibody, antidouble stranded DNA antibody, and serum C3 and C4 were normal. Kidney biopsy revealed diffuse tubular injury and a lymphocytic interstitial infiltrate along with an immune complex-mediated GN with cellular crescents and necrosis.[50] Immunofluorescence microscopy revealed diffuse granular mesangial staining for IgA, C3, and kappa and lambda light chains. Electron microscopy revealed hump-like subepithelial deposits with no subendothelial deposits. The final diagnosis was ATI with acute postinfectious, IgA-dominant GN.[50] As this patient had no signs of infection, had a normal C3, and had a lymphocytic infiltrate on biopsy, the AKI was felt to be caused by the ICI. Nivolumab was discontinued and glucocorticoids were initiated. The patient transiently needed hemodialysis, but after 6 months of glucocorticoid therapy, kidney function recovered.

MCD has also been reported in the setting of ICI therapy. In a letter to the editor, Kidd et al. described the first case of MCD associated with ICI therapy. They report on a 55-year-old man with metastatic melanoma treated with ipilimumab who presented with 2 weeks of lower extremity edema, found to have AKI with serum creatinine 2.97 mg/dL (baseline 1.2 mg/dL) with nephrotic range proteinuria (9 g per day) and a serum albumin of 2.2 g/dL. Kidney biopsy revealed an eosinophilic interstitial infiltrate and edema and unremarkable glomeruli on light microscopy. However, electron microscopy revealed marked foot process effacement consistent with MCD. Treatment with steroids improved kidney function and proteinuria to baseline.[37]

Kitchlu et al. also reported two patients who developed nephrotic syndrome secondary to MCD in the setting of ICI therapy. A 43-year-old man with Hodgkin lymphoma treated with pembrolizumab presented with AKI and edema, and was found to have nephrotic range proteinuria of 10.3 g/day. Kidney biopsy revealed focal tubular injury with positive linear basement staining for IgG but negative for IgM, IgA, C3, and C1q. On electron microscopy, marked foot process effacement was seen without deposits, consistent with MCD. Pembrolizumab was discontinued and treatment with a prednisone and taper, followed by dexamethasone and more prednisone, resulted in partial kidney improvement.[43] A 45-year-old man with metastatic melanoma treated with ipilimumab developed nephrotic syndrome 18 months into treatment. Kidney function remained normal; however, hypoalbuminemia (albumin 2.6 g/dL) and proteinuria quantified at 9.5 g/day were noted. Kidney biopsy revealed mesangial staining for IgM on immunofluorescence and diffuse foot process effacement, consistent with MCD. Ipilimumab was discontinued, and prednisone was initiated, with improvement in nephrotic syndrome. Two years later he was retrialed on ipilimumab, however, and developed recurrence of nephrotic syndrome.[43] Like the majority of patients with ICI-mediated AIN, MCD caused by ICI therapy appears to be responsive to glucocorticoid therapy.

FSGS has also been described in the setting of ICI use. Ghosh et al. described a 42-year-old man receiving nivolumab for lung cancer who developed an AKI, 2 weeks after the first dose. Nephrotic range proteinuria with 30.8 g/day developed and high-dose intravenous (IV) steroids were administered. Kidney function continued to worsen despite this regimen and biopsy revealed collapsing FSGS involving 20 out of 46 glomeruli. Hemodialysis was initiated for advanced kidney failure and, despite cessation of nivolumab therapy and steroid taper, the patient remained dialysis dependent.[45] Daanen et al. described a 62-year-old man with renal cell carcinoma treated with nivolumab who developed AKI and generalized edema with nephrotic range proteinuria (17 g/day) after four cycles of treatment. Corticosteroid therapy was initiated and kidney biopsy was ultimately obtained for worsened kidney function despite this treatment. Biopsy revealed FSGS. Nivolumab was discontinued and pulse methylprednisolone was given followed by oral prednisone. Mycophenolate mofetil (MMF) was added because of the poor kidney response to glucocorticoids; partial improvement was achieved, although nephrotic syndrome recurred with steroid tapering 5 months later.[44]

Lin et al. reported on a 75-year-old male with metastatic melanoma treated with nivolumab who presented with signs of nephrotic syndrome after his fifth treatment. Laboratory tests revealed the following: albumin of 1.4 mg/dL, normal serum creatinine, and nephrotic proteinuria quantified at 12 g/day. Nivolumab was discontinued and prednisone was started empirically. Kidney biopsy revealed granular IgG capillary wall staining on immunofluorescence and subepithelial dense deposits and podocyte effacement on electron microscopy consistent with membranous nephropathy. After drug discontinuation and steroid treatment, the patient achieved partial recovery of nephrotic syndrome.

Although ICI therapy is a relatively uncommon cause of AKI, its prevalence will likely increase as ICI therapy continues to expand. Because patients who develop AKI are generally asymptomatic, routine monitoring of kidney function with intermittent serum creatinine measurements and urinalysis is essential. It is prudent to make a definitive diagnosis of the cause of AKI and/or proteinuria/nephrotic syndrome in patients receiving ICIs before administering glucocorticoids as not all lesions (ATI/ATN, etc.) respond to steroids.[3] Once other causes of kidney disease have been excluded, current oncology-driven recommendations for the management of ICI-mediated nephrotoxicity are based on the gradation of the AKI (Table 18.2).[51,52] For grade 1 kidney injury, which is defined as serum creatinine 1 to 1.5 times baseline or greater than 1 to 1.5 times the upper limit of normal, 1+ proteinuria on urinalysis, or urinary protein less than 1.0 g/day, the recommendation is to monitor the serum creatinine weekly and continue immunotherapy. If the serum creatinine worsens and the patient progresses to a higher grade (2, 3, or 4), the recommendations change.

Grade 2 kidney injury is defined as serum creatinine 1.5 to 3.0 times baseline or greater than 1.5 to 3.0 times the upper limit of normal, 2+ proteinuria on urinalysis, or urinary protein quantified between 1.0 to 3.4 g/day. Grade 3 kidney injury is defined as serum creatinine greater than 3.0 times baseline or greater than 3.0 to 6.0 times the upper limit of normal, or urinary protein quantified greater than 3.5 g/day. For both grade 2 and 3 kidney injury, the recommendation is to monitor serum creatinine at least every 2 to 3 days and to withhold ICI therapy. Therapy can be resumed if kidney injury and associated symptoms are mild, resolve, or return to baseline. In addition, it is recommended to administer IV methylprednisolone 0.5 to 1.0 mg/kg/day or equivalent until there is improvement of kidney function to mild severity. Glucocorticoid taper over the course of a month is additionally recommended. Lastly, grade 4 kidney injury is defined by a serum creatinine 6.0 times the upper limit of normal. Recommendations are to monitor the serum creatinine daily, and consider nephrology consultation with potential for kidney biopsy. ICI therapy should be permanently discontinued and IV methylprednisolone should be administered at 1 to 2 mg/kg/day or equivalent, until there is improvement to mild severity. Glucocorticoids should be tapered over a month at the minimum.[3,51,52]

From a nephrology perspective, we recommend a slightly different approach to patients developing AKI and proteinuria in the setting of ICI therapy. Patient who develop the Kidney Disease: Improving Global Outcomes (KDIGO) stage 1 AKI can be monitored and evaluated for reversible causes, such as volume depletion and NSAID or contrast-related kidney injury. Those who progress to a higher AKI stage, or present with stage 2 or 3 AKI, should have a nephrology consultation to evaluate for the cause of kidney injury and the possible role of kidney biopsy. The same applies for persistent proteinuria that develops

Table 18.2 Oncologic Recommendations for Management of Nephrotoxicity (CTCAE v4.0 grade)

Grade of Kidney Injury	Definition (Serum Creatinine)	Definition (Proteinuria)	Treatment Recommendations
Grade 1	1–1.5 × BL or > 1–1.5 × ULN	1+ proteinuria on UA or urinary protein < 1.0 g/day	Monitor sCr weekly and continue immunotherapy If sCr worsens and patient progresses to higher grade, recommendations change
Grade 2	1.5–3.0 × BL or > 1.5–3.0 × ULN	2+ proteinuria on UA or urinary protein between 1.0–3.4 g/day	Monitor sCr every 2–3 days and withhold ICI therapy Resume therapy if AKI and symptoms are mild, resolve, or return to BL Treat with IV methylprednisolone 0.5–1.0 mg/kg/day or equivalent until improvement of AKI Taper glucocorticoids over a month
Grade 3	3.0 × BL or > 3.0–6.0 × ULN	urinary protein > 3.5 g/day	Same as grade 2 treatment earlier
Grade 4	6.0 × ULN		Monitor sCr daily Discontinue ICI therapy permanently Consider nephrology consult for kidney biopsy IV methylprednisolone at 1–2 mg/kg/day or equivalent until improvement. Taper glucocorticoids over a month

AKI, Acute kidney injury; *BL*, baseline; *ICI*, immune checkpoint inhibitor; *IV*, intravenous; *sCr*, serum creatinine; *UA*, urinalysis; *ULN*, upper limit of normal.
Data from Boutros C, Tarhini A, Routier E, et al. Safety profiles of anti-CTLA-4 and anti-PD-1 antibodies alone and in combination. *Nat Rev Clin Oncol.* 2016;13:473-486; and Weber JS, Kähler KC, Hauschild A. Management of immune-related adverse events and kinetics of response with ipilimumab. *J Clin Oncol.* 2012;30:2691-2697.

following ICI therapy, especially if proteinuria exceeds 1 g/day. General workup should include complete blood count, chemistry, kidney ultrasonography (exclude obstruction), urinalysis, and urine microscopy. Proteinuria noted on urinalysis should be quantified with a spot urine protein:creatinine ratio or 24-hour urinary collection. Urine microscopy revealing sterile pyuria and WBC casts are suggestive of an inflammatory kidney lesion (AIN or GN) and should prompt a kidney biopsy. Because serum and urine tests lack both sensitivity and specificity for AIN, stage 2 or 3 AKI without an obvious cause would benefit from kidney biopsy to define the underlying lesion. This information will help guide therapy, as ICI-induced AIN is generally glucocorticoid responsive, whereas other AKI lesions (ATI/ATN, TMA, FSGS, etc.) are not. This will limit unnecessary and potentially harmful steroid exposure in patients with cancer (and may allow ongoing ICI therapy). In addition to glucocorticoid therapy, patients with biopsy-proven AIN should have the ICI discontinued in most cases (KDIGO stage 2 and 3 AKI or Oncology grade 2–4 toxicity).

Reinitiation of ICI therapy in patients who have developed AKI is an important and currently unresolved issue. In general, it is considered reasonable to reinitiate ICI therapy if AKI is grade 2 or less and the patient has responded well to treatment with glucocorticoids. Grade 3 to 4 AKI following ICI exposure requires a discussion with the oncology team regarding the risks and benefits of restarting therapy.[3] Of note, two patients reported by Cortazar et al. who developed grade 3 to 4 AKI were rechallenged on these drugs after AKI improved following glucocorticoid therapy. Neither one developed recurrent AKI.[39] A third patient who developed AKI from ICI therapy and was treated conservatively with drug cessation, and no glucocorticoid therapy, did not have any worsening in his kidney function upon drug reexposure. These findings exemplify the importance of having individualized discussions with the patient, nephrologist, and oncologist regarding the risks and benefits of ICI reinitiation.

Given the increasing use of ICI therapy for various cancers, and the potential for nephrotoxicity, nephrologists need to be aware of the different mechanisms of injury. In addition, it is important to be familiar with guidelines for drug discontinuation, glucocorticoid treatment, and reinitiation of ICI therapy. By far the most common pathology of ICI-mediated AKI is AIN, whereas proteinuria (+/- AKI) may occur because of drug-induced membranous nephropathy, immune complex GN, TMA, MCD, and FSGS. We believe it is critical to obtain a kidney biopsy in patients suspected of having ICI-induced AKI or proteinuria to facilitate our understanding of the mechanism of injury, frequency of lesion types, and the likelihood of response to glucocorticoid therapy.

Chimeric Antigen Receptor T-Cells

There is tremendous promise in the field of oncology with the expanding use of CAR T-cell therapy. CAR T-cells are autologous T-cells that have been modified to evoke an immune response targeted at specific tumor antigens alone. They have had the most success in hematologic malignancies

thus far, although studies are ongoing looking at their use in solid malignancies.[53]

In a proof-of-concept clinical trial, Till et al. described the use of autologous, modified CD20-specific T-cells to treat eight patients with relapsed or refractory B-cell non-Hodgkin lymphoma (NHL) or mantle cell lymphoma.[54] Subsequent trials have used CD19-specific CAR T-cells to target follicular lymphoma[55] and chronic lymphocytic leukemia (CLL).[56] Next, CD19-specific CAR T-cells were used to treat refractory, relapsed pre-B-cell acute lymphoblastic leukemia (ALL).[57] In a subsequent clinical trial in 2014, this therapy was successfully used in the treatment of ALL achieving sustained remission for up to 24 months.[58]

As of August 2017, CAR T-cell therapy has been approved in the treatment of pediatric patients with B-cell ALL who did not have an initial response to therapy or had relapsed.[59] Subsequently, CAR T-cells were approved for the treatment of certain types of B-cell lymphomas in adults after two or more treatments have failed. These B cell lymphomas include diffuse large B-cell lymphoma (DLCBCL), primary mediastinal large B-cell lymphoma, high grade B-cell lymphoma, and DLCBCL that arises from follicular lymphoma.[30] Clinical trials are now focusing on the use of CAR T-cells for the treatment of solid organ malignancies. At present, trials are ongoing examining the use of CAR T-cell therapy in glioblastoma multiforme, ovarian cancer, pancreatic cancer, and mesothelioma.[60]

Despite the promise and success of CAR T-cell therapy thus far, the systemic toxicity, as well as the potential nephrotoxicity, that comes from harnessing the immune system can present significant problems. By far the most common systemic toxicity patients face is the cytokine release syndrome (CRS), a systemic inflammatory response syndrome, which occurs with the activation and proliferation of CAR T-cells and the destruction of tumor cells.[61–63] This immune system activation leads to the release of high systemic levels of cytokines and inflammatory markers—specifically IL-6, IL-10, IFN-γ, C-reactive protein, and ferritin (Fig. 18.4). The CRS typically occurs within 1 to 14 days of CAR T-cell infusion and initially presents with fever, which can be as high as 105°F.[61] In this setting, patients commonly develop associated myalgias and tachycardia. The syndrome can progress to vasodilatory shock and capillary leak with subsequent multiorgan failure (Fig. 18.5).

Capillary leak syndrome involves multiple organ systems, including cardiovascular, with the potential for tachycardia, hypotension, arrhythmias, and depressed ejection fraction, as well as pulmonary, with potential for dyspnea, hypoxia, pulmonary edema, and pneumonitis. The gastrointestinal system can be affected, with elevation in transaminases and hyperbilirubinemia, as well as nausea, emesis, and diarrhea. Potential neurologic effects include headaches, hallucinations, or altered levels of consciousness, and hematologic effects are vast and include cytopenias, febrile neutropenia, and B-cell aplasia, as well as the potential for coagulopathy. Musculoskeletal toxicities include myalgias and elevated creatinine kinase, and renal toxicity involves AKI, electrolyte abnormalities, and tumor lysis syndrome (TLS).[53] CRS can be life-threatening and thus must be promptly recognized.[62] The CRS can be self-limited or may require therapy with anticytokine

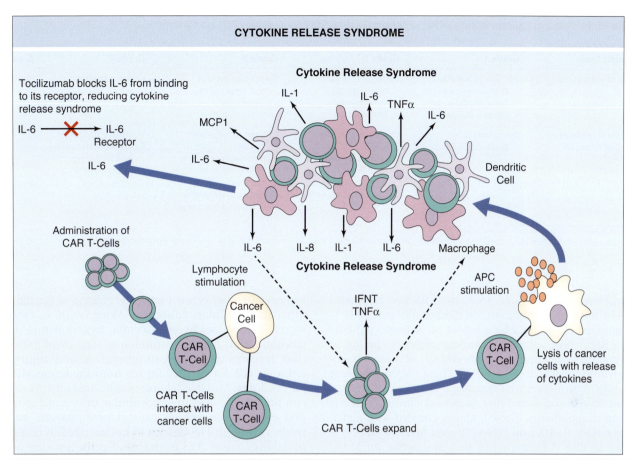

CYTOKINE RELEASE SYNDROME

Tocilizumab blocks IL-6 from binding to its receptor, reducing cytokine release syndrome

Administration of CAR T-Cells

Lymphocyte stimulation

CAR T-Cells interact with cancer cells

CAR T-Cells expand

APC stimulation

Lysis of cancer cells with release of cytokines

Fig. 18.4 Chimeric antigen receptor (CAR)-T cell infusion leads to cytokine release syndrome. Following infusion of CAR T-cells, the cells interact with cancer cells, expand further, and release interferon gamma (IFN-γ) and tumor necrosis factor alpha (TNF-α). These stimulate macrophage activation. CAR T-cells also cause lysis of cancer cells, which leads to release of cytokines and activation of macrophages and dendritic cells. Interleukin-1 (IL-1), IL-6, and IL-8 are released, as well as TNF-α and monocyte chemoattractant 1 (MCP1). IL-6 is the most significant cytokine in the cytokine release syndrome. As shown previously, tocilizumab blocks IL-6 from binding to its receptor, reducing the effects of cytokine release syndrome.

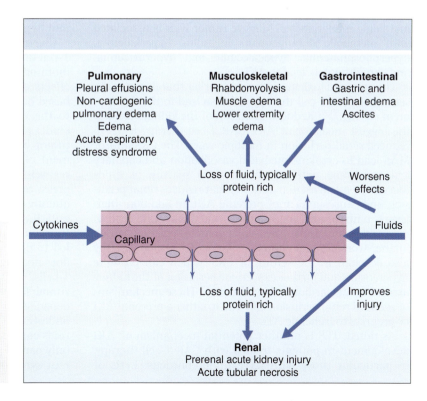

Fig. 18.5 Capillary leak syndrome resulting from chimeric antigen receptor (CAR) T-cell therapy or interleukin (IL)-2 therapy. CAR T-cell therapy and IL-2 therapy are associated with release of numerous cytokines, including IL-1, IL-6, IL-8, tumor necrosis factor alpha (TNF-α), and interferon gamma (IFN-γ). These cytokines promote leaky vascular endothelium that leads to loss of protein-rich fluid from the capillaries in multiple organ systems as shown previously. The administration of intravenous fluids as a therapy for this syndrome benefits the acute kidney injury but worsens the pulmonary, musculoskeletal, and gastrointestinal side effects and precipitates volume overload.

Table 18.3   National Cancer Institute 2014 Consensus Grading Scale for Cytokine Release Syndrome

2014 NCI Consensus Grading Scale	Grade 1	Grade 2	Grade 3	Grade 4	Grade 5
Scale of symptoms	Symptoms not life-threatening, i.e., fever, myalgia, fatigue, headache	Symptoms require and respond to moderate intervention	Symptoms require and respond to aggressive intervention	Life-threatening symptoms	Death
Specific therapeutics/ grade of organ toxicity	Symptomatic treatment only	Oxygen requirement < 40% Hypotension responsive to IV fluids or low-dose vasopressors Grade 2 organ toxicity	Oxygen requirement > 40% Hypotension requiring high-dose or multiple vasopressors Grade 3 organ toxicity or grade 4 transaminitis	Ventilator support Grade 4 organ toxicity (not including transaminitis)	

IV, Intravenous; *NCI,* National Cancer Institute.
Data from Lee DW, Gardner R, Porter DL, et al. Current concepts in the diagnosis and management of cytokine release syndrome. *Blood.* 2014;124:188-195.

agents.[61] As seen in Table 18.3, the CRS can be graded 1 to 4 by severity of symptoms and therapeutics required.[64]

Namuduri et al. describe a subset of pediatric patients with CRS, whose clinical syndrome presents similar to macrophage activation syndrome (MAS) or hemophagocytic lymphohistiocytosis (HLH).[65] These patients present with liver dysfunction and hepatosplenomegaly, increased ferritin levels, and sometimes decreased fibrinogen levels causing coagulopathy. These findings, coupled with elevations of IL-6, IL-10, and IFN-γ, suggest MAS or HLH secondary to CRS.[65] Fitzgerald et al. also describe an MAS/HLH clinical picture that developed in the setting of CRS in 12/39 patients who received CAR T-cell therapy for ALL.[62]

Another systemic toxicity that can be seen in the setting of CAR T-cell therapy is the TLS. TLS can occur in the setting of therapy, particular in patients with CLL.[56,65] Treatment with CAR T-cells can lead to TLS because of rapid lysis of large tumor burdens, with some of these hematologic malignancies. Massive tumor lysis is associated with metabolic derangements including hyperkalemia, hyperphosphatemia, hypocalcemia, and hyperuricemia, and can ultimately lead to AKI.

The systemic toxicities described earlier that occur in the setting of CAR T-cell therapy can also lead to the development of AKI.[53,62] Reduced perfusion of the kidneys is likely the biggest mediator of AKI. CAR T-cell therapy leads to reduced renal perfusion in multiple ways. The CRS and/or MAS lead to cytokine-mediated vasodilation and capillary leak syndrome with significant third spacing of fluids (decreased intravascular volume) that reduces renal perfusion and causes a form of prerenal AKI. In addition, high fevers, nausea, and vomiting associated with CRS lead to insensible losses and intravascular volume depletion, which further worsen renal perfusion. An acute cardiomyopathy also develops in the setting of CRS, which can promote hypotension and further exacerbate perfusion of the kidney akin to acute cardiorenal syndrome.[53] These mechanisms of reduced renal perfusion can lead to either a prerenal AKI or progress to ischemic ATI.

As noted, TLS is another potential mechanism of AKI development in patients treated with CAR T-cell therapy, in particular those with large tumor burdens. Lysis of

tumor cells is associated with the release of purines and other intracellular contents. Along with a cytokine storm, TLS causes hyperuricemia, hyperkalemia, hypocalcemia, and hyperphosphatemia. The cytokine storm that develops with TLS can promote kidney injury and enhance risk for further injury from the released cellular products. Massive release of uric acid and phosphate can potentially lead to intratubular uric acid deposition and calcium phosphate crystal precipitation, respectively. Although TLS has yet to be described, it remains a possible cause of AKI from CAR T-cells. Another potential mechanism of AKI is MAS targeting the kidneys, which can cause AIN or acute GN. Although these kidney lesions have been described with MAS from other causes, they have not been described with CAR T-cells and remain speculative. In addition to AKI, electrolyte derangements have been described in the setting of CAR T-cell therapy, including hyponatremia, hypokalemia, and hypophosphatemia.

Given the severity of the adverse effect profile of CAR T-cell therapy, clinicians must be extremely vigilant when monitoring patients following infusion. Risk for adverse effects of the therapy can be anticipated before therapy based on tumor burden and likely response of the tumor to the CAR T-cells. Prevention in high-risk patient includes pretreatment with chemotherapy (to decreases the tumor burden) and steroids (to reduce the CRS). Treatment of CAR T-cell related nephrotoxicity uses IV fluid resuscitation and vasopressors to maintain systemic blood pressure and perfusion of the kidneys. In addition, a frequently used therapy for CRS is tocilizumab, a monoclonal anti–IL-6 receptor antibody.[61,62] Given the high levels of IL-6 found in patients with CRS, use of this therapy has led to dramatic improvement in patients. In addition, it does not negatively impact the therapeutic benefit of CAR T-cells.[62] Fitzgerald et al. recommend the use of tocilizumab for patients with grade 4 CRS and catecholamine-dependent vasodilatory shock to improve blood pressure and prevent multiorgan failure.[62] In addition, corticosteroids can be used as second-line therapy for patients with only partial response to tocilizumab or who develop recurrent symptoms. Corticosteroids are not used as first-line therapy, because there is thought they could decrease the efficacy of CAR T-cell therapy.[62]

CAR T-cells currently offer great promise in the field of oncology. At present, the nephrotoxicity associated with this therapy primarily relates to decreased renal perfusion in the form of prerenal AKI or ischemic ATI caused by CRS or MAS. The nephrotoxicity from TLS remains a possibility, whereas there is a theoretical risk of AIN from MAS. However, neither of these nephrotoxicities has been reported. Clinicians should remain vigilant in monitoring the volume status of patients receiving CAR T-cell infusions and proactive in managing complications with IV hydration, vasopressors, and tocilizumab.

Interferon

The IFNs are cytokines that were named for the ability to *interfere* with viral replication. There are three main types of IFNs: α, β, and γ: IFN-α is mainly synthesized by leukocytes other than lymphocytes, whereas IFN-β is mainly fibroblast-derived and IFN-γ originates from T cells and natural killer cells. IFN-α and IFN-β are produced primarily by cells infected with viruses, act via common receptors, and induce changes in neighboring cells that block viral replication. IFN-γ acts to stimulate macrophage activation and MHC expression. Collectively, the IFNs are a critical component of the innate immune system that protects against viral infection. The IFNs are indicated for the treatment of multiple medical conditions, with cancer being an important therapeutic target. IFN-α was approved by the U.S. Food and Drug Administration (FDA) in 1986 for the treatment of HCL. It was later approved for the treatment of acquired immunodeficiency syndrome-related Kaposi sarcoma in 1988 and both metastatic melanoma and CML in 1995. The drug was then approved for use in treating follicular NHL. Nononcologic indications for IFN-α include the treatment of hepatitis B and hepatitis C (HCV), as well as condyloma acuminate.[66] IFN-β is approved for multiple sclerosis (MS). IFN-γ is approved for chronic granulomatous disease and malignant osteopetrosis. It used to be recommended as treatment for idiopathic pulmonary fibrosis, although this is no longer recommended.[67]

Although IFN-α maintains significant promise in the treatment of the noted malignancies and nononcologic conditions, there have been reports of several different adverse kidney effects from the IFNs, in particular IFN-α. As seen in Table 18.4, the major sites of kidney injury are the podocyte, with MCD and FSGS (Fig. 18.6) the major

Table 18.4 Kidney Lesions Associated With Interferon Therapy

Reference	Patients (n)	Onset of AKI After Initiation of Interferon	Kidney Presentation	Kidney Biopsy	Treatment	Outcome
Markowitz et al. (2010)						
	11	4 months (median), 12.6 months (mean)	AKI, nephrotic range proteinuria	cFSGS	Drug discontinuation, ± corticosteroids	Kidney function: 4 CR, 5 PR Proteinuria: 1 CR, 2 PR
Kayar et al. (2016)						
	1	3 months	AKI, nephrotic range proteinuria	FSGS	Drug discontinuation, corticosteroids	Kidney function: CR Proteinuria: CR
Ozturk et al. (2016)						
	1	6 years	Proteinuria	FSGS	Drug discontinuation	Proteinuria: CR
Markowitz et al. (2015)						
	32	NA	AKI, nephrotic range proteinuria	8 MCD 10 FSGS 14 cFSGS	Drug discontinuation ± corticosteroids	Kidney function: CR or PR in all MCD Improved in all FSGS but < 50% CR or PR
Zuber et al. (2002)						
	29	32.1 ± 7.9 months (8 patients) 34.0 ± 7.1 months (21 patients)	AKI, hypertension, proteinuria	TMA	Drug discontinuation ± corticosteroids, FFP, and plasma exchange	Kidney function: 7 CR or PR, 9 required chronic dialysis, 13 died
Kundra et al. (2017)						
	68	35 months (IFN-α for CML) 12 months (IFN-α for HCV) 68.6 months (IFN-β for MS)	AKI	TMA	Plasma exchange ± corticosteroids, FFP ± corticosteroids, or rituximab, or drug dose reduction or discontinuation	Kidney function: 27 CR, 28 CKD, 12 died

AKI, Acute kidney injury; *cFSGS*, collapsing focal segmental glomerulosclerosis; *CKD*, chronic kidney disease; *CML*, chronic myelogenous leukemia; *CR*, complete remission; *FFP*, fresh frozen plasma; *FSGS*, focal segmental glomerulosclerosis; *HCV*, hepatitis C virus; *IFN*, interferon; *MCD*, minimal change disease; *MS*, multiple sclerosis; *NA*, not applicable; *PR*, partial remission; *TMA*, thrombotic microangiopathy.

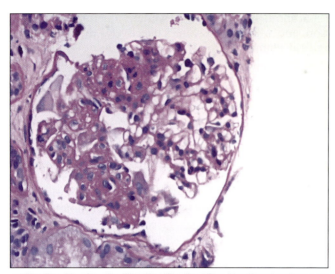

Fig. 18.6 Focal segmental glomerulosclerosis secondary to inter-feron therapy. Interferon therapy can cause nephrotic syndrome and acute kidney injury by inducing the glomerulopathy focal segmental glomerulosclerosis. In this image, a segmental sclerosing lesion is seen affecting the glomerulus (periodic acid-Schiff stain).

histopathologic lesions,[67,68] and endothelium, with TMA observed on kidney biopsy.[31,69,70]

FOCAL SEGMENTAL GLOMERULAR SCLEROSIS

FSGS is a kidney lesion that manifests with podocyte injury and segmental glomerular tuft sclerosis. Markowitz et al. described a cohort of 11 patients between 1999 and 2008 who developed kidney injury in the setting of IFN therapy that was noted to be biopsy-proven collapsing FSGS.[67] Five patients were under therapy with IFN-α for HCV infection and one for metastatic melanoma. IFN-β was used for MS in three patients and two were treated with IFN-γ for idiopathic pulmonary fibrosis. It is notable that 10 of 11 patients in this cohort were African American, raising the possibility that the patient had a genetic predisposition (APOL-1 mutation) to podocyte injury from IFN. The median duration of IFN therapy at time of kidney biopsy was 4 months with a mean of 12.6 months. Notably, the mean duration of therapy was shorter for those patients on IFN-α, totaling 3.3 months. Ten of 11 patients developed AKI and the mean serum creatinine concentration was 3.5 mg/dL. In addition, nine of 11 patients had nephrotic range proteinuria, with the mean 24-hour urine protein totaling 9.7 g/day.[67] Urinalyses of five patients revealed hematuria, and one patient had leukocyturia, but no patients had red blood cell (RBC) casts. Biopsy revealed collapsing FSGS in all 11 patients.

Clinical follow-up was available for 10 of the 11 patients included, with a mean follow-up time of 23.6 months. All 10 patients stopped IFN therapy following biopsy and diagnosis of FSGS. Six were treated with steroids, including one who received both steroids and cytoxan for MS. During the follow-up period, nine of 10 patients had a decrease in serum creatinine from a mean of 3.9 mg/dL to a mean of 1.9 mg/dL.[67] Of these, seven of nine patients reached a final serum creatinine concentration of 1.7 mg/dL or less and four patients normalized their serum creatinine concentration. Follow-up quantitative urinary protein data

available in seven of nine patients noted a decline in proteinuria from a mean of 9.9 g/day to a mean of 3.0 g/day. Of these seven, one met criteria for complete recovery, two had partial recovery, and four had improvement in proteinuria but did not meet criteria for either partial or complete recovery. Of note, the authors found that treatment with steroids did not affect kidney recovery rates, and therefore could not recommend any intervention other than discontinuation of IFN therapy.[67] In summary, this cohort represents a presentation of IFN nephrotoxicity manifested as AKI and nephrotic syndrome, with biopsy-proven collapsing FSGS. It is interesting to note that 10 of 11 patients in this cohort were African American, suggesting a potential genetic predisposition to this particular nephrotoxicity.

Kayar et al. described a case of biopsy-proven FSGS occurring in the setting of IFN-α therapy used in a 39-year-old male with Behcet disease.[71] After 3 months of treatment, the patient developed volume overload and kidney failure, with a serum creatinine of 3.1 mg/dL, hypoalbuminemia with albumin of 1.2 g/dL, and proteinuria of 7.6 g/day. Biopsy revealed FSGS. IFN was discontinued and methylprednisolone, a statin, and an angiotensin-converting enzyme inhibitor were initiated for the kidney lesion. Serum creatinine concentration improved to 1 mg/dL and proteinuria declined to 0.4 g/day, 3 months later.[71]

Ozturk et al. described a 32-year-old gentleman who developed proteinuria while receiving IFN-β for MS for 6 years.[72] Serum creatinine concentration was 0.75 mg/dL and quantitative urine protein was 1.6 g/day, which increased to 3 g/day within a month. IFN therapy was stopped at this point and kidney biopsy revealed FSGS. Over the next 6 months, proteinuria declined to 363 mg/day with cessation of IFN and angiotensin receptor blocker therapy, without corticosteroid administration.[72]

In a review of the literature in 2015, Markowitz et al. observed that IFN-α was linked to collapsing FSGS in nine patients, as described in detail earlier, and in nine patients with FSGS-NOS (non-otherwise specified).[68] IFN-β therapy was associated with collapsing FSGS in three patients, whereas IFN-γ was associated with collapsing FSGS in two patients and FSGS-NOS in one patient. In this review, the authors noted that the majority of patients with variants of FSGS improved after cessation of IFN therapy, although less than 50% sustained either a complete or partial recovery. A large portion of patients received treatment with corticosteroids, although it is not clear that this therapy was beneficial.[68]

MINIMAL CHANGE DISEASE

Another podocytopathy that complicates IFN therapy is MCD. In a review of the literature by Markowitz et al., six cases of MCD associated with exposure to IFN-α were described. In addition, two cases of MCD caused by IFN-β were reported.[68] IFN was discontinued in all patients, and most patients were treated with corticosteroids with achievement of either partial or complete kidney recovery.[68]

THROMBOTIC MICROANGIOPATHY

In addition to glomerular epithelial cell injury, the IFNs have been observed to cause endothelial cell injury with an associated TMA lesion in the kidney. In 2002, Zuber et al. published a report of eight patients with TMA associated with IFN-α therapy, as well as 21 cases of IFN-α induced TMA, previously reported in the literature.[31] All eight patients in the Zuber publication were receiving high-dose IFN-α therapy for CML, over a treatment time of 32.1 ± 7.9 months. Five patients developed hypertension before the diagnosis of TMA; however, seven of eight were hypertensive at the time of diagnosis. Five out of eight patients manifested distal ischemic lesions, whereas two patients had neurologic disturbances described as severe headaches. The mean serum creatinine concentration was 3.0 mg/dL ± 1.1 mg/dL and mean proteinuria was 4.2 g/day ± 1.3 g/day. Systemic manifestations of TMA included microangiopathic hemolytic anemia in six patients and moderate thrombocytopenia (platelet count between $50–140 \times 10^3/mm^3$) in three patients. Only one patient had no hematologic features of TMA.[31] All patients underwent kidney biopsy, which revealed typical findings of TMA involving the glomeruli and small arterioles. Five patients had diffuse involvement of the glomeruli and arterioles, two had less than 50% involvement, and one had less than 20% involvement.

IFN-α therapy was immediately discontinued in seven of eight patients; the eighth patient remained on therapy because of the absence of AKI, but the drug was ultimately withdrawn. Cessation of therapy improved kidney function in three patients, all of whom manifested only mild to moderate kidney injury. Four patients had severe clinical presentations and required intensive therapy including plasmapheresis, fresh frozen plasma (FFP) infusions, and immunosuppressive therapy. Despite intensive therapy, only two patients showed small improvement in their kidney function and dialysis was necessary for the other two. Four patients ultimately died.[31]

Of the 21 other cases reviewed, 18 were receiving IFN therapy for CML, one for HCL, and two for HCV. In this cohort, patients were treated with high-dose IFN-α therapy for 34.0 ± 7.1 months. Patients' clinical presentation were similar to that of the cohort of eight outlined previously, with hypertension noted in 12 of 21, AKI in the majority of patients, and proteinuria in over 50%. IFN-α therapy was discontinued in 18 of 21 patients. Multiple treatment modalities were used as therapy including plasmapheresis, steroids, cyclophosphamide, and FFP. Despite these interventions, seven patients required chronic dialysis and ultimately nine patients died.[31]

In 2017 Kundra and Wang performed a literature review and described 68 cases of IFN therapy associated TMA between 1993–2016.[70] Twenty-nine patients were treated with IFN-α for CML, 20 with IFN-β for MS, and 17 with IFN-α for HCV infection. One patient was treated for HCL and one for Sezary syndrome with IFN-α. Total duration of treatment varied by therapy: those treated with IFN-β for MS were treated for a mean of 68.6 months, whereas those treated with IFN-α for CML were treated for a mean of 35 months, and those treated for HCV infection were treated for a mean of 12 months. The majority of patients presented with anemia, thrombocytopenia, AKI, and symptoms of neurologic dysfunction.[70] Treatment options varied for these patients. Some 56% of patients were treated with plasma exchange with or without steroids, 19% were treated with steroids with or without plasma infusion, and 25% were treated with other modalities, including IFN discontinuation or dose reduction, rituximab, hypertension therapy, or hemodialysis. After treatment, 40% of patients had complete kidney recovery, 42% developed chronic kidney disease, and 18% died.[70]

In 2016 Kavanaugh et al. sought to prove a causal association between IFN therapy and TMA.[69] They generated transgenic mice models that produced varying levels of IFN in the brain. On histopathologic analysis, they noted a dose-dependent spectrum of microvascular disease across anatomic regions consistent with TMA. They felt these findings were caused by transcriptional activation of the IFN response through the type 1 IFN receptor. These data, along with the described patient reports of TMA in the setting of IFN therapy, support a causative role for IFN therapy in the pathogenesis of TMA.[69]

Although IFN may be a useful treatment modality for a variety of different conditions, clinicians must keep in mind the potential for adverse kidney effects. FSGS lesions with kidney failure and high-grade proteinuria have been reported as early as 3 months into therapy and as late as 6 years into therapy. Patients tend to respond poorly to cessation of IFN therapy and corticosteroids generally are not helpful. MCD with AKI and high-grade proteinuria may also occur and patients tend to respond to cessation of therapy with a definite benefit of corticosteroid use. Finally, TMA has been described to occur on average 35 months after therapy with IFN-α or as late as 68.6 months out with IFN-β. Cessation of therapy can be helpful and the role of plasmapheresis, plasma infusion, and/or corticosteroids is less known. Given the vast range of time to development of kidney disease, clinicians must remain vigilant in monitoring for signs and symptoms of kidney injury throughout the entire duration of IFN therapy. Prompt cessation of therapy is critical, as well as administration of adjuvant therapy as clinically indicated.

Interleukin-2

The FDA approved the use of high-dose IL-2 therapy in 1992 for patients with metastatic renal cell carcinoma. There were seven phase II trials spanning 21 academic medical centers that led to its approval. In these studies, patients received high dose IL-2 every 8 hours for 14 doses over a 5-day period. After a washout period of 5 to 9 days, the patients received an additional cycle barring any side effects. The courses of two cycles were repeated if patients showed disease response or stabilization.[73,74] In these trials, the most common toxicity was hypotension, which occurred in 96% of patients, with grade III/IV hypotension occurring in 74% of patients.[74]

As with metastatic renal cell carcinoma, high dose IL-2 was also one of the most effective treatment regimens for metastatic melanoma. IL-2 gained FDA approval in 1998 after eight clinical trials revealed its clinical efficacy. These trials used high dose IL-2 every 8 hours with a maximum of 14 doses over 5 days.[75] The toxicity profile in these studies was similar to that seen in the metastatic renal cell carcinoma trials. Hypotension was the most common side effect, occurring in 64% of patients, with grade III/VI hypotension occurring in 45% of patients.[75]

Although very effective, high-dose IL-2 tends to cause a multitude of systemic toxicities, as a result of the activated immune response leading to a cytokine-driven capillary leak syndrome. This causes intravascular volume depletion, edema formation, the formation of ascites and pleural effusions, and acute kidney dysfunction (see Fig. 18.5).[76,77] Kidney injury is thought to occur because of reversible renal hypoperfusion;[78] however, an intrinsic mechanism of injury is also invoked.[77]

In 1994, Guleria et. al. described a cohort of 199 patients who received high-dose IL-2 therapy for metastatic melanoma or renal carcinoma. In this study, the majority of patients developed hypotension, oliguria, edema, and weight gain. AKI also occurred and 13% of patients had their IL-2 therapy discontinued as a result of serum creatinine concentration elevation.[78] All patients had a serum creatinine concentration less than 1.9 mg/dL before treatment and peak serum creatinine was 2.1 ± 0.09 mg/dL (range 0.8–9.1) on approximately day 3. Urinalyses of patients revealed proteinuria graded as > 3+ in 11% of patients. The majority of patients had WBCs and RBCs in their urinalyses and approximately 30% of patients formed coarse or fine granular casts during therapy, suggestive of ATI. Nearly all of these abnormal urine study findings returned to baseline after discontinuation of therapy. In addition, the majority of serum creatinine concentration elevations returned to baseline with discontinuation of therapy. The resolution of abnormal urine studies, and the return of serum creatinine to baseline with cessation of IL-2, suggests that the majority of AKI is caused by prerenal physiology in the setting of the capillary leak syndrome. Although there is clearly some intrinsic injury given the granular cast formation, the quick resolution suggests that the majority of serum creatinine elevation comes from renal hypoperfusion in the setting of vascular leak. It should be noted, however, that the patients in this study routinely received indomethacin to reduce fevers and chills, thus this may have worsened AKI is some of the observed cases.

Guleria et al. provide the largest cohort; however, many studies of IL-2 both before and after confirm the reversible renal dysfunction seen. Belldegrun et al. described 99 patients with different metastatic cancers who were treated with IL-2 or IL-2 with lymphokine-activated killer cells.[79] More than 90% of patients in this cohort developed some degree of AKI. Patients had a mean pretreatment serum creatinine concentration of 1.06 ± 0.03 mg/dL and peak serum creatinine was 3.44 ± 0.19 mg/dL with most peaks occurring on day 3. Apart from elevations in serum creatinine, patients were also noted to have a 77.5% decrease in mean total daily urine volume. In addition, the majority had fractional excretions of sodium (FeNa) less than 1% with mean 0.068 ± 0.012 %. Like in Guleria's cohort, the majority of patients (84.3%) had complete recovery to baseline serum creatinine concentration within 2 weeks of therapy discontinuation and 95.2% had complete recovery to baseline kidney function within 30 days, suggesting a prerenal mechanism of injury. In fact, those with baseline serum creatinine concentration less than 1.5 mg/dL had swifter recovery.[79]

Memoli et al. described nine patients with metastatic renal cell carcinoma who had undergone unilateral nephrectomy and were treated with two cycles of high-dose IL-2. In the first cycle, they were treated with IL-2 alone and in the second they were treated with IL-2 and concomitant continuous IV dopamine infusion.[80] In the IL-2 only group, patients developed increases in serum creatinine concentration, decreases in glomerular filtration rate (GFR), and reductions in absolute urinary sodium excretion. Urine output and FeNa also decreased, all consistent with a prerenal insult occurring in the setting of capillary leak.[80] When the same group received a continuous IV dopamine infusion starting on the third of 5 days of IL-2 therapy, the patients all had rapid improvement in serum creatinine concentration, improvement in creatinine clearance, and immediate improvements in urinary output and FeNa.[80]

Shalmi et al. examined a cohort of 10 patients receiving IL-2 therapy for metastatic carcinoma to understand the pathophysiology driving the kidney injury.[77] In this study, the average pretreatment serum creatinine concentration was 1.0 ± 0.1 mg/dL with a blood urea nitrogen (BUN) of 18 ± 1.7 mg/dL and on day 4, the average serum creatinine concentration was 1.9 ± 0.3 mg/dL with a BUN of 24 ± 4.6 mg/dL. The BUN to creatinine ratio was observed to be reduced during the study course because of disproportionate increases in serum creatinine relative to BUN. By the third or fourth day of the study, eight out of 10 patients developed trace to 1+ proteinuria, two had sterile leukocyturia, and the authors noted occasional hyaline or granular casts in the urine. They did observe urinary RBCs or muddy brown casts. GFR decreased in nine out of 10 patients, as did the estimated renal plasma flow (ERPF) in some patients, although it only dropped by 30% or less in five patients and four patients actually had increases in ERPF.[77] Because of the decreased BUN to serum creatinine ratio, and the more prominent reduction in GFR as compared with EPRF, the authors felt this more likely reflected an intrinsic renal process (ATI, renal inflammation, etc.) rather than a prerenal process.[77]

In a 2017 review of the IL-2 toxicity, Marabondo et al. confirmed much of the older findings regarding the nephrotoxicity of IL-2 therapy. They caution that the kidney injury is mediated by a prerenal component, secondary to hypotension, which may also progress to ATI/ATN. In addition, an intrinsic kidney lesion may also develop from the effects of cytokine release.[76,81] Patients receiving therapy with IL-2 should be monitored for urine output and have daily BUN and serum creatinine checked. Mild creatinine increases or oliguria that develop during IL-2 therapy can be challenged with fluid administration. In addition, most increases in serum creatinine concentration reverse within 3 to 5 days with no long-term effects, suggesting a lack of true structural injury. Occasionally, patients with underlying kidney disease and other risk factors may develop ATI/ATN. If serum creatinine concentration rises higher than 4.0 mg/dL, it is recommended that IL-2 therapy is discontinued.[81]

These data suggest that although IL-2 therapy is associated with the development of AKI, the vast majority of patients appear to have prerenal azotemia because of capillary leak syndrome. As such, patients receiving IL-2 therapy should have regular monitoring of BUN, serum creatinine, and urine output. Although the majority of AKI will resolve posttreatment, some may take longer to recover if ATI occurs.

Summary

In conclusion, anticancer drug-induced kidney disease is a problem commonly encountered by nephrologists. The nephrotoxic medications used by oncologists have increased significantly over the past several decades. Novel immunotherapies offer effective cancer treatment but have also increased acute and chronic kidney disease in cancer patients. The ICIs are associated with AIN and other less common kidney lesions. IFN and high-dose IL-2 are older immunotherapies that have well-known nephrotoxicities. In addition, CAR T-cells are a new immunotherapy recently approved to treat B-cell ALL that causes cytokine release syndrome and associated hemodynamic AKI.

Key Points

- Anticancer drug-induced kidney disease is a common problem that is associated with acute and chronic kidney disease.
- Novel immunotherapies offer new, effective cancer treatment, but are also associated with nephrotoxicity in cancer patients.
- Immunotherapies are agents that exploit various properties of immune cells to augment immune system-mediated killing of tumor cells.
- Interferon and high-dose interleukin-2 are older immunotherapies that have well-known nephrotoxicities.
- The immune checkpoint inhibitors, which have changed the treatment paradigm for several malignancies, are associated with acute interstitial nephritis and other forms of kidney disease.
- Chimeric antigen receptor (CAR) T-cells are a new immunotherapy that are associated with cytokine release syndrome and acute kidney injury.

References

1. Khalil DN, Smith EL, Brentjens RJ, Wolchok JD. The future of cancer treatment: immunomodulation, CARs and combination immunotherapy. *Nat Rev Clin Oncol.* 2016;13:273-290.
2. Hanahan D, Weinberg RA. Hallmarks of cancer: the next generation. *Cell.* 2011;144:646-674.
3. Murakami N, Motwani S, Riella LV. Renal complications of immune checkpoint blockade. *Curr Probl Cancer.* 2017;41:100-110.
4. Weber J. Immune checkpoint proteins: a new therapeutic paradigm for cancer—preclinical background: CTLA-4 and PD-1 blockade. *Semin Oncol.* 2010;37:430-439.
7. Parry RV, Chemnitz JM, Frauwirth KA, et al. CTLA-4 and PD-1 receptors inhibit T-cell activation by distinct mechanisms. *Mol Cell Biol.* 2005; 25:9543-9553.
25. Keir ME, Butte MJ, Freeman GJ, Sharpe AH. PD-1 and its ligands in tolerance and immunity. *Annu Rev Immunol.* 2008;26:677-704.
28. Pardoll DM. The blockade of immune checkpoints in cancer immunotherapy. *Nat Rev Cancer.* 2012;12:252-264.
29. Lee DW, Barrett DM, Mackall C, Orentas R, Grupp SA. The future is now: chimeric antigen receptors as new targeted therapies for childhood cancer. *Clin Cancer Res.* 2012;18:2780-2790.
31. Zuber J, Martinez F, Droz D, et al. Alpha-interferon-associated thrombotic microangiopathy: a clinicopathologic study of 8 patients and review of the literature. *Medicine (Baltimore).* 2002;81:321-331.
33. Krieg C, Létourneau S, Pantaleo G, Boyman O. Improved IL-2 immunotherapy by selective stimulation of IL-2 receptors on lymphocytes

and endothelial cells. *Proc Natl Acad Sci USA.* 2010;107:11906-11911.
37. Kidd JM, Gizaw AB. Ipilimumab-associated minimal-change disease. *Kidney Int.* 2016;89:720.
38. Champiat S, Lambotte O, Barreau E, et al. Management of immune checkpoint blockade dysimmune toxicities: a collaborative position paper. *Ann Oncol.* 2016;27:559-574.
39. Cortazar FB, Marrone KA, Troxell ML, et al. Clinicopathological features of acute kidney injury associated with immune checkpoint inhibitors. *Kidney Int.* 2016;90:638-647.
40. Perazella MA. Checkmate: kidney injury associated with targeted cancer immunotherapy. *Kidney Int.* 2016;90:474-476.
41. Shirali AC, Perazella MA, Gettinger S. Association of acute interstitial nephritis with programmed cell death 1 inhibitor therapy in lung cancer patients. *Am J Kidney Dis.* 2016;68:287-291.
42. Izzedine H, Mateus C, Boutros C, et al. Renal effects of immune checkpoint inhibitors. *Nephrol Dial Transplant.* 2017;32:936-942.
43. Kitchlu A, Fingrut W, Avila-Casado C, et al. Nephrotic syndrome with cancer immunotherapies: a report of 2 cases. *Am J Kidney Dis.* 2017;70:581-585.
44. Daanen RA, Maas RJH, Koornstra RHT, Steenbergen EJ, van Herpen CML, Willemsen AECAB. Nivolumab-associated nephrotic syndrome in a patient with renal cell carcinoma: a case report. *J Immunother.* 2017;40:345-348.
45. Ray A, Ghosh S, Ghosh M, Yarlagadda S. Nivolumab induced renal failure with collapsing focal segmental glomerulosclerosis (FSGS). *J Am Soc Nephrol.* 2016;27:102A.
46. Izzedine H, Gueutin V, Gharbi C, et al. Kidney injuries related to ipilimumab. *Invest New Drugs.* 2014;32:769-773.
47. Weber JS, Dummer R, de Pril V, Lebbé C, Hodi FS, Investigators M. Patterns of onset and resolution of immune-related adverse events of special interest with ipilimumab: detailed safety analysis from a phase 3 trial in patients with advanced melanoma. *Cancer.* 2013; 119:1675-1682.
48. Spain L, Diem S, Larkin J. Management of toxicities of immune checkpoint inhibitors. *Cancer Treat Rev.* 2016;44:51-60.
49. Fadel F, El Karoui K, Knebelmann B. Anti-CTLA4 antibody-induced lupus nephritis. *N Engl J Med.* 2009;361:211-212.
50. Jung K, Zeng X, Bilusic M. Nivolumab-associated acute glomerulonephritis: a case report and literature review. *BMC Nephrol.* 2016; 17:188.
51. Boutros C, Tarhini A, Routier E, et al. Safety profiles of anti-CTLA-4 and anti-PD-1 antibodies alone and in combination. *Nat Rev Clin Oncol.* 2016;13:473-486.
53. Brudno JN, Kochenderfer JN. Toxicities of chimeric antigen receptor T cells: recognition and management. *Blood.* 2016;127:3321-3330.
56. Porter DL, Levine BL, Kalos M, Bagg A, June CH. Chimeric antigen receptor-modified T cells in chronic lymphoid leukemia. *N Engl J Med.* 2011;365:725-733.
57. Grupp SA, Kalos M, Barrett D, et al. Chimeric antigen receptor-modified T cells for acute lymphoid leukemia. *N Engl J Med.* 2013;368:1509-1518.
58. Maude SL, Frey N, Shaw PA, et al. Chimeric antigen receptor T cells for sustained remissions in leukemia. *N Engl J Med.* 2014;371: 1507-1517.
61. Frey NV, Porter DL. Cytokine release syndrome with novel therapeutics for acute lymphoblastic leukemia. *Hematol Am Soc Hematol Educ Program.* 2016;567-572.
62. Fitzgerald JC, Weiss SL, Maude SL, et al. Cytokine release syndrome after chimeric antigen receptor T cell therapy for acute lymphoblastic leukemia. *Crit Care Med.* 2017;45:e124-e131.
63. Bonifant CL, Jackson HJ, Brentjens RJ, Curran KJ. Toxicity and management in CAR T-cell therapy. *Mol Ther Oncolytics.* 2016;3:16011.
65. Namuduri M, Brentjens RJ. Medical management of side effects related to CAR T cell therapy in hematologic malignancies. *Expert Rev Hematol.* 2016;9:511-513.
67. Markowitz GS, Nasr SH, Stokes MB, D'Agati VD. Treatment with IFN-{alpha}, -{beta}, or -{gamma} is associated with collapsing focal segmental glomerulosclerosis. *Clin J Am Soc Nephrol.* 2010;5: 607-615.
68. Markowitz GS, Bomback AS, Perazella MA. Drug-induced glomerular disease: direct cellular injury. *Clin J Am Soc Nephrol.* 2015;10:1291-1299.
69. Kavanagh D, McGlasson S, Jury A, et al. Type I interferon causes thrombotic microangiopathy by a dose-dependent toxic effect on the microvasculature. *Blood.* 2016;128:2824-2833.

70. Kundra A, Wang JC. Interferon induced thrombotic microangiopathy (TMA): analysis and concise review. *Crit Rev Oncol Hematol.* 2017; 112:103-112.

71. Kayar Y, Bayram Kayar N, Alpay N, et al. Interferon induced focal segmental glomerulosclerosis. *Case Rep Nephrol.* 2016: 6967378.

72. Ozturk M, Basoglu F, Yilmaz M, Ozagari AA, Baybas S. Interferon β associated nephropathy in a multiple sclerosis patient: a case and review. *Mult Scler Relat Disord.* 2016;9:50-53.

73. Dutcher JP. Current status of interleukin-2 therapy for metastatic renal cell carcinoma and metastatic melanoma. *Oncology (Williston Park).* 2002;16:4-10.

74. Fyfe G, Fisher RI, Rosenberg SA, Sznol M, Parkinson DR, Louie AC. Results of treatment of 255 patients with metastatic renal cell carcinoma who received high-dose recombinant interleukin-2 therapy. *J Clin Oncol.* 1995;13:688-696.

75. Atkins MB, Lotze MT, Dutcher JP, et al. High-dose recombinant interleukin 2 therapy for patients with metastatic melanoma: analysis of 270 patients treated between 1985 and 1993. *J Clin Oncol.* 1999; 17:2105-2116.

76. Webb DE, Austin HA, Belldegrun A, Vaughan E, Linehan WM, Rosenberg SA. Metabolic and renal effects of interleukin-2 immunotherapy for metastatic cancer. *Clin Nephrol.* 1988;30:141-145.

77. Shalmi CL, Dutcher JP, Feinfeld DA, et al. Acute renal dysfunction during interleukin-2 treatment: suggestion of an intrinsic renal lesion. *J Clin Oncol.* 1990;8:1839-1846.

78. Guleria AS, Yang JC, Topalian SL, et al. Renal dysfunction associated with the administration of high-dose interleukin-2 in 199 consecutive patients with metastatic melanoma or renal carcinoma. *J Clin Oncol.* 1994;12:2714-2722.

79. Belldegrun A, Webb DE, Austin HA, et al. Effects of interleukin-2 on renal function in patients receiving immunotherapy for advanced cancer. *Ann Intern Med.* 1987;106:817-822.

80. Memoli B, De Nicola L, Libetta C, et al. Interleukin-2-induced renal dysfunction in cancer patients is reversed by low-dose dopamine infusion. *Am J Kidney Dis.* 1995;26:27-33.

81. Marabondo S, Kaufman HL. High-dose interleukin-2 (IL-2) for the treatment of melanoma: safety considerations and future directions. *Expert Opin Drug Saf.* 2017;16:1347-1357.

82. Belliere J, Meyer N, Mazieres J, et al. Acute interstitial nephritis related to immune checkpoint inhibitors. *Br J Cancer.* 2016;115:1457-1461.

83. Lin JT, Schiff MA, Salvatore S, Shoushtari AN, Glezerman I. Membranous nephropathy related to the checkpoint inhibitor nivolumab. *J Am Soc Nephrol.* 2016;27:102A.

A full list of references is available at Expertconsult.com

19 Chemotherapy in Chronic Kidney Disease and Dialysis

SABINE KARAM, VICTORIA GUTGARTS, AND ILYA GLEZERMAN

Malignancy remains a major cause of morbidity and mortality in the United States. It is estimated that up to 1,735,350 new cases of cancer will be diagnosed in 2018, with 609,640 deaths from cancer predicted for that year. On the other hand, survival in cancer patients has improved dramatically, with a 5-year survival of 66.9% in 2008 to 2014.[1] Many of these cases will be diagnosed in patients with chronic kidney disease (CKD) because the prevalence of cancer is higher in these patients. For example, the prevalence of cancer in 2010 in the general population older than 65 years of age was 10.4%, whereas in the same age group in CKD patients, the prevalence was 17.9%. The discrepancy is even greater in younger individuals (age 20–64 years), with prevalences of 2.0% and 13.7%, respectively.[2] Given these statistics, nephrologists and oncologists need to be aware of dosage adjustments and overall safety of use of anticancer therapies in patients with CKD. Unfortunately, most clinical trials in oncology exclude patients with moderate to severe CKD and most of the data on the use of anticancer therapies in these patients come from case reports and case series. This chapter will summarize current recommendations for management of CKD patients undergoing conventional, novel, and biologic anticancer therapies.

Conventional Chemotherapy

ALKYLATING AGENTS

Nitrogen Mustards

Mechlorethamine (Nitrogen Mustard)

Mechlorethamine is the prototype anticancer chemotherapeutic drug. Successful clinical use of mechlorethamine gave birth to the field of anticancer chemotherapy. It is used mostly in Hodgkins lymphoma and as palliative treatment for malignant effusions of metastatic carcinomas. The dosage is based on ideal dry weight and the drug is rapidly metabolized with minimal urinary excretion, hence no adjustment is needed in kidney failure.[3] There are no data available regarding its use in hemodialysis (HD) or in peritoneal dialysis (PD).

Cyclophosphamide

The oxazaphosphorine alkylating agent, cyclophosphamide, is used across a wide range of tumor types and was introduced to clinical practice in 1958. The drug may be administered either parenterally or orally. Systemic availability after oral administration is greater than 75%.[4] Cyclophosphamide

is inactive until it undergoes hepatic transformation to form 4-hydroxycyclophosphamide, which then breaks down to form the ultimate alkylating agent, phosphoramide mustard and other inactive products.[5] The drug is minimally protein bound but some of its metabolites are more than 60% protein bound. The metabolites and up to 25% of the unchanged parent compound are ultimately eliminated by the kidneys.[3,6] Pharmacokinetics studies of cyclophosphamide in kidney failure have yielded conflicting results. Some authors have not found any alterations in the presence of hepatic or renal insufficiency,[5,7] leading them to not recommend any adjustment of the dose in the presence of kidney failure, whereas others have reported a significantly decreased clearance of the drug in the presence of severe renal insufficiency.[8,9] Myelosuppression is usually the dose-limiting toxicity; however, in the setting of bone marrow transplantation, escalation beyond that dosage range is limited by cardiac toxicity.[5] Synergistic hematopoietic toxicity may occur with concomitant use of allopurinol.[4] Both unchanged cyclophosphamide and its metabolites are extensively cleared by HD.[10] For optimal dosing, the use and timing of HD should be considered. There are no data in PD.

Ifosfamide

Ifosfamide, an isomer of cyclophosphamide, is extensively used in the treatment of solid tumors in children and in soft tissue sarcoma.[11] Other indications include refractory germ cell cancer, as a third-line agent,[12,13] osteosarcoma, bladder cancer, small cell lung cancer,[14] cervical cancer, ovarian cancer,[15] and non-Hodgkin lymphoma. Like cyclophosphamide, it should be coadministered with 2-mercaptoethane sulfonate sodium (MESNA) to prevent hemorrhagic cystitis. It is extensively metabolized, principally in the liver, to active and inactive metabolites and principally excreted in the urine.[16] The terminal half-life is 4 to 8 hours on average in adults. The drug itself is not directly toxic to the kidney, but its metabolite chloracetaldehyde, has been shown to be toxic to renal tubular cells in vitro and in vivo.[17] Both acute and reversible kidney damage along with chronic toxicity may develop. Proximal tubular dysfunction is the commonest presentation, and may lead to a Fanconi syndrome, including hypophosphataemic rickets and proximal renal tubular acidosis (RTA).[18] Other manifestations include distal RTA and nephrogenic diabetes insipidus. Younger age at exposure and cumulative ifosfamide dose are considered the major determinants of nephrotoxicity.[19,20] Nephrotoxicity is also associated with previous or concurrent cisplatin therapy along with preexisting kidney impairment.[16,21] Neurotoxicity is another major side effect that is increased

183

in patients with compromised kidney function and is characterized by confusion, auditory and/or visual hallucinations, mutism, and encephalopathy, which may progress to stupor and coma.[13] Despite the lack of pharmacokinetic data, in a small case series, ifosfamide use in HD has been shown to be feasible.[22] Dose could be adjusted based on degree of myelosuppression and neurotoxicity. In vitro studies suggest that HD can decrease ifosfamide concentrations by 87% and chloracetaldehyde by 77%[23] and HD has been used to treat ifosfamide toxicity.[24] There are no data about its use in PD.

Melphalan

Melphalan was synthesized in 1953, and it has been an important therapy for multiple myeloma (MM) for 50 years despite the introduction of many novel agents. It acts both as cytotoxic agent through damage to deoxyribonucleic acid, and as immunostimulatory drug by inhibiting interleukin-6, as well as interacting with dendritic cells, and immunogenic effects in tumor microenvironment.[25] The absorption of melphalan is incomplete and prone to large interindividual variations, leading to a poorly predictable response.[26] It is eliminated renally and the kidney function has an effect on its pharmacokinetics with an increased median half-life (t1/2) and area under the concentration curve (AUC) when creatinine clearance (CrCl) is less than 40 mL/min.[27] Hence a dose reduction of 25% has been recommended for patients with CrCl between 10 and

40 mL/min and a further reduction to 50% if the clearance is less than 10 mL/min.[28] However, high unadjusted melphalan doses followed by stem cell transplantation has been safely used in patients on HD.[29,30] There are no data regarding its use in PD (Table 19.1).

Chlorambucil

Chlorambucil is mostly used to treat chronic lymphocytic leukemia (CLL) but also Hodgkin and non-Hodgkin lymphoma, breast, ovarian and testicular cancers, Waldenstrom macroglobulinemia, and choriocarcinoma. It is well absorbed orally and is metabolized by a microsomal β-oxidation process to phenylacetic acid mustard, which by itself has antineoplastic activity.[31] Less than 1% of both the unchanged drug and its phenylacetic acid metabolite are excreted unchanged in the urine.[32] Hence dosage reduction is not recommended in renal failure, even if some authors have advocated reducing the dose by 50% if the CrCl is less than 50 mL/min and by 75% if it is less than 10 mL/min.[28] The dose should also be reduced by 50% in PD.

Ethylenimines and Methylmelamines

Altretamine (Hexamethylmelamine)

Altretamine undergoes rapid hepatic metabolism and less than 1% of the drug is retrieved in the urine 24 hours after administration.[33,34] Hence no dose reduction is necessary in renal failure. There are no data about its use in HD or PD.

Table 19.1   Cytotoxic Drugs That Need Adjustment in Chronic Kidney Disease and in End-Stage Kidney Disease

Name	Renal Excretion	Dosage Adjustment in CKD	Dosage Adjustment in ESKD
ALKYLATING AGENTS			
Melphalan	35%	75% of the dose for CrCl between 10 and 40 mL 50% of the dose if CrCl < 10 mL/min	Full Dose in HD No data for PD
Chlorambucil		50% of the dose if the CrCl is < 50 mL/min 25% of the dose if CrCl < 10 mL/min	No data for HD 50% of the dose in PD
NITROSOUREAS			
Carmustine (BCNU)	43%	80% of the dose for CrCl < 60 mL/min 75% for CrCl is < 45 mL/min Avoid use for CrCl < 30 mL/min	Not dialyzable. Doses escalated and reduced depending on white cell count No data for PD
Lomustine (CCNU); Semustine (methyl-CCNU)	50% for CCNU and 47% for (methyl-CCNU)	75% of the dose for CrCl < 60 mL/min 50% of the dose for CrCl < 45 mL/min Avoid use if CrCl < 30 mL/min	No data for HD and PD
Streptozocin	15%–20%	75% of the dose for CrCl < 50 mL/min 50% of the dose for CrCl < 10 mL/min	No Data for HD or PD
TRIAZENES			
Dacarbazine (DTIC)	40%	75% of the dose for CrCl < 60 mL/min 50% of the dose for a CrCl between 10 and 30 mL/min Avoid for CrCl < 10 mL/min	Dialyzable to be given after HD
ANTIMETABOLITES			
Methotrexate	> 90%	50% of the dose for CrCl < 50 mL/min Avoid use for CrCl < 50 mL/min	Eliminated by high flux HD only 50% of the dose post-HD Minimally removed by PD
Pemetrexed	Almost entire renal elimination	Avoid if CrCl < 40 mL/min	Not removed by HD Avoid in PD

Table 19.1   Cytotoxic Drugs That Need Adjustment in Chronic Kidney Disease and in End-Stage Kidney Disease—cont'd

Name	Renal Excretion	Dosage Adjustment in CKD	Dosage Adjustment in ESKD
PYRIMIDINE ANALOGS			
Capecitabine		75% of the dose for CrCl between 30 and 50 mL/min Avoid for CrCl < 30 mL/min	Used safely in HD with no formal recommendations No data for PD
Cytosine arabinoside (ARA-C)	10%–30%	60% of the dose for CrCL < 60 mL/min, 50% for CrCl < 45 mL/min Avoid use if the CrCl is < 30 mL/min when doses of 1–3 g/m² are administered	Removable by HD Dose reduction recommended in PD
PURINE ANALOGS AND RELATED INHIBITORS			
Pentostatin	> 90%	75% of the dose if CrCl between 41 and 60 mL/min, 50% of the dose in patients with a CrCl between 21 and 40 mL/min	Administered in HD at a dose ranging between 1 and 3 mg/m² with no serious adverse events reported with HD done 1–2 hours after drug administration No data for PD
Fludarabine	60%	80% of the dose if the CrCl is between 30 and 70 mL/min 60% of the dose for CrCl < 30 mL/min	In HD, drug clearance is 25% of normal One case described of fludarabine use in CAPD, where the drug was used at reduced dose (20 mg/m² twice) and was well tolerated[107]
Cladribine	51%	75% of the dose for CrCl of < 50 mL/min 50% of the dose for CrCl of < 10 mL/min	Limited clearance by HD reported in one pediatric case[109] No data for PD
EPIPODOPHYLLOTOXINS			
Etoposide	20%–40%	75% of the dose for CrCl between 10 and 50 mL/min 50% of the dose for CrCl < 10 mL/min	Safe in HD even when administered at full doses[115–117] Not removed by either HD or PD[118] Pharmacokinetics not affected by dialysis timing[117,119]
CAMPTOTHECINS			
Topotecan	49%	75% of the dose if CrCl between 30 and 60 mL/min, 50% if CrCl between 10 and 30 mL/min Avoid for CrCl < 10 mL/min	50% of the dose in HD and PD
ANTHRACYCLINS			
Bleomycin	45%–66%	70% of the dose for CrCl < 50 mL/min 50% for CrCL < 30 mL/min	No data for HD or PD
Mitomycin C	< 20%	75% of the dose for CrCl between 30–60 mL/min, 50% for CrCl between 10–30 mL/min Avoid for CrCl < 10 mL/min	Used in HD at a dose of 4.7 mg/m² and administered after HD[158] No data for PD
PLATINUM COORDINATION COMPLEXES			
Cisplatin	30%–75%	50% of the dose for CrCl < 60 mL/min, 25% of the dose for CrCl < 45 mL/min Use contraindicated for CrCl < 30 mL/min	50% of the dose post-HD Nominal clearance only by PD
Carboplatin	70%	Dosing calculated using the Calvert formula where the GFR is calculated using CKD-EPI without adjusting for the BSA	3 h after HD, using the Calvert formula where GFR is 0 Used in PD with doubling of the half-life compared with patients with normal renal function
Oxaliplatin		Dose reduction if CrCl < 20 mL/min	Dose reduction of 30% in HD with administration of the drug after HD sessions or on nondialysis days OR Standard dose with performance of a HD session immediately after the infusion No data for PD

BSA, Body surface area; *CAPD*, continuous ambulatory peritoneal dialysis; *CKD*, chronic kidney disease; *CKD-EPI*, Chronic Kidney Disease Epidemiology; *CrCl*, creatinine clearance; *ESKD*, end-stage renal disease; *GFR*, glomerular filtration rate; *HD*, hemodialysis; *PD*, peritoneal dialysis.

Thiotepa

Thiotepa is rapidly metabolized by cytochrome P450 to triethylene phosphoramide (TEPA), which is the main and active metabolite with similar alkylating properties. Less than 2% of the administered dose of thiotepa is eliminated unchanged in the urine. Elimination of TEPA by the kidneys accounts for approximately 11% of the administered dose.[35,36] Many experts recommend no dosage adjustment in kidney failure; however, a pharmacokinetics study done in a patient with moderate renal insufficiency showed increased exposure to thiotepa and especially TEPA with subsequent toxicity, leading the authors to recommend reduced dosing in similar cases.[37] There are no data available about its use in HD or PD.

Alkyl Sulfonates

Busulfan

Busulfan is an alkylating agent used primarily in hematologic malignances as a preparative regimen before hematopoietic stem cell transplantation (HSCT). Busulfan is primarily eliminated by conjugation with glutathione, and less than 2% of an oral dose is eliminated unchanged in the urine[38] and dose reduction is usually not necessary in renal failure. Busulfan is effectively removed by HD but according to a report, a standard HD period (i.e., 4 hours) does not significantly affect busulfan apparent clearance.[39] There are no data regarding the use of busulfan in PD.

Nitrosoureas

Carmustine, Lomustine, and Semustine

Carmustine (BCNU), lomustine (CCNU), and semustine (methyl-CCNU) cross the blood-brain barrier and are mostly used for the treatment of gliomas. Urinary excretion of BCNU, CCNU, and methyl-CCNU is significant with 43%, 50%, and 47% of the drugs, respectively, retrieved in the urine 24 hours following drug administration.[40,41] Dose adjustment is recommended in kidney failure. For BCNU, it has been recommended to administer 80% of the dose if the CrCl is less than 60 mL/min, 75% if the CrCl is less than 45 mL/min, and to avoid its use for a CrCl of less than 30 mL/min.[42] For CCNU, the dose should be reduced by 25% if the CrCl is less than 60 mL/min and by 50% if the CrCl is less than 45 mL/min. The drug should also be avoided if the CrCl is less than 30 mL/min.[43] No formal recommendations exist for methyl-CCNU, but likely the same dose reductions apply. BCNU is not dialyzable; however, there have been documented cases when BCNU was used with a dose reduction in patients on HD with the doses escalated and reduced depending on white cell count.[44] There is no documentation of its use in PD. Moreover, there is no documentation about the use of either CCNU or methyl-CCNU in HD or PD.

Streptozocin

Streptozocin is active against pancreatic neuroendocrine tumors and pancreatic adenocarcinomas.[45] Only 15% to 20% of streptozocin is excreted in the urine.[46,47] It has been recommended to reduce the dose by 25% for a CrCl of less than 50 mL/min and by 50% for a CrCl of less than 10 mL/min.[28] However, the drug is known to have a dose-related nephrotoxic effect and to induce Fanconi syndrome.[48,49] It might be advisable to avoid it in the setting of advanced renal failure or deteriorating renal function. There are no reports of its use in HD or PD.

Triazenes

Dacarbazine

Dacarbazine (DTIC) is a cell cycle nonspecific antineoplastic alkylating agent used in the treatment of metastatic malignant melanoma and Hodgkin lymphoma. Up to 40% of the drug is excreted unchanged in the urine through tubular secretion.[50-52] It has been recommended to decrease the dose by 25% for a CrCl of less than 60 mL/min, to administer 50% of the dose for a CrCl between 10 and 30 mL/min, and to avoid with CrCl less than 10 mL/min.[53] DTIC is dialyzable[54] and has been safely used in HD.[55]

There is no report of use in PD.

Temozolomide

Temozolomide (TMZ) is used for the treatment of brain tumors and melanoma. The most important factor influencing the clearance of TMZ is body surface area (BSA) with increased BSA associated with increased clearance[56] and clearance by the kidneys playing an insignificant role.[57] TMZ has been safely administered in HD at full dose.[58] There is no reported use in PD.

ANTIMETABOLITES

Folic Acid Analogs

Methotrexate

Methotrexate (MTX) is a drug widely used in the treatment of malignancies and rheumatologic disorders. Because of almost exclusive renal elimination (> 90%)[59] and a known possible nephrotoxic effect at high doses (> 1 g/m^2), its use is usually relatively contraindicated in severe kidney failure. Clearance by the kidneys is under the influence of both tubular secretion and reabsorption.[60,61] Drug–drug interactions may play an important role in MTX excretion. Previous cisplatin use alters its elimination and may increase MTX toxicity,[62] as well as concomitant use of piperacillin-tazobactam.[63]

MTX has a high molecular weight and is highly protein bound, with 50% plasma protein binding at therapeutic plasma concentrations; hence conventional HD with a low flux filter does not result in a substantial removal of the drug. PD alone results in a minimal decrease in plasma MTX concentrations.[64] The use of high-flux HD can decrease plasma MTX concentration significantly (median, 75.7%; range, 42%–94%).[65,66] However, the major limitation of dialysis-based methods is the marked rebound in plasma MTX concentrations that can occur when the dialysis is stopped. Sequential use of charcoal hemoperfusion and single-pass albumin dialysis with albumin dialysate at 44 g/L, using a continuous renal replacement therapy machine, was recently reported as successful in treating MTX-induced oligoanuric acute kidney injury (AKI) with reversal of the toxicity and recovery of the kidney function.[67]

Pemetrexed

Pemetrexed belongs to a new generation of multitargeted antifolate cytotoxic agents. It was first approved in 2004 by the U.S. Food and Drug Administration in combination with cisplatin for nonresectable pleural mesotheliomas. It is also currently approved for the treatment of locally advanced or metastatic non-small cell lung cancer. Pemetrexed is eliminated almost entirely in the urine by both tubular secretion and glomerular filtration in the original drug form.[68] Accumulation may occur in case of pleural or peritoneal effusion, and cumulative side effects may appear. HD does not seem to be efficient for eliminating pemetrexed and hence cannot be used in case of acute toxicity.[69] Clinical trials with pemetrexed excluded patients with CrCl less than 45 mL/min but subsequent studies showed that standard dose of 500 mg/m^2 can be given to patients with CrCl greater than 40 mL/min. Pemetrexed should be avoided in patients with more significant renal dysfunction because of the potential for drug retention leading to severe myelosuppression.[70] There are no reports on pemetrexed use in PD.

Pyrimidine Analogs

5-Fluorouracil

5-fluorouracil (5-FU) is one of the major components of different folinic acid, fluorouracil, and oxaliplatin (FOLFOX) regimens used for the treatment of metastatic colorectal cancer. 5-FU undergoes extensive metabolic degradation to several catabolites, which are excreted mainly by the kidneys. More than 80% of an intravenous (IV) dose is inactivated by dihydropyrimidine dehydrogenase (DPD), mainly in the liver but also in other tissues.[71] Fluorouracil plasma clearance varies greatly among patients, partly because of dose- and time-dependent kinetics[72] and partly as a result of genetic polymorphism of DPD.[73] In general, 5-FU and its initial catabolite dihydrofluorouracil do not accumulate in renal failure, but the final 5-FU catabolite alpha-fluoro-beta-alanine (FBAL) does and it might increase its toxicity.[74] Usually no dose reduction is necessary in patients with kidney failure;[53] however, it has been recommended to reduce the dose by 50% in patients on HD.[28]

In the case of PD, 5-FU penetrates the intraperitoneal cavity, but the contribution of PD to drug clearance is negligible and the overall clearance of the drug is decreased and in this setting 50% dose reduction is appropriate.[75]

Capecitabine

Capecitabine is an orally administered precursor of 5'-deoxy-5-fluorouridine (5'-DFUR), which is preferentially activated to 5-FU in tumors. It is currently used in breast and colorectal cancers. Renal impairment has no effect on the pharmacokinetics of capecitabine or 5-FU, but leads to an increase in the systemic exposure to 5'-DFUR and FBAL with the AUC of 5'-DFUR correlating with safety.[76] Hence because of concern for increased incidence of adverse events (AEs) with renal failure, it is recommended that patients with moderate renal impairment corresponding to a CrCl between 30 and 50 mL/min to be treated with a reduced dose corresponding to 75% of the usual recommended standard starting dose. This should maintain both the tolerability and antitumor activity of capecitabine. It should generally be avoided if the CrCl is less than 30 mL/min.[77] However, with close monitoring of their clinical and laboratory data, and with dose modification based on reported AEs, capecitabine has been safely administered to patients with severe renal impairment, including patients on HD.[78] Capecitabine use has not been reported in PD.

Cytarabine (Cytosine Arabinoside)

Cytosine arabinoside (ARA-C), a deoxycytidine analog, is an S-phase specific antimetabolite drug that, for more than 40 years, has served as the backbone of acute myeloid leukemia (AML) therapy.[79] It is also used in the treatment of acute lymphoblastic leukemia (ALL) and lymphomas. Once administered, ARA-C has two fates: rapid deamination by deoxycytidine deaminase (DCD) into inactive metabolites or entry into a cell via specific membrane transport protein. As a result of its short half-life and the rapid inactivation by DCD outside of target cells, ARA-C is administered via continuous IV infusion (usually 0.1–0.2 g/m^2/day) or in high-dose infusions given over 1 to 3 hours (usually 2–3 g/m^2 every 12 hours for 2–3 days).[80] After IV administration, the drug is rapidly metabolized by deamination mainly in the liver to an inactive product, uracil arabinoside (ARA-U).[81] Approximately 10% to 30% of cytarabine and 80% of its inactive metabolite are eliminated by urinary excretion.[3] ARA-C use is associated with a wide range of adverse reactions, including severe neurologic and gastrointestinal toxicities that are dose dependent. Central nervous system toxicity, which may or may not be reversible, manifests as cerebral or cerebellar dysfunction following high-dose ARA-C therapy with an overall incidence of 5% to 20%.[82,83] No formal guidelines exist regarding dosage in renal insufficiency; however, in a series of 256 patients treated for AML, the following protocol was applied and was found to decrease the neurotoxicity of the drug: for patients with a serum creatinine (sCr) level of 1.5 to 1.9 mg/dL during treatment, or an increase in sCr during treatment of 0.5 to 1.2 mg/dL, ARA-C was decreased to 1 g/m^2 per dose. For patients with sCr 2.0 mg/dL (or higher) or a change in sCr greater than 1.2 mg/dL, the dose was reduced to 0.1 g/m^2/day.[84] Other authors recommend to administer 60% of the dose when the CrCL is less than 60 mL/min, 50% when the CrCl is less than 45 mL/min, and to avoid the use if the CrCl is less than 30 mL/min when doses of 1 to 3 g/m^2 are administered.[42] There is no pharmacokinetic rationale or clinical evidence to support dose reduction of standard dose cytarabine (100–200 mg/m^2/24 hours). HD is very effective in clearing ARA-C and its main metabolite ARA-U from the plasma in renal failure, and this maneuver could easily be used routinely to prevent ARA-U accumulation and minimize adverse effects in patients with kidney failure.[85,86] In patients receiving continuous ambulatory peritoneal dialysis (CAPD), plasma cytarabine concentrations may be considerably higher than those in patients with normal kidney function and in this case, dose reduction has been recommended.[87]

5-Azacitidine

Azacitidine is one of the hypomethylating agents available for the treatment of elderly patients with myelodysplastic syndromes (MDS) or AML. Even though urinary excretion is the main route of elimination of azacitidine and its metabolites, initial dosage modification for kidney dysfunction is not recommended. However, 5-azacytidine should be used with caution when the kidney function is unstable or impaired because of the nephrotoxicity of this agent.[42] If an unexplained increase of blood urea nitrogen or sCr occurs after the drug is given, the start of the next cycle must be held until values return to baseline, and the dosage has to be reduced by 50% for the next treatment course.[81] The adverse nephrotoxic effects include proximal and tubular dysfunction in addition to polyuria with salt wasting.[88] Azacitidine has been used at a standard dose in HD without serious adverse events.[89] There are no reports of its use in PD.

Gemcitabine

Gemcitabine, a nucleoside analog, is used to treat a variety of solid tumors. Gemcitabine pharmacokinetics appears to be linear over a dose range of 87 to 2500 mg/m^2 administered as a 30-minute infusion.[90] The majority of gemcitabine is rapidly inactivated in the liver and to a lesser extent in the blood by deamination into 2′,2′-difluoro-deoxyuridine (dFdU), through a reaction catalyzed by cytidine deaminase.[91] In addition, 10% of unchanged gemcitabine can undergo renal filtration, and within 1 week, more than 90% of the injected dose is usually recovered in the urine, either as parent gemcitabine (1%) or dFdU (99%).[92] Pharmacokinetics studies have reported conflicted findings regarding the impact of mild to moderate renal insufficiency on gemcitabine pharmacokinetics and toxicity in patients with advanced cancer.[90,93–96] It has been suggested to reduce the dose only if the CrCl is less than 30 mL/min.[43] Studies of gemcitabine use in dialysis have reported normal pharmacokinetics of the drug administered without any dose reduction with, however, significant retention of dFdU, which was effectively removed by dialysis performed 6 to 12 hours after drug administration.[97–99] There are no reports of its use in PD.

Purine Analogs and Related Inhibitors

Pentostatin

Pentostatin (2′-deoxycoformycin) is a potent tight-binding inhibitor of adenosine deaminase, a key enzyme in the purine salvage pathway. The terminal elimination half-life is approximately 6 hours following doses ranging from 2 to 30 mg/m^2 administered either as single doses or multiple daily doses over 3 to 5 days. The percentage of the intact drug recovered in the urine varies greatly according to studies and ranges between 32% to 48% at 48 hours and 95.9% at 24 hours.[100,101] Neurotoxicity and kidney toxicity are usually dose-limiting.[102] In a study of 13 patients, pentostatin was used safely with the dose reduction of 25% in patients with a CrCl between 41 and 60 mL/min and 50% in patients with a CrCl between 21 and 40 mL/min.[103] Pentostatin has been administered in HD at a dose ranging between 1 and 3 mg/m^2 with no serious adverse events reported with HD, 1 to 2 hours after drug administration, to remove any drug remaining in the system.[104] There is no experience of pentostatin use in PD.

Fludarabine

Fludarabine is a purine analog and is used in a variety of low-grade hematologic malignancies. After IV infusion, the parent drug is rapidly dephosphorylated to an active metabolite (F-ARA-A), which is to a large extent eliminated in the urine (60% within the first 24 h) at a rate dependent on the CrCl.[100] Hence the dose of fludarabine should be adjusted according to the kidney function. In a study where 22 patients with varying levels of kidney function received a single IV dose of fludarabine (25 mg/m^3), followed 1 week later by five daily doses that were adjusted according to three predefined CrCl levels, fludarabine dose adjustments provided reasonably equivalent F-ARA-A exposure with acceptable safety. Patients received 80% of the dose if the CrCl was between 30 and 70 mL/min and 60% of the dose if the CrCl was lower than that.[105] Fludarabine is dialyzable and it has been estimated that with HD, the drug clearance is 25% of the clearance in patients with normal kidney function. Fludarabine treatment can be considered in patients requiring dialysis, if dose reduction and adequate removal of the drug by HD is provided.[106] There is one case described of fludarabine use in CAPD where the drug was used at reduced dose (20 mg/m^2 twice) and was well tolerated.[107]

Cladribine

Cladribine is a purine nucleoside analog used in hematologic malignancies and multiple sclerosis. Cladribine is a prodrug and needs intracellular phosphorylation to active nucleotides. The renal clearance of cladribine is 51% of total clearance and 21% to 35% of an intravenously administered dose is excreted unchanged in the urine.[108] It has been suggested to administer 75% of the dose for a CrCl of less than 50 mL/min and 50% of the dose for a CrCl of less than 10 mL/min.[53] Limited data exist regarding its use in HD with one pediatric case. Only limited clearance was observed and no specific recommendation could be made regarding dose adjustment.[109] There are no data regarding its use in PD.

NATURAL COMPOUNDS

Epipodophyllotoxins

Etoposide

The urinary excretion of etoposide varies between 20% and 40% according to studies[110–113] and CrCl is the strongest predictor of etoposide clearance, followed by albumin concentration, because the drug is strongly bound to protein.[110] Patients with renal impairment are also at an increased risk of hematologic toxicity, therefore dose adjustments are recommended in kidney failure,[114] with some authors advocating dose reduction of 20% to 25% if the CrCl is between 10 and 50 mL/min and by 50% if the CrCl is less than 10 mL/min.[28,42] However, etoposide has been used in HD at variable doses and has been found to be safe even when administered at full doses.[115–117] Etoposide is not removed by either HD or PD[118] and the pharmacokinetics are not affected by dialysis timing.[117,119]

Vinca Alkaloids

Vinblastine, Vincristine, Vindesine, and Vinorelbine

The vinca alkaloids vinblastine, vincristine, vindesine, and vinorelbine are not excreted significantly in the urine. Vinblastine and its active metabolite desacetylvinblastine, along with vincristine, have kidney clearances that account for less than 12% of their respective dose.[120–123] Kidney clearance of vindesine is also low and accounts for less than 14% of the dose[121] and 24 hours following administration of vinorelbine, less than 11% of the dose is found in the urine.[124–126] No dose adjustment is necessary for vinca alkaloids in patients with renal impairment. However, despite a mostly hepatic metabolism, a reduction of 50% of the dose of vinorelbine has been advocated in HD because of increased risk of toxicity.[127] No data are available for the other vinca alkaloids, but the same consideration likely applies.[23] Their use in PD has not been reported.

Taxanes

Paclitaxel

Paclitaxel is used for treatment of a number of solid tumors. It inhibits mitosis and cell proliferation, resulting in the death of rapidly proliferating tumor cells.[128] Paclitaxel is a high molecular weight drug with a very low solubility in water[129] and is highly bound (90%) to plasma proteins.[130] It is metabolized in the liver with minimal renal excretion (< 10%)[131] and no dose adjustment is required in kidney failure. Paclitaxel has been used in HD[132–135] and several pharmacokinetic studies have shown similar curves for paclitaxel plasma concentrations in patients undergoing HD and those with a normal renal function for a given dosage.[133–135] Furthermore, because paclitaxel is not dialyzable, it may be used before or after HD sessions.[133] Paclitaxel has also been used in CAPD in combination with carboplatin. In this case plasma pharmacokinetics of paclitaxel were unaltered, with negligible urinary and peritoneal clearance.[136]

Docetaxel
Docetaxel is a semisynthetic analog of paclitaxel. Like paclitaxel, it is primarily cleared via hepatic metabolism with less than 10% excreted in the urine[137] and does not require adjustment in renal failure.[138] Docetaxel can be safely administered in HD at unadjusted doses,[139–141] with no differences seen in the plasma concentration-time curves of the drug administered before or after dialysis.[139] It has also been used in CAPD with unaltered pharmacokinetic parameters compared with normal kidney function.[142]

Camptothecins
Topotecan
Topotecan is a semisynthetic analog of camptothecin that inhibits the nuclear enzyme topoisomerase I. In adults with normal kidney function, approximately 49% of an intravenously administered dose is recovered in the urine as parent drug.[143] Significant correlation exists between CrCl and the plasma clearance of both total topotecan and its main metabolite topotecan lactone.[144] It is recommended to give 75% of the full dose if the CrCl is between 30 and 60 mL/min, 50% if the CrCl is between 10 and 30 mL/min, and to avoid the drug for lower clearances.[53] Neutropenia is the dose limiting toxicity and life-threatening myelosuppression has been described in patients with renal impairment caused by increased systemic exposure. Some authors have recommended to decrease the dose in patients with renal failure not only on the basis of their renal function, but also on the extent of prior myelosuppressive therapy.[145] In their opinion, no dose adjustments should be made for patients who have a CrCl higher than 40 mL/min if they have not received extensive prior chemotherapy. However, for patients with extensive prior chemotherapy or radiotherapy who are at increased risk of myelosuppression, the dose should be reduced by one-third if the CrCl is between 40 and 59 mL/min and by 50% if the CrCl is between 20 and 39 mL/min, with no recommendations made below that level of kidney function. Topotecan has been administered at a dose reduced by 50% in HD with tolerable hematologic toxicity.[146,147] The plasma clearance was increased fourfold by HD and 60% of the dose was removed, even as some rebound effect was reported.[146] Topotecan was also safely used in PD with the dose reduction of 50% and was found to be removable to a certain extent by this modality as well.[148]

Irinotecan
Irinotecan is a water-soluble camptothecin derivative that also inhibits topoisomerase I. After administration, irinotecan is converted by carboxylesterases to an active metabolite, SN-38. Urinary excretion of irinotecan and SN-38 after IV administration accounts for 15% to 30% of the elimination of the administered dose.[149–151] It is usually not recommended to adjust the dose of irinotecan in kidney failure.[53,152] Irinotecan can be administered in HD patients; however, based on the occurrence of severe adverse events in three HD patients,[153,154] the dose should be reduced because even though irinotecan is partially dialyzable, SN-38 is not.[153] It should be administered after HD sessions or on nondialysis days. There are no reports of use of irinotecan in PD.

ANTIBIOTICS
Anthracyclins
Daunorubicin
Daunorubicin (DNR) is produced by strains of streptomyces and acts pharmacologically through interference with cellular nucleic acid metabolism.[155] Urinary excretion of DNR and its main metabolite daunorubicinol accounts for 15%[156] and 23%[157] of the dose, respectively, and dose reduction is usually not needed in kidney failure. However, certain authors recommend administering 50% of the dose if the sCr level is less than 3 mg/dL or twice the upper limit of normal.[53] DNR is not dialyzable[23] and therefore has been used in HD at reduced doses. In one report, 66% of the dose was given as a consolidation treatment in a HD patient with acute promyelocytic leukemia[158] and 50% of the dose in another.[159] There are no available data related to the use of DNR in PD.

Doxorubicin
Less than 3% of an administered dose of doxorubicin appears in the urine as doxorubicinol.[160,161] Nonetheless, it has been recommended to administer 75% of the dose if the CrCl is less than 10 mL/min.[152] There are two reports on reduced-dose (10% and 50%, respectively) doxorubicin use in lymphoma patients on chronic HD.[162,163] Indeed in HD patients, the AUC of doxorubicin and its metabolite doxorubicinol were found to be increased 1.5-fold to threefold compared with patients who were not on HD.[164] There is also report of one case of doxorubicin administration in a pediatric patient with Wilms tumor on PD at reduced dose, with no adverse events reported.[148]

Epirubicin and Idarubicin
Epirubicin is a second-generation anthracycline from the same family as doxorubicin. Kidney elimination is poor and is around 9%.[165] Dose reduction is usually not recommended except at a very low glomerular filtration rate (GFR).[53] Epirubicin has been safely used in HD; however, there are no data available about its pharmacokinetics in that setting.[166] It has intermediate dialyzability in vitro[54] and should not be administered just before dialysis. There are no data available about its use in PD.

Idarubicin also has poor kidney elimination with a dose reduction advocated only if the sCr level is greater than 2.5 mg/dL.[53] There is one report of its use in HD where two-thirds of the usual dose was administered.[158] There are no data available about its use in PD.

Bleomycin
Bleomycin is a hydrophilic polypeptide antibiotic with a broad range of action. It is largely eliminated by the kidneys

with a urinary excretion varying between 45% and 66% of the dose in patients with normal kidney function. In several reports, a correlation was reported between CrCl and the rate of bleomycin clearance from the plasma.[167–170] Many studies have shown a relationship between renal function decline and increased bleomycin pulmonary toxicity especially in the setting of concomitant use of cisplatin.[171–173] Some authors have recommended administering 70% if the CrCl is less than 50 mL/min[53] and decrease it further to 50% for CrCL of 30 mL/min or below, whereas others advocate withholding it altogether at this later stage.[173] Moreover, serial measurements of pulmonary function should be performed before each dose administration. To our knowledge, there is no report of its use in end-stage renal disease (ESRD).

Mitomycin C

Mitomycin-C is metabolized by the liver and is rapidly cleared from plasma with less than 20% of the drug excreted in the urine.[174–176] It has been recommended to give 75% of the full dose if the CrCl is between 30 and 60 mL/min, 50% if the CrCl is between 10 and 30 mL/min and to avoid it if the CrCl is less than 10 mL/min.[53] Furthermore, this drug should be discontinued with the development of signs and symptoms of hemolytic uremic syndrome, as mitomycin has been associated with this syndrome when cumulative dose exceeds 40 mg/m^2.[177] Mitomycin C has been used in HD at a dose of 4.7 mg/m^2 and was administered after HD.[158] There are no data regarding its use in PD.

PLATINUM COORDINATION COMPLEX

Cisplatin

Cisplatin (*cis*-diamminediachloroplatinum) is one of the most widely used drugs to treat various human malignancies and is highly effective for the treatment of testicular tumors and tumors of the head and neck, ovary, lung, cervix, endometrium, and bladder.[178,179] Cisplatin is rapidly bound to plasma and tissue proteins and only 10% of the drug remains free in the circulation at 2 h. Pharmacokinetic studies showed that cisplatin elimination is biphasic with initial $t_{1/2}$ of 48 min for kidney clearance of free platinum and second $t_{1/2}$ of 53 to 73 h for total protein bound platinum.[180] Nephrotoxicity is its main dose-limiting adverse effect, with an incidence of around 31%.[181] Hence the dose should be reduced by 50% for a CrCl of less than 60 mL/min, by 75% for a CrCl of less than 45 mL/min and its use is contraindicated if the CrCl is less than 30 mL/min.[53] However, because of its significant potential for nephrotoxicity, most oncologists avoid cisplatin use in patients with CrCl less than 60 mL/min.[3] Several studies have demonstrated good efficacy and tolerance of cisplatin in HD patients.[182–185] However, it is recommended to reduce the dose to decrease potential dose-related adverse effects, such as anemia and neuropathy. The initial doses of cisplatin in HD patients must be reduced by 50%, at a recommended dose of 25 to 50 mg/m^2 every 3 to 6 weeks. Only free cisplatin is dialyzable and because only free platinum exerts antitumor activity, cisplatin should be given following HD sessions or on nondialysis days.[186] Administration of cisplatin in PD has been reported in three patients[75,187,188] with only

nominal clearance in dialysate, suggesting that dose reduction is indicated in PD.

Carboplatin

Carboplatin is another platinum complex used to treat a wide range of solid tumors.[189] Carboplatin is mainly cleared (70%) by kidney excretion, with most of the drug excreted unchanged in the urine over the first 24 hours,[190] hence determination of GFR is important for accurate dosing. The carboplatin dose needed to achieve a target AUC has historically been calculated using the Calvert formula: Dose (mg) = target AUC ([mg/mL]·min) × (GFR + 25) (mL/min), where the constant of 25 mL/min represents the non-GFR clearance of carboplatin.[191] In the original Calvert et al. study, GFR was measured using the ^{51}CrEDTA method. However, it is cumbersome and impractical for use in the clinical setting. Several formulas have been used to calculate the GFR in carboplatin administration with various degrees of accuracy. Recently, Janowitz et al. studied 2471 cancer patients who had chromium-51 labeled ethylenediamine tetraacetic acid (^{51}CrEDTA) measured GFR and proposed a novel GFR calculation formula. Seven other GFR or CrCl calculators were compared and BSA adjusted Chronic Kidney Disease Epidemiology (CKD-EPI) formula appeared to correlate best with measured GFR in this patient population.[192] It should be noted that the use of CKD-EPI in Calvert's formula requires removal of BSA indexing as follows: estimated GFR (eGFR) (mL/min) = eGFR (mL/min/1.73 m^2) × BSA (m^2)/1.73.[193] Both measured and calculated GFR are prone to errors and may over- or underestimate carboplatin dose, leading to increased toxicity or decreased efficacy (Fig. 19.1).[193]

Carboplatin has been used in anuric patients undergoing renal replacement therapy.[132,134,194–197] It is easily dialyzed because of its low protein binding capacity and intermediate molecular weight.[198] The plasma concentration is affected by the dose and timing of treatment in addition to the duration of HD. One pharmacokinetics study of carboplatin suggested that HD should be performed when the protein-binding ratio of the drug is low, with the optimal time being 3 hours following administration to maintain a stable concentration.[198] It has also been suggested for patients on HD to calculate the dose using Calvert's formula by setting the GFR at zero in the formula, provided that HD is started within 24 hours after the start of infusion.[199] Carboplatin has also been used in PD with doubling of the half-life compared with patients with normal renal function. Of the administered carboplatin dose, up to 20% was cleared via the dialysate, whereas only up to 8% was cleared via the urine.[136]

Oxaliplatin

Oxaliplatin (cis-[(1R,2R)-1,2-cyclohexanediamine-N,N'] oxalato(2-)-O,O'] platinum) is a cisplatin analog. The major dose-limiting side effects of oxaliplatin are acute and chronic peripheral neuropathies.[200] Oxaliplatin is not nephrotoxic. After its administration, the drug binds rapidly and irreversibly to plasma proteins (predominantly serum albumin) and erythrocytes. Thereafter, it is rapidly cleared from plasma by covalent binding to tissues and kidney elimination. Urinary excretion is the predominant route of elimination and there is a strong negative correlation between free drug plasma availability and kidney

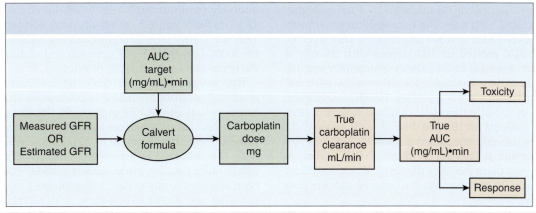

Fig. 19.1 Factors determining carboplatin exposure and outcomes. Calvert's formula is used to calculate carboplatin dose. The two variables in this formula are glomerular filtration rate (GFR) and area under the curve versus time (AUC). Although GFR is either calculated or measured, AUC depends on intrinsic patient and tumor characteristics. *Blue-shaded boxes* represent quantities determined by clinicians and *red-shaded boxes* represent actual carboplatin exposure and outcomes. Modified from Beumer JH, Inker LA, Levey AS. Improving carboplatin dosing based on estimated GFR. *Am J Kidney Dis.* 2018;71(2):163-165.

function.[201,202] However, in a pharmacokinetics study, there was no relationship between moderate renal impairment and the acute toxicity associated with oxaliplatin.[202] Moreover, in another study where oxaliplatin was administered at the dose of 130 mg/m^2 every 3 weeks, oxaliplatin-induced side effects were no more common or severe in patients with mild to moderate renal dysfunction, leading the authors to deduce that dose reductions, when the drug is administered as a single agent, are not necessary in patients with a CrCL greater than 20 mL/min.[203] There are several reports of oxaliplatin use in HD and the dialysis removal rate is more than 80%.[204,205] Although some experts have advocated for an empiric dose reduction of 30% in HD with administration of the drug after HD sessions or on nondialysis days,[186] others have recommended administering a standard dose with performance of an HD session immediately after the infusion.[206] There are no data regarding the use of oxaliplatin in PD.

Novel and Biological Therapies

During the past decade, there has been a large growth in the number of available targeted therapies that interfere with specific molecules involved in tumor growth. Although these therapies have demonstrated efficacy and clinical benefits, patients with CKD and on dialysis have largely been excluded from clinical trials. Because the prevalence of kidney disease is high in cancer patients, it is essential to examine the limited data and case series that are available, so that these patients can be given the benefit of targeted therapy when faced with disease.

VASCULAR ENDOTHELIAL GROWTH FACTOR PATHWAY

Vascular endothelial growth factor (VEGF) is produced by podocytes and binds to VEGF specific tyrosine kinase receptors present on glomerular, peritubular, and mesangial cells. Local production maintains the normal functioning of these cells and disruption of the pathway can result in

hypertension (HTN), proteinuria, and thrombotic microangiopathy (TMA). Several medications are used to target this pathway, because the formation of new blood capillaries may increase tumor dissemination and oxygen delivery promoting tumor survival.[207]

Bevacizumab is a monoclonal antibody that binds directly to VEGF. It is used in colorectal, kidney, ovarian, lung, cervical cancers, and glioblastoma. Kidney toxicity can include proteinuria seen in 2.2% of patients. When combined with chemotherapy, the relative risk of proteinuria increases to 4.79%. The highest risk of developing proteinuria is seen with renal cell carcinoma.[208] This association may be secondary to increased glomerular filtration, because these patients often have solitary kidney because of nephrectomy. Preexisting renal disease is also a risk factor for proteinuria.[209] Other renal toxicities include HTN caused by a variety of mechanisms, including decreased nitric oxide synthesis leading to vasoconstriction.[210] TMA limited to the kidneys has been shown in studies where the VEGF podocyte specific gene was knocked out in murine models as well as in clinical reports.[211]

VEGF binding antibody is not excreted via the kidneys, so no dosage adjustments are recommended in patients with chronic kidney disease. In 2007 Garnier-Viougeat et al. reported a case of bevacizumab use in a patient with renal cell carcinoma (RCC) on dialysis. The dose was initiated at 5 mg/kg every 2 weeks, which is half the recommended routine dose. Blood samples were taken before and after dialysis and the pharmacokinetic parameters were equivalent to patients with normal renal function.[212]

Sunitinib, sorafenib, axitinib, and regorafenib are all examples of VEGF tyrosine kinase inhibitors (TKIs). Tyrosine kinases are responsible for protein phosphorylation, which is necessary for proper signal transduction. TKIs block the intracellular domain of the VEGFR. Similarly to VEGF ligand inhibitors, VEGF TKIs can cause HTN, proteinuria, and TMA. In addition, focal segmental glomerular sclerosis has been reported in a large retrospective series.[213]

Although the kidneys excrete roughly 20% to 25% of VEGF TKIs, no dosage adjustment is necessary in renal impairment. In a large cohort, use of VEGF TKI in patients with eGFR less than 60 or 60 mL/min/1.73 m^2 or higher was not associated with a decline in long-term renal function and appeared safe in CKD patients.[214] Talwar et al. described an RCC patient on HD treated with 25 mg of sunitinib every 4 weeks, half of the recommended routine dose. The patient was managed for 16 months with improved clinical parameters, suggesting that this medication can be used in ESRD patients.[215] Axitinib has also been given to RCC patients on HD at a dose of 6 mg twice daily, and was tolerated with controlled disease.[216] A recent systematic review on the safety of sorafenib, in RCC in dialysis patients, suggests there may be an increased risk of toxicity in these patients. They recommend a reduced starting dose of 400 mg/day.[217]

Human Epidermal Growth Factor Receptor 2 and Epidermal Growth Factor Receptor Inhibitors

Human epidermal growth factor receptors (HER) contain an extracellular ligand binding domain and an intracellular tyrosine kinase domain. There are four members in the HER family, which include HER 1 (also known as *epidermal growth factor receptor* [*EGFR*]), HER 2, HER 3, and HER 4. Although these receptors play a critical role in cell development, overexpression or mutations in EGFR and HER 2 has been shown in breast and gastric cancers.[218]

HER 2 is the preferred dimerization partner of the HER receptors. Dimerization causes autophosphorylation of the tyrosine residues and downstream activation of signaling pathways, including mitogen activated protein kinase (MAPK) and phosphoinositide 3 kinase (PI3K). In patients that are HER 2 positive, there is a link to more aggressive disease, making it a negative prognostic indicator.[219] Trastuzumab and pertuzumab are two recombinant humanized monoclonal antibodies that target HER 2. Trastuzumab is directed against HER 2 specifically and pertuzumab targets the extracellular dimerization of HER 2. Lapatinib is a TKI that can inhibit the HER 2 and EGFR pathways.

Trastuzumab rarely causes adverse kidney effects, but when combined with chemotherapy, the incidence of nephrotoxicity is 0.3%.[220] HTN is another adverse effect, seen with the combination of trastuzumab and anastrazole yielding, in one study, a rate of HTN of 6.8% versus 3.8% in the group treated with anastrazole alone.[221] HER 2 inhibiting antibodies are primarily cleared through the reticuloendothelial system, where only 2% of lapatinib is excreted by the kidneys.[222] Thus far, there are no studies for specific recommendations for dosage adjustment for patients with CKD or on dialysis, and caution should be exercised. However, given physicochemical properties and pharmacokinetics of these agents, dose adjustments are unlikely to be needed in patients with CKD. One case report by Micallef et al. describes trastuzumab administered to two patients at the dose of 6 mg/kg during the last 90 minutes of dialysis, with good clinical outcome.[223] Piacentini et al. described lapatinib use in a breast cancer patient on HD, in combination with letrozole, with minimal residual disease.[224]

EGFR inhibition is another target for therapy particularly in non-small cell lung cancer (NSCLC). EGFR is activated by its ligands, EGF and transforming growth factor. EGFR dimerization stimulates downstream activation via the MAPK and c-Jun N-terminal kinase pathways. Chimeric monoclonal antibody, cetuximab, and fully humanized monoclonal antibody, panitumumab, bind EGFR directly, whereas EGFR TKIs include gefitinib, erlotinib, and afatinib. The EGFR TKIs are highly protein bound and are mainly excreted via the feces. Less than 5% of gefitinib and afatinib is excreted via urine and less than 10% of erlotinib.[222]

Hypomagnesemia is a frequent adverse event with cetuximab and panitumumab. One hypothesis for the mechanism suggests that the EGFRs present on the distal convoluted tubule become affected, and magnesium cannot be reabsorbed.[225] The development of hypomagnesemia correlates with the duration of treatment and age of the patient, where older patients are more susceptible.[226] Gefetinib has been reported to cause fluid retention with an incidence of 6.6% in the INTEREST (Iressa NSCLC Trial Evaluating Response and Survival versus Taxotere) study,[227] one case of AKI,[228] and one case of nephrotic syndrome.[229]

Patients with CKD and ESRD have not been included in the clinical trials for direct EGFR and EGFR TKI. There is one case report of a patient with stage 3 CKD who was given doses of cetuximab similar to patients with normal kidney function, with no difference in pharmacokinetics of the drug.[230] Several case reports demonstrate safe cetuximab usage in dialysis patients.[231] Panitumumab has also successfully been used in dialysis patients with colon cancer at routine doses.[232]

Several case reports also recommend EGFR TKI use in CKD and dialysis patients. Rossi et al. described two patients with NSCLC and CKD who were treated with gefitinib at routine doses.[233] Gefitinib has also been safely administered for patients on dialysis, where 90% of the drug remained in the plasma during HD.[234] Afatinib was used for a patient on dialysis and proved to be efficacious although was started at a 25% reduced dose.[235] The pharmacokinetics of erlotinib for patients on dialysis was investigated and found to be comparable to patients in a control group with normal kidney function.[236]

Immune Checkpoint Inhibitors

Programmed cell death proteins are another target in the treatment of cancer. The two main proteins are programmed death-1 (PD-1), which is expressed on the surface of immune cells, and programmed death ligand-1 (PD-L1), which is expressed on cancer cells.[218] PD-1 is expressed on T-cells, B-cells, monocytes, and natural killer T-cells. Its ligands include PD-ligand 1 (PD-L1) and PD-ligand 2 (PD-L2). When either of these ligands bind to PD-1, the immune cells involved become inactivated. Drugs that target PD-1, such as monoclonal antibodies, nivolumab and pembrolizumab, prevent the interaction between PD-1 and its ligand, thereby preventing the immune cells from undergoing apoptotic cell death, so that they remain active against tumor cells.[237]

PD-1 inhibitors have been used in the treatment of melanoma, lung cancer, renal cancer, and hematologic malignancies.[238] During initial trials, an elevated creatinine was seen in patients given nivolumab versus chemotherapy alone, 13% versus 9%, respectively.[239] Nivolumab caused acute interstitial nephritis (AIN), reported in four biopsy-proven case series.[240] Pembrolizumab also caused AIN in three patients who recovered after treatment with high-dose steroids.[218]

Dosage information for PD checkpoint inhibitors is described in Table 19.2. Clinical trials excluded patients with

Table 19.2 Dosing of Novel and Biologic Anticancer Agents in Patients With Chronic Kidney Disease and End-Stage Kidney Disease

Target for Inhibition	Name	Recommended Dosing	Renal Excretion	Dose Adjustment in CKD	Dose Adjustment in Dialysis (based on case series)
VEGF INHIBITORS					
VEGF	Bevacizumab	Cervical cancer, NSCLC: *15 mg/kg every 3 weeks* Colorectal cancer: *5 mg/kg every 2 weeks* Glioblastoma, ovarian cancer, RCC: *10 mg/kg every 2 weeks*	No	No	Garnier-Viougeat et al.[212] *RCC: 5 mg/kg every 2 weeks*
VEGF - TKI	Sunitinib	Gastrointestinal stromal tumor, RCC, thyroid cancer: *50 mg every 4 weeks* Pancreatic neuroendocrine tumors, soft tissue sarcoma: *37.5 mg once daily*	< 20%	No	Talwar et al.[215] *RCC: 25 mg every 4 weeks*
	Sorafenib	Hepatocellular carcinoma, RCC, thyroid cancer: *400 mg twice daily*	< 20%	No	Leonetti et al.[217] *RCC: 400 mg/day*
	Axitinib	Thyroid cancer, RCC: *5 mg twice daily*	< 25%	No	Thiery-Vuillemin et al.[216] *RCC: 6 mg twice daily*
	Regorafenib	Colorectal cancer, gastrointestinal stromal tumor, hepatocellular carcinoma: *160 mg daily*	< 25%	No	No data
EGFR INHIBITOR					
EGFR	Cetuximab	Colorectal cancer, NSCLC, head and neck cancer, squamous cell skin cancer: *400 mg/m² loading dose* *250 mg/m² maintenance dose weekly*	No	Krens at al.,[230] Osteosarcoma GFR: 35 mL/min *400 mg/m²*	Fontana et al.[231] Colorectal cancer *400 mg/m² loading dose* *250 mg/m² maintenance dose weekly*
	Panitumumab	Colorectal cancer, metastatic: *6 mg/kg every 14 days*	No	No	Kobayashi et al.[232] Colorectal cancer *5 mg/kg every 14 days*
EGFR - TKI	Erlotinib	NSCLC: *150 mg daily* Pancreatic cancer: *100 mg daily*	< 10%	No	Togashi et al.[236] NSCLC *150 mg daily*
	Gefitinib	NSCLC: *250 mg daily*	< 5%	Rossi et al.[233] NSCLC, *250 mg daily*	Del Conte et al.[234] NSCLC, *250 mg daily*
	Afatinib	NSCLC: *40 mg daily*	< 5%	eGFR 15 to 29 mL/min/1.73 m²: *30 mg daily*	Bersanelli et al.[235] Lung adenocarcinoma: *30 mg daily*
HER2 INHIBITORS					
HER2	Trastuzumab	Breast cancer, adjuvant treatment, HER2+: *4 mg/kg loading dose* *2 mg/kg maintenance dose weekly* Breast cancer, metastatic, HER2+: *4 mg/kg loading dose* *2 mg/kg maintenance dose weekly* Gastric cancer, metastatic, HER2+: *8 mg/kg loading dose* *6 mg/kg maintenance dose every 3 weeks*	No	No	Micallef et al.[223] Breast cancer: *8 mg/kg loading dose* *6 mg/kg maintenance every 21 days*

Continued

Table 19.2   Dosing of Novel and Biologic Anticancer Agents in Patients With Chronic Kidney Disease and End-Stage Kidney Disease—cont'd

Target for Inhibition	Name	Recommended Dosing	Renal Excretion	Dose Adjustment in CKD	Dose Adjustment in Dialysis (based on case series)
	Pertuzumab	Breast cancer adjuvant treatment, HER2+: 840 mg loading dose 420 mg maintenance dose every 3 weeks Breast cancer, metastatic, HER2+: 840 mg loading dose 420 mg maintenance dose every 3 weeks	No	No	No data
HER 2 - TKI	Lapatinib	Breast cancer, metastatic, HER2+: 1000–1500 mg daily depending on prior/current other therapy	< 2%	No	Piacentini et al.[224] Breast cancer: 1250 mg daily
PD INHIBITORS					
PD-1	Nivolumab	Colorectal cancer, metastatic, hepatocellular cancer, melanoma, NSCLC, RCC, urothelial carcinoma: 240 mg every 2 weeks Head and neck squamous cancer, Hodgkin lymphoma: 3 mg/kg every 2 weeks	No	No	Carlo et al.[243] Tabei et al.[242] No dose adjustment
PD-L1	Pembrolizumab	Gastric, head and neck, Hodgkin lymphoma, melanoma, NSCLC metastatic, urothelial cancer: 200 mg every 3 weeks	No data	No	Chang et al.[244] No dose adjustment
BRAF INHIBITORS					
BRAF	Vemurafenib	Melanoma, NSCLC: 960 mg every 12 hours	< 5%	No	No data
	Dabrafenib	Melanoma, NSCLC: 150 mg every 12 hours	< 25%	No	No data
PROTEASOME INHIBITORS					
	Bortezomib	Multiple myeloma: 1.3 mg/m² on select days of a 42-day treatment cycle Mantle cell lymphoma: 1.3 mg/m² on select days of a 21-day treatment cycle	No	No	No
	Carfilzomib	Multiple myeloma: Cycle 1: 20 mg/m² on select days of a 2- day cycle Cycles 2 to 12: 27 mg/m² on select days of a 28-day cycle Cycles 13 and beyond: 27 mg/m² on select days of a 28-day cycle	No	No	No
ALK TKI					
	Crizotinib	NSLCL: 250 mg twice daily	No	CrCl < 30 mL/min: 250 mg daily	No data

ALK, Anaplastic lymphoma kinase; *BRAF*, B-Raf kinase; *CKD*, chronic kidney disease; *eGFR*, estimated glomerular filtration rate; *EGFR*, epithelial growth factor receptor; *GFR*, glomerular filtration rate; *HER2*, human epithelial growth factor receptor 2; *NCSLC*, non-small cell lung cancer; *PD-1*, programmed cell death protein 1; *RCC*, renal cell carcinoma; *TKI*, tyrosine kinase inhibitor; *VEGF*, vascular endothelial growth factor.

impaired kidney function and dosing for these patients is based on case studies. In 2016 Herz et al. described four patients with metastatic melanoma and impaired kidney function (baseline Cr 1.7–2.5 mg/dL) treated with routine doses of nivolumab or pembrolizumab.[241] One of the patients was a kidney transplant recipient who was on tacrolimus and

prednisolone in addition. Kidney function tests remained stable for all four patients while treated with checkpoint inhibitors, suggesting that CKD should not limit the use.

For patients with ESRD, based on case reports, dosage adjustment may not be necessary.[242] Two separate case reports by Carlo et al. and Tabei et al. each describe a patient with RCC and ESRD after nephrectomy, treated with routine doses of nivolumab, while continuing dialysis.[243] Both authors hypothesized that because of its high molecular weight, nivolumab was not cleared by dialysis. Pembrolizumab has also been used in HD patients with melanoma and was successfully treated.[244]

Cytotoxic T-lymphocyte antigen 4 (CTLA 4) is another immune pathway targeted by checkpoint inhibitors.[237] Ipilimumab, a monoclonal antibody that blocks CTLA 4, has also been shown to cause AIN.[245] Ipilimumab was well tolerated by patients with CKD (baseline sCr 1.79–2.59 mg/dL).[241] Two ESRD patients received ipilimumab with durable oncologic response. One of them, however, developed grade 3 skin toxicity and ipilimumab was held after two doses because of recurrent infections.[246]

V-Raf Murine Sarcoma Viral Oncogene Homolog B (BRAF) Inhibitors

The MAPK pathway is dysregulated in roughly 50% of all human malignancies.[247] The MAPK pathway is responsible for promotion of cell growth. It becomes triggered by mitogen-activated protein kinase enzyme (MEK), which is activated by kinases, such as B-Raf. Mutations in the *BRAF* oncogene are present in 5% to 10 % of all human malignancies.[248] Melanoma, colorectal cancer, papillary thyroid cancer, NSCLC, and ovarian cancer may have BRAF mutations resulting in persistent gene transcription. Since the discovery of this mutation, BRAF inhibitors vemurafenib and dabrafenib have been approved for treatment.

BRAF inhibitors are highly protein bound, metabolized in the liver, primarily excreted through the feces. One percent of vemurafenib is excreted in the urine, whereas 23% of dabrafenib is excreted in the urine.[249] No dose adjustment is recommended for patients with GFR greater than 30 mL/min, but for more severe renal impairment, caution should be exercised, because data are limited.[218] Iddawela et al. report a patient with ESRD on PD who was given routine doses of vemurafenib and developed asymptomatic QTC prolongation, which was managed with dose reduction.[218] Given the increased prevalence for electrolyte disturbances in general with these medications, additional monitoring of electrolytes and electrocardiogram should be undertaken for dialysis patients.

New onset kidney injury has been reported with BRAF, with biopsies consistent with acute tubular necrosis, and kidney injury typically resolves after discontinuing the drug. BRAF inhibitors may also inhibit creatinine tubular secretion, leading to sCr elevation.[250]

Proteasome Inhibitors

Proteasome is a protein degradation machinery, which plays a critical role in homeostasis by preventing the accumulation of misfolded proteins.[251] Both normal and transformed cells depend on proteasomes for cell survival. Proteasome inhibitors have been used primarily in MM, mantle cell lymphoma, and amyloidosis.[252] Three proteasome inhibitors that are used include bortezomib, carfilzomib, and ixazomib.

Bortezomib is mainly metabolized via cytochrome p450 isoforms, with some excretion via the bile and kidney. In a multicenter study, Chanan-Khan et al. investigated the use of bortezomib in 24 MM patients with advanced kidney failure, because approximately 30% of patients with MM present with baseline kidney dysfunction. All patients, except one, were beginning dialysis at the time of bortezomib initiation and received an average of five cycles of 1.3 mg/m^2 in combination with dexamethasone, thalidomide, and doxorubicin. Overall response rate was comparable to those of MM patients with normal kidney function and three patients became independent of dialysis.[253] Although bortezomib has been shown to be effective in patients with renal impairment, there is a higher incidence of severe AEs, including thrombocytopenia and diarrhea.[254]

Carfilzomib binds selectively and irreversibly to the chymotrypsin catalytic subunit of the 20S proteasome, with suggested less off-target activity compared with bortezomib.[255] Pharmacokinetic studies showed that kidney clearance plays minor role in plasma clearance of carfilzomib.[256] Badros et al. investigated the pharmacokinetics in patients with renal impairment and saw that at 15 mg/m^2 proteasome inhibition did not differ between patients with no renal impairment, any CKD, and those on HD.[257]

Anaphylactic Lymphoma Kinase Tyrosine Kinase Inhibitors

The *anaplastic lymphoma kinase (ALK)* gene encodes the ALK receptor tyrosine kinase enzyme. Rearrangements in the *ALK* gene have been shown in a small subset of NSCLC.[258] Crizotinib is the first-generation ALK inhibitor approved in ALK-positive NSCLC. Adverse kidney effects reported with this drug include AKI, renal cyst formation and progression, hyponatremia, hypokalemia, and hypophosphatemia.[218] Along with NSCLC, crizotinib has also been used in other ALK positive cancers, such as anaplastic large cell lymphoma. Kothari et al. reported a case of a patient with renal impairment successfully treated with a dose of 250 mg once daily.[259] Published data regarding use of crizotinib in dialysis patients are not available.

Summary

Numerous case reports and cases series describe mostly empiric experience of anticancer therapy use in CKD patients. However, more pharmacokinetic studies and inclusion of patients with moderate to severe CKD in ongoing oncology clinical trials, are needed to further our understanding of safety and efficacy of anticancer drugs in CKD.

Key Points

- Growing numbers of patients with abnormal kidney function are exposed to anticancer therapies.
- Most of the data regarding dosing of anticancer therapy in patients with kidney dysfunction come from case reports and case series.
- Most of the conventional chemotherapy agents can be safely administered to patients with kidney disease with dose modification when appropriate.
- A growing body of evidence shows that most novel and biological anticancer therapies do not require significant dose adjustments when administered to patients with kidney dysfunction.

References

3. Flombaum CD. Nephrotoxicity of chemotherapy agents and chemotherapy administration in patients with renal disease. In: Cohen E, ed. *Cancer and the kidney: the frontier of nephrology and oncology.* New York, NY: Oxford University Press; 2011.

6. Bagley CM Jr, Bostick FW, DeVita VT Jr. Clinical pharmacology of cyclophosphamide. *Cancer Res.* 1973;33(2):226-233.

10. Wang LH, Lee CS, Majeske BL, Marbury TC. Clearance and recovery calculations in hemodialysis: application to plasma, red blood cells, and dialysate measurements for cyclophosphamide. *Clin Pharmacol Ther.* 1981;29(3):365-372.

16. Dechant KL, Brogden RN, Pilkington T, Faulds D. Ifosfamide/mesna. A review of its antineoplastic activity, pharmacokinetic properties and therapeutic efficacy in cancer. *Drugs.* 1991;42(3):428-467.

22. Latcha S, Maki RG, Schwartz GK, Flombaum CD. Ifosfamide may be safely used in patients with end stage renal disease on hemodialysis. *Sarcoma.* 2009;2009:575629.

23. Sauer H, Füger K, Blumenstein M. Modulation of cytotoxicity of cytostatic drugs by hemodialysis in vitro and in vivo. *Cancer Treat Rev.* 1990;17(2-3):293-300.

27. Osterborg A, Ehrsson H, Eksborg S, Wallin I, Mellstedt H. Pharmacokinetics of oral melphalan in relation to renal function in multiple myeloma patients. *Eur J Cancer Clin Oncol.* 1989;25(5):899-903.

28. Aronoff GA. *Drug prescribing in renal failure: dosing guidelines for adults and children.* 5th ed. Philadelphia, PA: ACP Press; 2007.

30. Batalini F, Econimo L, Quillen K, et al. High-dose melphalan and stem cell transplantation in patients on dialysis due to immunoglobulin light-chain amyloidosis and monoclonal immunoglobulin deposition disease. *Biol Blood Marrow Transplant.* 2018;24(1):127-132.

32. Newell DR, Hart LI, Harrap KR. Estimation of chlorambucil, phenyl acetic mustard and prednimustine in human plasma by high-performance liquid chromatography. *J Chromatogr.* 1979;164(1):114-119.

37. Ekhart C, Kerst JM, Rodenhuis S, Beijnen JH, Huitema AD. Altered cyclophosphamide and thiotepa pharmacokinetics in a patient with moderate renal insufficiency. *Cancer Chemother Pharmacol.* 2009; 63(2):375-379.

39. Ullery LL, Gibbs JP, Ames GW, Senecal FM, Slattery JT. Busulfan clearance in renal failure and hemodialysis. *Bone Marrow Transplant.* 2000;25(2):201-203.

42. Kintzel PE, Dorr RT. Anticancer drug renal toxicity and elimination: dosing guidelines for altered renal function. *Cancer Treat Rev.* 1995;21(1):33-64.

43. TNLC Network. *Dosage Adjustment for Cytotoxics in Renal Impairment.* 2009 [July 16, 2018]. Available at: http://www.londoncancer.org/media/65600/renal-impairment-dosage-adjustment-for-cytotoxics.pdf.

44. Boesler B, Czock D, Keller F, et al. Clinical course of haemodialysis patients with malignancies and dose-adjusted chemotherapy. *Nephrol Dial Transplant.* 2005;20(6):1187-1191.

53. Hendrayana T, Wilmer A, Kurth V, Schmidt-Wolf IG, Jaehde U. Anticancer dose adjustment for patients with renal and hepatic dysfunction: from scientific evidence to clinical application. *Sci Pharm.* 2017; 85(1):pii: E8.

57. Dhodapkar M, Rubin J, Reid JM, et al. Phase I trial of temozolomide (NSC 362856) in patients with advanced cancer. *Clin Cancer Res.* 1997;3(7):1093-1100.

59. Bleyer WA. The clinical pharmacology of methotrexate: new applications of an old drug. *Cancer.* 1978;41(1):36-51.

65. Wall SM, Johansen MJ, Molony DA, DuBose TD Jr, Jaffe N, Madden T. Effective clearance of methotrexate using high-flux hemodialysis membranes. *Am J Kidney Dis.* 1996;28(6):846-854.

67. Chan WK, Hui WF. Sequential use of hemoperfusion and single-pass albumin dialysis can safely reverse methotrexate nephrotoxicity. *Pediatr Nephrol.* 2016;31(10):1699-1703.

70. Adjei AA. Pharmacology and mechanism of action of pemetrexed. *Clin Lung Cancer.* 2004;5(suppl 2):S51-S55.

74. Rengelshausen J, Hull WE, Schwenger V, Göggelmann C, Walter-Sack I, Bommer J. Pharmacokinetics of 5-fluorouracil and its catabolites determined by 19F nuclear magnetic resonance spectroscopy for a patient on chronic hemodialysis. *Am J Kidney Dis.* 2002;39(2):E10.

78. Jhaveri KD, Flombaum C, Shah M, Latcha S. A retrospective observational study on the use of capecitabine in patients with severe renal impairment (GFR ,30 mL/min) and end stage renal disease on hemodialysis. *J Oncol Pharm Pract.* 2012;18(1):140-147.

97. Kiani A, Köhne CH, Franz T, et al. Pharmacokinetics of gemcitabine in a patient with end-stage renal disease: effective clearance of its

main metabolite by standard hemodialysis treatment. *Cancer Chemother Pharmacol.* 2003;51(3):266-270.

121. Owellen RJ, Root MA, Hains FO. Pharmacokinetics of vindesine and vincristine in humans. *Cancer Res.* 1977;37(8 Pt 1):2603-2607.

133. Woo MH, Gregornik D, Shearer PD, Meyer WH, Relling MV. Pharmacokinetics of paclitaxel in an anephric patient. *Cancer Chemother Pharmacol.* 1999;43(1):92-96.

146. Herrington JD, Figueroa JA, Kirstein MN, Zamboni WC, Stewart CF. Effect of hemodialysis on topotecan disposition in a patient with severe renal dysfunction. *Cancer Chemother Pharmacol.* 2001; 47(1):89-93.

152. Superfin D, Iannucci AA, Davies AM. Commentary: oncologic drugs in patients with organ dysfunction: a summary. *Oncologist.* 2007; 12(9):1070-1083.

153. Vénat-Bouvet L, Saint-Marcoux F, Lagarde C, Peyronnet P, Lebrun-Ly V, Tubiana-Mathieu N. Irinotecan-based chemotherapy in a metastatic colorectal cancer patient under haemodialysis for chronic renal dysfunction: two cases considered. *Anticancer Drugs.* 2007;18(8):977-980.

164. Yoshida H, Goto M, Honda A, et al. Pharmacokinetics of doxorubicin and its active metabolite in patients with normal renal function and in patients on hemodialysis. *Cancer Chemother Pharmacol.* 1994;33(6):450-454.

183. Gorodetsky R, Vexler A, Bar-Khaim Y, Biran H. Plasma platinum elimination in a hemodialysis patient treated with cisplatin. *Ther Drug Monit.* 1995;17(2):203-206.

186. Janus N, Thariat J, Boulanger H, Deray G, Launay-Vacher V. Proposal for dosage adjustment and timing of chemotherapy in hemodialyzed patients. *Ann Oncol.* 2010;21(7):1395-1403.

191. Calvert AH, Newell DR, Gumbrell LA, et al. Carboplatin dosage: prospective evaluation of a simple formula based on renal function. *J Clin Oncol.* 1989;7(11):1748-1756.

192. Janowitz T, Williams EH, Marshall A, et al. New model for estimating glomerular filtration rate in patients with cancer. *J Clin Oncol.* 2017;35(24):2798-2805.

193. Beumer JH, Inker LA, Levey AS. Improving carboplatin dosing based on estimated GFR. *Am J Kidney Dis.* 2018;71(2):163-165.

212. Garnier-Viougeat N, Rixe O, Paintaud G, et al. Pharmacokinetics of bevacizumab in haemodialysis. *Nephrol Dial Transplant.* 2007; 22(3):975.

217. Leonetti A, Bersanelli M, Castagneto B, et al. Outcome and safety of sorafenib in metastatic renal cell carcinoma dialysis patients: a systematic review. *Clin Genitourin Cancer.* 2016;14(4):277-283.

223. Micallef RA, Barrett-Lee PJ, Donovan K, Ashraf M, Williams L. Trastuzumab in patients on haemodialysis for renal failure. *Clin Oncol (R Coll Radiol).* 2007;19(7):559.

231. Fontana E, Pucci F, Ardizzoni A. Colorectal cancer patient on maintenance dialysis successfully treated with cetuximab. *Anticancer Drugs.* 2014;25(1):120-122.

232. Kobayashi M, Endo S, Hamano Y, et al. Successful treatment with modified FOLFOX6 and panitumumab in a cecal cancer patient undergoing hemodialysis. *Intern Med.* 2016;55(2):127-130.

235. Bersanelli M, Tiseo M, Artioli F, Lucchi L, Ardizzoni A. Gefitinib and afatinib treatment in an advanced non-small cell lung cancer (NSCLC) patient undergoing hemodialysis. *Anticancer Res.* 2014;34(6):3185-3188.

236. Togashi Y, Masago K, Fukudo M, et al. Pharmacokinetics of erlotinib and its active metabolite OSI-420 in patients with non-small cell lung cancer and chronic renal failure who are undergoing hemodialysis. *J Thorac Oncol.* 2010;5(5):601-605.

241. Herz S, Höfer T, Papapanagiotou M, et al. Checkpoint inhibitors in chronic kidney failure and an organ transplant recipient. *Eur J Cancer.* 2016;67:66-72.

246. Cavalcante L, Amin A, Lutzky J. Ipilimumab was safe and effective in two patients with metastatic melanoma and end-stage renal disease. *Cancer Manag Res.* 2015;7:47-50.

253. Chanan-Khan AA, Kaufman JL, Mehta J, et al. Activity and safety of bortezomib in multiple myeloma patients with advanced renal failure: a multicenter retrospective study. *Blood.* 2007;109(6):2604-2606.

257. Badros AZ, Vij R, Martin T, et al. Carfilzomib in multiple myeloma patients with renal impairment: pharmacokinetics and safety. *Leukemia.* 2013;27(8):1707-1714.

259. Kothari S, Ud-Din N, Lisi M, Coyle T. Crizotinib in anaplastic lymphoma kinase-positive anaplastic large cell lymphoma in the setting of renal insufficiency: a case report. *J Med Case Rep.* 2016;10:176.

A full list of references is available at Expertconsult.com

20 *Radiation Nephropathy*

ERIC P. COHEN

Definition

Radiation nephropathy is the kidney parenchymal injury and loss of function caused by radiation exposure to the kidneys. Its typical form is caused by external beam ionizing radiation, by x-rays or gamma-rays. It may also be caused by radioisotope therapies that irradiate kidneys internally. It is not common in current clinical practice but remains a risk of accidental or belligerent radiation exposures. The term *nephropathy* is preferred instead of nephritis, because radiation nephropathy does not have major inflammatory features.[1]

Historical Recognition

Radiation nephropathy was first recognized in 1927.[2] Earlier descriptions of kidney injury in irradiated subjects may have been caused by tumor lysis syndromes rather than true radiation injury to kidneys.[3] The best cohort studies are those of Luxton and colleagues, in which radiation nephropathy is described in men who had undergone external beam x-irradiation for treatment of seminoma.[4,5] After delivery of 20 Gy or more x-irradiation in fractionated doses, over a period of 4 weeks, approximately 20% of thus-treated subjects developed radiation nephropathy of varying severity. Similar presentations were reported in case reports and smaller series over the next 25 years, in both adults and children.[6–8] Structural and ultrastructural features were well-described.[7]

Epidemiology

There are two modern congeners of radiation nephropathy. The first occurs in subjects that have undergone hematopoietic stem cell transplantation (HSCT) that is preceded by total body irradiation, as part of the conditioning regimen.[1,9] This has been called *bone marrow transplant nephropathy* (*BMT nephropathy*). The second may complicate the use of internal radioisotope therapies.[10]

The 2017 Annual Data Report of the United States Renal Data System reports that of 700,000 prevalent patients on chronic dialysis in the USA, 159 have radiation nephropathy as their indicated cause of end-stage renal disease (ESRD). Eighty-nine patients on chronic dialysis are reported as a complication of HSCT.[11] It is likely that these are underestimates, because the 2728 forms that indicate the diagnosis of ESRD are not reliable.[12]

Clinical Features

Radiation nephropathy presents typically at 3 or more months after sufficient irradiation, with azotemia and hypertension. There is nonnephrotic proteinuria. The more severe variants may develop thrombocytopenia and even microangiopathic hemolytic anemia, reminiscent of hemolytic uremic syndrome (HUS) or thrombotic thrombocytopenic purpura (TTP).

Urinalysis shows proteinuria and microhematuria. The proteinuria is generally below the nephrotic range.

Radiation nephropathy may occur in children and in adults, in men and in women. No racial predisposition is known. But Judele et al. have reported complement regulatory defects in subjects who developed thrombotic microangiopathy after radiation-based HSCT, defects that are the same ones that are associated with HUS.[13] It is not known whether these complement regulatory defects predispose to usual radiation nephropathy.

Previous or concurrent use of chemotherapy, such as cyclophosphamide or cis-platinum, may predispose to radiation nephropathy, much as some chemotherapies predispose to normal tissue radiation injury generally.[14] It is likely, but not proven, that underlying kidney disease predisposes to radiation nephropathy.[15]

Dose Considerations

EXTERNAL BEAM

The dose of radiation required to predictably cause noncancerous normal tissue radiation injury is well above that used in diagnostic radiology. Thus a computed tomography scan of the abdomen delivers 1 centiGray (or "rad") to both kidneys, which is 1000-fold lower than the single fraction dose of 10 Gy that may cause radiation nephropathy. Because there is tissue repair in between fractions, a total radiation dose of 10 Gy, given in multiple fractions over a week or more, is not likely to cause kidney injury. But a higher total dose, for example, 20 Gy, given over 4 weeks, may well cause radiation nephropathy, as described by Luxton and others (vide supra).

The aforementioned dose considerations are valid for radiation fields that only expose the kidneys, and for partial or total body irradiation.

Irradiation of a single kidney and not the other may cause unilateral kidney arterial and or parenchymal injury, scarring, and renin-dependent hypertension, but not radiation nephropathy per se.[16,17] Despite improvements in treatment planning, this remains a current clinical issue for people undergoing radiotherapy of the upper abdomen. When the irradiation fields include the kidneys, kidney scarring ensues.[18]

RADIOISOTOPE

Administration of therapeutic radioisotope, for instance yttrium 90 attached to octreotide, may cause kidney injury by glomerular filtration of the radioisotope conjugate and its reabsorption by the kidney tubules.[10,19] The radiation injury is then local, with damage to tubules and glomeruli. It is difficult to calculate the exact irradiation dose, because it is delivered continuously, over days to weeks.

Use of radioisotope therapies may increase in the future, for instance with delivery of antibodies conjugated to beta- or gamma-emitting radioisotopes. The antibody provides the specificity and the isotope damages the targeted cancer cells. The pharmacokinetics of the conjugate will determine its potential kidney toxicity. Dose-finding studies should be done to identify the potential kidney doses, which will define whether a conjugate is safe for use.

As for diagnostic x-ray, use of diagnostic nuclear medicine isotope scanning poses no kidney risk because the doses are well below those that may cause injury to the kidneys.

Histology

The light microscopic appearance of radiation nephropathy is characteristic, with decreased glomerular cellularity, increased mesangial matrix, and mesangiolysis (Fig. 20.1).

There is no evidence for an immunopathogenesis of radiation nephropathy, which makes immunofluorescence studies unhelpful.

Electron microscopy often shows glomerular endothelial injury and dramatic expansion of the subendothelial space with a somewhat electron-lucent material (Fig. 20.2).

There is tubulointerstitial scarring, as is expected for any chronic kidney disease.

Testing

There is no specific blood test that is diagnostic of radiation nephropathy. There is also no specific imaging feature, although kidney parenchymal volume loss may be more marked than is typical for other chronic kidney diseases.[20] Palestro et al. did report a transient kidney positivity after bone scanning of two subjects that had been irradiated 9 months before,[21] but neither developed signs of radiation nephropathy.

The serum lactate dehydrogenase may be elevated in the more severe variants that occur after HSCT. Assays that indicate TTP are negative, such as those for ADAMSTS13 (a disintegrin and metalloproteinase with a thrombospondin type 1 motif, member 13) level or activity. But abnormalities of complement regulatory components have been reported in the thrombotic microangiopathy that can complicate HSCT.[22]

Differential Diagnosis

Acute kidney injury (AKI) in total or partial-body-irradiated subjects has been described, but does not have the features as described earlier. In addition, AKI has not been reported in subjects that have undergone local kidney irradiation.

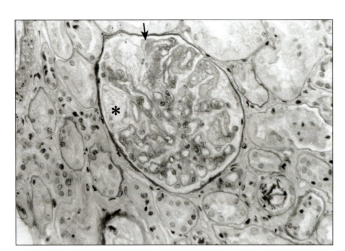

Fig. 20.1 Photomicrograph by light microscopy of a kidney biopsy specimen in a typical case of bone marrow transplant nephropathy. There is mesangiolysis (*asterisk*) and extreme widening of the space between the endothelium and glomerular basement membrane (*arrow*). The tubular epithelium is intact, but the tubules are separated by an expanded interstitium (PAS stain; magnification 250x). (Reproduced by permission from Cohen EP. Radiation nephropathy after bone marrow transplantation. *Kidney Int*. 2000;58(2):903-918; Figure 3.)

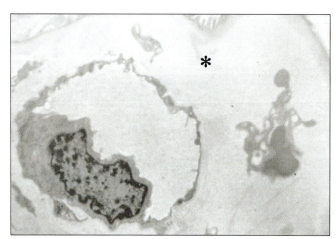

Fig. 20.2 Photomicrograph by electron microscopy of a kidney biopsy specimen in a typical case of bone marrow transplant nephropathy. Endothelial swelling and irregularity are present. There is extreme widening of the space between the endothelium and glomerular basement membrane (*asterisk*). No immune deposits are apparent, and the glomerular basement membrane itself does not appear abnormal. (Reproduced by permission from Cohen EP. Radiation nephropathy after bone marrow transplantation. *Kidney Int*. 2000;58(2):903-918; Figure 4.)

Thus the AKI in subjects that have undergone partial or total body irradiation appears more related to the multiorgan injury, volume depletion, and sepsis that such subjects may develop.[23]

In a subject who develops kidney disease after HSCT, there are multiple causes of both acute and chronic kidney disease. AKI within several weeks of irradiation is not likely to be caused by radiation nephropathy. Other causes of AKI should be sought, especially if the irradiation dose was below the usual thresholds. These include volume depletion, sepsis, and use of nephrotoxic therapies.

Medication use after allogeneic HSCT may include cyclosporine, tacrolimus, or sirolimus to prevent graftversus-host disease (GVHD). Each is potentially nephrotoxic, and the effects of the first two calcineurin inhibitors (CNIs) may be similar to radiation nephropathy. But withdrawal of the CNI should at least stabilize the loss of kidney function in cases of clear-cut CNI toxicity, whereas CNI withdrawal will not benefit radiation nephropathy. Sirolimus nephrotoxicity is less apt to cause hypertension, and more apt to cause significant proteinuria, and thus can be distinguished from radiation nephropathy.

GVHD after allogeneic HSCT can be complicated by kidney injury, in particular nephrotic syndrome. Kidney biopsy in these cases shows minimal change nephropathy, focal glomerulosclerosis, and even membranous nephropathy.[24] These features are not those of radiation nephropathy.

In a patient who has cancer, nephrotoxicities of chemotherapy must also be considered. Their cause and expression may be easy to recognize, as in the hypomagnesemic nephropathy caused by cis-platinum, or may be less specific, as in the interstitial nephritis caused by immunomodulators. Other chemotherapies, such as gemcitabine, may cause HUS-like syndromes that have clinical features similar to those of radiation nephropathy. The key differential feature is whether the patient has had kidney radiation exposure in a dose sufficient to cause injury.

Evolution

Luxton included milder forms of radiation nephropathy in his reports,[4] and it is possible that some kidney-irradiated patients merely develop proteinuria or hypertension without subsequent loss of kidney function. The modern congener of radiation nephropathy, "BMT nephropathy," appears however to be progressive, with loss of kidney function. We have described a biphasic loss of kidney function in such cases, with an initial rapid then a slower phase (Fig. 20.3). It is possible, but not established, that medical intervention causes the loss of function to become slower.

Pathophysiology: Experimental Models

There are well-established local kidney and total body irradiation models of radiation nephropathy.[25–27] Mice, rats, dogs, pigs, and monkeys have been used. The radiosensitivity of these species is not very different, although mice

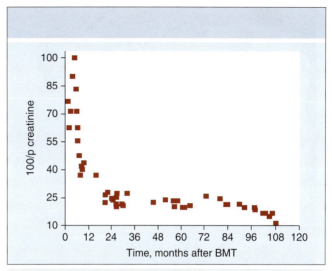

Fig. 20.3 Evolution of kidney function shown here as 100/plasma creatinine versus time in the patient that had the kidney biopsy as shown on Figs. 20.1 and 20.2. There is a biphasic pattern, with an initial rapid decline, then a plateau that culminated in end-stage kidney disease 9 years after bone marrow transplantation (BMT). (Reproduced by permission from Cohen EP. Radiation nephropathy after bone marrow transplantation. *Kidney Int.* 2000;58(2):903-918; Figure 5.)

can show a longer latency to expression of injury than do rats, pigs, and monkeys. The rat models are very useful because they show a similar radiation dose response, latency, and histopathology to the radiation nephropathy in humans. In addition to external beam models, there are also models of internal radioisotope radiation nephropathy in mice.[28]

TIME COURSE AND HISTOLOGY

In laboratory animals, single fraction local kidney or total body irradiation of 9 to 11 Gy causes a similar chronology of kidney injury.[29–31] Proteinuria occurs within 1 to 2 months after irradiation, followed by azotemia and hypertension. Histopathology studies show injury of all kidney tissues, including vasculature, glomeruli, tubular epithelium, and interstitium. The mesangiolysis of human radiation nephropathy is very evident in the rat model, less so in pigs or monkeys.

THE ROLE OF FIBROSIS

Progressive fibrosis of glomeruli and interstitium occurs in all models. An accentuation of peritubular fibrosis occurs at the origin of the proximal tubule in the rat, porcine, and monkey models of radiation nephropathy, and is called glomerulotubular neck stenosis[32,33] (Fig. 20.4). This feature has also been seen in BMT nephropathy, a modern congener of radiation nephropathy. It also occurs in other chronic progressive human kidney diseases.[34] It is likely to evolve to an atubular glomerulus,[35] which is a clear mechanism for how fibrosis itself can cause kidney function loss.[20]

THE RENIN ANGIOTENSIN SYSTEM

The rat model has been used to test whether radiation itself activates the renin-angiotensin system. There is

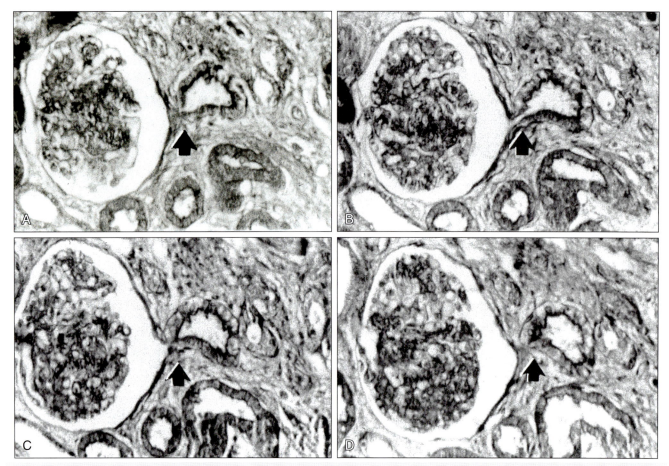

Fig. 20.4 A stenotic glomerulotubular neck in porcine radiation nephropathy. The *arrows* point to the stenotic neck, which appears to be constricted by surrounding fibrotic interstitium. The serial sections confirm that the neck stenosis is not an artefact. (Reproduced by permission from Cohen EP, Robbins ME, Whitehouse E, Hopewell JW. Stenosis of the tubular neck: a possible mechanism for progressive renal failure. *J Lab Clin Med.* 1997;129(5):567-573; Figure 4.)

thus far only scant evidence that the renin-angiotensin system is activated in radiation nephropathy. The benefit of angiotensin-converting enzyme inhibitors (ACEi) or angiotensin receptor blockers (ARB) to treat, prevent, and mitigate experimental radiation nephropathy may be via other mechanistic pathways.

Nonetheless, suppression of the renin-angiotensin system by a temporary high salt diet is associated with the significant mitigation benefit of the temporary high salt diet, when the latter is used in a rat model starting at 3 weeks after irradiation and ending at 10 weeks.[36]

OXIDATIVE STRESS

Although the initial effect of tissue irradiation is to cause double strand deoxyribonucleic acid breaks via immediate oxidative stress, the role of persistent chronic oxidative stress in radiation nephropathy is doubtful.[37] The antioxidants apocynin and genestein do not mitigate experimental radiation nephropathy.[38]

ENDOTHELIAL INJURY

Vascular injury has long been implicated in normal tissue radiation injury, including the kidneys. Human studies show reduction in kidney blood flow at doses as low as 400 rads

(cGy) and similar features are seen in laboratory animals.[39,40] Occlusion of blood vessels ranging from 10 to 100 microns in diameter occurs as a late effect in lung or kidney in rat models.[41] A high-dose 30 Gy local irradiation model in rats showed endothelial dysfunction with impaired endothelial dependent vasodilation.[42] More recently, we showed impaired endothelial-dependent vasodilation of preglomerular arterioles after an 11 Gy partial body irradiation single fraction exposure, also in a rat model.[43] This vascular effect was first evident at 3 weeks after irradiation and its severity increased at 6 then 12 weeks after irradiation. Impaired endothelial generation of epoxyeicosatrienoic acid (EET) metabolites correlates with this microvascular effect. Moreover, studies in the rat model of radiation nephropathy show the benefit of EET mimetics as mitigators.[44]

TREATMENT, PREVENTION, AND MITIGATION

Use of the radiation nephropathy model has enabled differentiation of treatment, prevention, and mitigation of normal tissue radiation injuries (Fig. 20.5). Although prevention of normal tissue radiation injuries may be possible with agents, such as amifostine, these are generally too toxic for human use. They would also not be useful for nonanticipated exposures, such as those caused by accident or terrorist events.

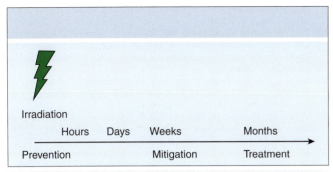

Irradiation

Hours   Days   Weeks   Months

Prevention   Mitigation   Treatment

Fig. 20.5 Diagram showing the concepts of prevention, mitigation, and treatment of radiation injury. Prevention is use of an agent starting before irradiation, whereas treatment is intervention once radiation injury has been expressed. In late responding normal tissues, such as lung or kidney, that is months after the initial irradiation. Mitigation is starting the mitigating agent after irradiation but before the tissue injury is evident.

Treatment of established normal tissue radiation injury was long felt to be limited to symptomatic management. We overturned this paradigm in 1992 by our report that the ACEi, captopril, could significantly slow the loss of kidney function in experimental radiation nephropathy.[45] We showed that the thiol group of captopril was not necessary for this benefit, because enalapril is similarly beneficial.[46] ARBs were subsequently shown to be effective.[47]

We established that ACE inhibitors were also effective in preventing radiation nephropathy, when these agents are started before irradiation.[30] Those studies also showed that the preventive benefit of captopril did not depend on maintaining normal blood pressure.

We then showed the effect of mitigation, which is starting an agent after irradiation but before the expression of tissue injury. Thus captopril and other ACE inhibitors can be started up to 3 weeks after irradiation and exert a beneficial effect on the later development of proteinuria, azotemia, and hypertension.[48] The mitigation paradigm has been extended to other normal tissue injuries, notably to lung and brain.[49–51] Use of an agent as a mitigator means that such agents can be used after radiation accidents or belligerent exposures. That is very significant for such non-planned events.

As stated earlier, EET mimetics have a significant and beneficial mitigation effect on experimental radiation nephropathy,[44] which is near to the benefit achieved by captopril. In addition, selenium compounds exert a mitigating benefit, but they have not been tested in direct comparison to ACEi.[52]

We also showed that a temporary high salt diet was effective to mitigate the later occurrence of radiation nephropathy in a rat model.[36] This benefit was associated with suppression of the renin-angiotensin system. Review of the literature has revealed past studies that tested dietary protein restriction and also dexamethasone in radiation nephropathy models in laboratory animals.[53,54] These reports have not been confirmed.

Clinical Prevention

Complete avoidance of kidneys during radiotherapy will prevent radiation nephropathy from occurring. The dose and volume constraints that apply to kidney irradiation may be summarized by the volume of kidneys that receive 20 Gy or more fractionated irradiation. If that volume is greater than 30%, there is a more than 5% risk of significant kidney radiation injury.[55]

It is not known whether diet or medication enable prevention of human radiation nephropathy.

Mitigation

Mitigation is the use of an agent after irradiation, but before the expression of tissue injury from irradiation. As reviewed previously, this approach has been successful in laboratory animals, for normal tissue radiation injuries to brain, lungs, and kidney. We translated these data in a prospective randomized double-blind controlled trial of captopril versus placebo in subjects that had undergone radiation-based HSCT.[56] We found that captopril reduced the occurrence of the BMT nephropathy syndrome, although this effect did not achieve statistical significance.

Treatment

Although the experimental results in laboratory animals support the use of ACE inhibitors or ARBs as the preferred agents to treat radiation nephropathy, there are no controlled data to justify that specific approach in human medicine. Instead, the general guidelines for treatment of hypertensive chronic kidney disease apply. In our experience, about 75% of subjects with the BMT nephropathy variant will need diuretics for control of their blood pressure.[1] Because of the tendency of these patients to develop hyperkalemia, using ACE inhibitors or ARBs may not be possible.

As noted earlier, reduction of dietary protein may mitigate radiation nephropathy in rats. It is not known whether dietary protein reduction is preferentially effective for human radiation nephropathy.

Prognosis

Radiation nephropathy may cause complete kidney failure, in which case dialysis or kidney transplant are needed. Survival of such patients on chronic dialysis is lower than average, perhaps because of their comorbidities that include past cancer and the immunosuppressive effect of their HSCT.[57] Some of these patients have undergone kidney transplantation; they are fully immunotolerant of the transplanted kidney if that kidney comes from the same donor as the HSCT.[58]

Key Points

- Radiation nephropathy is less common now than it was 60 years ago because radiation therapy is more precisely guided and because of other nonradiation therapies for cancer. It remains a possible occurrence after hematopoietic stem cell transplant and after use of radioisotope therapies.

- Radiation nephropathy is a chronic fibrosing kidney disease, without major inflammatory features.
- Studies in laboratory animals have identified the role of endothelial dysfunction, fibrosis, and also of the renin-angiotensin system in the pathogenesis of radiation nephropathy.
- It is possible to both mitigate and treat human radiation nephropathy.

References

1. Cohen EP. Radiation nephropathy after bone marrow transplantation. *Kidney Int.* 2000;58(2):903-918.
2. Domagk G. Die Roentgenstrahlung wirkung auf das Gewebe, im besonderen betrachtet an den Nieren. *Beitr z Path Anat u z allg Path.* 1927;77:525-575.
3. Warthen AS. The changes produced in the kidneys by Rontgen irradiation. *Am J Med Sci.* 1907;113:736-746.
4. Luxton RW. Radiation nephritis. A long-term study of 54 patients. *Lancet.* 1961;2(7214):1221-1224.
5. Luxton RW, Kunkler PB. Radiation nephritis. *Acta Radiol Ther Phys Biol.* 1964;2:169-178.
6. Rosen S, Swerdlow MA, Muehrcke RC, Pirani CL. Radiation nephritis; light and electron microscopic observations. *Am J Clin Pathol.* 1964;41:487-502.
7. Keane WF, Crosson JT, Staley NA, Anderson WR, Shapiro FL. Radiation-induced renal disease. A clinicopathologic study. *Am J Med.* 1976;60(1):127-137.
8. Cogan MG, Arieff AI. Radiation nephritis and intravascular coagulation. *Clin Nephrol.* 1978;10(2):74-78.
9. Antignac C, Gubler MC, Leverger G, Broyer M, Habib R. Delayed renal failure with extensive mesangiolysis following bone marrow transplantation. *Kidney Int.* 1989;35(6):1336-1344.
10. Lambert B, Cybulla M, Weiner SM, et al. Renal toxicity after radionuclide therapy. *Radiat Res.* 2004;161(5):607-611.
13. Rotz SJ, Luebbering N, Dixon BP, et al. In vitro evidence of complement activation in transplantation-associated thrombotic microangiopathy. *Blood Adv.* 2017;1(20):1632-1634.
14. Phillips TL, Wharam MD, Margolis LW. Modification of radiation injury to normal tissues by chemotherapeutic agents. *Cancer.* 1975;35(6):1678-1684.
15. Bodei L, Cremonesi M, Ferrari M, et al. Long-term evaluation of renal toxicity after peptide receptor radionuclide therapy with 90Y-DOTATOC and 177Lu-DOTATATE: the role of associated risk factors. *Eur J Nucl Med Mol Imaging.* 2008;35(10):1847-1856.
17. Staab GE, Tegtmeyer CJ, Constable WC. Radiation-induced renovascular hypertension. *AJR Am J Roentgenol.* 1976;126(3):634-637.
18. Tran LK, Maturen KE, Feng MU, et al. Renal remodeling after abdominal radiation therapy: parenchymal and functional changes. *AJR Am J Roentgenol.* 2014;203(2):W192-W198.
19. Cohen EP, Robbins ME. Radiation nephropathy. *Semin Nephrol.* 2003;23(5):486-499.
20. Cohen EP. Fibrosis causes progressive kidney failure. *Med Hypotheses.* 1995;45(5):459-462.
21. Palestro C, Fineman D, Goldsmith SJ. Acute radiation nephritis. Its evolution on sequential bone imaging. *Clin Nucl Med.* 1988;13(11):789-791.
23. Fliedner TM, D Dörr H, Meineke V. Multi-organ involvement as a pathogenetic principle of the radiation syndromes: a study involving 110 case histories documented in SEARCH and classified as the bases of haematopoietic indicators of effect. *BJR Suppl.* 2005;27:1-8.
25. Moulder JE, Fish BL. Late toxicity of total body irradiation with bone marrow transplantation in a rat model. *Int J Radiat Oncol Biol Phys.* 1989;16(6):1501-1509.
26. van Kleef EM, Zurcher C, Oussoren YG, et al. Long-term effects of total-body irradiation on the kidney of Rhesus monkeys. *Int J Radiat Biol.* 2000;76(5):641-648.
27. Unthank JL, Miller SJ, Quickery AK, et al. Delayed effects of acute radiation exposure in a murine model of the h-ars: multiple-organ injury consequent to <10 Gy total body irradiation. *Health Phys.* 2015;109(5):511-521.
28. Jaggi JS, Seshan SV, McDevitt MR, LaPerle K, Sgouros G, Scheinberg DA. Renal tubulointerstitial changes after internal irradiation with alpha-particle-emitting actinium daughters. *J Am Soc Nephrol.* 2005;16(9):2677-2689.
29. Robbins ME, Jaenke RS, Bywaters T, et al. Sequential evaluation of radiation-induced glomerular ultrastructural changes in the pig kidney. *Radiat Res.* 1993;135(3):351-364.
30. Cohen EP, Moulder JE, Fish BL, Hill P. Prophylaxis of experimental bone marrow transplant nephropathy. *J Lab Clin Med.* 1994;124(3):371-380.
31. Moulder JE, Cohen EP, Fish BL. Captopril and losartan for mitigation of renal injury caused by single-dose total-body irradiation. *Radiat Res.* 2011;175(1):29-36.
32. Cohen EP, Robbins ME, Whitehouse E, Hopewell JW. Stenosis of the tubular neck: a possible mechanism for progressive renal failure. *J Lab Clin Med.* 1997;129(5):567-573.
33. Cohen EP, Regner K, Fish BL, Moulder JE. Stenotic glomerulotubular necks in radiation nephropathy. *J Pathol.* 2000;190(4):484-488.
34. Cohen EP. Stenosis of the glomerulotubular neck. *Nephron.* 2002;92(2):259-262.
36. Moulder JE, Fish BL, Cohen EP. Dietary sodium modification and experimental radiation nephropathy. *Int J Radiat Biol.* 2002;78(10):903-911.
37. Cohen SR, Cohen EP. Chronic oxidative stress after irradiation: an unproven hypothesis. *Med Hypotheses.* 2013;80(2):172-175.
38. Cohen EP, Fish BL, Irving AA, Rajapurkar MM, Shah SV, Moulder JE. Radiation nephropathy is not mitigated by antagonists of oxidative stress. *Radiat Res.* 2009;172(2):260-264.
39. Avioli LV, Lazor MZ, Cotlove E, Brace KC, Andrews JR. Early effects of radiation on renal function in man. *Am J Med.* 1963;34:329-337.
40. Robbins ME, Campling D, Rezvani M, Golding SJ, Hopewell JW. Radiation nephropathy in mature pigs following the irradiation of both kidneys. *Int J Radiat Biol.* 1989;56(1):83-98.
41. Cohen EP, Molteni A, Hill P, et al. Captopril preserves function and ultrastructure in experimental radiation nephropathy. *Lab Invest.* 1996;75(3):349-360.
42. Juncos LI, Cornejo JC, Gomes J, Baigorria S, Juncos LA. Abnormal endothelium-dependent responses in early radiation nephropathy. *Hypertension.* 1997;30(3 Pt 2):672-676.
43. Imig JD, Hye Khan MA, Sharma A, Fish BL, Mandel NS, Cohen EP. Radiation-induced afferent arteriolar endothelial-dependent dysfunction involves decreased epoxygenase metabolites. *Am J Physiol Heart Circ Physiol.* 2016;310(11):H1695-H1701.
44. Hye Khan MA, Fish B, Wahl G, et al. Epoxyeicosatrienoic acid analogue mitigates kidney injury in a rat model of radiation nephropathy. *Clin Sci. (Lond).* 2016;130(8):587-599.
45. Cohen EP, Fish BL, Moulder JE. Treatment of radiation nephropathy with captopril. *Radiat Res.* 1992;132(3):346-350.
46. Moulder JE, Fish BL, Cohen EP. Treatment of radiation nephropathy with ACE inhibitors. *Int J Radiat Oncol Biol Phys.* 1993;27(1):93-99.
47. Moulder JE, Fish BL, Cohen EP. Angiotensin II receptor antagonists in the treatment and prevention of radiation nephropathy. *Int J Radiat Biol.* 1998;73(4):415-421.
48. Cohen EP, Fish BL, Moulder JE. Successful brief captopril treatment in experimental radiation nephropathy. *J Lab Clin Med.* 1997;129(5):536-547.
49. Kim JH, Brown SL, Kolozsvary A, et al. Modification of radiation injury by ramipril, inhibitor of angiotensin-converting enzyme, on optic neuropathy in the rat. *Radiat Res.* 2004;161(2):137-142.
50. Gao F, Fish BL, Moulder JE, Jacobs ER, Medhora M. Enalapril mitigates radiation-induced pneumonitis and pulmonary fibrosis if started 35 days after whole-thorax irradiation. *Radiat Res.* 2013;180(5):546-552.
52. Sieber F, Muir SA, Cohen EP, et al. Dietary selenium for the mitigation of radiation injury: effects of selenium dose escalation and timing of supplementation. *Radiat Res.* 2011;176(3):366-374.
53. Geraci JP, Mariano MS, Jackson KL. Amelioration of radiation nephropathy in rats by dexamethasone treatment after irradiation. *Radiat Res.* 1993;134(1):86-93.
54. Robbins ME, Bywaters T, Jaenke RS, et al. Influence of a low protein diet on radiation nephropathy in the pig. *Int J Radiat Biol.* 1993;64(4):407-416.

55. Dawson LA, Kavanagh BD, Paulino AC, et al. Radiation-associated kidney injury. *Int J Radiat Oncol Biol Phys.* 2010;76(suppl 3): S108-S115.
56. Cohen EP, Bedi M, Irving AA, et al. Mitigation of late renal and pulmonary injury after hematopoietic stem cell transplantation. *Int J Radiat Oncol Biol Phys.* 2012;83(1):292-296.
57. Cohen EP, Piering WF, Kabler-Babbitt C, Moulder JE. End-stage renal disease (ESRD) after bone marrow transplantation: poor survival compared to other causes of ESRD. *Nephron.* 1998;79(4): 408-412.
58. Butcher JA, Hariharan S, Adams MB, Johnson CP, Roza AM, Cohen EP. Renal transplantation for end-stage renal disease following bone marrow transplantation: a report of six cases, with and without immunosuppression. *Clin Transplant.* 1999;13(4):330-335.

A full list of references is available at Expertconsult.com

Paraneoplastic Glomerulopathies

21 Paraneoplastic Glomerular Diseases

JONATHAN J. HOGAN AND JAI RADHAKRISHNAN

Introduction

Paraneoplastic syndromes refer to manifestations of cancer that are not related to tumor burden, invasion, or metastatic disease.[1] The manifestations may be systemic or organ-limited and can involve virtually any organ system.[2] There is a paucity of literature on paraneoplastic kidney disease (PnKD), likely because of the rarity of these conditions. This narrative review will focus on PnKDs that occur in the setting of solid tumors and hematologic malignancies.

Because most of the literature on the epidemiology of PnKD comprises case reports and case series, the incidence and prevalence of PnKD are difficult to ascertain.[3] Some data have shown that the risk for cancer is higher in patients with glomerular disease than in the general population. For example, the Danish Kidney Biopsy Registry, which includes all kidney biopsies performed in Denmark since 1985, reported that the risk for cancer at 1 year and 1 to 4 years after the diagnosis of glomerulopathy was increased by 2.4- and 3.5-fold, respectively, compared with the general population.[4] In a population-based study in Tromsø, Norway (originally designed to evaluate cardiovascular disease), the albumin-creatinine ratio at baseline for patients with glomerular disease significantly correlated with the incidence of cancer during 10 years of follow-up. Further, those with albumin-creatinine ratios in the highest quintile were 8.3- and 2.4-fold more likely to be diagnosed with bladder cancer and lung cancer compared with the lowest quintile.[4,5]

The pathophysiology of PnKD is usually linked to products of tumor cells or from paraneoplastic autoimmune manifestations that cause kidney damage.[1,2] This mechanism is well-characterized in certain paraneoplastic neurologic syndromes. For example, anti-Hu (ANNA1) antibody in the setting of small cell lung cancer is associated with encephalomyelitis, sensory neuropathy, and paraneoplastic cerebellar degeneration, and anti-Yo (PCA1) antibody in ovarian and breast cancers is associated with paraneoplastic cerebellar degeneration.[6] However, with the exception of monoclonal gammopathies, the exact pathomechanisms linking tumor products and renal disease are poorly understood.

In patients diagnosed with PnKD, the temporal profile of the cancer diagnosis and kidney manifestations may be asynchronous. It is generally accepted that malignancies are present for up to several years before becoming clinically apparent. Patrone et al. applied a modified version of Collins' law,[7] which was originally used to estimate the time-to-recurrence of Pediatric Wilms tumors, in order to estimate the time-to-recurrence of adult solid tumors.[8] Further, if more than 6 years have elapsed since remission

of the cancer, it is unlikely that a glomerulopathy is related to the malignancy. To illustrate this point further, in the study by Lefaucher et al., the tumor was clinically evident in only 52% of the patients, underscoring the fact that cancers may be clinically silent and unless looked for systemically, may lead to unnecessary treatment of membranous nephropathy (MN).

The lack of published criteria for PnKD makes it challenging to distinguish between kidney disease occurring coincidentally in a patient with cancer and true PnKD. Box 21.1 summarizes "criteria" that have been suggested to help strengthen the link between cancer and kidney disease, when suspected.[9] There are several case reports that satisfy criteria 1 and 2, but criteria 3 is generally lacking. The exceptions are plasma cell dyscrasias and B-cell disorders, which produce monoclonal antibodies that are directly toxic to the kidney.[10]

Among the PnKD, and despite not meeting criteria 3, solid tumor-associated MN and Hodgkin lymphoma-associated minimal change disease (MCD) have become recognized as typical forms of paraneoplastic glomerulonephritides. Other glomerular diseases mentioned in this chapter are rarely associated with cancer, with the association between the kidney lesions and cancer infrequently fulfilling the criteria listed.

Finally, it is important to note that treatment paradigms for PnKD may be quite different from noncancer-related glomerular disease, in that the main strategy in PnKD is treatment of the underlying cancer. Patients with Hodgkin disease-associated podocytopathy[11] and solid cancer-associated MN[12] are frequently resistant to immunosuppressive regimens that are traditionally used in these entities but respond well to treatment of the cancer.

Paraneoplastic Kidney Diseases in Patients With Hematologic Malignancies

Paraprotein-associated disorders are caused by clonal plasma or B-cell populations that produce monoclonal immunoglobulins (Igs), which may cause kidney damage. These antibodies have physiochemical properties that lead to specific types of kidney injury, leading to a variety of histologic patterns on kidney biopsy (Box 21.2). An important point to emphasize is that the presence of end-organ damage may prompt treatment even if the underlying clone does not officially meet criteria for cancer. This necessitates familiarity with the criteria for overt multiple myeloma, smoldering multiple myeloma, and monoclonal gammopathy

Box 21.1   Criteria for Renal Paraneoplastic Syndromes

1. A renal syndrome and cancer that develop concurrently or within a few years of each other
2. The renal syndrome resolves or improves significantly after cancer treatment without immunotherapy and relapses with recurrence of cancer
3. A pathophysiologic link is present between the cancer and kidney disease

Data from Cambier JF, Ronco P. Onco-nephrology: glomerular diseases with cancer. *Clin J Am Soc Nephrol.* 2012;7(10):1701-1712.

Box 21.2   Kidney Diseases Caused by Pathogenic Monoclonal Immunoglobulins

Myeloma (light chain) cast nephropathy
Monoclonal immunoglobulin deposition disease
  Light chain deposition disease
  Heavy chain deposition disease
  Heavy and light chain deposition disease
Light chain proximal tubulopathy
Type I cryoglobulinemic glomerulonephritis
Paraprotein-associated C3 glomerulonephritis
Proliferative glomerulonephritis with monoclonal immunoglobulin deposits
Monoclonal immunoglobulin (AL/light chain, AH/heavy chain, ALH/light and heavy chain) amyloidosis
Immunotactoid glomerulopathy

Box 21.3   Criteria for Overt Multiple Myeloma, Smoldering Multiple Myeloma, and Monoclonal Gammopathy of Undetermined Significance

Multiple Myeloma

Clonal plasma cells in the bone marrow $\geq$ 10%, or biopsy-proven plasmacytoma, and any myeloma-defining event (hypercalcemia, renal insufficiency, anemia, bone lesions)
Any of the following:
- Clonal plasma cells in the bone marrow $\geq$ 60%
- Serum free light chain ratio of $\geq$ 100 (involved/uninvolved)
- More than 1 focal lesion on MRI

Smoldering Multiple Myeloma

Serum M protein (IgG or IgA) $\geq$ 30 g/L or urine M protein $\geq$ 500 mg/24 hours and/or 10%–60% clonal plasma cells in the bone marrow AND no evidence of myeloma defining events or amyloidosis

Monoclonal Gammopathy of Undetermined Significance

Presence of monoclonal gammopathy:
- serum concentration of IgM or non-IgM monoclonal protein < 30 g/L
- abnormal serum free light chain ratio (with increased level of involved light chain)
- urinary monoclonal protein < 500 mg/24 hours
< 10% clonal plasma cells on bone marrow biopsy
No evidence of myeloma defining event, amyloidosis, or systemic lymphoma[75]

Ig, Immunoglobulin; *M*, monoclonal; *MRI*, magnetic resonance imaging.
Modified from Rajkumar SV, Dimopoulos MA, Palumbo A, et al. International Myeloma Working Group updated criteria for the diagnosis of multiple myeloma. *Lancet Oncol.* 2014;15(12):e538-548.

of undetermined significance (MGUS) (Box 21.3). For example, the majority of patients with AL (light chain) amyloidosis have >10% clonal plasma cells found on bone marrow biopsy, and thus do not meet criteria for multiple myeloma. Nonetheless, the kidneys are commonly affected by AL amyloidosis, and the disease itself is associated with significant morbidity and mortality. Similarly, in other paraprotein diseases of the kidney, the presence and detection of renal involvement may be the factor that prompts treatment of the underlying clone. In this section, we will highlight selected paraprotein-mediated disorders. Many of these are discussed in Chapters 6-9.

MYELOMA CAST NEPHROPATHY

Although not a glomerular disease, myeloma cast nephropathy (MCN), also known as *myeloma kidney*, is a prototypical paraneoplastic renal disease. The pathogenesis of cast nephropathy is linked to the binding of Ig free light chains to uromodulin (Tamm-Horsfall protein), causing tubulointerstitial injury via precipitation of light chain casts in the distal nephron. This occurs via interaction or via the binding of free light chain complementary determining region-3 with the light chain binding domain of uromodulin.[13,14] The incidence of MCN is not known because the vast majority of patients with myeloma do not undergo a kidney biopsy. Severe renal failure (often requiring dialysis) is common in patients presenting with biopsy-proven MCN,[15] and compared with other kidney diseases associated

with monoclonal gammopathies, the diagnosis of MCN is supported if only a small percentage of total proteinuria is composed of albumin.[16] Having MCN on kidney biopsy portends a worse overall prognosis than having light chain deposition alone.[17]

The first principle of treating MCN is to rapidly lower serum free light chain levels by targeting the underlying plasma cell clone, which is associated with improved renal outcomes.[15] Antiplasma cell strategies have expanded greatly in the last 2 decades, including the proteasome inhibitor bortezomib (US Food and Drug Administration–approved for the treatment of multiple myeloma in 2003) and high-dose melphalan/autologous stem cell transplantation. Patients achieving renal response with treatment have improved overall and renal survival[18] (Table 21.1).

The use of adjunctive, extracorporeal therapies for additional light chain removal is controversial. Plasma exchange therapy has been used with mixed results in randomized controlled trials and retrospective case series.[19–22] The interpretation of these data is complicated by small patient numbers, the small percentage of patients undergoing a kidney biopsy to confirm the diagnosis of MCN, and their publication before the era of modern antiplasma cell therapies.

High cut-off hemodialysis has been advocated in MCN with the theoretical benefit of removing pathogenic light

Table 21.1 Candidate Renal Response Criteria in Multiple Myeloma

Renal Response	eGFR at Baseline (mL/min/1.73m^2)	Best Creatinine Clearance
Complete response	< 50	> 60 mL/min
Partial response	< 15	30–59 mL/min
Minor response	< 15	15–29 mL/min
	15–29	30–59 mL/min

eGFR, Estimated glomerular filtration rate based on the Modification of Diet in Renal Disease or Chronic Kidney Disease-Epidemiology Equation.
Data from Palladini G, Dispenzieri A, Gertz MA, et al. New criteria for response to treatment in immunoglobulin light chain amyloidosis based on free light chain measurement and cardiac biomarkers: impact on survival outcomes. J Clin Oncol. 2012;30(36):4541-4549.

chains from the circulation.[23] A recently published study randomized 98 patients in France with renal failure requiring dialysis and biopsy-proven MCN to treatment with intensive high cut-off hemodialysis versus conventional dialysis, in addition to standardized chemotherapy (bortezomib with dexamethasone).[24] Dialysis independence was not different between treatment arms at 3 months (primary endpoint, 41% vs. 33%, p=.42), although more patients treated with high cut-off dialysis were dialysis-free at 12 months (secondary endpoint, 61% vs. 38%, p=.02). The EuLite (EUropean trial of free LIght chain removal by exTEnded haemodialysis in cast nephropathy) study is another randomized controlled trial studying high cut-off dialysis in MCN, the results of which are forthcoming[25] (clinicaltrials.gov ID NCT00700531).

There has also been interest in treating cast nephropathy by inhibiting the interaction of free light chains with uromodulin in the nephron. A competitive inhibitor of this interaction prevents renal failure in a rat model of MCN.[14] No studies have been published to date exploring this approach in humans.

LIGHT CHAIN (AL) AMYLOIDOSIS

Light chain (AL) amyloidosis is a paraneoplastic disease where within an amyloidogenic monoclonal Ig light chains deposit organs and cause damage. Heavy chain (AH) and light/heavy chain (ALH) amyloidosis occur when the amyloidogenic protein is composed of heavy or light + heavy chains, respectively. These are much less common and are approached similarly to AL amyloidosis, and will not be discussed further. The majority of cases of AL amyloidosis are caused by plasma cell clones that do not meet criteria for multiple myeloma, with B or lymphoplasmacytic clones being rare. The kidney is one of the most common organs affected in AL amyloidosis, with up to 70% of patients demonstrating renal involvement, and which presents with proteinuria (commonly nephrotic syndrome) and renal insufficiency. It should also be noted that patients with vascular and interstitial renal AL amyloidosis (i.e., without glomerular involvement) can present with minimal proteinuria.[26]

Historically, the prognosis for patients with AL amyloidosis has been extremely poor. The median survival after diagnosis was 7 months until the 1990s, when treatment with melphalan and prednisone was shown to extend patient survival. Subsequently, the use of high-dose melphalan followed by autologous stem cell transplantation, and bortezomib-based chemotherapeutic regimens, have dramatically improved patient outcomes. The presence and degree of cardiac involvement are the main determinants of patient survival, and cardiac response (changes in N-terminal pro b-type natriuretic peptide levels) with treatment are associated with survival.[27] Baseline renal parameters (estimated glomerular filtration rate [eGFR] and proteinuria) and their response to therapy may be predictive of renal survival in AL amyloidosis. Renal progression ($\geq$ 25% decrease in eGFR) may be associated with worse renal prognosis, whereas renal response (> 30% decrease in proteinuria to < 0.5 g/day and nonprogression of eGFR) is associated with improved renal outcomes. Recent data suggest that patients with end-stage renal disease may benefit from treatment with high-dose melphalan followed by autologous stem cell transplantation, which then may allow them to undergo successful kidney transplantation.[28]

The renal response to therapy may be much slower than that observed for other glomerular diseases, possibly because the amyloid that has deposited in the kidneys may persist for years after treatment. Emerging adjunctive therapies include antiamyloid antibodies to improve organ function by removing amyloid deposits.[29,30]

The Monoclonal Immunoglobulin Deposition Diseases

The monoclonal immunoglobulin deposition diseases (MIDDs) comprise light chain deposition disease (LCDD), heavy chain deposition disease (HCDD), and light and heavy chain deposition disease (LHCDD). LCDD is the most common of the MIDDs, and the majority of cases occur in the setting of multiple myeloma or nonmyeloma plasma cell clones.[31] On kidney biopsy, immunofluorescence microscopy shows staining for kappa, or less commonly lambda, light chain, without staining for Ig heavy chain. Although glomerular involvement is common, the pathognomonic finding on kidney biopsy is the presence of light chain deposits in the tubular basement membranes. Extrarenal involvement may occur, with one recent series of patients with multiple myeloma and LCDD finding cardiac involvement in one-third of patients.[32]

HCDD is much less common than LCDD and is characterized by immunofluorescence staining for Ig heavy chain without light chain on kidney biopsy. IgG is the most common involved heavy chain with IgA HCDD being less common. The molecular characterization of HCDD is based on a deletion in the heavy chain constant domain 1 (CH1) region of the Ig, which results in the production and secretion of a truncated heavy chain by plasma cells that in turn deposits in the kidney. Indeed, virtually all patients with HCDD have this mutation, and HCDD can be reproduced in a mouse model by introducing the CH1 mutation.[33] Antiplasma cell therapy, including bortezomib-based regimens and high-dose melphalan/autologous stem cell transplantation, results in hematologic response rates in the majority of patients, and renal response is predicated on attaining hematologic response.[31,34]

LYMPHOPLASMACYTIC LYMPHOMA/ WALDENSTRÖM MACROGLOBULINEMIA

Lymphoplasmacytic lymphoma, also known as *Waldenström macroglobulinemia*, results in the production of IgM proteins that can cause end-organ damage. Renal disease is rare, with a recent case series describing 3% of patients with lymphoplasmacytic lymphoma developing kidney disease.[35] However, the presence of monoclonal IgM deposition on kidney biopsy should raise suspicion for lymphoplasmacytic lymphomas, because a recent retrospective series found that lymphoplasmacytic lymphoma was present in (74%) of patients with IgM-mediated kidney disease.[36] The IgM paraprotein in lymphoplasmacytic lymphoma may exhibit amyloidogenic or cryoglobulinemic properties, with kidney biopsy findings,[35] and a variety of histologies can be observed on kidney biopsy (amyloidosis, infiltration by the lymphoplasmacytic lymphoma, LCDD, light chain cast nephropathy). As with all paraprotein-mediated kidney diseases, management of monoclonal IgM-mediated kidney disease focuses on treatment of the underlying lymphoplasmacytic clone.

Type I Cryoglobulinemic Glomerulonephritis

Cryoglobulins are Igs that have the physiochemical property of precipitating at cold temperatures. Type I cryoglobulins are monoclonal Igs that have the properties of cryoglobulins, and these proteins are produced by underlying B- or plasma cell clones. Recent case series have described type I cryoglobulins comprising 10% to 22% of all detectable cryoglobulins, with the remaining containing mixed (including polyclonal) Igs. More than half of patients have cutaneous involvement, and renal disease occurs in 14% to 20% of patients, with glomerulonephritis being the most common finding on kidney biopsy.[37,38]

The kidney biopsies in patients with type I cryoglobulinemic renal disease usually show endocapillary or membranoproliferative glomerulonephritis on light microscopy. Cryoplugs (periodic acid–Schiff-positive, microvascular thrombi) and/or overt vasculitis may be present in some cases. Congo red staining is negative except in rare cases where the cryoglobulin also has amyloidogenic properties. Immunofluorescence microscopy exhibits staining for the involved monoclonal Ig. On electron microscopy, the cryoglobulins manifest as electron dense deposits in a subendothelial and mesangial distribution. These deposits may exhibit organized substructure in the form of large fibrils, tactoids, and microtubules.[39] Management of type I cryoglobulinemic glomerulonephritis focuses on diagnosis and treatment of the underlying clonal cell disorder. Plasma exchange therapy has been used in cases of severe, life-threatening vasculitis and rapidly progressive glomerulonephritis.

MONOCLONAL GAMMOPATHIES OF RENAL SIGNIFICANCE

The monoclonal gammopathies of renal significance (MGRS) do not meet criteria for multiple myeloma or systemic lymphoma. Histologically, these can result in many of the biopsy findings found in Box 21.2. These renal pathologies can be found in patients with myeloma or lymphoma, but the majority of cases do not meet criteria

for malignancy.[31,40,41] Similar to multiple myeloma and AL amyloidosis, the diagnosis and treatment focuses on the underlying clonal cell disorder, and recent data support that achieving a hematologic response is associated with renal outcomes in these patients.[31]

A specific challenge exists in MGRS cases where the workup does not reveal evidence of an underlying plasma or B-cell clone. This is the case for the majority of patients with proliferative glomerulonephritis with mononuclear immunoglobulin deposits, and these patients also commonly do not have a detectable paraprotein in the blood or urine. One hypothesis to explain this discrepancy is that these patients have low level clones and/or paraproteinemia that are not detectable by current screening methods, but this remains to be proven. Recent uncontrolled data suggest that these patients' renal outcomes may improve with empiric, chemotherapy-type regimens that target a hypothesized underlying clone.[42] These observations require reproduction and validation, particularly given that most nephrologists do not have access to these drugs, and they may cause severe adverse events.

Membranous Nephropathy

The prevalence of cancer in patients with MN is between 6% and 22%.[9,12,43] The risk of cancer in patients with MN increases with age. Patients exhibit symptoms of malignancy in about half of cases, with the remainder being asymptomatic. Cancers of the lung and prostate are the malignancies most frequently associated with MN. There are no clinical features on presentation that distinguish cancer-associated MN from idiopathic MN (iMN).[3]

Histologically, the light (glomerular basement membrane thickening) and immunofluorescence microscopy (granular staining for IgG, kappa, lambda and C3 in a subepithelial distribution) findings are indistinguishable from primary MN (Fig. 21.1A and B). However, there may be other histologic features that distinguish cancer-associated MN from iMN. One study found that having more than eight inflammatory cells per glomerulus was associated with cancer-associated MN versus iMN (sensitivity 92% and specificity 75%).[12] Analysis of the IgG subclasses of the immune deposits in cancer-associated MN shows a predominance of IgG1 and IgG2, rather than IgG4 predominance that is common in idiopathic MN.[44] Antibodies to the transmembrane glycoprotein M-type phospholipase A2 receptor (PLA2R) is typical of primary MN and is now thought to distinguish this autoimmune entity from secondary MN (e.g., in lupus).[45] However, in one study, serum anti-PLA2R antibodies were found to be present in three of 10 patients with MN in whom cancers were subsequently detected. The fact that anti-PLA2R antibodies persisted despite resection of the tumor and that IgG4 was the predominant Ig subclass suggests that these cases were likely coincidental primary MN rather than cancer-associated MN.[46]

In a more recent study, antibodies to thrombospondin type-1 domain-containing 7A (THSD7A) were discovered in a subset of patients with MN.[47] In a subsequent study using larger cohorts, eight of 40 patients with THSD7A MN developed a malignancy within a median time of 3 months from the time of diagnosis of MN.[48] In a single

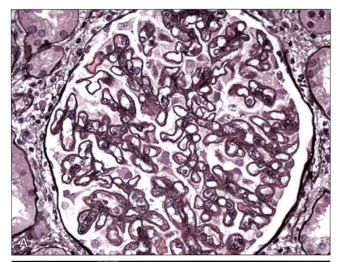

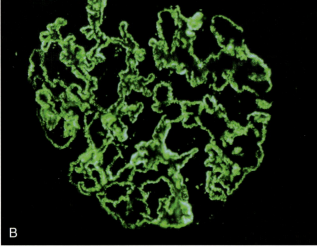

Fig. 21.1 A. Glomerular basement membrane thickening caused by spikes (H&E 400×). **B.** Immunofluorescence staining for immunoglobulin G reveals granular global capillary wall staining in the distribution of the subepithelial deposits (440×). (Images provided by Glen Markowitz, MD, Department of Pathology and Cell Biology, Columbia University Medical Center.)

IgG4 is a TH2 cell-related isotype (IL-4 and IL-13-driven). In paraneoplastic MN, both TH1 and TH2 cytokines may be activated by tumor antigens or other stimulants, resulting in the unique pattern of IgG subtype and increased numbers of inflammatory cells.[51]

A search for malignancy should be undertaken in older patients with newly diagnosed MN after excluding other secondary causes, although the exact age that should trigger screening is not known. The presence of anti-THSD7A antibody, absence of anti-PLA2R antibody, and/or predominant IgG1 and IgG2 deposits are other reasons to exclude malignancies thoroughly. Patients in these categories should be evaluated for cancer risk factors, prescribed gender- and age-appropriate screening (colonoscopy, prostate-specific antigen testing, and mammography), and low-dose chest computed tomography should be performed in smokers. If malignancy is not detected on initial screening, close follow-up for cancer should be undertaken.

Treatment is directed toward the primary cancer. In the series reported by Lefaucheur,[12] of 23 patients with cancer-associated MN, complete remission was observed in six cases. All remissions occurred in patients whose tumor was also in remission, whereas conversely, tumors were in remission in only three of 14 patients with persistent nephrotic-range proteinuria. Patients with cancer-associated MN appear to have a poorer prognosis[52] than those without cancer, with median patient survival time after the diagnosis of cancer-associated MN of only 13 months.[12]

Podocytopathies

MCD or focal glomerulosclerosis (FSGS) may occur in association with Hodgkin disease (HD)[53–56] and, less commonly, non-Hodgkin lymphoma or leukemia,[54] thymoma,[3,57] mycosis fungoides,[58] renal cell carcinoma,[59] and other solid tumors.[60–62]

Hodgkin disease is particularly associated with podocytopathies, most commonly MCD. In a series of 600 patients with HD, four patients were diagnosed with MCD.[53] In another case series of 21 patients from France, the onset of MCD preceded the diagnosis of HD in 38% of patients, 50% of whom patients had steroid-resistant nephrotic syndrome.[11] Treatment of HD was associated with remission of MCD.[11] Similarly, remission of proteinuria has been observed in patients with treatment of HD-associated FSGS with chemotherapy.[63]

Secretion of a cytokine may underlie glomerular injury in these disorders. Vascular endothelial growth factor (VEGF) may be one such cytokine; overexpression of VEGF in the podocyte is associated with podocytopathy in experimental models.[64] Serum VEGF levels were found to be elevated in one patient with rectal carcinoma and MCD, and resection of the cancer was associated with remission of nephrotic syndrome and corresponding reduction of VEGF levels. Moreover, VEGF was highly expressed in the cancer tissue.[65] C-Maf-inducing protein (C-Mip) was found to be expressed in podocytes and lymphoma tissue in patients with HD-associated MCD, but not in patients with HD without MCD, suggesting a potential involvement in the pathogenesis of HD-associated MCD.[66] In another patient who presented with nephrotic syndrome from FSGS, small

case report, a patient with THSD7A MN, a mixed adeno-neuroendocrine carcinoma of the gallbladder was noted. The primary gallbladder tumor and corresponding lymph-node metastases were positive for THSD7A on immunohistochemical analysis in association with serum anti-THSD7A antibodies. After chemotherapy, anti-THSD7A antibodies in plasma became undetectable, and urinary protein-creatinine ratio decreased from 5.0 to 0.7.[49]

The exact pathogenesis of the immune deposits in cancer-associated MN is unknown but several possible mechanisms have been postulated.[50] It is possible that antibodies are formed against a tumor antigen or podocyte antigen (which is similar to tumor antigen) that is localized in the subepithelial space.[49] Tumor antigens may also form circulating immune complexes that are subsequently trapped in glomerular capillaries. Lastly, exogenous factors, for example, oncogenic viruses, may be associated with both the malignancy and MN.[9] The predominance of IgG1 and IgG2 suggest T-helper (TH)-1 cell-related mechanisms (driven by interleukin [IL]-12 and interferon), whereas cell carcinoma of lung was found on testing. C-Mip was overexpressed in both podocytes and cancer cells but was not found in control kidney and lung tissue samples. Exposure of cultured podocytes to patient serum led to disorganization of the podocyte skeleton and expression of C-Mip that was not seen in control serum, or serum of HD patients after chemotherapy. The nephrotic syndrome resolved after remission of lung cancer.[11,63,67]

Immunoglobulin A Nephropathy

In older patients, IgA nephropathy may be associated with cancer. In one study, 23% (6 of 26) of patients aged 60 years or older diagnosed with IgA nephropathy had cancer compared with none of the 158 patients younger than age 60 years. Solid tumors, especially of the upper and lower respiratory tract, are associated with IgA nephropathy.[68] IgA nephropathy associated with renal cell carcinoma has also been described, which may improve after resection of the cancer.[69] Although IgA vasculitis (Henoch-Schönlein purpura) has also been reportedly associated with cancer, in most cases reviewed, the evidence of an association was not conclusive.[70]

Pauci-Immune, Crescentic Glomerulonephritis

In a review of 80 patients in the preantineutrophil cytoplasmic antibody era with idiopathic crescentic glomerulonephritis, seven patients had a concurrent malignancy (six carcinomas, one lymphoma) versus one of 80 patients with FSGS or MCD.[71] The incidence of malignancies was also reported to be higher in another study of pauci-immune vasculitis compared with systemic lupus or IgA vasculitis. In contrast, one study did not report a higher risk of malignancy preceding the onset of vasculitis.[72] Thus it is possible that the association of malignancy may be caused by immunosuppressive treatment.[73] In summary, the association of pauci-immune glomerulonephritis with malignancies, although suggestive, is not firmly established.

Thrombotic Microangiopathy

The occurrence of thrombotic microangiopathy is rare in cancer. The majority of such patients have metastatic disease and the predominant tumors are mucin-secreting adenocarcinomas. Some patients may exhibit carcinocythemia (carcinoma cell leukemia). The mechanism of endothelial dysfunction may be from the direct effects of mucin on the production and action of von Willebrand factor.[74]

Key Points

- Paraneoplastic glomerular diseases are caused by proteins and other molecules that are produced by tumors or by other cells of the body in response to the tumor (i.e., not as a result of direct invasion or metastasis).

- In some cases, such as paraprotein-mediated glomerular disease, the association is clear, whereas in other cases, the association is made based on the temporal association between disease presentations and/or responses to treatment.
- Certain clinical presentations and kidney biopsy features should prompt for the search for underlying malignancy.
- Management of paraneoplastic glomerular diseases most often focuses on the diagnosis and treatment of the underlying malignancy. In some cases, therapy may be used specifically to target the ongoing kidney injury.
- To properly manage paraneoplastic glomerular disease, nephrologists must understand the current approach to diagnosis, staging, and treatment of the associated malignancy.

References

1. Jhaveri KD, Shah HH, Calderon K, Campenot ES, Radhakrishnan J. Glomerular diseases seen with cancer and chemotherapy: a narrative review. *Kidney Int*. 2013;84(1):34-44.
2. Bilynsky BT, Dzhus MB, Litvinyak RI. The conceptual and clinical problems of paraneoplastic syndrome in oncology and internal medicine. *Exp Oncol*. 2015;37(2):82-88.
3. Lien YH, Lai LW. Pathogenesis, diagnosis and management of paraneoplastic glomerulonephritis. *Nat Rev Nephrol*. 2011;7(2):85-95.
4. Birkeland SA, Storm HH. Glomerulonephritis and malignancy: a population-based analysis. *Kidney Int*. 2003;63(2):716-721.
9. Cambier JF, Ronco P. Onco-nephrology: glomerular diseases with cancer. *Clin J Am Soc Nephrol*. 2012;7(10):1701-1712.
10. Bridoux F, Leung N, Hutchison CA, et al. Diagnosis of monoclonal gammopathy of renal significance. *Kidney Int*. 2015;87(4):698-711.
11. Audard V, Larousserie F, Grimbert P, et al. Minimal change nephrotic syndrome and classical Hodgkin's lymphoma: report of 21 cases and review of the literature. *Kidney Int*. 2006;69(12):2251-2260.
12. Lefaucheur C, Stengel B, Nochy D, et al. Membranous nephropathy and cancer: epidemiologic evidence and determinants of high-risk cancer association. *Kidney Int*. 2006;70(8):1510-1517.
14. Huang ZQ, Sanders PW. Localization of a single binding site for immunoglobulin light chains on human Tamm-Horsfall glycoprotein. *J Clin Invest*. 1997;99(4):732-736.
15. Hutchison CA, Cockwell P, Stringer S, et al. Early reduction of serum-free light chains associates with renal recovery in myeloma kidney. *J Am Soc Nephrol*. 2011;22(6):1129-1136.
16. Leung N, Gertz M, Kyle RA, et al. Urinary albumin excretion patterns of patients with cast nephropathy and other monoclonal gammopathy-related kidney diseases. *Clin J Am Soc Nephrol*. 2012;7(12):1964-1968.
17. Zand L, Nasr SH, Gertz MA, et al. Clinical and prognostic differences among patients with light chain deposition disease, myeloma cast nephropathy and both. *Leuk Lymphoma*. 2015;56(12):3357-3364.
18. Dimopoulos MA, Terpos E, Chanan-Khan A, et al. Renal impairment in patients with multiple myeloma: a consensus statement on behalf of the International Myeloma Working Group. *J Clin Oncol*. 2010; 28(33):4976-4984.
19. Leung N, Gertz MA, Zeldenrust SR, et al. Improvement of cast nephropathy with plasma exchange depends on the diagnosis and on reduction of serum free light chains. *Kidney Int*. 2008;73(11): 1282-1288.
20. Clark WF, Stewart AK, Rock GA, et al. Plasma exchange when myeloma presents as acute renal failure: a randomized, controlled trial. *Ann Intern Med*. 2005;143(11):777-784.
21. Zucchelli P, Pasquali S, Cagnoli L, Ferrari G. Controlled plasma exchange trial in acute renal failure due to multiple myeloma. *Kidney Int*. 1988;33(6):1175-1180.
22. Johnson WJ, Kyle RA, Pineda AA, O'Brien PC, Holley KE. Treatment of renal failure associated with multiple myeloma. Plasmapheresis, hemodialysis, and chemotherapy. *Arch Intern Med*. 1990;150(4): 863-869.
23. Hutchison CA, Bradwell AR, Cook M, et al. Treatment of acute renal failure secondary to multiple myeloma with chemotherapy and

extended high cut-off hemodialysis. *Clin J Am Soc Nephrol.* 2009; 4(4):745-754.

24. Bridoux F, Carron PL, Pegourie B, et al. Effect of high-cutoff hemodialysis vs conventional hemodialysis on hemodialysis independence among patients with myeloma cast nephropathy: a randomized clinical trial. *JAMA.* 2017;318(21):2099-2110.

27. Palladini G, Dispenzieri A, Gertz MA, et al. New criteria for response to treatment in immunoglobulin light chain amyloidosis based on free light chain measurement and cardiac biomarkers: impact on survival outcomes. *J Clin Oncol.* 2012;30(36):4541-4549.

28. Batalini F, Econimo L, Quillen K, et al. High-dose melphalan and stem cell transplantation in patients on dialysis due to immunoglobulin light-chain amyloidosis and monoclonal immunoglobulin deposition disease. *Biol Blood Marrow Transplant.* 2018;24(1):127-132.

31. Cohen C, Royer B, Javaugue V, et al. Bortezomib produces high hematological response rates with prolonged renal survival in monoclonal immunoglobulin deposition disease. *Kidney Int.* 2015;88(5): 1135-1143.

32. Mohan M, Buros A, Mathur P, et al. Clinical characteristics and prognostic factors in multiple myeloma patients with light chain deposition disease. *Am J Hematol.* 2017;92(8):739-745.

33. Bonaud A, Bender S, Touchard G, et al. A mouse model recapitulating human monoclonal heavy chain deposition disease evidences the relevance of proteasome inhibitor therapy. *Blood.* 2015;126(6): 757-765.

34. Bridoux F, Javaugue V, Bender S, et al. Unravelling the immunopathological mechanisms of heavy chain deposition disease with implications for clinical management. *Kidney Int.* 2017;91(2):423-434.

35. Vos JM, Gustine J, Rennke HG, et al. Renal disease related to Waldenström macroglobulinaemia: incidence, pathology and clinical outcomes. *Br J Haematol.* 2016;175(4):623-630.

36. Chauvet S, Bridoux F, Ecotière L, et al. Kidney diseases associated with monoclonal immunoglobulin M-secreting B-cell lymphoproliferative disorders: a case series of 35 patients. *Am J Kidney Dis.* 2015;66(5): 756-767.

37. Sidana S, Rajkumar SV, Dispenzieri A, et al. Clinical presentation and outcomes of patients with type 1 monoclonal cryoglobulinemia. *Am J Hematol.* 2017;92(7):668-673.

38. Harel S, Mohr M, Jahn I, et al. Clinico-biological characteristics and treatment of type I monoclonal cryoglobulinaemia: a study of 64 cases. *Br J Haematol.* 2015;168(5):671-678.

40. Stokes MB, Valeri AM, Herlitz L, et al. Light chain proximal tubulopathy: clinical and pathologic characteristics in the modern treatment era. *J Am Soc Nephrol.* 2016;27(5):1555-1565.

41. Chauvet S, Frémeaux-Bacchi V, Petitprez F, et al. Treatment of B-cell disorder improves renal outcome of patients with monoclonal gammopathy-associated C3 glomerulopathy. *Blood.* 2017;129(11): 1437-1447.

42. Gumber R, Cohen JB, Palmer MB, et al. A clone-directed approach may improve diagnosis and treatment of proliferative glomerulonephritis with monoclonal immunoglobulin deposits. *Kidney Int.* 2018; 94(1):199-205.

44. Ohtani H, Wakui H, Komatsuda A, et al. Distribution of glomerular IgG subclass deposits in malignancy-associated membranous nephropathy. *Nephrol Dial Transplant.* 2004;19(3):574-579.

46. Qin W, Beck LH Jr, Zeng C, et al. Anti-phospholipase A2 receptor antibody in membranous nephropathy. *J Am Soc Nephrol.* 2011; 22(6):1137-1143.

48. Hoxha E, Beck LH Jr, Wiech T, et al. An indirect immunofluorescence method facilitates detection of thrombospondin type 1 domain-containing 7A-specific antibodies in membranous nephropathy. *J Am Soc Nephrol.* 2017;28(2):520-531.

49. Hoxha E, Wiech T, Stahl PR, et al. A mechanism for cancer-associated membranous nephropathy. *N Engl J Med.* 2016;374(20):1995-1996.

52. Bjørneklett R, Vikse BE, Svarstad E, et al. Long-term risk of cancer in membranous nephropathy patients. *Am J Kidney Dis.* 2007;50(3): 396-403.

53. Plager J, Stutzman L. Acute nephrotic syndrome as a manifestation of active Hodgkin's disease. Report of four cases and review of the literature. *Am J Med.* 1971;50(1):56-66.

55. Sherman RL, Susin M, Weksler ME, Becker EL. Lipoid nephrosis in Hodgkin's disease. *Am J Med.* 1972;52:699-706.

57. Ishida I, Hirakata H, Kanai H, et al. Steroid-resistant nephrotic syndrome associated with malignant thymoma. *Clin Nephrol.* 1996; 46:340-346.

62. Thorner P, McGraw M, Weitzman S, Balfe JW, Klein M, Baumal R. Wilms' tumor and glomerular disease. Occurrence with features of membranoproliferative glomerulonephritis and secondary focal, segmental glomerulosclerosis. *Arch Pathol Lab Med.* 1984;108:141-146.

63. Mallouk A, Pham PT, Pham PC. Concurrent FSGS and Hodgkin's lymphoma: case report and literature review on the link between nephrotic glomerulopathies and hematological malignancies. *Clin Exp Nephrol.* 2006;10(4):284-289.

64. Eremina V, Sood M, Haigh J, et al. Glomerular-specific alterations of VEGF-A expression lead to distinct congenital and acquired renal diseases. *J Clin Invest.* 2003;111(5):707-716.

65. Taniguchi K, Fujioka H, Torashima Y, Yamaguchi J, Izawa K, Kanematsu T. Rectal cancer with paraneoplastic nephropathy: association of vascular endothelial growth factor. *Dig Surg.* 2004;21(5-6): 455-457.

66. Audard V, Zhang SY, Copie-Bergman C, et al. Occurrence of minimal change nephrotic syndrome in classical Hodgkin lymphoma is closely related to the induction of c-mip in Hodgkin-Reed Sternberg cells and podocytes. *Blood.* 2010;115(18):3756-3762.

68. Mustonen J, Pasternack A, Helin H. IgA mesangial nephropathy in neoplastic diseases. *Contrib Nephrol.* 1984;40:283-291.

70. Pertuiset E, Lioté F, Launay-Russ E, Kemiche F, Cerf-Payrastre I, Chesneau AM. Adult Henoch-Schönlein purpura associated with malignancy. *Semin Arthritis Rheum.* 2000;29(6):360-367.

73. Wester Trejo MAC, Bajema IM, van Daalen EE. Antineutrophil cytoplasmic antibody-associated vasculitis and malignancy. *Curr Opin Rheumatol.* 2018;30(1):44-49.

74. Izzedine H, Perazella MA. Thrombotic microangiopathy, cancer, and cancer drugs. *Am J Kidney Dis.* 2015;66(5):857-868.

75. Rajkumar SV, Dimopoulos MA, Palumbo A, et al. International Myeloma Working Group updated criteria for the diagnosis of multiple myeloma. *Lancet Oncol.* 2014;15(12):e538-e548.

A full list of references is available at Expertconsult.com

22 *Paraneoplastic Glomerulonephritis*

DIVYA SHANKARANARAYANAN AND SHERON LATCHA

Introduction

Paraneoplastic syndrome refers to "clinical manifestations that are not directly related to tumor burden, invasion or metastasis, but are caused by secretion of tumor cell products, such as hormones, growth factors, cytokines and tumor antigens."[1] The idea that the kidneys could manifest paraneoplastic disease was first proposed in 1922 by Galloway who noticed the presence of an "unusual protein" in the urine of his patient afflicted with Hodgkin lymphoma.[2] It has been proposed that the diagnosis of paraneoplastic syndrome should be suspected when: (1) there is no obvious alternate etiology for the associated syndrome; (2) a temporal relationship exists between the diagnosis of the syndrome and cancer; (3) clinical (and histologic) remission occurs after complete surgical removal of the tumor or full remission is achieved by chemotherapy; and (4) recurrence of the tumor is associated with increase of associated symptoms.[3] Since the early 1920s, various animal studies and retrospective studies have provided evidence for paraneoplastic glomerulopathy (PNGN), but there still remains some skepticism about its existence. In addition to malignancies, benign tumors, such a pheochromocytoma, carotid body tumors, benign ovarian teratomas, and spinal cord tumors have also been reported to cause glomerular disease.[3–5] This chapter will focus on the reported incidence and purported mechanisms of PNGN in solid tumors.

Epidemiology of Paraneoplastic Glomerulopathy in Solid Tumors

PNGN is likely a rare clinical entity. Less than 1% of adult cancer patients develop PNGN with overt renal disease.[6] The true incidence of PNGN remains ill-defined for a number of reasons. First, patients with cancer can have various urinary abnormalities that are not routinely investigated, and urinalysis is not performed routinely among inpatients and outpatients with cancer.[7] Sometimes, patients with malignancy can have subclinical glomerulonephritis (GN) manifested by presence of immune complex (IC) deposits caused by defects in the immune-regulatory mechanisms without significant renal damage.[8] In addition, many of the reports on PNGN are based on retrospective data and case reports, which have their inherent reporting biases. The case reports of PNGN do not seem to reflect the relative incidence or prevalence of cancer in the general population. According to the American Cancer Society, lung cancer is the second most common cancer among men and women,

whereas prostate is the most common cause among males and breast cancer among females. However, based on the available published reports, the solid tumors most commonly associated with a PNGN are of renal, gastrointestinal, (GI) and lung origin (Fig. 22.1). Whereas solid tumors have been reported most commonly in association with membranous glomerulonephritis (MN) (Fig. 22.2), a wide spectrum of glomerular lesions have been described.

Notwithstanding the issues of reporting bias and the relative rarity of this clinical entity, several clinical and laboratory features have been recognized to associate with paraneoplastic disease in the kidney. In a population based longitudinal study of 5425 nondiabetics without any previous diagnosis of cancer, Jorgensen et al. found that elevated albumin to creatinine ratio was associated with higher incidence of cancer, even after adjustment for age, gender, body mass index, physical activity, and smoking.[9] Age greater than 60 years and a history of tobacco smoking has been associated with higher risk for cancer in patient with nephrotic syndrome (NS).[1,10]

PATHOPHYSIOLOGY

A causal link between neoplasia and PNGN remains ill defined, but there are several purported pathogenetic mechanisms. In a study of three patients with gastric cancer presenting with NS, glomerular eluates reacted specifically with the surface of the cancer cells from the same host seen under immunofixation (IF).[11] Thus one hypothesis is that there is deposition of circulating tumor antigen-antibody complexes in the glomeruli with subsequent activation of inflammatory pathways, which eventually produces glomerular disease. In addition, antibodies could be directed toward specific endogenous glomerular antigens. Couser et al.[12] report a case of a patient with MN who was found to have elevated carcinoembryonic antigen following the diagnosis of NS. The patient was subsequently diagnosed with colon cancer and underwent colon resection. The authors of the report demonstrated that an antibody in the serum of the patient reacted with an antigen on the glomerular basement membrane (GBM). This antibody was removed by adsorption of serum with homogenates of the patient's serum but not by the homogenates of normal colon, liver, or spleen.

Another possible pathogenetic mechanism is that tumors elaborate cytokines and/or permeability factors, which triggers glomerular injury. In a study on a patient with rectal adenocarcinoma associated minimal change disease (MCD), Taniguchi et al. demonstrated high levels of vascular endothelial growth factor (VEGF) in the tumor. After resection of the tumor, VEGF levels returned to normal and the

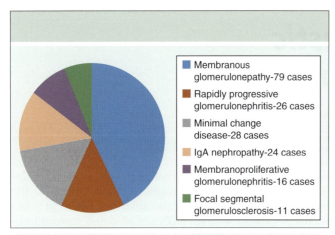

Fig. 22.1 Number of reported cases of paraneoplastic glomerulonephritis in solid tumors arranged by glomerular lesion.

- ■ Membranous glomerulonepathy-79 cases
- ■ Rapidly progressive glomerulonephritis-26 cases
- ■ Minimal change disease-28 cases
- ■ IgA nephropathy-24 cases
- ■ Membranoproliferative glomerulonephritis-16 cases
- ■ Focal segmental glomerulosclerosis-11 cases

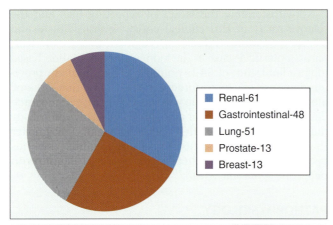

Fig. 22.2 Number of reported cases of various solid tumors reported with paraneoplastic glomerulonephritis.

- ■ Renal-61
- ■ Gastrointestinal-48
- ■ Lung-51
- ■ Prostate-13
- ■ Breast-13

proteinuria resolved. The authors hypothesized that the overexpression of VEGF by certain tumor cells was linked to the onset of proteinuria, and thus when the VEGF levels decreased after tumor resection, the proteinuria resolved.[3,10,13]

Intrinsic viral oncogenic activity has been offered as an additional pathogenetic mechanism for PNGN. Viral activity may interfere with the renal clearance of the prooncogenic biological mediators released from the body. Alternatively, viral infections could lead to both malignancy and a PNGN through a common pathway.[3,14] The possible role of viral oncogenic activity and PNGN is discussed in more detail in the chapter on Paraneoplastic Glomerulopathy in Hematologic Malignancies.

The cellular and humoral immune systems may also have a role in the pathogenesis of PNGN.[15] In an animal study that was performed by injecting rat colon cancer cells into immunocompetent and T-cell deficient F344 rats, the T-cell deficient rat's kidneys did not show any morphologic abnormalities and did not have any immunoglobulin (Ig)G deposition. Thus it can be hypothesized that the presence of an intact cellular and humoral immunity is required for development of PNGN.

The various histologic patterns of PNGN may be dependent on several factors, including: (1) the duration of the neoplasm; (2) degree of tumor differentiation, which may dictate the elaboration of specific and nonspecific antigens; (3) type of tumor antigen and other products expressed; (4) type and extent of host response to these antigens via cell-mediated and antibody-mediated mechanisms; and/or (5) physiochemical characteristics of the circulating IC that render them pathogenic or nephritogenic.[15]

Membranous Nephropathy

MN is the most common PNGN associated with solid tumors.[1,7] Paraneoplastic MN has been reported more often in males, in those at age greater than 60 years, and in patients with a history of heavy tobacco use.[1,10,16] The most commonly associated cancers are those of lung, GI, and renal origin (Table 22.1). Prostate cancer is increasingly being reported with paraneoplastic MN,[3,17] which may reflect the increased use of prostate-specific antigen as a screening test. In most reports, patients who were diagnosed with idiopathic MN were diagnosed with a neoplasia within 12 months.[10] However, the PNGN can present years after the neoplasia is evident.[15]

HISTOPATHOLOGY

On light microscopy (LM), the GBMs in MN appear thickened. On electron microscopy (EM), subepithelial deposits are evident. The presence of subendothelial or mesangial deposits should raise concern for a secondary or paraneoplastic process. There are several features on histopathology that have been associated with a paraneoplastic MN. Patients with paraneoplastic MN have an increased number of infiltrating inflammatory cells in the glomeruli (> 8 cells per glomeruli).[16] Also, whereas IgG4 is the predominant subclass found in idiopathic MN, IgG1, IgG2, and IgG3 are predominantly found in cases of secondary MN.[10] Circulating antiphospholipase A2 receptor is seen in up to 89% cases of idiopathic membranous nephropathy. It is worth noting that circulating antiphospholipase A2 receptor is occasionally present with secondary, including paraneoplastic membranous.[18,19]

PATHOGENETIC MECHANISM

Heymann nephritis is an experimental rat model for active and passive immune-mediated nephritis. Megalin, which is the target antigen, localizes to the podocytes in the rat model. However, in humans, megalin is found in the

Table 22.1 Number of Reported Cases of Paraneoplastic Membranous Nephropathy in Solid Tumors

Organ	Number of Cases
Gastrointestinal	26
Lung	27
Renal	12
Prostate	9
Breast	5

proximal tubule and not in podocytes. Hence investigators have sought to find an equivalent antigen present in the podocytes to explain paraneoplastic membranous glomerulonephritis (MGN). The finding of thrombospondin type-1 domain-containing 7A (THSD7A) antibody in a patient with MGN with a neoplasm, and the disappearance of the antibody and urinary protein after the malignancy was treated, suggests a potential causal relationship between THSD7A expression and MGN.[20] Other factors may exist, but they have yet to be fully defined. There are a number of isolated case reports in which eluates from the glomeruli of patients with known malignancy showed reactivity with the patient's serum and the tumor homogenates, but not with normal kidney.[21]

Immunoglobulin A Nephropathy

IgA nephropathy (IgAN) is the most common form of primary GN worldwide. There is geographic variation in the frequency of the disease and the prevalence of IgAN is highest in Japan and lowest in the USA. The clinical presentation ranges from gross hematuria at the time of an upper respiratory tract infection, isolated persistent hematuria, and varying degrees of proteinuria, rarely reaching nephrotic ranges.

IgAN is usually diagnosed around the second and third decade of life in the adult population. When IgA is initially diagnosed in patients older than 60 years, the prevalence of malignancy is 23%.[22] Table 22.2 shows the prevalence of IgAN among solid tumors listed according to tumor type. Paraneoplastic IgAN has been most often reported with renal cell carcinoma (RCC), followed by cancers of the GI and the respiratory systems. Based on histologic examination of native kidney specimens in patients with RCC who underwent a nephrectomy, the prevalence of IgAN was 18% in 60 patients with RCC.[23] A study of autopsy specimens of 129 patients with solid tumors found that glomerular deposits were more frequently observed in patients with GI carcinoma and that 36% of these specimens had demonstrable IgA mesangial deposits.[24]

HISTOPATHOLOGY

Patients with IgAN have increased levels of abnormally galactosylated IgA1 subtype. On LM, IgAN is characterized by mesangial expansion with cellular proliferation and increased mesangial matrix. There can also be segmental or global endocapillary proliferation, presence of crescents, and segmental sclerosis. Immunofixation (IF) study is required for the diagnosis of IgAN because optically normal glomeruli on LM will have IgA as the principal and sole Ig on IF.

Table 22.2 Number of Reported Cases of Paraneoplastic Immunoglobulin A Nephropathy in Solid Tumors

Organ	Number of Cases
Renal carcinoma	17
Gastrointestinal carcinoma	1
Respiratory system carcinoma	7

It is not known whether IgA in the deposits is the antigen or the antibody that fixes C3. On the EM reveals granular electron dense mesangial and paramesangial deposits.

PATHOGENETIC MECHANISM

There are major differences between mice and human IgA systems. Therefore a good animal model for IgAN is lacking. One hypothesis is that the invasion of the mucosa by the malignancy leads to increased circulating IgA, leading to mesangial IgA deposits.[22] In human models of RCC, elevated levels of interleukin-6 (IL-6) have been found in the serum and cell lines[25] on cancer patients. In murine models, it has been shown that IgA production is stimulated by IL-6.[26] Therefore one postulate is that elevated levels of IL-6 in RCC stimulates IgA production, leading to increased circulating levels of IgA, which in turn deposit in the mesangium. Alternatively, it is possible that tumors could stimulate secretion of abnormal IgA1-like particles that could then induce an IgG response in the host, which in turn could lead to formation of ICs that deposit in the mesangium.[27]

Minimal Change Disease

The classic presentation of MCD is sudden onset nephrotic range proteinuria, hypoalbuminemia, hypercholesterolemia, and pitting edema. MCD is the most common cause of childhood NS and accounts for NS in 90% of cases of children less than 10 years old and for 50% of cases more than 10 years old. In adults with NS, MCD is the underlying diagnosis in 10% to 15% cases.[28] Paraneoplastic MCD is most commonly associated with lymphoid malignancy, specifically Hodgkin lymphoma (Table 22.3). Solid tumors are not as commonly associated with paraneoplastic MCD.

Table 22.3 Number of Reported Cases of Paraneoplastic Minimal Change Disease in Solid Tumors

Organ	Tumor Type	Number of Cases
Thymus	Thymoma	26
Gastrointestinal	Colorectal carcinoma	6
	Pancreatic carcinoma	2
	Esophageal carcinoma	1
Respiratory system	Lung/bronchus carcinoma	8
	Mesothelioma	1
	Small cell carcinoma	1
Renal	Renal cell carcinoma	7
Genitourinary	Urothelial carcinoma	2
	Bladder carcinoma	1
	Vaginale testis mesothelioma	1
Ovarian	Ovarian carcinoma	1
Breast	Breast carcinoma	2
Other	Sarcoma	1
	Angiomyolipoma	1
	Neurilemmoma	1
	Undifferentiated carcinoma	1
	Melanoma	1

HISTOPATHOLOGY

MCD is characterized by normal looking glomeruli on LM with abundant proximal tubular protein reabsorption droplets. Staining for complement and Ig is negative on IF. The distinct histopathologic finding diffuse foot process effacement is seen on EM.

PATHOGENETIC MECHANISM

It has long been postulated that acquired podocytopathies are the consequence of immune factors, specifically a dysregulation of T-cell regulation. The Buffalo/Mna rat, which is a spontaneous model for thymoma and myasthenia gravis, has been studied for MCD-like glomerular disease. In these rats, NS presents at 1 month of age and the renal biopsy shows typical MCD features. In a retrospective study of 21 patients[29] with thymoma, all patients with type B2 grade of malignant thymoma had MCD. Sixty-seven percent (14 out of 21) of the cases of thymoma had MCD on renal biopsy. Various T-cell related cytokines, such as IL-2, IL-4, and IL-13 may act as permeability factors and contribute to nephrotic range proteinuria.[3] IL-13 levels are increased in the serum and T-cells of patients with MCD. Wistar rats that transfected with a vector, which resulted in overexpression of IL-13, developed significant proteinuria, hypoalbuminemia, and hypercholesterolemia when compared with control rats. The glomeruli of the transfected rats were optically normal on LM and had diffuse foot process fusion on EM. Further analysis revealed that there was downregulation of the proteins necessary to maintain the integrity of the GBM (nephrin, podocin, and dystroglycan), and upregulation of expression of IL-13 receptors.[30] VEGF may also act as a permeability factor in patients with MCD. Increased secretion of VEGF has been observed in RCC.[15]

Focal Segmental Glomerulosclerosis

FSGS and MCD are both manifestations of podocyte injury and may thus share similar pathogenetic mechanisms. FSGS accounts for 40% of cases of NS in adults. It is the most common primary glomerular disease leading to end-stage renal disease in the United States. The prevalence of paraneoplastic FSGS according to the cancer type is shown in Table 22.4. As with MCD, FSGS is more commonly reported with hematologic malignancies. Of the solid tumors, it has been most commonly reported with thymomas and RCC.

HISTOPATHOLOGY

Histologically, on LM, the lesion is characterized by segmental obliteration of the glomerular capillary, glomerular sclerosis, capsular adhesion, and hyaline deposition. As a result of proteinuria, increased proximal tubular reabsorption droplets can be found. On EM, there is extensive effacement of epithelial foot processes and absence of electron dense immune deposits. IF typically shows coarsely granular

Table 22.4   Number of Reported Cases of Paraneoplastic Focal Segmental Glomerulosclerosis in Solid Tumors

Organ	Tumor Type	Number of Cases
Renal	Renal cell carcinoma	6
Thymus	Thymoma	4
Gastrointestinal	Gastrointestinal carcinoma	2
Respiratory system	Lung/bronchus carcinoma	1
	Mesothelioma	1
Others	Breast carcinoma	1
	Melanoma	1
	Sarcoma	1
	Pheochromocytoma	1
	Hydatidiform mole	1

staining for IgM and C3 in the mesangial areas. These findings are generally caused by nonspecific trapping of IgM and C3, particularly in areas of sclerosis.

PATHOGENETIC MECHANISM

As is the case with MCD, a potential paraneoplastic link between thymoma and podocyte dysfunction in FSGS was studied in the Buffalo/Mna rat model because of their association with spontaneous thymoma.[31] Data showed that the thymic disease did not cause proteinuria, because thymectomy had no effect on proteinuria. In the Buffalo/Mna rats, two autosomal recessive genes were located on chromosome 13, which seems to confer susceptibility to glomerulosclerosis.[32] This chromosome corresponds to the long arm of human chromosome 1, where the *Nephs2* gene coding for podocin has been located. This gene colocalization suggests that perhaps there is a genetic predisposition to paraneoplastic FSGS.[32] As is the case with MCD, the cytokine milieu of malignancy may produce the ultrastructural changes seen in paraneoplastic FSGS. Increased production of macrophage associated cytokines, particularly tumor necrosis factor alpha (TNF-α) and cytokines associated with Th2-cells, have also been shown to produce an FSGS pattern of glomerular injury.[33]

Membranoproliferative Glomerulonephritis

Paraneoplastic membranoproliferative glomerulonephritis (MPGN) is more commonly associated with lymphoproliferative disorders than with solid tumors. Tumors of the respiratory tract and kidney have been reported in association with paraneoplastic MPGN (Table 22.5). There are additional case reports describing patients with RCC and a transitional cell carcinoma of the bladder who presented with NS. In these cases the renal biopsy showed MPGN and the proteinuria improved following resection of the tumor.[34,35] The paucity of reported cases and studies with solid tumors and MPGN makes it difficult to discern any causal pathogenicity for a PNGN.

Table 22.5 Number of Reported Cases of Paraneoplastic Membranoproliferative Glomerulonephritis in Solid Tumors

Organ	Tumor Type	Number of Cases
Respiratory system	Lung/bronchus carcinoma	5
	Pulmonary carcinoid	1
Renal	Renal cell carcinoma	4
Thymus	Thymoma	1
Gastrointestinal	Gastric carcinoma	2
Breast	Breast carcinoma	3
Genitourinary	Prostate carcinoma	1
	Bladder carcinoma	1
	Ovarian germinal carcinoma	1
Others	Carcinoma of unknown type	4
	Hydatidiform mole	1
	Desmoplastic round cell tumor	1
	Melanoma	3
	Angiosarcoma	1

Table 22.6 Number of Reported Cases of Paraneoplastic Rapidly Progressive Glomerulonephritis in Solid Tumors

Organ	Tumor Type	Number of Cases
Renal	Renal cell carcinoma	10
Gastrointestinal	Gastric carcinoma	6
	Esophageal carcinoma	1
	Hepatic carcinoma	1
	Colorectal carcinoma	1
Respiratory system	Larynx/pharynx carcinoma	2
	Lung/bronchus carcinoma	4
Genitourinary	Prostate carcinoma	3
	Bladder carcinoma	1
Breast	Breast carcinoma	3
Others	Solid without details	10
	Skin squamous cell carcinoma	1
	Kaposi sarcoma	1
	Thyroid carcinoma	1
	Ovarian carcinoma	1

Rapidly Progressive Glomerulonephritis

Rapidly progressive glomerulonephritis (RPGN) is characterized by acute renal failure, azotemia, hypertension, proteinuria, and hematuria. The urinary sediment can reveal red blood cell and white blood cell casts, cellular debris, and pigmented casts. RPGN is generally classified into: (1) antiglomerular basement membrane disease (anti-GBM); (2) immune complex vasculitis; and (3) antineutrophil cytoplasmic antibody (ANCA) vasculitis. Paraneoplastic RPGN has only rarely been reported, and when it has been, it has been associated most often with RCC. A summary of the case reports is shown in Table 22.6. There may be a higher prevalence of malignancy in patients with ANCA-associated vasculitis. One retrospective study found that the odds ratio of developing RCC was 8.73 ($p=.046$, 95% confidence interval 1.04–73.69) with ANCA positive granulomatosis with polyangiitis when compared with rheumatoid arthritis (control group).[36] For bladder cancer, the standard incidence ratio (SIR) was 4.8 and for squamous cell cancer, the SIR was 7.3.[37] The study may reflect the risk of malignancy related to exposure to cyclophosphamide for treatment of GPA. Henoch-Schönlein purpura (HSP) is a form of small vessel vasculitis, which displays a proliferative GN with crescents and IgA deposits containing immune complexes. Again, an increased risk of malignancy was reported in HSP patients when compared with normal population but not when compared with systemic lupus erythematosus.[38] HSP patients presenting with malignancy tend to be older than HSP patients without malignancy. Unfortunately, these observational studies do not provide any insights into the pathogenetic mechanism of a paraneoplastic RPGN.

HISTOPATHOLOGY

Immunologically mediated injury and inflammation of the small blood vessels and capillaries appear to be fundamental components in the pathogenesis of ANCA-mediated crescentic GN.[37] On LM, RPGN is characterized by segmental necrotizing features with crescents or extracapillary epithelial proliferation. ANCA-associated GN or pauci-immune crescentic GN is the most common form of RPGN. Although the glomerular disease is mediated by an immunologic mechanism, staining is negative for immune deposits on IF.

Key Points

- Paraneoplastic glomerulonephritis (GN) is described based on many case reports and observational studies, but there is significant paucity of human and animal model studies to elicit the exact pathogenic mechanisms.
- Paraneoplastic GN has been reported in both benign and malignant solid tumors.
- The most common paraneoplastic glomerulopathy in solid tumors is membranous glomerulopathy. The presence of proteinuria in patients greater than age 60 years with no other cause for proteinuria should raise concern for a paraneoplastic GN.
- Various tumoral cytokines may act as permeability factors in the pathogenesis of paraneoplastic minimal change disease and focal segmental glomerulosclerosis.
- Solid tumors most commonly associated with paraneoplastic glomerulopathy are those that originate from respiratory tract, gastrointestinal tract, and renal cell carcinoma.

References

1. Ronco PM. Paraneoplastic glomerulopathies: new insights into an old entity. *Kidney Int.* 1999;56(1):355-377.

3. Bacchetta J, Juillard L, Cochat P, Droz JP. Paraneoplastic glomerular diseases and malignancies. *Crit Rev Oncol Hematol.* 2009;70(1):39-58.

10. Beck Jr LH. Membranous nephropathy and malignancy. *Semin Nephrol.* 2010;30(6):635-644.

11. Wakashin M, Wakashin Y, Iesato K, et al. Association of gastric cancer and nephrotic syndrome. An immunologic study in three patients. *Gastroenterology.* 1980;78(4):749-756.

13. Taniguchi K, Fujioka H, Torashima Y, Yamaguchi J, Izawa K, Kanematsu T. Rectal cancer with paraneoplastic nephropathy: association of vascular endothelial growth factor. *Dig Surg.* 2004;21(5-6):455-457.

14. Birkeland SA, Storm HH. Glomerulonephritis and malignancy: a population-based analysis. *Kidney Int.* 2003;63(2):716-721.

15. Tojo A. Paraneoplastic glomerulopathy associated with renal cell carcinoma. *Renal Tumor.* IntechOpen, 2013.

16. Lefaucheur C, Stengel B, Nochy D, et al. Membranous nephropathy and cancer: Epidemiologic evidence and determinants of high-risk cancer association. *Kidney Int.* 2006;70(8):1510-1517.

17. Lien YH, Lai LW. Pathogenesis, diagnosis and management of paraneoplastic glomerulonephritis. *Nat Rev Nephrol.* 2011;7(2):85-95.

18. Beck Jr LH, Bonegio RG, Lambeau G, et al. M-type phospholipase A2 receptor as target antigen in idiopathic membranous nephropathy. *N Engl J Med.* 2009;361(1):11-21.

19. Qin W, Beck Jr LH, Zeng C, et al. Anti-phospholipase A2 receptor antibody in membranous nephropathy. *J Am Soc Nephrol.* 2011;22(6):1137-1143.

20. Hoxha E, Wiech T, Stahl PR, et al. A Mechanism for cancer-associated membranous nephropathy. *N Engl J Med.* 2016;374(20):1995-1996.

21. Alpers CE, Cotran RS. Neoplasia and glomerular injury. *Kidney Int.* 1986;30(4):465-473.

22. Mustonen J, Pasternack A, Helin H. IgA mesangial nephropathy in neoplastic diseases. *Contrib Nephrol.* 1984;40:283-291.

23. Magyarlaki T, Kiss B, Buzogány I, Fazekas A, Sükösd F, Nagy J. Renal cell carcinoma and paraneoplastic IgA nephropathy. *Nephron.* 1999;82(2):127-130.

24. Beaufils H, Jouanneau C, Chomette G. Kidney and cancer: results of immunofluorescence microscopy. *Nephron.* 1985;40(3):303-308.

25. Tsukamoto T, Kumamoto Y, Miyao N, Masumori N, Takahashi A, Yanase M. Interleukin-6 in renal cell carcinoma. *J Urol.* 1992;148(6):1778-1781, discussion 1781-1772.

26. Beagley KW, Eldridge JH, Lee F, et al. Interleukins and IgA synthesis. Human and murine interleukin 6 induce high rate IgA secretion in IgA-committed B cells. *J Exp Med.* 1989;169(6):2133-2148.

27. Novak J, Julian BA, Tomana M, Mesteck J. Progress in molecular and genetic studies of IgA nephropathy. *J Clin Immunol.* 2001;21(5):310-327.

29. Karras A, de Montpreville V, Fakhouri F, et al. Renal and thymic pathology in thymoma-associated nephropathy: report of 21 cases and review of the literature. *Nephrol Dial Transplant.* 2005;20(6):1075-1082.

30. Lai KW, Wei CL, Tan LK, et al. Overexpression of interleukin-13 induces minimal-change-like nephropathy in rats. *J Am Soc Nephrol.* 2007;18(5):1476-1485.

32. Kemp DS, Vellaccio F Jr. Letter: anomalously large steric inhibition of intramolecular O,N-acyl transfer to amino acid esters. *J Org Chem.* 1975;40(23):3464-3474.

33. Le Berre L, Hervé C, Buzelin F, Usal C, Soulillou JP, Dantal J. Renal macrophage activation and Th2 polarization precedes the development of nephrotic syndrome in Buffalo/Mna rats. *Kidney Int.* 2005;68(5):2079-2090.

34. Ahmed M, Solangi K, Abbi R, et al. Nephrotic syndrome, renal failure, and renal malignancy: an unusual tumor-associated glomerulonephritis. *J Am Soc Nephrol.* 1997;8(5):848-852.

35. Reshi AR, Mir SA, Gangoo AA, Shah S, Banday K. Nephrotic syndrome associated with transitional cell carcinoma of urinary bladder. *Scand J Urol Nephrol.* 1997;31(3):295-296.

36. Tatsis E, Reinhold-Keller E, Steindorf K, Feller AC, Gross WL. Wegener's granulomatosis associated with renal cell carcinoma. *Arthritis Rheum.* 1999;42(4):751-756.

37. Rutgers A, Sanders JS, Stegeman CA, Kallenberg CG. Pauci-immune necrotizing glomerulonephritis. *Rheum Dis Clin North Am.* 2010;36(3):559-572.

38. Pankhurst T, Savage CO, Gordon C, Harper L. Malignancy is increased in ANCA-associated vasculitis. *Rheumatology (Oxford).* 2004;43(12):1532-1535.

A full list of references is available at Expertconsult.com

23 *Hematologic Malignancies*

MOHIT GUPTA AND SHERON LATCHA

Paraneoplastic Glomerulopathy in Hematologic Malignancies

Paraneoplastic syndromes in the context of hematologic malignancies have been reported among multiple organ systems, including the nervous system, skin, bone marrow, and kidneys. Paraneoplastic glomerular injury has been demonstrated to be the result of tumoral production of cytokines, monoclonal and amyloid proteins, cryoglobulins, and the development of autoimmune diseases. Direct leukemic or lymphomatous infiltration of the kidney will not be included in this discussion, because paraneoplastic glomerulopathy (PNGN) refers to renal disease that is not a direct result of tumor burden, invasion, or metastasis.[1]

Box 23.1 illustrates the 2016 World Health Organization classification of hematologic malignancies. The major subtypes are grouped by lineage into lymphoid, myeloid, and histiocytic/dendritic neoplasms. This chapter will focus on the lymphoid and myeloid lineages, because there are no reports of PNGN with the latter subgroup. The prevalence and types of PNGN can vary significantly among the two major subtypes.[2] Overall, the reported incidence of PNGN related to hematologic malignancies is quite rare, with the total number of case reports in the literature only slightly in excess of 200. When compared with myeloid neoplasias, PNGN has been reported relatively more frequently in patients with the lymphoid malignancies, specifically Hodgkin lymphoma (HL), non-Hodgkin lymphoma (NHL), and chronic lymphocytic leukemia (CLL). Among the lymphoid neoplasias, paraneoplastic minimal change disease (MCD) and focal segmental glomerular sclerosis (FSGS) are more frequently reported with diseases of the T-cell lineage like HL, whereas paraneoplastic membranoproliferative glomerulonephritis (MPGN) and membranous nephropathy (MN) are more commonly reported with B-cell lineage tumors like CLL.

Lymphoid Malignancies

The frequency of renal involvement with lymphoid neoplasia ranges from 16% to 33%, depending upon the case series.[3,4] Varied patterns of glomerular lesions have been reported with the lymphoid malignancies, but there seems to be predilection for specific lesions. The following subsections present the paraneoplastic lesions associated with lymphoid neoplasia in their order of reported relative frequency. Fig. 23.1 illustrates the relative distribution of the patterns of PNGN based on case reports and case series in the literature. MCD and FSGS, which are glomerular lesions characterized by podocyte injury, account for more than 50% of case reports. Proliferative lesions like MPGN

account for about one-third of the reported cases. Most of the discussion in this section will focus on HL, NHL, and CLL because most of the cases of PNGN have been linked with these diseases. Lymphoid neoplasias that have been less frequently associated with a PNGN are discussed in the final portion of this section.

LYMPHOID MALIGNANCIES: MINIMAL CHANGE DISEASE AND FOCAL SEGMENTAL GLOMERULAR SCLEROSIS

MCD and FSGS are discussed together in this section because both entities present with podocyte injury, proteinuria, and minimal immune deposits. PNGN in patients with HL has been reported in up to 0.4% of cases. MCD is the most commonly reported glomerular lesion with HL. It is more frequently seen in the classic form of HL, including the mixed cellularity and the nodular sclerosing subtypes. The secondary MCD associated with HL exhibits a high degree of steroid and cyclosporine resistance, but generally goes into remission with successful treatment of the HL. The occurrence of nephrotic syndrome (NS) can precede the development of malignancy by several years, and recurrence of NS can often herald relapse of the lymphoma. The incidence of paraneoplastic FSGS is about one-tenth that of MCD. This form of secondary FSGS will also respond to chemotherapy administered for treatment of the primary lymphoma. Among patients with NHL, mantle cell lymphoma (MCL) has been reported in association with FSGS in two cases, and in both, the glomerular disease responded well to chemotherapy for the MCL.[5,6]

The pathogenesis of paraneoplastic MCD and FSGS remains poorly defined. Both lesions are essentially the sequela of injury and dysfunction of the glomerular podocyte. As such, paraneoplastic MCD and FSGS may result from abnormal tumoral expression of proteins, which are involved with cytoskeleton organization and podocyte signaling. There are several tumoral proteins of interest in this regard. Paraneoplastic MCD in patients with HL may be related to the increased production of the T-helper 2 cell (Th2) cytokine interleukin (IL)-13. In patients with HL, T-cells tend to expand towards the Th2 cell, and IL-13 levels are increased in the serum of patients with MCD.[7] In a rat model, increased production of IL-13 produces an MCD-type nephropathy.[2] Another putative protein is c-mip (c-maf inducing protein). Increased expression of c-mip switches off the interaction between nephrin and tyrosine kinase-fyn.[8] This in turn leads to defects in cytoskeleton organization and proximal podocyte signaling that may lead to the development podocyte disease. Increased production of vascular endothelial growth factor (VEGF) has also been associated with the development of podocyte

Box 23.1   Revised World Health Organization Classification of Lymphoid and Myeloid Malignancies (2016)

Lymphoid Neoplasia

- Hodgkin lymphoma
- Non-Hodgkin lymphoma, which includes
  - Mature B-cell neoplasms
  - Mature T and natural killer cell neoplasms
  - Posttransplant lymphoproliferative disorders

Myeloid Neoplasia

- Myeloproliferative neoplasms
  - Chronic myeloid leukemia
  - Polycythemia vera
  - Primary myelofibrosis
  - Essential thrombocythemia
- Myeloid/lymphoid neoplasms with eosinophilia and rearrangement
- Myelodysplastic/myeloproliferative neoplasms
  - Chronic myelomonocytic leukemia
- Myelodysplastic syndrome
- Acute myeloid leukemia and related neoplasms
- B- and T-cell lymphoblastic leukemia

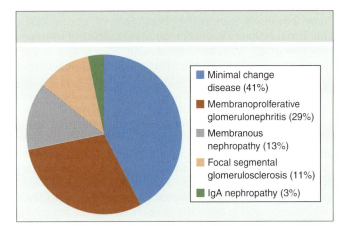

Fig. 23.1 Relative percentages of paraneoplastic glomerular lesions reported with lymphoid malignancies.

- Minimal change disease (41%)
- Membranoproliferative glomerulonephritis (29%)
- Membranous nephropathy (13%)
- Focal segmental glomerulosclerosis (11%)
- IgA nephropathy (3%)

dysfunction.[9] There are cases of paraneoplastic FSGS with HL and NHL in which altered T-cell function led to abnormal secretion of VEGF, which in turn led to increased glomerular permeability. A similar pattern of podocyte injury has been observed with the tumoral cytokine, transforming growth factor beta (TGF-β).[10,11]

LYMPHOID MALIGNANCIES: MEMBRANOPROLIFERATIVE GLOMERULONEPHRITIS

Among the lymphoid neoplasias, paraneoplastic MPGN has been reported most often in association with the B-cell lineage diseases, specifically NHL and CLL. The most common etiology for NS in patients with CLL is MPGN, followed by MCD and MN.[7,9,12] The T-cell lineage HL has seldom been associated with the development of paraneoplastic MPGN.[13]

There are several different mechanisms that have been suggested for the development of paraneoplastic MPGN with lymphoid neoplasia. One theory is that the glomerular lesion is caused by monoclonal immunoglobulins (Igs) that are secreted by B-cell clones.[14] Alternatively, the tumor may produce another monoclonal Ig, specifically cryoglobulins.[8] Chronic hepatitis C viral infection (HCV), with or without circulating cryoglobulins, is a significant infectious etiology of MPGN. It has been postulated that the HCV, which directly infects circulating peripheral blood mononuclear cells and bone marrow cells, stimulates the B lymphocytes to synthesize the type II mixed cryoglobulin. Using reverse transcriptase/polymerase chain reaction technique, investigators could detect IgM producing clonal B-cells in 38 patients with HCV infection, with and without type II mixed cryoglobulinemia.[15,16] They hypothesize that monoclonal B-cell clones may arise in a minority of patients with more severe lymphocyte dysfunction and a greater impairment of the immunoregulatory mechanisms. These clones then drive the development of both paraneoplastic MPGN and lymphoproliferative disorders. In one series of 119 consecutive HCV positive patients diagnosed with mixed cryoglobulinemia, 16 patients had mixed cryoglobulins and MPGN.[17] Bone marrow biopsies performed on patients with MPGN and those without MPGN showed a higher prevalence of lymphoma in the group with MPGN. This leads to the speculation that MPGN in this setting may represent a PNGN because of an occult B-cell lymphoma. These investigators also observed that all patients with MPGN died of infection and/or cardiovascular disease, suggesting severe lymphocyte and dysfunction in this group.[17] Although HCV is the major cause of mixed cryoglobulinemia, there is no evidence to suggest that viral infection is required for the pathogenesis of paraneoplastic MPGN.

LYMPHOID MALIGNANCIES: MEMBRANOUS NEPHROPATHY

Membranous nephropathy is relatively uncommon in patients with lymphoid malignancies. MN has been described relatively more frequently in association with the B-cell lineage diseases, such as CLL and NHL, compared with the T-cell lineage neoplasias.[18-23] There is a solitary case of MN in association with MCL.[16] In a case of MN in association with CLL, the glomerulopathy responded to treatment with fludarabine.[24]

LESS COMMON REPORTS OF PARANEOPLASTIC GLOMERULOPATHY WITH LYMPHOID NEOPLASIA

Waldenström Macroglobulinemia

Waldenström macroglobulinemia (WM) is a type of NHL. This B-cell lymphoid disorder constitutes about 2% of hematologic malignancies and is associated with a monoclonal IgM protein. The most common renal manifestations include hematuria and proteinuria.[25] In a case series of 1391 patients with WM, the reported incidence of WM-associated nephropathy at 5 years was 5.1%.[26] The diagnosis of both WM and renal disease was made concurrently in 54% of cases. Some of the lesions that were thought to be directly related to WM included, in order of frequency, light chain (AL) amyloidosis, monoclonal IgM deposition/cryoglobulinemia and lymphoplasmacytic lymphoma infiltration were the most common pathologies noted on the kidney biopsy. Lesions that were less commonly observed, and which may have represented a paraneoplastic process, included thrombotic microangiopathy (TMA), MN, and MCD.[26] Precipitation of IgM in the capillaries, infiltration of the interstitium with malignant cells, and proliferative glomerulonephritis are some additional glomerular abnormalities described on the renal biopsy reports in patients with WM.[1,27,28]

AMYLOID AND LYMPHOID MALIGNANCIES

Amyloidosis has historically been associated with HL, with most of the cases noted before 1970.[1] The majority of these cases of amyloidosis with HL were AA or secondary amyloid, and this finding may be related to the later inflammatory stages of the disease.[1] This is supported by the observation that, with advances in the treatment of HL, the incidence of Amyloid A (AA) amyloid has decreased.[1] In contrast to patients with HL, patients with NHL generally present with primary, or AL-type, amyloid.[29,30] Still, there are rare case reports of NHL with AA-type amyloidosis.[29] AL-amyloid has been reported in patients with monoclonal gammopathy in B-cell lymphomas and WM, where a single light chain type has been localized within fibrillar amyloid deposits.[31]

OTHER LYMPHOID MALIGNANCIES

Although most of the paraneoplastic glomerular lesions have been reported in HL, NHL, and CLL, there are scattered case reports of PNGN more rarely associated with other lymphoid neoplasia. In patients with MCL, glomerular involvement can be seen in the form of proliferative glomerulonephritis[32] and immune complex mediated glomerulonephritis.[33] Among patients with small lymphocytic lymphoma, antineutrophil cytoplasmic antibody-mediated crescentic glomerulonephritis (about than eight cases till date),[34] as well as focal necrotizing glomerulonephritis,[35] has been reported. B-cell lymphomas have also presented with extracapillary proliferative glomerulonephritis in association with granulomatosis and polyangiitis.[36] Isolated MPGN with C3 deposits has been reported in patients with HCL.[37] With angiotrophic lymphomas, which are characterized by the presence of primarily B-lymphocytes in small vessels, neoplastic lymphoid cells have been shown to infiltrate the glomeruli and peritubular capillaries.[38] Large cell lymphoma has been shown to cause extensive deposition of IgM kappa monoclonal Ig in the glomerular capillary lumen and can lead to the finding of amorphous material on renal biopsies.[38–41] Patients generally present with NS and may have enlarged kidneys on renal ultrasound. This could be related to the production of a local lymphocyte factor also referred to as a *vascular permeability factor* and altered glomerular hemodynamics.[42,43] "Crystal-storing histiocytosis" whose renal involvement is characterized by mesangial infiltration with mononuclear/multinuclear cells with rhomboid shaped crystals can be seen in the setting of a low-grade lymphoproliferative disorder.[44] IgA nephropathy

has been described in association with cutaneous T-cell lymphomas.[45]

Myeloid Neoplasia

Myeloid neoplasia constitutes a heterogeneous group of clonal hematopoietic stem cell disorders, which can be subdivided into acute and chronic myeloid neoplasia based on peripheral blood findings or bone marrow findings. Based on the 2016 World Health Organization classification (see Box 23.1), the myeloid neoplasms are further subdivided into myeloproliferative neoplasias (MPN), myeloid/lymphoid neoplasms with eosinophilia with various rearrangements, myelodysplastic syndrome (MDS), and myelodysplastic/ myeloproliferative neoplasms (MDS/MPN). The MPN are further subcategorized into chronic myeloid leukemia (CML), polycythemia vera (PV), essential thrombocythemia (ET), and primary myelofibrosis.[7,46]

In comparison with the lymphoid malignancies, the reported incidence of PNGN among patients with myeloid malignancies is much less common. Fig. 23.2 illustrates the relative percentages of paraneoplastic glomerular lesions reported with the types of PNGN among myeloid malignancies. Overall, mesangioproliferative glomerulonephritis is the lesion that has been most commonly reported on renal biopsy, followed by FSGS. In MDS, the incidence of PNGN has been reported to be from 0.5% to 4% with a wide variety of presentations, including mesangioproliferative glomerulonephritis, MN, IgA nephropathy, and rapidly progressive glomerulonephritis (RPGN).[7,47,48] Among patients with myeloproliferative neoplasia, the incidence of PNGN has been reported to be around 3.6%.[7] The pattern of renal involvement in patients with MPN is quite variable and is referred to as *MPN-related glomerulopathy*.[7,49,50] Some of the pathologic findings include mesangial/segmental sclerosis, hypercellularity, chronic TMA, and intracapillary hematopoietic cell infiltration.[47] The differential diagnosis of MPN-related glomerulopathy includes primary FSGS, diabetic glomerulosclerosis, smoking related glomerulopathy, TMA, and MPGN.[50–52]

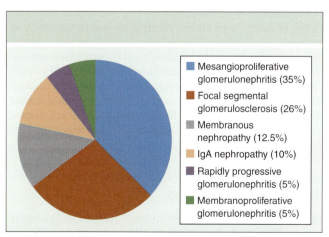

■ Mesangioproliferative glomerulonephritis (35%)
■ Focal segmental glomerulosclerosis (26%)
■ Membranous nephropathy (12.5%)
■ IgA nephropathy (10%)
■ Rapidly progressive glomerulonephritis (5%)
■ Membranoproliferative glomerulonephritis (5%)

Fig. 23.2 Relative percentages of paraneoplastic glomerular lesions reported with myeloid malignancies.

In patients with acute myeloid leukemia (AML) who were biopsied for the evaluation of nephrotic range proteinuria, FSGS, MPGN, mesangioproliferative glomerulonephritis, and MCD have been identified.[47] In patients with CML and nephrotic range proteinuria, the renal biopsy showed a range of glomerular lesions similar to those observed with AML, with the exception of FSGS. Owing to the indolent nature of CML, the development of PNGN may be coincidental.[7,47] In isolated case studies where MCD and RPGN were diagnosed in the setting of CML, the glomerular lesion was treated effectively with immunosuppression without any effect on the underlying CML.[53]

Several pathogenic mechanisms for glomerular injury have been postulated for PNGN associated with myeloid neoplasias. Increased concentrations of lysozyme in the urine of patients with chronic myelomonocytic leukemia has been described to produce nephrotic range proteinuria. This has been referred to as *pseudonephrotic syndrome*.[53] Other possible etiologies include splenomegaly-induced immunosuppression, autoimmune dysregulation, and increased production of platelet derived growth factor (PDGF) and TGF-β.[47,51]

MYELOID NEOPLASIA: MESANGIOPROLIFERATIVE GLOMERULOPATHY

Among the myeloproliferative neoplasms, mesangioproliferative glomerulopathy is more commonly associated with primary myelofibrosis as compared with ET, PV, or CML. The presence of MPN-related glomerulopathy is generally detected late in the course of the disease and is characterized by the development of proteinuria that is refractory to the usual treatments for proteinuria.[7,52] Histologically speaking, mesangioproliferative glomerulopathy is characterized by the presence of mesangial hypercellularity and duplication of the glomerular basement membrane with a subendothelial electron lucent layer. These features are similar to those seen with chronic TMA. Rarely, nodular mesangial sclerosis has been observed. There are no immune complexes on electron microscopy and immunofixation studies are also negative. On occasion, intracapillary hematopoietic cells can be seen.[47,52,54] Increased levels of TGF-β, and PDGF, are thought to be responsible for this mesangioproliferative pattern by promoting mesangial cell expansion and extracellular matrix proliferation. Upregulation of PDGF-A within the mesangial cells and PDGF-D have been demonstrated in animal models of anti-Ty 11 mesangioproliferative glomerulonephritis. Blockade of these pathways has been shown to reduce mesangial cell proliferation and tubulointerstitial fibrosis.[55] Concurrent to the aforementioned findings, rat models have also demonstrated an upregulation in PDGF receptor messenger ribonucleic acid between days 3 and 5 of disease induction, which corresponds to the time of mesangial cell proliferation.[56]

MYELOID NEOPLASIA: FOCAL SEGMENTAL GLOMERULAR SCLEROSIS

In patients with myeloproliferative neoplasia, the pathogenesis of FSGS may be related to alterations in lymphocyte function, which may in turn lead to increased production of "permeability factors." Purported permeability factors include cytokines such as TGF β-1, PDGF, basic fibroblast growth factor (BFGF), VEGF, epidermal growth factor (EGF), endothelial cell growth factor, and IL-1. These cytokines have been related to both the development of myelofibrosis and FSGS. In addition to these systemic cytokines, locally produced cytokines such as PDGF, tumor necrosis factor (TNF), and IL-1β are also associated with FSGS. PDGF is a major cytokine, whose synthesis can be induced by PDGF itself, EGF, and TGF-β. Under hypoxic conditions, the glomerular endothelial cells are stimulated to produce PDGF. Under conditions of hyperfiltration, hepatocyte growth factor and TGF-β are ultrafiltered in the glomerulus and stimulate the production of PDGF. In concert with other cytokines such as TGF-β, PDGF promotes extracellular matrix synthesis and mesangial cell contraction, leading to alterations in the glomerular hemodynamics.[55,57] In animal models, PDGF and TGF-β play an important role in the development of glomerulosclerosis, promoting podocyte apoptosis, and the development of FSGS-like lesions. These strong profibrotic stimuli act in concert with other members of the TGF family, including thrombospondin 1 and phosphorylated Smad2/Smad3.[58–61] Increased expression of BFGF in addition to VEGF has also been implicated in the development of FSGS among these patients.[62]

In the setting of MPN, increased production of PDGF, Platelet-Activating Factor (PAF), and TGF-β has been shown to stimulate intense fibrosis in the mesangial cells.[63] In patients with ET, there is increased production and abnormal function of platelets. The increased intraglomerular accumulation of platelets has been associated with the release of TGF-β which, in addition to producing fibrosis, also serves as a mitogen for glomerular cell proliferation.[58] In patients with PV, alterations in glomerular hemodynamics including renal vasodilatation and an increase in effective renal blood flow have been observed. Patients with PV can also develop hyperviscosity, which predisposes to the development of microvascular thrombi. Both of these processes can lead to endothelial cell injury, activation of macrophages, and extension of the extracellular matrix.[64–67]

MYELOID NEOPLASIA: MEMBRANOUS NEPHROPATHY AND MEMBRANOPROLIFERATIVE GLOMERULONEPHRITIS

Both MN and MPGN have only rarely been reported in association with the myeloproliferative disorders. They are relatively much more commonly seen with lymphoid neoplasias.[2,9,19] MN has been described in association with AML and chronic myelomonocytic leukemia (CMML).[68,69] Because of the indolent nature of CMML, the association of membranous nephropathy may or may not be related to the neoplasia. Patients have shown response to treatment with imatinib and mycophenolate mofetil in rare cases.[70] MPGN has been described in association with CML as well as PV.[49,50]

Key Points

■ The overall reported incidence of paraneoplastic glomerulopathy (PNGN) in relation to hematologic malignancies is quite rare, with the total number of cases being slightly in excess of 200.

- The observed rate of PNGN is higher in lymphoid malignancies as compared with myeloid neoplasia.
- Among the lymphoid malignancies, minimal change disease and (FSGS) focal segmental glomerular sclerosis are most commonly seen with Hodgkin lymphoma.
- Among the myeloid neoplasia, mesangioproliferative glomerulonephritis is the most commonly reported paraneoplastic lesions, followed by FSGS.
- A wide variety of putative mechanisms have been described in relation to the pathogenesis of different forms of PNGN, but more studies are needed to further define the pathogenetic mechanisms.

References

1. Ronco PM. Paraneoplastic glomerulopathies: new insights into an old entity. *Kidney Int.* 1999;56(1):355-377.
2. Lien YH, Lai LW. Pathogenesis, diagnosis and management of paraneoplastic glomerulonephritis. *Nat Rev Nephrol.* 2011;7(2):85-95.
3. Vankalakunti M, Rohan A, Vishwanath S, et al. Spectrum of renal involvement in hematolymphoid neoplasms: renal biopsy findings of 12 cases. *Indian J Nephrol.* 2015;25(4):201-205.
6. Hindocha S, Gopaluni S, Collins GP, Shenbagaraman P. Focal segmental glomerulosclerosis in a patient with mantle cell lymphoma. *BMJ Case Rep.* 2015;2015. pii: bcr2015211765.
8. Cambier JF, Ronco P. Onco-nephrology: glomerular diseases with cancer. *Clin J Am Soc Nephrol.* 2012;7(10):1701-1712.
9. Bacchetta J, Juillard L, Cochat P, Droz JP. Paraneoplastic glomerular diseases and malignancies. *Crit Rev Oncol Hematol.* 2009;70(1):39-58.
10. Newcom SR, Gu L. Transforming growth factor beta 1 messenger RNA in Reed-Sternberg cells in nodular sclerosing Hodgkin's disease. *J Clin Pathol.* 1995;48(2):160-163.
13. Büyükpamukçu M, Hazar V, Tinaztepe K, Bakkaloğlu A, Akyüz C, Kutluk T. Hodgkin's disease and renal paraneoplastic syndromes in childhood. *Turk J Pediatr.* 2000;42(2):109-114.
14. Favre G, Courtellemont C, Callard P, et al. Membranoproliferative glomerulonephritis, chronic lymphocytic leukemia, and cryoglobulinemia. *Am J Kidney Dis.* 2010;55(2):391-394.
15. Franzin F, Efremov DG, Pozzato G, Tulissi P, Batista F, Burrone OR. Clonal B-cell expansions in peripheral blood of HCV-infected patients. *Br J Haematol.* 1995;90(3):548-552.
16. Zakharova E, Stolyarevich E, Nikitin E. Mantle cell lymphoma associated with membranoproliferative and membranous glomerulonephritis: report of two cases. *Cancer Sci Res Open Access.* 2016;3(1):1-7.
17. Mazzaro C, Panarello G, Tesio F, et al. Hepatitis C virus risk: a hepatitis C virus related syndrome. *J Intern Med.* 2000;247(5):535-545.
19. Da'as N, Polliack A, Cohen Y, et al. Kidney involvement and renal manifestations in non-Hodgkin's lymphoma and lymphocytic leukemia: a retrospective study in 700 patients. *Eur J Haematol.* 2001;67(3):158-164.
20. Moulin B, Ronco PM, Mougenot B, Francois A, Fillastre JP, Mignon F. Glomerulonephritis in chronic lymphocytic leukemia and related B-cell lymphomas. *Kidney Int.* 1992;42(1):127-135.
24. Butty H, Asfoura J, Cortese F, Doyle M, Rutecki G. Chronic lymphocytic leukemia-associated membranous glomerulopathy: remission with fludarabine. *Am J Kidney Dis.* 1999;33(2):E8.
25. Salviani C, Guido G, Serriello I, Giannakakis K, Rocca AR. Renal involvement in Waldenström's macroglobulinemia: case report and review of literature. *Ren Fail.* 2014;36(1):114-118.
26. Vos JM, Gustine J, Rennke HG, et al. Renal disease related to Waldenström macroglobulinaemia: incidence, pathology and clinical outcomes. *Br J Haematol.* 2016;175(4):623-630.
27. Veltman GA, van Veen S, Kluin-Nelemans JC, Bruijn JA, van Es LA. Renal disease in Waldenström's macroglobulinaemia. *Nephrol Dial Transplant.* 1997;12(6):1256-1259.
30. Cohen LJ, Rennke HG, Laubach JP, Humphreys BD. The spectrum of kidney involvement in lymphoma: a case report and review of the literature. *Am J Kidney Dis.* 2010;56(6):1191-1196.
31. Latcha S, Seshan SV. *Paraneoplastic glomerulopathy.* Amsterdam, Netherlands: Elsevier; 2013:209-249.
32. Karim M, Hill P, Pillai G, Gatter K, Davies DR, Winearls CG. Proliferative glomerulonephritis associated with mantle cell lymphoma—natural history and effect of treatment in 2 cases. *Clin Nephrol.* 2004;61(6):422-428.
33. Abeysekera RA, Wazil AW, Nanayakkara N, Ratnatunga N, Fernando KM, Thinnarachchi J. Mantle cell lymphoma first presenting as immune complex-mediated glomerulonephritis: a case report. *J Med Case Rep.* 2015;9:115.
34. Henriksen KJ, Hong RB, Sobrero MI, Chang A. Rare association of chronic lymphocytic leukemia/small lymphocytic lymphoma, ANCAs, and pauci-immune crescentic glomerulonephritis. *Am J Kidney Dis.* 2011;57(1):170-174.
35. Pollock CA, Ibels LS, Levi JA, Eckstein RP, Wakeford P. Acute renal failure due to focal necrotizing glomerulonephritis in a patient with non-Hodgkin's lymphoma. Resolution with treatment of lymphoma. *Nephron.* 1988;48(3):197-200.
36. Wills Sanín B, Bolivar YR, Carvajal JJ, Quintero GE, Andrade R. Polyangiitis with granulomatosis as a paraneoplastic syndrome of b-cell lymphoma of the lacrimal gland. *Case Rep Hematol.* 2014;2014:713048.
37. Abboud I, Galicier L, De Labarthe A, Dossier A, Glotz D, Verine J. A paraneoplastic membranoproliferative glomerulonephritis with isolated C3 deposits associated with hairy cell leukaemia. *Nephrol Dial Transplant.* 2010;25(6):2026-2028.
38. Cossu A, Deiana A, Lissia A, et al. Nephrotic syndrome and angiotropic lymphoma report of a case. *Tumori.* 2004;90(5):510-513.
40. Oyama Y, Komatsuda A, Ohtani H, et al. Extensive intraglomerular thrombi of monoclonal IgM-kappa in a patient with malignant lymphoma. *Am J Kidney Dis.* 2000;35(3):E11.
41. Nishikawa K, Sekiyama S, Suzuki T, et al. A case of angiotropic large cell lymphoma manifesting nephrotic syndrome and treated successfully with combination chemotherapy. *Nephron.* 1991;58(4):479-482.
42. Kakumitsu H, Higuchi M, Tanaka K, Shibuya T. Nephrotic syndrome in a patient with intravascular lymphomatosis. *J-Stage.* 2003;42(1):98-101.
43. D'Agati V, Sablay LB, Knowles DM, Walter L. Angiotropic large cell lymphoma (intravascular malignant lymphomatosis) of the kidney: presentation as minimal change disease. *Hum Pathol.* 1989;20(3):263-268.
44. Sethi S, Cuiffo BP, Pinkus GS, Rennke HG. Crystal-storing histiocytosis involving the kidney in a low-grade B-cell lymphoproliferative disorder. *Am J Kidney Dis.* 2002;39(1):183-188.
45. Bajel A, Yin Lin M, Hill PA, et al. IgA nephropathy associated with cutaneous T cell lymphoma. *Leuk Lymphoma.* 2009;50(12):2083-2085.
46. Barbui T, Thiele J, Gisslinger H, et al. The 2016 WHO classification and diagnostic criteria for myeloproliferative neoplasms: document summary and in-depth discussion. *Blood Cancer J.* 2018;8(2):15.
47. Luciano RL, Brewster UC. Kidney involvement in leukemia and lymphoma. *Adv Chronic Kidney Dis.* 2014;21(1):27-35.
48. Ko KI, Lee MJ, Doh FM, et al. Membranous glomerulonephritis in a patient with myelodysplastic syndrome-refractory cytopenia with multilineage dysplasia. *Kidney Res Clin Pract.* 2013;32(3):134-137.
51. Rajasekaran A, Ngo TT, Abdelrahim M, et al. Primary myelofibrosis associated glomerulopathy: significant improvement after therapy with ruxolitinib. *BMC Nephrol.* 2015;16:121.
53. Sudholt BA, Heironimus JD. Chronic myelogenous leukemia with nephrotic syndrome. *Arch Intern Med.* 1983;143(1):168-169.
56. Iida H, Seifert R, Alpers CE, et al. Platelet-derived growth factor (PDGF) and PDGF receptor are induced in mesangial proliferative nephritis in the rat. *Proc Natl Acad Sci U S A.* 1991;88(15):6560-6564.
57. Kaygusuz I, Koc M, Arikan H, et al. Focal segmental glomerulosclerosis associated with idiopathic myelofibrosis. *Ren Fail.* 2010;32(2):273-276.
58. Floege J, Burns MW, Alpers CE, et al. Glomerular cell proliferation and PDGF expression precede glomerulosclerosis in the remnant kidney model. *Kidney Int.* 1992;41(2):297-309.
60. Kim JH, Kim BK, Moon KC, Hong HK, Lee HS. Activation of the TGF-beta/Smad signaling pathway in focal segmental glomerulosclerosis. *Kidney Int.* 2003;64(5):1715-1721.
62. Schrijvers BF, Flyvbjerg A, De Vriese AS. The role of vascular endothelial growth factor (VEGF) in renal pathophysiology. *Kidney Int.* 2004;65(6):2003-2017.

63. Au WY, Chan KW, Lui SL, Lam CC, Kwong YL. Focal segmental glomerulosclerosis and mesangial sclerosis associated with myeloproliferative disorders. *Am J Kidney Dis.* 1999;34(5):889-893.

65. Gulcan E, Yildirim R, Uludag K, Keles M, Uyanik A. Development of focal segmental glomerulosclerosis in a patient with polycythemia vera: can polycythemia vera be a cause of focal segmental glomerulosclerosis? *Nefrologia.* 2012;32(6):852-854.

68. Sahiner S, Ayli MD, Yüksel C, Oneç K, Abayli E. Membranous nephropathy associated with acute myeloid leukemia. *Transplant Proc.* 2004;36(9):2618-2619.

69. Enriquez R, Sirvent AE, Marin F, Perez M, Alpera MR, Amorós F. Severe renal complications in chronic myelomonocytic leukemia. *J Nephrol.* 2008;21(4):609-614.

70. Dwyer JP, Yates KM, Sumner EL, et al. Chronic myeloid leukemia-associated membranoproliferative glomerulonephritis that responded to imatinib mesylate therapy. *Clin Nephrol.* 2007;67(3):176-181.

A full list of references is available at Expertconsult.com

24 Cancer Screening Recommendations

SHERON LATCHA

Paraneoplastic glomerulopathy remains a rare clinical entity. Please refer to Chapters 22 and 23 for a more detailed discussion on the reported prevalence and some of the purported mechanisms for paraneoplastic glomerular diseases. Arguably, the data supporting the relationship between neoplasia and paraneoplastic glomerulopathy are most convincing for membranous nephropathy with solid tumors, and minimal change disease with Hodgkin lymphoma. Nonetheless, diverse patterns of glomerular diseases have been reported in association with a number of malignancies. Because glomerular disease can be the initial clinical manifestation of an underlying malignancy, the nephrologist may have a crucial role in initiating the evaluation for an underlying malignancy, and in doing so, avoid delays in the proper identification and treatment of a neoplasia. If paraneoplastic glomerulopathy is properly identified and treated, treatment of the tumor should lead to remission of the renal disease and thus spare the patient exposure to unnecessary immunosuppressive therapy for an incorrect diagnosis of a primary glomerular disease. Moreover, if an antecedent occult tumor is not properly identified, the development of that tumor may be subsequently ascribed to the immunosuppressive therapy that was used to treat the initial presenting glomerular disease.

As detailed in Chapters 22 and 23, a number of reports support an increased prevalence in cancer among patients with primary glomerular diseases. Tumors of the lung, colorectal system, prostate, breast, and the hematologic and lymphatic tissue have been most frequently reported in association with paraneoplastic glomerulopathy.[1-4] Paraneoplastic glomerular disease can present before, after, or concurrent with the detection of an associated neoplasia. Based on analysis of Danish registry data, the risk of cancer was 2.5 and 3.5 times higher than in the general population at 1 and 2 years, respectively, after diagnosis of the glomerular disease.[2] In another case series of 24 patients with paraneoplastic membranous nephropathy, in 21 cases the cancer was detected at the time of the renal biopsy, and in the remaining three, within 1 year after the renal biopsy.[1] Given the lack of any clear pattern or time course between detecting the paraneoplastic glomerular disease and malignancy, the clinician should maintain a constant level of suspicion for this underlying, albeit rare, clinical entity.

There is no clear consensus on whether all patients who present with a glomerular disease should be screened for an underlying malignancy. In addition, there are no clear guidelines on what an appropriate cancer screening program should entail. Moreover, the duration of cancer screening after the glomerular disease is recognized as uncertain. Based on prospective and retrospective reports, populations who may be at risk for paraneoplastic glomerulopathy include older patients, those with a history of heavy tobacco use,[1] unexplained proteinuria,[5] those exposed to immunosuppressive medications,[6,7] and patients with membranous nephropathy on the renal biopsy. In addition, there are specific findings on the renal biopsy that may serve as a signal for underlying malignancy.[3,8]

Unexplained microalbuminuria, especially in a patient with other risk factors for bladder and lung cancer, may be a hint to an underlying paraneoplastic glomerulopathy. In a prospective analysis of 5425 Norwegians with no underlying history of diabetes, cancer, or macroalbuminuria, when compared with individuals with the lowest quintile of albumin to creatinine ratio, those with a ratio at the highest quintile were 8.3 times more likely to develop bladder cancer, and 5.4 times more likely to develop lung cancer.[5] Risk factors for bladder cancer include age older than 65 years, smoking history, male gender, Caucasian race, cyclophosphamide exposure, and occupational exposures (rubber, textiles, paint).[9]

Individuals exposed to some of the immunosuppressive therapies used to treat primary glomerular diseases, autoimmune diseases, and for protection against renal transplant rejection are at increased risk for later development of specific malignancies and may warrant additional scrutiny for an underlying cancer. Cyclophosphamide exposure is linked to the bladder tumors and hematologic malignancies. Cyclophosphamide itself and acrolein, an inactive metabolite of cyclophosphamide, may have oncogenic effects on the bladder urothelium. The risk of malignancy is dose related. Individuals who had received greater than 36 grams of cyclophosphamide had a standardized incidence ratio (SIR) of bladder cancer of 9.6 when compared with those who received lower doses of the drug or no drug at all.[10] Patients with lupus who were treated with cyclophosphamide had a higher risk of lymphoma and those with granulomatous polyangiitis who had received greater than 36 grams of cyclophosphamide had a SIR of 59 for acute myeloid leukemia when compared with the general population.[6] Long-term use of chlorambucil for treatment of polycythemia vera[11] and ovarian cancer[12] is associated with an increased risk for acute leukemia. It is not known if the increased risk of acute leukemia is related to cumulative dose of the drug. Long-term exposure to azathioprine in organ transplant recipients is linked to increased risk for skin cancer, lymphoma, and urinary tract cancers.[13-15] In patients with multiple sclerosis, the risk of cancer correlated with cumulative doses of greater than 600 grams of azathioprine and treatment duration of greater than 10 years.[16]

Azathioprine has been largely replaced by the calcineurin inhibitors (CNIs), cyclosporine and tacrolimus, for prevention of graft rejection in transplant recipients and for treatment of some primary glomerular diseases. When compared with azathioprine, the CNIs are associated with earlier development of cancers.[7] As is the case with azathioprine, the risk of cancer increases with increased total dose and duration of CNI exposure.[17] Recipients of solid organ transplants are exposed to CNIs, in addition to other classes of immunosuppressants. When compared with the general population, the SIR for virus related cancer in recipients of solid organ transplants is 7.54 for non-Hodgkin lymphoma (NHL), 3.58 for Hodgkin lymphoma (HL), 6.15 for Kaposi sarcoma, up to 7.6 for human papilloma virus–related cancers, 4.65 for kidney, and 1.97 for lung cancer.[18] The SIR for nonmelanoma skin cancer in this group is 50 at 4 years posttransplant and increases greater than 100-fold at 10 years from transplant.[19]

There are several specific findings on the renal biopsy in patients with membranous nephropathy that may serve as a clue for a paraneoplastic process. Because idiopathic membranous nephropathy is not associated with electron dense deposits in the mesangium and subendothelium, the presence of such deposits should raise concern for a secondary or paraneoplastic process. In addition, inflammatory cells are rarely seen in idiopathic membranous nephropathy. In one report, the presence of more than eight leukocytes per glomerulus had a sensitivity and specificity of 75% and 92%, respectively, for identifying a paraneoplastic glomerulopathy.[1] Idiopathic membranous nephropathy is most often associated with immunoglobulin (Ig)G4 deposits, whereas IgG1, IgG2, and IgG3 are seen more frequently with secondary membranous nephropathy.[20] Circulating antiphospholipase A2 receptor is seen in up to 89% cases of idiopathic membranous nephropathy. Nonetheless, in patients who are not responding appropriately to directed therapy against membranous nephropathy, it is noteworthy that circulating antiphospholipase A2 receptor is occasionally present with secondary, including paraneoplastic, membranous nephropathy.[21,22] Furthermore, there are some clinical findings in patients with membranous nephropathy that should raise the suspicion for a paraneoplastic process. Membranous nephropathy and cancer are both associated with increased risk for thromboembolic events, and the risk of thromboembolic events increases in the presence of cancer. Up to 25% of patients with cancer associated membranous nephropathy developed a thromboembolic event in one report.[23] Along with patients with membranous nephropathy, another population that may warrant closer scrutiny are those with mixed cryoglobulinemia without evidence for hepatitis C viral infection, because studies have revealed a fourfold increased risk of developing B-cell and NHL.[24]

None of the national or international nephrology groups have offered or endorsed any cancer screening guidelines in patients with suspected paraneoplastic glomerulopathy. Screening guidelines require data from large randomized controlled trials, and it is unlikely that such data can be obtained in the population under consideration. In general, cancer screening is performed with the intent of early detection and early treatment of cancers to improve life expectancy. Any such benefit for cancer screening in patients with paraneoplastic glomerulopathy is unknown. Additional

unknown factors include the financial cost of cancer screening in this population, potential complications of cancer screening, test performance (sensitivity, specificity, positive predictive value), or whether there is any benefit of early detection of cancers that have no mortality benefit when detected early. Because paraneoplastic glomerulopathy can predate the discovery of a tumor, it is unclear if a paraneoplastic glomerulopathy associates with early (in situ) or advanced malignancies. If one finds an in situ cervical cancer as part of the workup for a paraneoplastic glomerulopathy, there is no way of being certain that this early lesion is linked to the glomerular abnormality or if ongoing screening is required. With these cautions and limitations in mind, the general recommendations that follow are thus opinion based.

At a minimum, all patients with glomerular disease should have a complete personal history, family history, physical examination, smoking history, medication history (with attention to chemotherapy, radiation treatment, and immunosuppressive drugs), and routine serum chemistry and a urinalysis. If a hematologic malignancy is suspected, testing of the serum, urine bone marrow, and peripheral blood are essential for confirmation. Patients with age and other specific risk factors for malignancy should have appropriate screening. In a patient who was previously treated with cyclophosphamide or who has a history of tobacco use, it may be reasonable to check a urinalysis to evaluate for hematuria. Table 24.1 lists the current recommendations for cancer screening from the U.S. Preventive Services Task Force.[25] For patients who have been treated with azathioprine and for recipients of solid organ transplants, it may be prudent to screen for skin cancers, because these cancers can be very aggressive in these populations. For

Table 24.1 US Preventive Services Task Force Cancer Screening Recommendations

Cancer	Screening Method	Population	Grade of Recommendation
Breast	Mammogram	Women age 50–74 years	B
Cervical	PAP, HPV DNA	Women age 21–65 years	A
Colorectal	Colonoscopy, sigmoidoscopy, fecal occult blood test	Age 50–75 years	A
Lung	Low dose CAT scan	Age 55–80 years heavy smokers	B
Prostate	PSA	Men, any age	D
Skin	Whole body scan	Any age	I

Grade A: The USPSTF recommends the service. High certainty of substantial benefit.
Grade B: The USPSTF recommends the service. Moderate certainty of substantial benefit.
Grade C: The USPSTF recommends selectively offering based on professional judgment and patient preferences.
Grade D: The USPSTF recommends against the service.
Grade I: The USPSTF concludes that evidence is insufficient, conflicting, and the balance of benefits and harms cannot be determined.
CAT, Computed tomography; *DNA,* deoxyribonucleic acid; *HPV,* human papilloma virus; *PAP,* Papanicolau; *PSA,* prostate specific antigen.

Table 24.2   Cancer Screening Recommendations for Solid Organ Transplant Recipients

Cancer	AST-Kidney	CST & CSN	EBPG	KDIGO	KHA-CARI	NKF	RA	Comments
Breast	Every 1–2 years	G	R	G	NS	NS	G	Same as general population
Cervical	Yearly	Yearly	Yearly	G	Yearly	NS	G	More frequently than in general population
Colorectal	G	G	R	G	NS	NS	G	Same as general population
Lung	NR	NS	NS	NS	NS	NS	NS	
Prostate	Yearly	NR	Yearly	NR	NS	NS	NR	Same as general population
Skin	Yearly	Yearly	NS	Yearly	Yearly	Yearly	R	Modify based on risk factors

AST-Kidney, American Society of Transplantation 2000; *CST & CSN*, Canadian Society of Transplantation and Canadian Society of Nephrology 2000; *EBPG*, European Best Practice Guidelines 2009; *G*, same as general population; *KDIGO*, Kidney Disease Improving Global Outcome 2009; *KHA-CARI*, Kidney Health Australia-Caring for Australasians with Renal Impairment; *NKF*, National Kidney Foundation; *NR*, not recommended; *NS*, not specified; *R*, recommended; *RA*, Renal Association Clinical Practice Guidelines 2011.

recipients of solid organ transplants, a recent review article summarized the recommendations from national and international transplantation societies. Some of those findings are presented in Table 24.2.[26] Screening for malignancy may also be considered in those individuals who fail to respond appropriately to the standard therapy for their primary glomerulopathy. In a study where eight out of 21 patients had minimal change disease diagnosed months before the diagnosis of HL, two of eight were resistant to steroid therapy or cyclosporine. The minimal change disease responded to treatment for their HL.[27]

Because the risk of a paraneoplastic glomerulopathy is not restricted to the onset of the renal disease or the time period immediately surrounding this presentation, ongoing surveillance using urinalysis and/or renal function tests may be useful to uncover new onset of renal disease, despite quiescence or remission of the malignancy.[28] The duration of surveillance remains ill defined. If a specific tumor is suspected, known circulating tumor markers may be helpful in identifying the underlying malignancy.

The treatment of paraneoplastic glomerulopathy requires a multidisciplinary approach and requires dialogue among the nephrologist, oncologist, surgeon, and other members of the health care team. It is generally agreed upon that the treatment of paraneoplastic glomerulopathy is standard and specific therapy for the primary malignancy.[29] Some severe glomerular lesions in the setting of solid tumors, such as crescentic glomerulonephritis secondary to antineutrophil cytoplasmic antibodies vasculitis, may need aggressive therapy to block the glomerular inflammatory process. In the setting of nephrotic syndrome, in addition to standard chemotherapy, directed drug therapy against proteinuria and hyperlipidemia may also be required. Although almost all the renal lesions associated with lymphoid malignancies mainly require specific antineoplastic therapy to induce partial or complete remission, therapy is somewhat varied in paraneoplastic glomerulopathy with myeloid malignancies and thymomas, most probably related to the diverse cell types involved.[29]

Key Points

■ None of the national or international nephrology groups have offered or endorsed any cancer screening guidelines in patients with suspected paraneoplastic glomerulopathy.

■ Glomerular disease can be the initial clinical manifestation of an underlying malignancy, and as such, the nephrologist may have a crucial role in initiating the evaluation for an underlying malignancy.

■ Paraneoplastic glomerular disease can present before, after, or concurrent with the detection of an associated neoplasia.

■ Populations who may be at risk for paraneoplastic glomerulopathy include older patients, those with a history of heavy tobacco use, unexplained proteinuria, those exposed to immunosuppressive medications, and patients with membranous nephropathy on the renal biopsy.

■ There are several specific findings on the renal biopsy in patients with membranous nephropathy that may serve as a clue for a paraneoplastic process.

References

1. Lefaucheur C, Stengel B, Nochy D, et al. Membranous nephropathy and cancer: epidemiologic evidence and determinants of high-risk cancer association. *Kidney Int.* 2006;70(8):1510-1517.
2. Birkeland SA, Storm HH. Glomerulonephritis and malignancy: a population-based analysis. *Kidney Int.* 2003;63(2):716-721.
3. Bjørneklett R, Vikse BE, Svarstad E, et al. Long-term risk of cancer in membranous nephropathy patients. *Am J Kidney Dis.* 2007;50(3):396-403.
4. Rihova Z, Honsova E, Merta M, et al. Secondary membranous nephropathy—one center experience. *Ren Fail.* 2005;27(4):397-402.
5. Jørgensen L, Heuch I, Jenssen T, Jacobsen BK. Association of albuminuria and cancer incidence. *J Am Soc Nephrol.* 2008;19(5):992-998.
6. Bernatsky S, Ramsey-Goldman R, Joseph L, et al. Lymphoma risk in systemic lupus: effects of disease activity versus treatment. *Ann Rheum Dis.* 2014;73(1):138-142.
7. Penn I. Post-transplant malignancy: the role of immunosuppression. *Drug Saf.* 2000;23(2):101-113.
8. Glassock RJ. Prophylactic anticoagulation in nephrotic syndrome: a clinical conundrum. *J Am Soc Nephrol.* 2007;18(8):2221-2225.
9. Sanli O, Dobruch J, Knowles MA, et al. Bladder cancer. *Nat Rev Dis Primers.* 2017;3:17022.
10. Faurschou M, Sorensen IJ, Mellemkjaer L, et al. Malignancies in Wegener's granulomatosis: incidence and relation to cyclophosphamide therapy in a cohort of 293 patients. *J Rheumatol.* 2008;35(1):100-105
11. Tefferi A, Rumi E, Finazzi G, et al. Survival and prognosis among 1545 patients with contemporary polycythemia vera: an international study. *Leukemia.* 2013;27(9):1874-1881.

12. Kaldor JM, Day NE, Pettersson F, et al. Leukemia following chemotherapy for ovarian cancer. *N Engl J Med.* 1990;322(1):1-6.

13. Penn I, Starzl TE. Malignant tumors arising de novo in immunosuppressed organ transplant recipients. *Transplantation.* 1972;14(4):407-417.

14. Frascà GM, Sandrini S, Cosmai L, et al. Renal cancer in kidney transplanted patients. *J Nephrol.* 2015;28(6):659-668.

15. Pasternak B, Svanström H, Schmiegelow K, Jess T, Hviid A. Use of azathioprine and the risk of cancer in inflammatory bowel disease. *Am J Epidemiol.* 2013;177(11):1296-1305.

16. Casetta I, Iuliano G, Filippini G. Azathioprine for multiple sclerosis. *J Neurol Neurosurg Psychiatry.* 2009;80(2):131-132, discussion 132.

17. Carenco C, Assenat E, Faure S, et al. Tacrolimus and the risk of solid cancers after liver transplant: a dose effect relationship. *Am J Transplant.* 2015;15(3):678-686.

18. Engels EA, Pfeiffer RM, Fraumeni JF Jr, et al. Spectrum of cancer risk among US solid organ transplant recipients. *JAMA.* 2011;306(17):1891-1901.

19. Krynitz B, Edgren G, Lindelöf B, et al. Risk of skin cancer and other malignancies in kidney, liver, heart and lung transplant recipients 1970 to 2008—a Swedish population-based study. *Int J Cancer.* 2013;132(6):1429-1438.

20. Ponticelli C, Glassock RJ. Glomerular diseases: membranous nephropathy—a modern view. *Clin J Am Soc Nephrol.* 2014;9(3):609-616.

21. Beck LH Jr, Bonegio RG, Lambeau G, et al. M-type phospholipase A2 receptor as target antigen in idiopathic membranous nephropathy. *N Engl J Med.* 2009;361(1):11-21.

22. Qin W, Beck LH Jr, Zeng C, et al. Anti-phospholipase A2 receptor antibody in membranous nephropathy. *J Am Soc Nephrol.* 2011;22(6):1137-1143.

23. Glassock RJ. Attending rounds: an older patient with nephrotic syndrome. *Clin J Am Soc Nephrol.* 2012;7(4):665-670.

24. Saadoun D, Sellam J, Ghillani-Dalbin P, Crecel R, Piette JC, Cacoub P. Increased risks of lymphoma and death among patients with non-hepatitis C virus-related mixed cryoglobulinemia. *Arch Intern Med.* 2006;166(19):2101-2108.

25. *Cancer Screening Guidelines.* Available at: https://www.uspreventiveservicestaskforce.org/Page/Document/UpdateSummaryFinal/cervical-cancer-screening.

26. Acuna SA, Huang JW, Scott AL, et al. Cancer screening recommendations for solid organ transplant recipients: a systematic review of clinical practice guidelines. *Am J Transplant.* 2017;17(1):103-114.

27. Audard V, Larousserie F, Grimbert P, et al. Minimal change nephrotic syndrome and classical Hodgkin's lymphoma: report of 21 cases and review of the literature. *Kidney Int.* 2006;69(12):2251-2260.

28. Karras A, de Montpreville V, Fakhouri F, Grünfeld JP, Lesavre P. Renal and thymic pathology in thymoma-associated nephropathy: report of 21 cases and review of the literature. *Nephrol Dial Transplant.* 2005;20(6):1075-1082.

29. Lien YH, Lai LW. Pathogenesis, diagnosis and management of paraneoplastic glomerulonephritis. *Nat Rev Nephrol.* 2011;7(2):85-95.

Renal Tumors

25 *Renal Cell Cancer*

NITI MADAN AND ROBERT H. WEISS

Introduction

Kidney cancer, or renal cell carcinoma (RCC), is the most common malignancy seen in the practice of nephrology. It is one of the relatively few cancers whose incidence is increasing despite our growing knowledge of the associated risk factors, yet the study of this disease within nephrology pedagogy and continuing education is woefully lacking.[1] Although there are many subtypes of RCC, the most common by far is clear cell RCC (ccRCC) and the vast majority of these are characterized by mutations in the von Hippel-Lindau (*VHL*) gene. Because this subtype is also the most studied, both in the clinic and in the laboratory, it will be the major subject of this chapter. Indeed, because of the various genetic and consequent metabolic abnormalities seen in all types of kidney cancer, this disease has been labeled the "*internist's tumor*"[2] and "*a metabolic disease.*"[3] Evaluating the various signs and symptoms of the disease in light of its genetics and biology (see later) allows a better understanding of its behavior and provides insight into new therapeutic approaches. After reading this chapter, it is hoped that practicing nephrologists are not only more aware of the biology of RCC, but also understand the profound effect of its presence in the setting of chronic kidney disease (CKD) and the consequence of its treatment on the incidence and progression of CKD.

Basic Science Considerations

The finding that ccRCC is, to a greater extent than other malignancies, characterized by metabolic reprogramming—in which "normal" metabolism is altered for the benefit of the cancer—has led to advances in therapeutic design, which are based on this finding.[3,4] Indeed, many of the paraneoplastic effects that are commonly seen with the clinical presentation (Table 25.1) are a result of this altered metabolism. Another characteristic of the varieties of kidney cancer is that most are associated with genetic mutations, which in many cases contribute to the metabolic derangements.[5] For these reasons, an understanding of the biologic underpinnings of kidney cancer is essential for anyone who deals with this disease, both in the clinical and research settings.

BASIC BIOLOGY OF CLEAR CELL RENAL CELL CARCINOMA

RCC is the most common malignancy that originates from the renal cortex.[6] Each of the known mutated genes from the various subtypes of kidney cancer have been shown to

have some effect upon cellular metabolism,[7] a now commonly recognized property of classic oncogenes,[8] such as oxygen and/or iron sensing, the tricarboxylic acid (TCA) cycle, glutamine metabolism, and tumor energetics;[3] hence the appellation "*metabolic disease.*"[2,5,9] Indeed, ccRCC has also been shown to be characterized by alterations in metabolism, as is evidenced by nonstandard pathways in amino acids degradation, as well as energy production and protection from oxidative stress; this phenomenon of metabolic reprogramming[10] was first described by Warburg early in the 20th century[11] and has become evident in a variety of malignancies, including RCC. In fact, such findings have been put to use in developing new biomarkers and therapeutic paradigms.[3]

ccRCC is by far the most common subtype, comprises 70% to 85% of all RCCs, and is one of the most lethal subtypes. The loss of *VHL* suppressor gene[12] is common in ccRCC,[13–15] and this mutation, to a large degree, dictates its biological behavior by causing activation of hypoxia pathways even in the absence of true hypoxia and characterizes ccRCC as a malignancy with "Warburg metabolism" (i.e., aerobic glycolysis).[11] Activation of downstream events by the VHL system, including neoangiogenesis and paraneoplastic phenomena, enable ccRCC cells to thrive as their surroundings become progressively more deprived of oxygen.[16]

RENAL CELL CARCINOMA IS A METABOLIC DISEASE

ccRCC arises from the proximal tubular epithelium and, in its metastatic form, is associated with high mortality. Recent studies involving different genomic platforms,[17] also described in proteomic[18,19] and metabolomic[20] studies, identified a profound metabolic shift in aggressive ccRCCs involving the TCA, pentose phosphate, and phosphoinositide 3-kinase pathways among others. Additional research has identified reprogrammed pathways in ccRCC, for example in both the tryptophan and glutamine metabolic pathways, which have been, or can soon be, exploited for novel therapeutic approaches that have the potential to transform the treatment of this disease.[3,20,21] The reader is referred to several recent reviews on this topic.[3,4,9,22]

THE BIOLOGY AND RATIONALE OF CURRENT THERAPEUTICS

Prior therapeutic approaches exploited the high level of immunogenicity of RCC and used immunotherapy with interferon and interleukin-2 (IL-2), but these were associated with severe and unpleasant adverse effects with only

Table 25.1 Paraneoplastic Manifestations Are Present in Up to 13%–20% of Patients With Renal Cell Carcinoma

Endocrine	Nonendocrine
Hypertension	Kidney failure
Polycythemia	Anemia
Hepatic dysfunction (not caused by metastasis)	Coagulopathy
Hypercalcemia	Neuropathy and myopathy
Cushing syndrome	Vasculopathy
Glucose metabolism alterations	Amyloidosis
Galactorrhea	

modest success. More recently, therapies targeting newly elucidated biochemical pathways have a better response, and fewer adverse effects, and there are even more pipeline therapies based on metabolic reprogramming as with tryptophan[23] and arginine[24] reprogramming. Most recently, the immune checkpoint inhibitors have shown considerable promise in treating ccRCC and studies are currently underway to find optimal combinations use these new drugs.[25] However, the marked inter- and intratumoral heterogeneity in ccRCC[26] has made it difficult to study this disease as a single entity with respect to therapeutic response. Clinical issues related to the various therapeutic approaches will be discussed in detail later on this chapter.

Clinical Presentation

RCCs, which originate within the renal cortex, constitute 80% to 85% of primary renal neoplasms. Transitional cell carcinoma of the renal pelvis is the next most common (8%). Other parenchymal epithelial tumors, like oncocytomas, collecting duct tumors, and renal sarcomas are rare. Nephroblastoma or Wilms tumor is common in children.

Patients are frequently asymptomatic at presentation and the diagnosis is often made in the renal clinic during imaging for workup of CKD.[1] Indeed, approximately one-third of patients have metastatic disease at diagnosis, at which point the prognosis is markedly poor.[27] In symptomatic cases, the most common presenting symptoms are flank pain, hematuria, a palpable abdominal mass, and weight loss.[28,29] The fact that fewer patients are presenting with symptoms and more with radiologic incidental diagnosis may contribute to better outcomes in RCC, as the disease-specific 5-year survival is better in patients who are diagnosed incidentally, likely because the tumor is less advanced in these cases (76% incidental vs. 44% symptomatic).[30] Several online (although unvalidated) "calculators" for renal survival are available, for example: http://www.lifemath.net/cancer/renalcell/outcome/index.php. There have also been published reports of nomograms and other such tools for calculating survival.[31,32]

Hematuria is generally observed with tumor invasion into the collecting system. When severe, such bleeding can cause clots and "colicky" abdominal discomfort. Scrotal varicoceles, mostly left-sided, are observed in as many as

11% of men with RCC.[33] This finding occurs when the tumor obstructs the gonadal vein where it enters the renal vein. Inferior vena cava involvement can produce a variety of symptoms, such as lower extremity edema, ascites, hepatic dysfunction (Budd-Chiari syndrome), and pulmonary emboli. Metastasis occurs most commonly in lung, lymph nodes, bone, liver, and brain, and in many cases the initial diagnosis of RCC is made via biopsy of accessible metastasis or by finding a renal mass on abdominal imaging.

Paraneoplastic syndromes can develop in some patients in the form of systemic symptoms (see Table 25.1)[34–36] and can arise from ectopic production of hormones like erythropoietin, parathyroid hormone-related protein (PTHrP), gonadotropins, human chorionic somatomammotropin, an adrenocorticotropic hormone (ACTH)-like substance, renin, glucagon, and insulin. Anemia, hepatic dysfunction, fever, cachexia, hypercalcemia, erythrocytosis, thrombocytosis, and AA amyloidosis can also be present. Erythrocytosis occurs because of overproduction of erythropoietin caused by impaired degradation of hypoxia-inducible transcription factors under normoxic conditions.[37] Hypercalcemia occurs because of lytic bone lesions, overproduction of PTHrP,[38] increased prostaglandins production, and bone resorption. Tumor nephrectomy will naturally correct many of these symptoms, but needs to be undertaken cautiously, especially in patients with CKD (see later).

Screening

Screening of asymptomatic individuals is not recommended because of the low prevalence of RCC in the general population. However, high risk individuals should undergo periodic screening with abdominal ultrasound, computed tomography (CT), or magnetic resonance imaging (MRI) to detect early disease. Candidates for screening include patients with any of the following conditions:[39]
1. Prior kidney irradiation[39–41]
2. Inherited conditions associated with increased incidence of RCC or other renal tumors, including von Hippel-Lindau syndrome and tuberous sclerosis
3. End-stage renal disease (ESRD), especially younger subjects without serious comorbidities, who have been on dialysis for 3 to 5 years, because they can develop acquired cystic disease of the kidney
4. A strong family history of RCC

Diagnosis

Patients with signs or symptoms suggestive of RCC should get imaging evaluation for the presence of a renal mass. Historically, patients were diagnosed with RCC after presenting with flank pain, gross hematuria, and a palpable abdominal mass, but this triad is noted only in the minority of patients with disease. Incidental diagnosis of RCC is becoming more common because of frequent use of radiologic investigations done for unrelated problems, most notably for acute kidney injury (AKI) or hematuria workup in the renal clinic.[2] As previously mentioned, unexplained paraneoplastic syndromes can prompt an RCC investigation; this is the origin of the moniker *the internist's tumor*.[2] Most paraneoplastic symptoms disappear after tumor resection.[42]

Typical radiologic features of ccRCC include exophytic growth, intratumoral necrosis or hemorrhage, and high uptake of contrast agents (Fig. 25.1).[43] CT is more sensitive in detecting a renal mass, but renal ultrasound is useful in distinguishing a simple benign renal cyst from a more complex cyst or a solid tumor. Criteria for a simple renal cyst include: round shape, sharply demarcated lesion with smooth walls, no echogenicity within the cyst, and hyperechoic posterior wall, indicating good transmission through a cyst. By contrast, if the cyst has thickened irregular walls or septa and enhances after intravenous contrast, this suggests further investigation for malignancy. MRI can be helpful if ultrasonography and CT are nondiagnostic or contrast cannot be given. CT or MR angiography is preferable to renal arteriography for preoperative mapping of the vasculature, in preparation for possible nephron-sparing surgery. [18]Fluorodeoxyglucose positron emission tomography ([18]FDG-PET) scanning, although useful for screening and staging other malignancies, has been problematic for RCC,[44] although newer PET techniques evaluating evidence of metabolic reprogramming such as ^{18}F-glutamine-PET, although currently experimental, might ultimately prove more clinically useful.[45]

Tissue diagnosis can be obtained from total or partial nephrectomy or by biopsy of a metastatic lesion before treatment (see later). Adjacent noncancerous tissue should also be evaluated by the pathologist because concurrent renal disease and even CKD is frequently present in patients with RCC (because of shared risk factors, Fig. 25.2) and in many cases, is undiagnosed. A phone call to the pathologist before total or partial nephrectomy should be done to ensure that the pathologist evaluates the noncancerous kidney tissue for other unsuspected renal diseases (e.g., diabetes, immunoglobulin A nephropathy, thin basement membrane disease), which would allow for optimal long-term management and follow-up of CKD by the nephrologist. Percutaneous biopsy of a small renal mass can be considered if there is a high index of suspicion of metastatic lesion to the kidney, lymphoma, or a focal kidney infection. Biopsy can also be considered if the patient is not a surgical candidate and before initiating medical treatment. The risk of tumor seeding with RCC biopsy has been largely debunked[46] and as such, this technique should be used without hesitation if there is any doubt about the histology, to avoid unnecessary surgery.

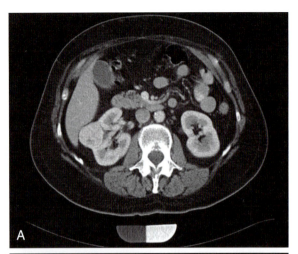

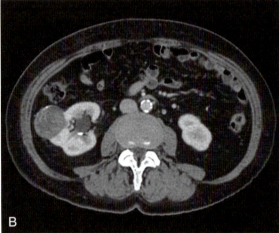

Fig. 25.1 Computed tomography scans of clear cell renal cell carcinoma: a solid mass on the right kidney is visualized on these noncontrast scans (Courtesy Dr. Marc Dall'Era, UC Davis).

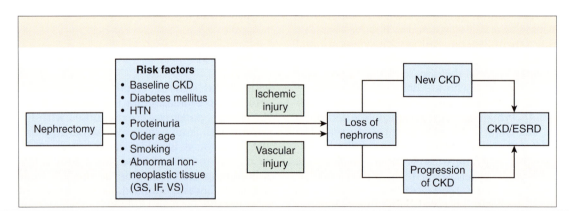

Fig. 25.2 New-onset chronic kidney disease (CKD) or progression of CKD and end-stage renal disease may develop following nephrectomy because of nephron loss in patients with underlying risk factors (from[2] with permission). *GS:* glomerulosclerosis; *HTN:* hypertension; *IF:* interstitial fibrosis; *VS:* vascular sclerosis.

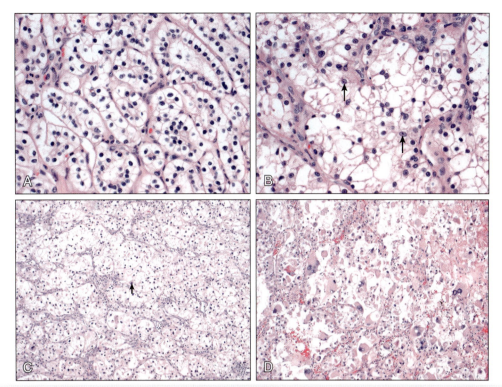

Fig. 25.3 Clear cell renal cell carcinoma: the World Health Organization/International Society of Urologic Pathologists grading system (recently supplanted Fuhrman nuclear grading). (Courtesy Dr. Morgan Darrow, UC Davis).
A. Grade 1: Nucleoli are absent or inconspicuous at 400× (400× photo)
B. Grade 2: Nucleoli (*arrows*) are conspicuous and eosinophilic at 400× (400× photo)
C. Grade 3: Nucleoli (*arrow*) are conspicuous and eosinophilic at 100× (100× photo)
D. Grade 4: Extreme nuclear pleomorphic and/or multinuclear giant cells and/or rhabdoid and/or sarcomatoid differentiation. This photo shows cells with extreme nuclear pleomorphism and rhabdoid features (large eccentric nuclei, large prominent nucleoli, and abundant eosinophilic cytoplasm) (100× photo).

In staging RCC, the extent of local and regional involvement is best determined by abdominal CT, which can also detect renal vein invasion, nodal metastasis, perinephric invasion, and adjacent organ invasion. Distant metastases can be detected by bone scan, CT of the chest, MRI, and PET/CT. In addition to radiologic diagnosis, tissue diagnosis provides information about the histopathologic type of RCC and adjacent noncancerous kidney tissue, which has important implications for prognosis and treatment. Biopsy of the metastatic site is often easier and thus may be preferable. If the patient is diagnosed with metastatic disease and therefore requires systemic therapy, most modern drugs for the disease are associated with renal-relevant adverse effects, which are best managed by the nephrologist in concert with the oncologist and/or urologist (see later).

CLINICAL ISSUES WITH RENAL CELL CARCINOMA SUBTYPES

Clear Cell Renal Cell Carcinoma

The ccRCC histologic subtype is most common (see Fig. 25.3) and is one of the most lethal subtypes.[17] It arises from the proximal tubular epithelium and, in its metastatic form, is associated with a high mortality. The large majority of cases of ccRCC are sporadic and only 2% to 3% of ccRCC are linked to hereditary disease, most commonly von Hippel-Lindau syndrome.[47]

Papillary Renal Cell Carcinoma

The second most common subtype, papillary RCC (pRCC), (Fig. 25.4) is also of proximal tubule origin but has been studied less extensively.[48] There are two subtypes, type 1 pRCC and type 2 pRCC, the latter with a worse prognosis.

Chromophobe Renal Cell Carcinoma

This rare (5%) kidney cancer (Fig. 25.4) originates from the collecting duct and is similar to the benign oncocytoma.[49,50] It is more common in young females and is the least aggressive of all the RCC types, unless characterized by sarcomatous transformation.

Cystic Diseases and Renal Cell Carcinoma

The link between cystic disease and RCC was described in the 1800s by Brigidi and Severi.[51] Cortical cystic disease can range from simple cysts to complex cysts with increasing[52] risk for malignancy as defined by the Bosniak classification[53–55] (Table 25.2). However, CKD-associated cystic diseases, including acquired cystic kidney disease (ACKD) and autosomal dominant polycystic kidney disease (ADPKD), have different characteristics from that of the general population and deserve further consideration, as will be discussed in the following sections.

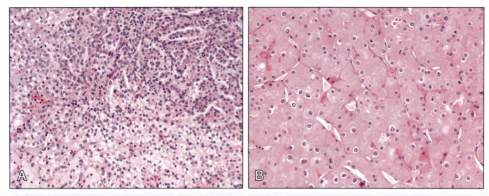

Fig. 25.4 A. Papillary renal cell carcinoma, type 1 (200×). Cells arranged in compact tubulopapillary structures. The presence of macrophages with foamy cytoplasm (lower left) is characteristic. The cells of type 1 papillary RCC have pale clear to basophilic cytoplasm and line papillary structures as a single uniform layer. **B.** Chromophobe renal cell carcinoma (200×). The cells are large with distinct cell borders, are arranged in solid sheets, and have an oncocytic appearance (abundant granular eosinophilic cytoplasm). The nuclei are irregular and have clear perinuclear "halos." (Photomicrographs courtesy Dr. Morgan Darrow, UC Davis.)

Table 25.2 Bosniak Classification of Cystic Renal Masses

	Septa	Wall	Solid	Enhancement	Cyst Size
Category I Simple benign	No	Hairline thin wall	No	No	
Category II	Yes, few hairline thin septa	Fine calcification	No	Perceived but nonenhancing	< 3 cm smooth margin
Category II F Minimally complicated	Multiple thin septa, thick nodular calcification	Thick nodular calcification	No	Perceived but nonenhancing	> 3 cm
Category III Complex	Thick irregular or smooth	Thick irregular or smooth	No	Measurable	> 3 cm
Category IV Malignant	Thick irregular or smooth	Thick irregular or smooth	Soft tissue components	Measurable	> 3 cm

Acquired Cystic Kidney Disease and Renal Cell Carcinoma

ESRD is associated with a relatively high risk of RCC, possibly because of the cystic transformation seen in many of these kidneys. The incidence of RCC in the ESRD population ranges from 1% to 7% in various studies, a rate higher than that of the general population, in whom the incidence is 1.6%.[56–59] Fourfold to fivefold increase in rate of RCC was seen in dialysis patients as compared with the general population.[59] The prognosis of RCC in patients with ESRD-associated renal cystic disease, independent of the renal disease prognosis, is equivalent or better compared with the general population. These patients are more likely to have papillary tumors, be younger with a better performance status, have fewer symptoms, smaller tumor size, and lower tumor grade and stage.

The development of ACKD has been described among 7% to 22% of CKD patients, but this escalates among dialysis-dependent ESRD patients (10%–44% within 1–3 years of onset of renal replacement therapy) and increases further with prolonged duration of dialysis (> 90% after 5–10 years of renal replacement therapy).[57,60–62] Although the presence of ACKD leading to RCC has also been described among

transplant recipients (23%), this incidence is far less than that observed in ESRD patients on dialysis (80%),[57] which is surprising in light of the immunosuppression accompanying transplant.

The diagnosis of ACKD is made by the presence of greater than three cysts collectively in both kidneys.[60,62] ACKD cysts tend to be smaller in size (typically < 0.6 cm in diameter, but can range up to 2–3 cm) compared with cysts in ADPKD or other cystic diseases. In addition to ESRD duration, risk factors for the development of ACKD, and likely progression to RCC, include male sex, younger age at ESRD onset, and glomerulonephritis as primary kidney disease. Diabetic nephropathy has been associated with lower incidence of ACKD among Japanese dialysis patients.[63] Although race and dialysis modality have not been shown to be definitively associated with ACKD incidence, ACKD has been reported to be less common with peritoneal dialysis.[56,60,64]

The appearance and progression of acquired renal cysts may stem from a reparative response to uremic metabolites, chronic acidosis, and ischemia.[56,60] Cyst fluid content has been found to be higher in creatinine content, suggesting some filtering or secretory capacity, unlike simple or ADPKD cysts (which have similar cyst and plasma creatinine levels). ACKD cysts often regress after transplantation, once normal filtration is restored.[60,65]

The association of ACKD with both RCC and ESRD may explain causality for the increased risk of RCC in ESRD.[57] Indeed, there are many shared risk factors between CKD and RCC (see Fig. 25.1), which may at least in part explain this association. The annual incidence of RCC in a Japanese ACKD cohort followed for 20 years was 0.151% per year for those on dialysis less than 10 years, and 0.340% per year with dialysis duration for more than 10 years.[55,60] pRCC is the predominant histologic subtype among ACKD and dialysis-associated tumors, in contrast to ccRCC, which is typically seen in the general population.

Polycystic Kidney Disease and Renal Cell Carcinoma

The prevalence of RCC in ADPKD appears to be no greater than that in the general population according to small case series and observational studies,[39,66–69] although there is some controversy in the literature on this subject. As in the general population, the histologic diagnosis of RCC in ADPKD tends to be ccRCC in a recent case series,[67] although in another study, tubulopapillary pathology was also observed (42%).[68] RCC in ADPKD presents at a younger mean age (50–60 years) than spontaneous RCC, but often with advanced disease where a third of patients have bilateral kidney involvement or metastatic disease. The diagnosis in these patients may be delayed because of the complexity of diagnostic images in the presence of multiple benign cysts in ADPKD. Symptomatic diagnosis rather than incidental discovery of RCC is more common in this select population.[66,67,69]

Prognosis of Renal Cell Carcinoma in End-Stage Renal Disease

The prognosis of RCC in the ESRD population is equivalent or better compared with the general population.[70–74] Five-year survival and cancer-specific mortality were markedly better in ESRD as compared to the general population. In ESRD, the majority of patients (87%) were incidentally diagnosed, and these patients had more favorable characteristics like younger age, better performance status, fewer symptoms, smaller tumor size, lower tumor grade and stage, and were more likely than the general population to have papillary histology. The higher survival in ESRD group is attributed to the incidental finding, thus leading to earlier diagnosis.

Acquired Cystic Kidney Disease, Renal Cell Carcinoma, and Renal Transplantation

Screening for RCC in renal transplant candidates who have ESRD is controversial and not currently recommended despite the use of powerful immunosuppression drugs, which increase cancer risk in general.[57,75,76] Most studies have found that the prevalence of native kidney RCC in renal transplant recipients (3%–5%) was no different from non-transplant ESRD population but still 100-fold greater than the general population.[77–79] ACKD is less commonly described among transplant recipients (23%–33%) but can be as high as 57%,[80] which is still far less than that observed in ESRD patients on dialysis (80%).[57] As expected, RCC is more common in transplant patients with ACKD than those without ACKD. In general, transplant patients have much better prognosis than nontransplant ESRD and the general population because more such individuals are diagnosed at a younger age, have smaller tumor size and less metastatic disease, more are at stage T1, papillary subtype and undergo more frequent surveillance. The 10-year cancer-specific survival of 88% to 95% in transplant recipients is higher than the general population (75%).[81] Five-year cancer-specific survival in transplant patients was 97% as compared with the nontransplanted ESRD group of 77%. The overall patient and graft survival between those with and without RCC have been comparable. Given the minimal gain of life expectancy, screening for ACKD in the entire ESRD population is not recommended. However, screening may be considered in younger, healthier patients. The malignancy risk of most cystic lesions can be assessed using these criteria and prognosis is determined with staging and grading tools (see Table 25.2).[54]

Clinical judgment and risk analysis should be applied in determining the benefit of RCC screening. Although survival did not reportedly improve with ACKD screening, according to a decision analysis performed in dialysis patients,[75] screening among potential transplant recipients in our opinion seems quite reasonable, given the noninvasiveness of the imaging. Furthermore, a more favorable prognosis in the transplant candidate population group than in a dialysis group in general (which was the focus of that study) suggests that screening may be more beneficial in the former group because of younger age at diagnosis, earlier discovery of tumor (better prognostic characteristics, stage and size), and longer life expectancy. However, in the ESRD population with a high risk for RCC, the benefit of periodic screening has not been established.

TUMOR NODE METASTASIS STAGING

Tumor node metastasis (TNM) staging for RCC was first established in 1997 by the Union Internationale Contre le Cancer and the American Joint Committee on Cancer, and was most recently updated in 2017 (Table 25.3).[82] T-staging (T1-T4) is classified by the extent and size of the tumor, which differentiates cancer-specific survival. T1 tumors are limited to the kidney and are 7 cm or smaller; T2 tumors are larger than 7 cm but totally within the kidney; T3 tumors extend beyond the kidney, but within Gerota's fascia, and may involve neighboring veins (renal vein or inferior vena cava); and T4 tumors invade Gerota's fascia or extend to the ipsilateral adrenal gland. T1-T2 are further subdivided according to renal mass size, and T3 is subdivided depending on venous involvement. T-staging imposes the greatest discrimination of 5-year cancer-specific survival, where T1a tumors have survival as high as 98%, which declines to 10% with stage T4. Nodal invasion minimally alters outcomes, but distant metastases

Table 25.3   Kidney Cancer Tumor, Node, Metastasis Staging American Joint Committee on Cancer Union for International Cancer Control 2017

Primary Tumor (T)

T Category	T Criteria
Tx	Primary tumor cannot be assessed
T0	No evidence of primary tumor
T1a	Tumor < 4 cm in greatest dimension, limited to kidney
T1b	Tumor > 4 cm but < 7 cm in greatest dimension, limited to kidney
T2a	Tumor > 7 cm in greatest dimension, limited to kidney
T2b	Tumor > 10 cm, limited to kidney
T3a	Tumor extends into renal vein, branches, invades pelvicalyceal system and perirenal/renal sinus fat but not beyond Gerota's fascia
T3b	Tumor extends into the vena cava below the diaphragm
T3c	Tumor extends into the vena cava above the diaphragm or invades the wall of the vena cava
T4	Tumor invades beyond Gerota's fascia including contiguous extension into the ipsilateral adrenal gland

Regional lymph nodes (N) N category	N criteria
Nx	Regional lymph nodes cannot be assessed
N0	No regional lymph node metastasis
N1	Metastasis in regional lymph node(s)

Distant metastasis (M) M category	
M0	No distant metastasis
M1	Distant metastasis

Prognostic Stage Groups

When T is...	When N is...	When M is...	Stage is....
T1	N0	M0	I
T1	N1	M0	III
T2	N0	M0	II
T2	N1	M0	III
T3	NX, N0	M0	III
T3	N1	M0	III
T4	Any N	M0	IV
Any T	Any N	M1	IV

including ipsilateral adrenal gland invasion worsens prognosis considerably.[83] More recently, renal sinus fat involvement has been found to be associated with lower survival.[84] Composite prognostic staging (I-IV) summarizes the TNM findings. Tumors with stage I-II have kidney limited lesions only. The prognostic stage is elevated to III when there is any nodal involvement regardless of kidney size or T-staging, and is escalated to stage IV when Gerota's fascia invasion, adrenal gland, or distant metastasis occurs.

Grading, in contrast to staging, guides prognosis based on nuclear features. Of the grading systems, the World Health Organization/International Society of Urologic Pathologists grading system has supplanted the older Fuhrman categorization and is most universally used for prognostic assessment despite some limitations. The nuclear size, irregularity, and nucleoli prominence differentiate RCC into 4 grades (see Fig. 25.3). Five-year cancer-specific survival is highest for grade 1 (51%–93%), and lowest in grade 4 (10%–28%).[83] Although this grading system is reliably used for ccRCC, it has not been adequately validated for pRCC or chromophobe RCC subtypes.[84,85]

Independent of TNM staging, higher grade and larger tumor size predict poorer survival, with histologic subtype also playing a role. The most common and sporadic form of RCC, ccRCC (60%–90% prevalence vs. 6%–14% for papillary, and 6%–14% for chromophobe), has inferior outcomes as compared with pRCC or chromophobe RCC.[85] Other features, such as the presence of sarcomatoid or rhabdoid (eccentric large nuclei and eosinophilic cytoplasm) differentiation and microscopic coagulative tumor necrosis, add to the worse prognosis. Sarcomatoid differentiation, seen in only 4% of all RCCs, reflects extreme dedifferentiation and is associated with a dismal prognosis. All tumors with a sarcomatoid component were classified as nuclear grade 4.[86] Each 10% increase in sarcomatoid changes is associated with a 6% increased risk of death from RCC and with poor survival. Cancer-specific survival rates at 2 and 5 years after nephrectomy were 33.3% and 14.5%, respectively. The presence of distant metastases at the radical nephrectomy and histologic tumor necrosis were significantly associated with death from RCC among patients with sarcomatoid RCC. Patients with ccRCC (conventional) and chromophobe RCC were more likely to have tumors with a sarcomatoid component (5.2% and 8.7%, respectively) compared with patients with pRCC (1.9%).

Rhabdoid differentiation is even rarer with similarly poor survival.[83,84]

Various integrated staging systems based on variables often including TNM staging, tumor size, clinical symptoms, histologic subtype, grading, and other prognostic pathologic findings have been devised and can be used to predict outcomes both preoperatively and postoperatively. Accuracy of these tools are high for RCC recurrence (66%–80%), distant metastases (78%–85%), and RCC cancer-specific survival (64%–89%). Such algorithms are particularly helpful for patients with advanced disease (metastatic RCC) who are in the highest mortality range and therefore are poorly differentiated by TNM staging alone. Therapeutic effectiveness of choice of antineoplastic treatment (cytokine or targeted therapy) has been examined using these staging systems to select optimal treatment regimens.[83,87]

Treatment

The nephrologist, although traditionally excluded in this area, should play a significant role in the management of renal masses.[2] More than half of patients are diagnosed with RCC incidentally, and often in the renal clinic, and many have CKD in addition to RCC because of shared risk factors (see Fig. 25.1). The evolution of both medical and surgical treatment for this "nephrologist's tumor"[2] is currently occurring rapidly, and input of the nephrologist in treatment decisions, especially (but not only) when CKD becomes part of the equation, is essential.

GENERAL PRINCIPLES FOR RENAL CELL CARCINOMA MANAGEMENT (FIG. 25.5)

Surgical Management

The initial approach is based on extent of disease, patient's age, and comorbidity. Surgery by radical or partial nephrectomy remains the mainstay of curative treatment for patients who present with early stage RCC. However, a significant proportion of patients develop metastatic disease after RCC surgery, which results in high mortality, and these individuals generally require systemic therapies. The incidence of metastasis depends on tumor stage and grade. In those individuals who present late with advanced and metastatic disease, the overall clinical course of RCC varies; approximately 50% of patients survive less than 1 year and

10% survive for more than 5 years. Surgery is curative in the majority of patients who have localized disease; however, surgical treatment with radical or partial nephrectomy is based upon the extent of disease, patient age, and comorbidities. In selected patients with resectable primary tumor and a concurrent single metastasis, surgical resection of metastasis plus radical nephrectomy can be curative. In patients with small renal masses, advanced CKD, and who are high-risk surgical candidates, ablative therapies can be considered.

Partial Nephrectomy

Before surgery, laboratory data need to be obtained for risk assessment for CKD. Partial nephrectomy is useful for preservation of kidney function,[89–91] as a nephron sparing procedure, and should be considered for all patients. The goal of partial nephrectomy is to completely remove the primary tumor, while preserving the maximal amount of healthy renal tissue. Partial nephrectomy is indicated for patients with T1 tumor with normal contralateral kidney, and in patients with a solitary kidney or those with conditions that affect kidney function. Minimizing nephron mass loss, for small renal masses in particular, should be prioritized with either partial nephrectomy or thermal ablation to lower the risk of CKD or its progression. Partial nephrectomy has equivalent/comparable oncologic and overall survival and greater renal preservation. Data were pooled from systematic review and meta-analysis of partial versus radical nephrectomy. According to pool estimates, partial nephrectomy correlated with a 19% risk reduction in all-cause mortality, 29% risk reduction in cancer specific mortality, and 61% risk reduction in severe chronic kidney disease. For these reasons, it is nephrologist's role to advocate for the partial nephrectomy approach in all referred patients with small renal masses (<4 cm) and no metastasis. Although such a survival benefit was not clearly seen in the sole randomized controlled trial, the European Organization for Research and Treatment of Cancer study, renal protection was apparent, with fewer reaching estimated glomerular filtration rate less than 60 mL/min/1.73 m² after partial nephrectomy versus radical nephrectomy.[91,92] The American Urological Association recommends nephrology referral for high CKD risk patients including those with known CKD, including proteinuria, with diabetes mellitus, or poor blood pressure control, a recommendation with which we concur.[93]

Nephrectomy scoring systems (radius, exophytic or endophytic, nearness to collecting system or sinus, anterior or posterior, and location relative to polar lines [R.E.N.A.L] and preoperative aspects and dimensions used for anatomic classification [PADUA]) have been proposed to predict the complexity of the partial nephrectomy procedure and to predict perioperative outcomes according to anatomic and topographic tumor characteristics.[94,95] The PADUA and RENAL nephrometry assign numerical values to a focused set of morphologic variables readily ascertainable with conventional contrast material–enhanced CT or MRI, such as tumor size and location. Overall, the performance of these metrics has been deemed favorable, with multiple studies demonstrating predictive strength with respect to operative complications.

Laparoscopic and robot-assisted partial nephrectomy are the main alternatives to classic open partial nephrectomy.

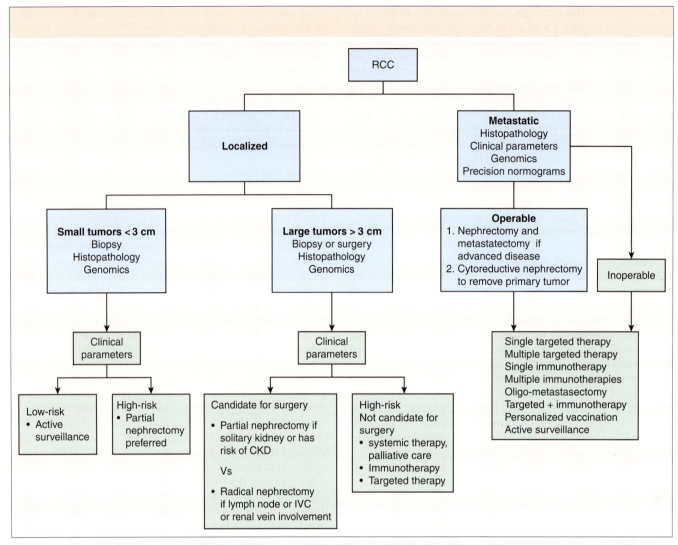

Fig. 25.5 Treatment algorithm for renal cell carcinoma (RCC). *CKD*, Chronic kidney disease; *IVC*, inferior vena cava.

Laparoscopic technique should be reserved for small tumors and with no complexity features. Hematuria, perirenal hematoma, and urinary fistulas are most common complications, and less frequent issues include AKI and infection.[96]

Radical Nephrectomy

Classical radical nephrectomy consists of removal of the affected kidney, perirenal fat tissue, adrenal gland, and regional lymph nodes. However, if the tumor is smaller than 5 cm and is located at the inferior pole, the adrenal gland can be spared. The regional lymph node dissection is reserved for patients with clinically positive nodes detected either by CT or during the surgical procedure. Radical nephrectomy should be considered for a patient with multiple small tumors and in cases where the tumor extends into vasculature. The laparoscopic approach for radical nephrectomy is currently performed for stage I and stage II tumors, whereas an open surgical approach remains the gold standard for the treatment for more complex cases. The robot-assisted approach can be considered as a potential alternative to open surgery in cases with venous tumor thrombus.

Cytoreductive Nephrectomy

As mentioned earlier, many RCCs are silent until the disease is locally advanced and therefore unresectable or metastatic. In these cases systemic therapy with immunotherapy, molecularly targeted agents, and surgery and radiation, all might have a role depending upon extent of disease, sites of involvement, and other patient-specific factors. Many centers offer cytoreductive nephrectomy in metastatic disease, if there is a substantial disease volume at the primary site, but only a low burden of metastatic disease. The median overall survival is 17.1 months in cytoreductive nephrectomy cases versus 7.7 months in the noncytoreductive nephrectomy group, even while they receive systemic targeted therapies.[97]

Active Surveillance and Ablative Therapies

Active surveillance or ablative procedures, like cryotherapy and radiofrequency ablation, can be considered in patients with small renal masses who are not surgical candidates, for example elderly patients, those with CKD or other competing health risks, and limited life expectancy. No definite surveillance protocol exists, but the most common approach is to perform renal ultrasonography or MRI every 3 months for 1 year and then every 6 months for a year and then annually thereafter. Intervention should be considered for tumor growth to greater than 3 to 4 cm or by more than 0.4 to 0.5 cm per year.[98] Active surveillance is an option for patients with small asymptomatic lesions.

Adjuvant Therapy

Adjuvant systemic therapy has not been shown to have a role after complete surgical resection outside of a formal clinical trial. Sunitinib, an antiangiogenic kinase inhibitor, has been approved for adjuvant therapy based on improvements in disease-free survival compared with placebo in high-risk disease,[99] but the phase 3 trial failed to show survival benefit and was associated with significant toxicity.

Radiation therapy (RT) is helpful mainly for bone metastases, brain metastases, and painful recurrences in the renal bed. Although RCCs are characterized as radioresistant tumors, conventional and stereotactic RT is frequently useful to treat a single or limited number of metastases. In these settings, the utility of RT is similar to that in metastases from other tumor types. RT has been used as an adjuvant therapy following nephrectomy in patients at high risk of local recurrence but its role in this setting remains unproven and is generally discouraged.[100,101]

Systemic Therapy

The evolution of drugs for metastatic RCC in recent years is illustrated in Table 25.4 with terminology aptly described.[102] The so-called "Dark Age" was before 2005 and median survival was 15 months. Then followed the "Modern Age" (2005–2014) and median survival improved to 30 months with newer drugs. Currently, in the "Golden Age," the median survival is expected to be 5 years. The ultimate goal of the future "Diamond Age" is long-term survival.[102] The current therapies are associated with various adverse events, which are shown in Table 25.5.

Immunotherapy: Interleukin 2, Interferon-Alpha

Cytokines, such as interferon-alpha and high-dose IL-2, that enhance antitumor immune activity have been used since the 1990s to treat metastatic RCC. Both these drugs benefit only a small subset of patients with intrinsic favorable disease biology and are associated with substantial

toxicity of flu-like adverse events, particularly with high-dose IL-2,[103] so their use is limited. In addition, such therapies may enhance the intrinsic antiimmunity of many RCCs.[23]

Targeted Therapy

Targeted therapy, which is becoming increasingly essential for RCC treatment, affects the cancer's specific genes, proteins, metabolism, or the tissue environment that contributes to cancer growth and survival. These treatments block the growth and spread of cancer cells, while generally limiting damage to healthy cells. Given the highly vascular nature of RCCs, it is not surprising that several therapies are available to exploit this feature.

Most ccRCCs have mutations in the *VHL* gene that cause the cancer to appear hypoxic and thus overproduce vascular endothelial growth factor (VEGF), a growth factor that causes neoangiogenesis. Most tyrosine kinase inhibitors (TKIs) block VEGF and other chemical signals that promote the development of new blood vessels (angiogenesis). Approved agents are sorafenib, sunitinib, pazopanib, axitinib, lenvatinib, and cabozantinib.[104–109] The anti-VEGF TKIs sunitinib, pazopanib, and the combination of bevacizumab and interferon-alpha are approved first-line options, whereas axitinib and cabozantinib are approved as second-line options. The anti-VEGF monoclonal antibody, bevacizumab, is approved for use with interferon-alpha.[110,111] The mammalian target of rapamycin (mTOR) inhibitors everolimus and temsirolimus are approved in the second-line setting and the first-line setting in patients with poor risk status.[112,113]

Checkpoint Inhibitor Immunotherapy

Immunotherapy targets the immune system to recognize and eradicate cancer cells. Modern immunotherapy has focused on "checkpoint" proteins, such as cytotoxic T-lymphocyte-associated-protein-4 (CTLA-4) and programmed death-1 protein (PD-1), which are receptors on the surface of immune cells that act like a brake, or checkpoint, preventing the development of autoimmunity.[114] CTLA-4 receptor has homology to the T-cell activator molecule CD-28 and prevents T-cell activation by outcompeting CD-28 for its ligand.[115] The binding of PD-1 with programmed death ligand (PDL-1) results in T-cell anergy.[116]

Table 25.4 The Evolution of System Therapy for ccRCC

Year	1992–2004 Dark Age	2005 Modern Age	2006 Modern Age	2007 Modern Age	2008 Modern Age
Drug	Immunotherapy 1. Interferon-alpha	Sorafenib **TKIs**	Sunitinib	Temsirolimus **(mTORC1) inhibitors**	Everolimus (mTORC1) inhibitors
Drug	2. High-dose IL-2				
Year	2009 Modern Age	2010 Modern Age	2012 Modern Age	2015-2025 Golden Age	After 2025 Diamond Age
Drug	Bevacizumab and Interferon-alpha	Pazopanib TKIs	Axitinib TKIs	TKIs: Cabozantinib Lenvatinib	Drug combinations Vaccinations
Drug				**CPIs:** Nivolumab	Drug sequences

CPI, Checkpoint inhibitor; *IL-2*, interleukin 2; *mTORC1*, mammalian target of rapamycin complex 1; *TKI*, tyrosine kinase inhibitor.

Table 25.5   Adverse Events Associated With Systemic Therapy for Clear Cell Renal Cell Carcinoma

Adverse Events	Sorafenib (TKIs)	Sunitinib (TKIs)	Pazopanib (TKIs)	Bevacizumab + IFN-alpha (anti-VEGF)
Hepatic			++	
Gastrointestinal	++ Diarrhea	++ Diarrhea	++ Diarrhea	
Hypertension	++	++	++	++
Renal				
Proteinuria				++
Skin	++ Hand-foot	++ Hand-foot	++ Hand-foot	
Respiratory				
Cardiovascular				
Infections				
Bleeding				++
Endocrine				

Adverse Events	Temsirolimus (mTOR inhibitor)	Everolimus (mTOR inhibitor)	Nivolumab (Checkpoint inhibitors) PD-1	Ipilimumab (Checkpoint inhibitors) CTLA4
Hepatic			++	
Gastrointestinal			++ Colitis	
Hypertension				
Renal			AIN, hyponatremia	Podocytopathy AIN, hyponatremia
Proteinuria				
Skin	++ Stomatitis	++ Stomatitis	++	
Respiratory		++ Pneumonitis	++ Pneumonitis	
Cardiovascular				
Infections				
Bleeding			++	
Endocrine	++ Hyperglycemia, hypercholesterolemia	++ Hyperglycemia, hypercholesterolemia	++	

AIN, Acute tubulointerstitial nephritis; *CTLA4*, cytotoxic T-lymphocyte-associated-protein-4; *IFN*, interferon; *mTOR*, mammalian target of rapamycin; *PD-1*, programmed death 1 protein; *TKI*, tyrosine kinase inhibitor; *VEGF*, vascular endothelial growth factor.

Immune checkpoint inhibitors (CPIs), monoclonal antibodies that target inhibitory proteins, such as CTLA-4, PD-1, and PDL-1,[117] represent a novel immunotherapy. CPIs enhance tumor killing by blunting the braking mechanism that blocks T-cell activation, thereby augmenting the immune response. Although CPIs are considered the most innovative and promising agents in the treatment of cancer,[118,119] their pathophysiology is still not fully understood, but may be similar to that of autoimmune disease, wherein activated lymphocytes target self-antigens.

Antibodies against PDL-1 include avelumab and atezolizumab and antibodies against PD-1 include nivolumab and pembrolizumab. PD-1 negatively regulates T-cell function and its ligand PDL-1 is highly expressed by cancer cells. Blockade of this PD-1–PDL-1 axis promotes T-cell activation and immune killing of the cancer. Ipilimumab, an antibody and which binds CTLA4, thus promotes T cell activation.[120,121] Combination therapies of anti-VEGF (axitinib and bevacizumab) and checkpoint inhibitors (nivolumab) are also used.

By the end of 2014, nivolumab[122,123] and pembrolizumab, both PD-1 inhibitors, also were approved. Nivolumab was approved in the United States and the European Union after the CheckMate 025 RCT showed an overall survival benefit compared with everolimus in patients who have failed therapy with sunitinib and pazopanib. However, the response rate was only 25% and most patients did not have significant tumor shrinkage.

Immune-related adverse events complicate the use of CPIs. Their pathophysiology may be similar to that of autoimmune disease, wherein activated lymphocytes target self-antigens.[124] The most specific immune-related adverse effects of ipilimumab are colitis, hypothyroidism, and hypophysitis. Adverse events associated with pembrolizumab and nivolumab are pneumonitis and hypothyroidism.[124]

CPI-related renal toxicity is not common. AKI and hyponatremia, are the most frequently reported renal events.[125] Acute tubulointerstitial nephritis (AIN) is the most common pathophysiology of AKI, and the nephrologist should be aware of this complication, because it generally responds to steroids and drug withdrawal.[125–128] The overall incidence of AKI was 2.2%, and occurred more frequently in patients who received combination therapy with ipilimumab and nivolumab (4.9%) than patients who received monotherapy. The incidence of grade III or IV AKI, defined as an increase in creatinine greater than threefold above baseline, an increase in creatinine to a level greater than 4.0 mg/dL, or need for renal replacement therapy, was 0.6%.[127] A recent metaanalysis analyzed eight randomized clinical trials involving CPIs, amounting to 4070 patients. All grade immune-related renal toxicity ranged from 0.7% to 6%, whereas high-grade immune-related renal toxicity ranged from 0% to 2%.[128]

MECHANISM OF RENAL INJURY

The mechanism of CPI-induced AIN is as yet not completely understood, but it has been speculated that there are two possible mechanisms. First, CTLA-4 and PD-1 pathways normally operate to limit autoimmunity and interference with these pathways can lead to unwanted immune effects. PD-1 signaling limits T-cell mediated inflammatory injury, and PD-1 knockout mice spontaneously develop interstitial nephritis and lupus-like-glomerulonephritis.[129,130] Second, CPI-induced AIN may be caused by the loss of tolerance to endogenous kidney antigens, as opposed to the delayed-type hypersensitivity response characteristic of more conventional AIN.[131] Patients can have hematuria (16%), new or worsened hypertension (11%),[127,132] and subnephrotic range proteinuria. Nephrotic syndrome is a rare finding only associated with ipilimumab.[133,134] Increased serum creatinine and pyuria are the only clinical clues in a large majority of cases. As with traditional AIN, white blood cell casts are only rarely seen. CPI-induced AIN has a more heterogeneous time course from drug exposure to the development of AKI. It could be 3 to 64 weeks based on the drug used.[127,132] Also there are extrarenal immune adverse effects seen with these drugs. Pathologic diagnosis by renal biopsy is definitive, and reveals tubulitis and interstitial inflammation, consisting of activated lymphocytes, macrophages, and eosinophils.[127,135] Noncaseating granulomatous interstitial nephritis may also occur.[127]

MANAGEMENT OF CHECKPOINT INHIBITORS-INDUCED ACUTE TUBULOINTERSTITIAL NEPHRITIS

First, the CPI should be discontinued, then if necessary, immunosuppression including high-dose steroids, Mycophenolate Mofetil, and potentially, tumor necrosis factor alpha inhibitors can be used.[128] Later, the patient can be given the same or an alternate CPI if renal function is stable after initial discontinuation.[127] Development of grade 3 or 4 toxicity, defined as AKI with increase in creatinine more than threefold above baseline, an increase in creatinine to a level more than 4.0 mg/dL, or need for renal replacement therapy, necessitates permanent discontinuation of the drug.[136]

HYPONATREMIA

Ipilimumab can cause hyponatremia from hypocortisolemia via immune-related injury to the pituitary gland. Loss of ACTH-secreting corticotrophs leads to a loss of corticotropin-releasing hormone that causes adrenal insufficiency. Studies show that upon drug withdrawal, MRI findings of hypophysitis resolved after treatment with hydrocortisone.[137,138]

The PD-1 inhibitors (nivolumab, pembrolizumab) are also associated with thyroid dysfunction.[139] Hypophysitis is also seen with nivolumab but the incidence is less than 1%.[139,140] Another adverse effect reported for nivolumab is adrenalitis resulting in primary adrenal failure presenting with hyponatremia, which has failed to resolve with hydrocortisone but responded to fludrocortisone.[141]

First-Line Systemic Therapy

Immunotherapy with CPIs and molecularly targeted therapies are the primary systemic modalities for the management of patients whose disease is not controlled by definitive locoregional therapy.[142] If the combination of nivolumab and ipilimumab is not available then anti-angiogenic targeted therapy (pazopanib and sunitinib) are the preferred agents. A recently published trial[143] showed an efficacy and overall survival benefit of two CPIs used concurrently, nivolumab plus ipilimumab, over sunitinib in the first-line treatment of intermediate or poor-risk advanced ccRCC.

Second-Line Therapy

The standard of care for systemic treatment of RCC is rapidly changing because of the advent of new drugs and results of clinical trials. As of this writing, there is less general agreement regarding patients who have progressed on first-line therapy with CPI immunotherapy. Treatment with VEGF TKI will be the next option. Options include axitinib, cabozantinib, sunitinib, and pazopanib. Patients who have progressed following immunotherapy and one or two courses of antiangiogenic therapy may benefit from alternative VEGF or mechanistic mTOR targeted agent.

Nivolumab is approved for use after failure of VEGF TKI therapy; however, nivolumab has been shown to have about a 20% overall response rate in this setting. For those who respond, the response can be durable in some cases.

Axitinib and cabozantinib, both next-generation multikinase inhibitors, are also approved for use after progression on pazopanib/sunitinib. The mTOR inhibitors also are approved for use in the second-line setting (and in fact there is one trial that suggests a benefit to giving lenvatinib, another multikinase inhibitor, with everolimus in this setting), but they are generally used more in the third-line setting.

At this point it is unclear how to treat patients after progression on CPI therapy. None of the VEGF TKIs, such as cabozantinib or axitinib, or the mTOR inhibitors, were studied in patients who had previously received nivolumab therapy, but this is usually the next step. Clinical trials are currently underway.

Key Points

- Clear cell renal cell carcinoma (ccRCC) is a metabolic disease characterized by many examples of metabolic reprogramming.
- ccRCC is often asymptomatic at presentation and is often accompanied by paraneoplastic phenomena, which can aid in its diagnosis.
- ccRCC is frequently discovered during the workup of other kidney diseases.
- New therapeutic approaches have recently been introduced, including immune checkpoint inhibitors and therapies based on metabolic reprogramming.

References

1. Hu SL, Weiss RH. The role of nephrologists in the management of small renal masses. *Nat Rev Nephrol.* 2018;14(4):211-212.
2. Hu SL, Chang A, Perazella MA, Okusa MD, Jaimes EA, Weiss RH. The nephrologist's tumor: basic biology and management of renal cell carcinoma. *J Am Soc Nephrol.* 2016;27(8):2227-2237.
3. Wettersten HI, Aboud OA, Lara PN Jr, Weiss RH. Metabolic reprogramming in clear cell renal cell carcinoma. *Nat Rev Nephrol.* 2017;13(7):410-419.
4. Wettersten HI, Weiss RH. Applications of metabolomics for kidney disease research: from biomarkers to therapeutic targets. *Organogenesis.* 2013;9(1):11-18.
5. Linehan WM, Srinivasan R, Schmidt LS. The genetic basis of kidney cancer: a metabolic disease. *Nat Rev Urol.* 2010;7(5):277-285.
9. Linehan WM, Ricketts CJ. The metabolic basis of kidney cancer. *Semin Cancer Biol.* 2013;23(1):46-55.
10. Ward PS, Thompson CB. Metabolic reprogramming: a cancer hallmark even Warburg did not anticipate. *Cancer Cell.* 2012;21(3):297-308.
14. Gnarra JR, Tory K, Weng Y, et al. Mutations of the VHL tumour suppressor gene in renal carcinoma. *Nat Genet.* 1994;7(1):85-90.
18. Perroud B, Ishimaru T, Borowsky AD, Weiss RH. Grade-dependent proteomics characterization of kidney cancer. *Mol Cell Proteomics.* 2009;8(5):971-985.
21. Hakimi AA, Reznik E, Lee CH, et al. An integrated metabolic atlas of clear cell renal cell carcinoma. *Cancer Cell.* 2016;29(1):104-116.
23. Trott JF, Kim J, Abu Aboud O, et al. Inhibiting tryptophan metabolism enhances interferon therapy in kidney cancer. *Oncotarget.* 2016;7(41):66540-66557.
24. Yoon CY, Shim YJ, Kim EH, et al. Renal cell carcinoma does not express argininosuccinate synthetase and is highly sensitive to arginine deprivation via arginine deiminase. *Int J Cancer.* 2007;120(4):897-905.
25. Quinn DI, Lara PN Jr. Renal-cell cancer—targeting an immune checkpoint or multiple kinases. *N Engl J Med.* 2015;373(19):1872-1874.
26. Gerlinger M, Rowan AJ, Horswell S, et al. Intratumor heterogeneity and branched evolution revealed by multiregion sequencing. *N Engl J Med.* 2012;366(10):883-892.
45. Abu Aboud O, Habib SL, Trott J, et al. Glutamine addiction in kidney cancer suppresses oxidative stress and can be exploited for real-time imaging. *Cancer Res.* 2017;77(23):6746-6758.
54. Bosniak MA. The Bosniak renal cyst classification: 25 years later. *Radiology.* 2012;262(3):781-785.
59. Port FK, Ragheb NE, Schwartz AG, Hawthorne VM. Neoplasms in dialysis patients: a population-based study. *Am J Kidney Dis.* 1989;14(2):119-123.
60. Ishikawa I. Acquired cystic disease: mechanisms and manifestations. *Semin Nephrol.* 1991;11(6):671-684.
61. Ishikawa I, Saito Y, Asaka M, et al. Twenty-year follow-up of acquired renal cystic disease. *Clin Nephrol.* 2003;59(3):153-159.
64. Savaj S, Liakopoulos V, Ghareeb S, et al. Renal cell carcinoma in peritoneal dialysis patients. *Int Urol Nephrol.* 2003;35(2):263-265.
65. Ishikawa I. Unusual composition of cyst fluid in acquired cystic disease of the end-stage kidney. *Nephron.* 1985;41(4):373-374.
66. Keith DS, Torres VE, King BF, Zincki H, Farrow GM. Renal cell carcinoma in autosomal dominant polycystic kidney disease. *J Am Soc Nephrol.* 1994;4(9):1661-1669.
67. Nishimura H, Ubara Y, Nakamura M, et al. Renal cell carcinoma in autosomal dominant polycystic kidney disease. *Am J Kidney Dis.* 2009;54(1):165-168.
68. Hajj P, Ferlicot S, Massoud W, et al. Prevalence of renal cell carcinoma in patients with autosomal dominant polycystic kidney disease and chronic renal failure. *Urology.* 2009;74(3):631-634.
69. Chang YL, Chung HJ, Chen KK. Bilateral renal cell carcinoma in a patient with autosomal dominant polycystic kidney disease. *J Chin Med Assoc.* 2007;70(9):403-405.
70. Hashimoto Y, Takagi T, Kondo T, et al. Comparison of prognosis between patients with renal cell carcinoma on hemodialysis and those with renal cell carcinoma in the general population. *Int J Clin Oncol.* 2015;20(5):1035-1041.
71. Ikezawa E, Kondo T, Hashimoto Y, et al. Clinical symptoms predict poor overall survival in chronic-dialysis patients with renal cell carcinoma associated with end-stage renal disease. *Jpn J Clin Oncol.* 2014;44(11):1096-1100.
72. Shrewsberry AB, Osunkoya AO, Jiang K, et al. Renal cell carcinoma in patients with end-stage renal disease has favorable overall prognosis. *Clin Transplant.* 2014;28(2):211-216.
73. Neuzillet Y, Tillou X, Mathieu R, et al. Renal cell carcinoma (RCC) in patients with end-stage renal disease exhibits many favourable clinical, pathologic, and outcome features compared with RCC in the general population. *Eur Urol.* 2011;60(2):366-373.
81. Breda A, Luccarelli G, Rodriguez-Faba O, et al. Clinical and pathological outcomes of renal cell carcinoma (RCC) in native kidneys of patients with end-stage renal disease: a long-term comparative retrospective study with RCC diagnosed in the general population. *World J Urol.* 2015;33(1):1-7.
89. Huang WC, Levey AS, Serio AM, et al. Chronic kidney disease after nephrectomy in patients with renal cortical tumours: a retrospective cohort study. *Lancet Oncol.* 2006;7(9):735-740.
90. Pignot G, Bigot P, Bernhard JC, et al. Nephron-sparing surgery is superior to radical nephrectomy in preserving renal function benefit even when expanding indications beyond the traditional 4-cm cutoff. *Urol Oncol.* 2014;32(7):1024-1030.
95. Crestani A, Rossanese M, Calandriello M, Sioletic S, Giannarini G, Ficarra V. Introduction to small renal tumours and prognostic indicators. *Int J Surg.* 2016;36(Pt C):495-503.
96. MacLennan S, Imamura M, Lapitan MC, et al. Systematic review of perioperative and quality-of-life outcomes following surgical management of localised renal cancer. *Eur Urol.* 2012;62(6):1097-1117.
97. Hanna N, Sun M, Meyer CP, et al. Survival analyses of patients with metastatic renal cancer treated with targeted therapy with or without cytoreductive nephrectomy: a national cancer data base study. *J Clin Oncol.* 2016;34(27):3267-3275.
98. Campbell SC, Novick AC, Belldegrun A, et al. Guideline for management of the clinical T1 renal mass. *J Urol.* 2009;182(4):1271-1279.
99. Motzer RJ, Ravaud A, Patar JJ, et al. Adjuvant sunitinib for high-risk renal cell carcinoma after nephrectomy: subgroup analyses and updated overall survival results. *N Engl J Med.* 2016;73(1):62-68.
100. Finney R. The value of radiotherapy in the treatment of hypernephroma— a clinical trial. *Br J Urol.* 1973;45(3):258-269.
104. Escudier B, Eisen T, Stadler WM, et al. Sorafenib in advanced clear-cell renal-cell carcinoma. *N Engl J Med.* 2007;356(2):125-134.
105. Motzer RJ, Hutson TE, Tomczak P, et al. Sunitinib versus interferon alfa in metastatic renal-cell carcinoma. *N Engl J Med.* 2007;356(2):115-124.
121. Hodi FS, O'Day SJ, McDermott DF, et al. Improved survival with ipilimumab in patients with metastatic melanoma. *N Engl J Med.* 2010;363(8):711-723.
122. Motzer RJ, Escudier B, McDermott DF, et al. Nivolumab versus everolimus in advanced renal-cell carcinoma. *N Engl J Med.* 2015;373(19):1803-1813.
123. Robert C, Long GV, Brady B, et al. Nivolumab in previously untreated melanoma without BRAF mutation. *N Engl J Med.* 2015;372(4):320-330.
125. Wanchoo R, Karam S, Uppal NN, et al. Adverse renal effects of immune checkpoint inhibitors: a narrative review. *Am J Nephrol.* 2017;45(2):160-169.
126. Kourie HR, Klastersky J. Immune checkpoint inhibitors side effects and management. *Immunotherapy.* 2016;8(7):799-807.

127. Cortazar FB, Marrone KA, Troxell ML, et al. Clinicopathological features of acute kidney injury associated with immune checkpoint inhibitors. *Kidney Int.* 2016;90(3):638-647.

128. Abdel-Rahman O, Fouad M. A network meta-analysis of the risk of immune-related renal toxicity in cancer patients treated with immune checkpoint inhibitors. *Immunotherapy.* 2016;8(5):665-674.

129. Waeckerle-Men Y, Starke A, Wuthrich RP. PD-L1 partially protects renal tubular epithelial cells from the attack of CD8+ cytotoxic T cells. *Nephrol Dial Transplant.* 2007;22(6):1527-1536.

130. Nishimura H, Nose M, Hiai H, Minato N, Honjo T. Development of lupus-like autoimmune diseases by disruption of the PD-1 gene encoding an ITIM motif-carrying immunoreceptor. *Immunity.* 1999;11(2):141-151.

131. Spanou Z, Keller M, Britschgi M, et al. Involvement of drug-specific T cells in acute drug-induced interstitial nephritis. *J Am Soc Nephrol.* 2006;17(10):2919-2927.

143. Motzer RJ, Tannir NM, McDermott DF, et al. Nivolumab plus ipilimumab versus sunitinib in advanced renal-cell carcinoma. *N Engl J Med.* 2018;378(14):1277-1290.

A full list of references is available at Expertconsult.com

26 Wilms Tumor and von Hippel Lindau Disease

JOSHUA A. SAMUELS

Introduction

Nephroblastoma, or Wilms tumor (WT), is the most common primary renal malignancy in childhood and represents 6% of all childhood cancers. WTs comprise over 95% of all kidney tumors in children younger than 15 years old.[1,2] Usually found in children 1 to 5 years old, the tumor is still a rare finding. Overall, the incidence of WT is 1 in 10,000 children under 5 years of age and only 7 per million children under age 15 years.[3,4] The Children's Oncology Group (COG) reports that in the United States, roughly 600 children are diagnosed with a primary renal tumor each year and that over 90% of these are WTs.

Named for Max Wilms, the disease is characterized by the presence of an embryonal tumor derived from the metanephros. Although historically a death sentence, WT is one of the greatest success stories of modern medicine: survival rates rose from less than 5% in 1900 to over 90% in modern times.[3] The increased survival is the result of both improved diagnosis and identification, in addition to better surgical and chemotherapeutic approaches. Much of this improvement in outcomes is attributable to large research organizations, such as the Children's Cancer Group, Société Internationale d'Oncologie Pédiatrique (SIOP), and the National Wilms' Tumor Study Group (NWTS) (replaced by the renal tumor section of the COG) in 2001. For decades, these organizations have collected systematic databases for analysis and have supported large controlled treatment trials.[5] This chapter will review the presentation, diagnosis, treatment, and outcomes of WT.

Diagnosis and Histology

Nephroblastoma usually presents as a single kidney nodule, although multifocal unilateral or even bilateral tumors are possible. Bilateral tumors typically account for only 5% to 7% of all diagnosed WT.[6] Clinical presentation may include hematuria or abdominal pain and roughly a quarter (25%) of patients present with hypertension. Grossly, WTs are often large masses, which can vary greatly in size (Fig. 26.1). By the time they are diagnosed, tumors usually disrupt renal architecture. Typical histology includes blastemal, epithelial, and stromal tissue, although the proportion of each tissue type varies considerably between tumors.[7] It is rare to see the classic histologic triad, and biphasic or even monophasic tumors are not uncommon.[8]

When epithelial tissue predominates, differential diagnosis includes renal cell carcinoma (RCC) (rare in childhood), metanephric adenoma, or hyperplastic nephrogenic rest. Pure blastemal tumors, the least differentiated and likely most malignant, may resemble other types of embryonal "small round blue cell" tumors, such as neuroblastoma, desmoplastic small round cell tumor, primitive neuroectodermal tumor (PNET), and even lymphoma. There are several patterns of blastemal tumor growth, including serpentine, diffuse, nodular, and basaloid.

Histopathology

Predisposing nephrogenic rests are areas of embryonal tissue of metanephric origin still present after 36-weeks' gestation. Only rarely will these nephrogenic rests develop clonal expansion to become malignant WTs.[8] Up to 30% of patients with sporadic WT will have nephrogenic rests, although they are found in well over 90% of patients with multifocal or bilateral disease.[9] The presence of multiple nephrogenic rests is referred to as *nephroblastomatosis*. WTs present with classic triphasic histopathologic components: blastemal, epithelial, and stromal. The proportion and degree of differentiation of these cell types is widely variant, such that each tumor is histologically unique. This significant histologic heterogeneity can make diagnosis challenging for pathologists. Nonetheless, morphologic appearance of WT is critical to appropriate staging and risk stratification. The blastemal cells are tightly packed with small, round nuclei and little cytoplasm (Fig. 26.2). Blastemal-predominant tumors, among the "small round blue cell" tumors, may be difficult to distinguish from neuroblastoma, PNET, and desmoplastic small round cell tumors. These blastemal WTs are more aggressive and have a poorer outcome. In addition to blastemal type, WTs with diffuse anaplasia are considered "high risk" and are more aggressively treated (see later). The epithelial component is heterogeneously differentiated from normal appearing glomeruli to poorly defined tubules. In contrast, the stromal component resembles anything from immature fibroblasts to muscle or neural tissue. There may be spindle cells (mesenchymal embryo) with myxoid cytoplasm.

Although classic triphasic WT is relatively easy to identify, many tumors are biphasic or monophasic in appearance.[10] Additional challenges to accurate diagnosis may also be introduced with preoperative chemotherapy, a cornerstone of SIOP treatment regimens. Because of this, there are separate classification schemes for pre- and post-chemotherapy appearance.

Blastemas represent the least differentiated tumors and are considered the most malignant. Histologic patterns of blastemal WT include diffuse, nodular, serpentine, and basaloid.[11] All four of these patterns may be present within

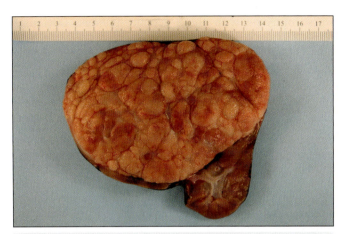

Fig. 26.1 Gross appearance of Wilms tumor. (Image courtesy Amanda Tchakarov, MD, Department of Pathology, McGovern Medical School at UTHealth.)

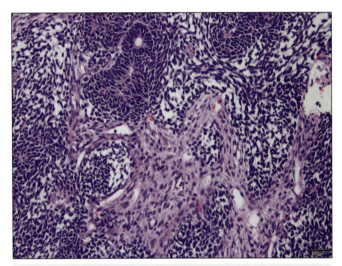

Fig. 26.2 Microscopic appearance of Wilms tumor. (Image courtesy Amanda Tchakarov, MD, Department of Pathology, McGovern Medical School at UTHealth.)

Table 26.1 Société Internationale d'Oncologie Pédiatrique Wilms Tumor Staging

Stage	Criteria
I	(a) Tumor is limited to kidney and is completely resected (resection margins "clear") (b) The tumor may be protruding into the pelvic system and "dipping" into the ureter (but it is not infiltrating their walls) (c) The vessels of the renal sinus are not involved (d) Intrarenal vessel involvement may be present
II	(a) The tumor extends beyond kidney or penetrates through the renal capsule and/or fibrous pseudocapsule into perirenal fat but is completely resected (resection margins "clear") (b) The tumor infiltrates the renal sinus and/or invades blood and lymphatic vessels outside the renal parenchyma but is completely resected (c) The tumor infiltrates adjacent organs or vena cava but is completely resected
III	(a) Incomplete excision of the tumor, which extends beyond the resection margins (b) Any abdominal lymph nodes are involved (c) Tumor rupture before or intraoperatively (regardless of other criteria for staging) (d) The tumor has penetrated through the peritoneal surface (e) Tumor thrombi present at resection margins of vessels or ureter, transected or removed piecemeal by surgeon (f) The tumor has been surgically biopsied (wedge biopsy) before preoperative chemotherapy or surgery
IV	Hematogenous metastases (lung, liver, bone, brain, etc.) or lymph node metastases outside the abdominopelvic region
V	Bilateral renal tumors at diagnosis

Box 26.1   The National Wilms Tumor Study Group/Children's Oncology Group Wilms Tumor Staging

Stage I

The tumor is limited to the kidney and has been completely resected
The tumor was not ruptured or biopsied before removal
No penetration of the renal capsule or involvement of renal sinus vessels

Stage II

The tumor extends beyond the capsule of the kidney but was completely resected with no evidence of tumor at or beyond the margins of resection
There is penetration of the renal capsule OR
There is invasion of the renal sinus vessels

Stage III

Gross or microscopic residual tumor remains postoperatively including inoperable tumor, positive surgical margins, tumor spillage surfaces, regional lymph node metastases, positive peritoneal cytology, or transected tumor thrombus
The tumor was ruptured or biopsied before removal

Stage IV

Hematogenous metastases or lymph node metastases outside the abdomen (e.g., lung, liver, bone, and brain)

Stage V

Bilateral renal involvement is present at diagnosis and each side may be considered to have a stage

the same tumor and pattern does not appear to affect prognosis. Diffusely growing blastemal WT may show significant infiltration and lack a pseudocapsule between affected and healthy kidney. Although these tumors may be aggressive, blastemal predominant tumors are usually considered "favorable histology" unless viable blastemal cells persist post standard chemotherapy (in the SIOP regimen).

Epithelial tumors also have a myriad of histologic presentations, from highly differentiated to primitive. These tumors may appear as nests of primitive rosette-like cells to fully formed tubules or glomeruli. Epithelial predominant tumors are also considered lower risk and thus "favorable histology."

Stromal tumors consist of mesenchymal cells and loose myxoid areas. As with the epithelial component, cells may appear with heterogeneous differentiation, including muscle, cartilage, fat, or even bone tissue. These stromal structures, particularly, are greatly affected by preoperative chemotherapy. These chemotherapy-induced changes (CIC) include necrosis, fibrosis, or bleeding. Frustratingly, the classification of WT is not standard between the many pediatric oncology research groups. SIOP and COG each has a unique criterion, which are described later (Table 26.1 and Box 26.1).[5]

Anaplasia, either focal or diffuse, is found in up to 10% of WTs.[10] This finding has both prognostic and treatment implications and identification of this pathologic entity is critical. As the presence of anaplastic tumor is strongly associated with recurrent disease, patients with anaplasia are referred to as having "unfavorable histology." Anaplasia is characterized by: (1) enlarged nuclei; (2) heterochromatic nuclei; and (3) multipolar mitotic figures. Patients with anaplastic tumors are often treated more aggressively.

Genetics of Wilms

Much work has been done on genetics of WT and the field continues to advance rapidly.[12] First cloned in 1990, *WT1* at 11p13 was the first tumor suppressor gene identified in WT. The *WT1* gene encodes a 55 kDa zinc finger transcription factor that helps control deoxyribonucleic acid (DNA) binding.[13] The gene may also regulate posttranscription gene expression through messenger ribonucleic acid binding. With 10 exon regions, there are multiple splicing events that are disrupted. The *WT1* gene is mutated in up to 12% of WTs. Other genes, such as *CTNNB1* (15%) and *WTX* (18%), have also been identified. *CTNNB1* on 3p21 encodes an 88 kDa beta-catenin protein heavily involved in Wnt/beta-catenin signaling pathway. In WT, mutated beta-catenin is found in approximately 15% of tumors.

WT on the X, also referred to as *WTX*, refers to mutations located on Xq11.1.[11] This gene contributes to stabilization of beta-catenin and acts as a tumor suppressor independent of the Wnt signaling pathway and WTX inactivation has recently been found in up to 30% of WT pathology specimens.

Taken together, genetic variations in one of these three genes (*WT1*, *CTNNB1*, and *WTX*) is found in up to one-third of the cases of WT.[11,12] In addition to these genes that are associated with the presence of WT, there are other genes that are markers of outcome. Disease progression in WT has been associated with expression of several genes, including *TP53*, *MYCN*, *CITED1*, *SIX2*, *TOP2A*, and *CRABP2*.[14] These genes are involved in renal development, chromatin remodeling, DNA methylation, and other cellular functions.[15] Mutations in p53 is the most frequent finding in human malignancy. Located on 17p13.1, the gene encodes TP53, a protein involved in many cellular events, such as DNA repair, apoptosis, and differentiation/proliferation. p53 in WT is associated with relapse, progression, anaplasia, and metastasis. Up to 75% of anaplastic WTs have been reported to have p53 mutations.[16]

Interestingly, not all of the genetic changes seen in WT are the result of genetic mutations. Large scale loss of heterozygosity (LOH) was the first aberration identified. LOH is a common finding in many types of cancer. Even when there exists the genetic loss of one allele, the remaining unaffected allele is able to "cover" protein synthesis and hide the defect. If some second "hit" damages or alters the function of this other allele, then a recessive trait, often a tumor suppressor, becomes manifest. This LOH can be the result of mitotic errors, gene conversion, faulty DNA repair or replication, or some other mishap. LOH for 1p and 16q was identified more frequently among subjects with adverse outcomes in the NWTS-4 trial. Given these findings of worse outcome with these genetic findings, COG uses these LOH markers as a molecular marker for risk stratification.[15] In recent COG protocols, patients having double positive tumors receive increased treatment intensity.

Epidemiology

First described by Max Wilms in 1899, WTs are one of the most common solid tumors in childhood. It is currently the third most common malignancy in children. WT comprises 95% of all renal cancers among children younger than 15 years old. The disease affects approximately 1 in 10,000 children and its incidence is 7 per million and there are roughly 600 children newly diagnosed annually in the United States. WT is usually a sporadic disease, although family history is present in up to 2% of cases. Approximately 10% of WTs are related to germline mutations or other congenital abnormalities that result in a syndromic inheritance (see later).

WT is the second most common solid abdominal tumor (behind neuroblastoma) in children. The mean age at diagnosis is just 3 years old. Presentation is usually an asymptomatic mass detected by parents, primary care providers, or more recently, incidentally found on abdominal imaging.

Syndromic Wilms Tumors

WTs are frequently seen as part of a generalized overgrowth syndrome. Many of these conditions are related to a chromosomal abnormality, most often identified on chromosome 11. Although occasionally isolated, several named syndromes are strongly associated with the development of WT. Although many of these syndromes are rare (for example Perlman syndrome, Simpson-Golabi-Behmel syndrome, and 9q22.3 microdeletion), several conditions are common enough to warrant specific discussion.

DENYS-DRASH AND FRASIER

Both Denys-Drash syndrome and Frasier syndrome are characterized by renal disease, intersex, and predisposition to develop tumors.[17] Each is also associated with WT1 mutations, with 96% of Denys-Drash and 100% of Frasier patients having constitutional heterozygosity mutations of the *WT1* gene. Before the age of molecular diagnostics, it was unclear if they actually represent separate entities or are in fact the same disorder, although there are notable differences in clinical presentation, not the least of which is risk of WT.

Denys-Drash syndrome consists of WTs, intersex, and the nephrotic syndrome. Characteristic glomerular damage leads to nephrotic syndrome at an early age, and progressive sclerosis leading to renal failure is inevitable. Most patients, although not all, develop early WT, usually before age 2 years. In general, XX chromosomal patients are phenotypic girls, whereas the XY patients often have ambiguous genitalia or male pseudo-hermaphroditism.

In contrast to Denys-Drash, Frasier syndrome is not associated with WT.[17] Patients with Frasier syndrome present in similar fashion to Denys-Drash, but have more gradual decline in kidney function and lack the risk for WT. Instead of kidney tumors, these patients are at increased risk of gonadal tumors, specifically gonadoblastoma. The disorder is caused by specific *WT1* mutations that disrupt gene splicing at the second alternative splice donor site. These mutations are located in intron 9 of the *WT1* gene and result in deficiency of the positive KTS isoforms of lysine, threonine, and serine (from 2:1 to 1:2). This minor change highlights the complicated epigenetics of this condition, because the WT1 protein is both normal in structure and binding ability. The lack of KTS positive isoforms in the affected cells leads to the clinical manifestation of Frasier syndrome without increasing tumorigenicity (the negative isoform is equally tumor suppressing for WT). This explains why Frasier patients do not develop WT.

BECKWITH-WIEDEMANN SYNDROME

Beckwith-Wiedemann syndrome (BWS) is a classic although rare genetic overgrowth syndrome. The syndrome has an estimated prevalence of approximately 1 per 10,000 live births. Although varying diagnostic criteria make generalizations difficult, patients mostly present in early childhood with macrosomia, macroglossia, and often abdominal wall defects, such as omphalocele or umbilical hernia, and visceromegaly. Patients with BWS are at high risk of developing multifocal WTs, with approximately 10% of children experiencing either a WT or a hepatoblastoma. Other nephrourologic complications are common, with 30% to 60% of patients having some anomaly (cysts and nephrocalcinosis top the list of non-WT complications). Not all patients with BWS present with all of the classic findings. Consensus recommendations now call for genetic testing in unclear cases.[18] Classic abnormalities at 11p15.5–11p15.4 are diagnostic. From a nephrologic standpoint, patients with BWS should be screened for both nephrocalcinosis/hypercalcuria and for WT. Given the doubling time of WT as 11 to 13 days, renal ultrasound is recommended every 3 months until age 7 years. After age 7 years, imaging may be spaced at greater intervals. Patients with certain molecular markers (IC1 Gain of Methylation [GOM] and segmental upd(11)pat molecular subgroups) are at highest risk for WT. Given the frequent screening for WT, patients with BWS are often discovered much earlier than in the general population.[18] As such, their tumors are more often smaller and less likely anaplastic or metastatic at diagnosis. Treatment is usually partial nephrectomy with or without chemotherapy.

WAGR SYNDROME

WT in association with aniridia, genitourinary abnormalities, and mental retardation has been dubbed the WAGR syndrome. This rare genetic condition involves deletion of 11p13 and is therefore associated with WTs. The aniridia (and probably the mental deficiencies) is caused by additional deletion of the neighboring *PAX6* ocular development gene.

Clinically, infants with WAGR usually present with sporadic aniridia. Such infants should always undergo screening for WAGR, because the presence of external genital abnormalities is not universal. Genetic testing for the characteristic 11p13 deletion can confirm diagnosis. A recent review of 54 cases of WAGR in patients ranging from 7 months to 42 years revealed that more than half (57%) had WT. Other genitourinary anomalies included cryptorchidism (60% of males), bicornuate uterus (17% of females), and ambiguous genitalia (10%).

Diagnosis and Staging of Wilms Tumors

Staging criteria of WTs are based on both prechemotherapy and postchemotherapy tumor burden and extent. Although there are slight differences, both SIOP and COG have similar staging criteria (see Table 26.1 and Box 26.1). Stage 1 WT presents with tumor confined to the kidney and completely resected without rupture or spillage into the abdomen during removal. Stage 2 involves tumors that spread beyond the capsule of the affected kidney into the renal sinus, vessels, or lymphatics. COG also specifies that the entire tumor is removed with no evidence of spread beyond resection. Stage 3 WTs include those not completely resected, with positive tumor margins, spillage into the abdomen, or rupture before removal. Because of the risk of spread, SIOP also includes tumors that have been biopsied prechemotherapy or surgery as Stage 3. Both groups classify Stage 4 tumors as those with hematogenous spread or lymph node involvement outside the abdomen. Stage 5 WT refers to tumors that are bilateral at the time of diagnosis.

Treatment

HISTORY

In the early 1900s, surgery was the only treatment option for children with nephroblastoma. As surgery and anesthesia advances were made in the 1930s and 1940s, survival improved from 0% to almost 25%. The addition of postoperative radiation therapy (pioneered by Sydney Farber and M.H. Wittenborg at Boston Children's Hospital in the 1950s) increased survival to around 50%. Real headway was made in the 1960s, with the addition of chemotherapy (first dactinomycin and then vincristine) increasing survival rates to over 80%.[7,19] The creation of large, multicenter studies in the late 1960s has improved survival even further (2-year survival is 97%) and continues to elucidate the optimal treatment. Major collaborative research consortiums have been formed on both sides of the Atlantic. The American Children's Oncology Group (which began as the National Wilms' Tumor Study group [NWTSG]) and the European International Society of Pediatric Oncology (SIOP) have advocated different approaches to WT.[5]

The COG protocol in the United States calls for immediate surgical resection of WTs, followed by postoperative management as dictated by the pathology. In contrast, SIOP calls for presurgical chemotherapy without a biopsy in most cases of WT. Once the tumor has shrunk, surgical resection without tumor spillage into the abdomen is conducted and further therapy dictated by pathology findings. SIOP, with its presurgical chemotherapy, recognizes a specific "blastemal subtype" of WT that is more chemoresistant.

These tumors, which require more intensive postsurgical treatment, are not classified in the surgery-first COG protocols.

Overall, survival does not appear to differ significantly between the two approaches (> 90%). Although discussion of the specific differences in approach is beyond the scope of this chapter, both regimens use surgical resection and chemotherapy for most patients. These treatment modalities, along with radiation, are discussed subsequently.

MODERN SURGICAL MANAGEMENT

Surgical management remains the most common definitive treatment modality.[20,21] Unilateral radical ureteronephrectomy with lymph node sampling is the current gold-standard surgical treatment for children with WT. Although surgical approaches vary, the transperitoneal approach described more than 70 years ago remains the standard operating technique. Other incisions, such as flank or paramedian, have been reported to have increased complications and poorer oncologic outcomes. Complete abdominal exploration is important, with specific focus on the liver, renal vein and inferior vena cava, and peritoneal surfaces. As imaging modalities have improved, assessment of the contralateral kidney is becoming less common.[22] Because most WTs do not invade other organs, there is no need to resect bowel or liver in most instances. Surgical resection of the ipsilateral adrenal gland is also dependent on several factors and is no longer considered vital to outcomes. Failure to sample at least seven lymph nodes is a common surgical oversight. Discovery of lymph involvement is important to assist in staging, plan postoperative therapy, and to provide more accurate prognostication of outcome.

Although radical nephrectomy remains the most common surgical approach, nephron sparing surgery is gaining popularity in recent years.[9,20,21,23] Minimally invasive surgery, both laparoscopic and robot assisted, is being performed more frequently. Care must be made to remove the kidney without peritoneal spillage. This approach is particularly attractive when bilateral disease is present. A meta-analysis comparing radical nephrectomy (RN) and partial nephrectomy (nephron sparing surgery, NSS) by Wilcox Vanden Berg and colleagues including 66 studies and more than 4000 patients suggested similar long-term survival regardless of complete nephrectomy versus nephron sparing partial nephrectomy.[23] Most studies were single center retrospective cohorts, and over 70% of included subjects were from Europe or the USA. The authors found that 2844 (74%) patients underwent radical nephrectomy, whereas 1040 (26%) received NSS. Outcomes did not differ between RN and NSS in terms of reported rupture rates (13% vs. 7%) during surgery, overall recurrence (12% vs. 11%), and survival (85% vs. 88%). Regardless of surgical modality, overall survival was greatly improved in more recent publications, with rates of 61% to 87% in the 1980s but over 90% in studies published since 2010.[23]

RADIATION

Postoperative (or even intraoperative) radiation is used in select high-risk patients. Once a mainstay of therapy, improvements in chemotherapy and in our understanding of

recurrence risk has lessened the need for radiation. Overall increased efficacy of surgical and chemotherapeutic approaches has decreased the need for adjuvant radiation. One study showed the overall proportion of patients receiving radiation fell from 73% in 1976 to 53% in 2008. Currently used only in high-risk children with unfavorable histology, total dose of radiation has decreased from 20 Gy to only 10 Gy. These advances have resulted in fewer treatment complications (notably growth retardation), without increasing patient risk.

CHEMOTHERAPY

Use of chemotherapy for WT is standard, although the timing differs between the different research groups. NWTSG/COG in the USA and SIOP have developed standardized protocols for treatment. The major differences between the protocols involves timing of surgical intervention in relation to chemotherapy.[5,9,24] Presurgical chemotherapy is considered standard practice outside the United States (notably through the European SIOP and the Indian Council of Medical Research). When preoperative chemotherapy is used, a 4-week regimen of vincristine and actinomycin D is standard in nonmetastatic disease, whereas 6 weeks is given for metastatic disease. Restaging is then completed, and surgical management is planned.

COG protocols differ and recommend immediate surgical resection followed by chemotherapy for most patients. One benefit of this COG approach is that small, Stage 1 tumors with favorable histology in children under 24 months are treated with surgery alone.

In both COG and SIOP regimens, postoperative chemotherapy regimen is dictated by staging based on pathology findings.[9] Most regimens in treatment of nephroblastoma include: actinomycin D, vincristine, doxorubicin, cyclophosphamide, ifosfamide, etoposide, and carboplatin.

Bilateral Wilms Tumors

WTs are synchronously bilateral at diagnosis in only 4% to 7% of cases. Bilateral tumors are more likely to be unfavorable histology (up to 10%) and to have associated genitourinary (GU) abnormalities.[6] Almost a quarter of patients presenting with bilateral WT have syndromic GU anomalies, aniridia, WAGR syndrome, Denys-Drash syndrome, or hemihypertrophy/overgrowth syndrome.

Not surprisingly, the cure rate among those with bilateral disease is worse than those with unilateral disease. Overall cure has been reported between 70% to 80% for those with bilateral disease.[6] In addition, there is an increased risk of chronic kidney disease (CKD) and need for either dialysis or kidney transplantation. Treatment aimed at nephron sparing is more important in bilateral disease.[25]

Adult Wilms Tumors

Because WT is rare in patients over 16 years of age, most adult kidney tumors are RCC.[26] Only 3% of WTs are in adults and this represents less than 1% of all adult renal tumors.[27,28] Diagnostic criteria for patients older than

15 years of age was described by Kilton and include primary renal neoplasm, histologic features of embryonic glomerulotubular structure, immature spindle or round cell stroma, and the absence of RCCs.[23] Most reported patients (< 500 in the literature) have advanced disease (Stage 3 and 4). After radical nephrectomy of the affected side, chemotherapy with vincristine, actinomycin-D, doxorubicin, and ifosfamide are common. Although more advanced disease is sometimes treated with cisplatin and etoposide, no standard therapy exists for adults and prognosis is poor compared both with children with WTs and with adults with RCC.[29]

Long-Term Survivors

As more patients are surviving childhood WT, adult complications of therapy are also becoming more common. Frequent complications include heart failure or second malignancies (likely related to chemotherapy or radiation toxicity), and long-term impairment of renal function.

Studies are varied but show that significant numbers of survivors have long-term renal dysfunction after successful treatment for WT.[30,31] Although difficult to quantify, in patients with unilateral nonsyndromic WT who underwent unilateral nephrectomy (the most common population), the rates of CKD range from 0.5% to as high as 19%. This degree of CKD does not appear to be increased above other children with solitary kidneys. Among 27 adults who underwent unilateral nephrectomy during childhood (including four caused by WT), Robitaille found an average creatinine clearance of 84 mL/min (75% of age matched controls).[32]

End-stage renal disease (ESRD) is a rare but serious complication. The NWTSG evaluated long-term follow-up in almost 8000 patients between 1969 and 2004. The cumulative incidence of ESRD at 20 years follow-up was less than 1%. Less severe forms of CKD, including proteinuria and mildly decreased glomerular filtration rate, appear in 10% to 15% in several studies. The risk is greater in patients who undergo radiation therapy. Because it is a newer treatment modality, outcomes in patients who undergo NSS is of great interest. Whether the long-term risk of kidney dysfunction is mitigated remains to be seen.

Patients with bilateral WT obviously have a higher risk of CKD following treatment.[25] NWTSG data from the 8000 patients mentioned earlier show a 3% risk of ESRD in those with bilateral disease. Although still low, this risk is almost sixfold higher than in patients with unilateral WT. There is also some evidence that survivors of childhood WT are at increased risk of RCC during early adult years.

Summary

Management of WT is one of modern medicine's great success stories. In the past 100 years, survival has increased from just 5% to well over 90% currently. This impressive improvement in outcomes is the result of several large, well designed multinational consortiums dedicated to WT. Based on these successes, perhaps nephrologists can adopt a similar collaborative approach to other common conditions and foster a "paradigm" shift in our collective management.

Von Hippel Lindau

von Hippel Lindau disease (VHL) is an autosomal dominant condition that results in multiple vascular neoplasms. The most common tumors are CNS hemangioblastomas and retinal tumors, pancreatic islet cell tumors, pheochromocytomas (PCCs), and clear cell renal carcinoma.[33] Nonmalignant renal and pancreatic cysts may also form.

Although Treacher Collins described a family with retinal hemangioblastomas in 1894, it was von Hippel who first characterized the familial retinal lesions (1904) and Lindau who then recognized the cerebellar lesions and renal tumors and cysts (1927).[34] The name von Hippel Lindau was first described in 1936. Current criteria were published by Melmon and Rosen in 1964.[34] The incidence of VHL is roughly 1 out of 36,000 births. Penetrance is high (> 90%) by age 65 years.[34]

Clinical Characteristics

The most typical presenting feature of VHL is benign CNS hemangioblastomas, present in 40% to 80% of cases. These tumors commonly occur in the cerebellum, spinal cord, and brain stem. Early symptoms are common, with many patients presenting in early childhood, although average age of presentation is 33 years. Location dependent, symptoms include weakness, pain in extremities, back or head, or dizziness. Polycythemia is a common laboratory finding. Hemangioblastomas are diagnosed by magnetic resonance imaging (MRI), which is recommended yearly for patients over the age of 10 years.

Retinal angiomas are histologically similar lesions that arise in more than half of VHL patients. Visual loss is not uncommon, with up to 35% of carriers experiencing impairment. Vision loss occurs in more than half of patients with retinal angiomas over the age of 50 years.

PCCs occur in a large subset of patients with VHL, perhaps as many as 30%. Often bilateral or extraadrenal, these tumors are usually catecholamine producing. Symptoms include hypertension, tachycardia, palpitations, and sweating with pallor. Mean age of diagnosis is 30 years. Diagnosis is based on imaging and laboratory findings, with plasma-free metanephrines the most laboratory sensitive (97%) test. Contrast MRI or meta-isobenzylguanidine scanning are most commonly used imaging techniques. Treatment of PCC in VHL centers on laparoscopic surgical resection after 10 to 14 days of perioperative blood pressure management with combination alpha and beta blockade. There are two clinical subtypes of VHL, depending on the risk of PCC.[35] Type 1 carries a low risk of PCC (< 10%), whereas type 2 is associated with a 40% to 60% risk of PCC. Within type 2 VHL, there are additional subtypes stratified by risk of RCC. Type 2b, the most common in European countries, has the highest risk of RCC (Table 26.2).

Renal manifestations of VHL include both renal cystic disease and clear cell carcinoma. Multiple, bilateral cysts are found in 50% to 70% of patients. Although bilateral, the effect of renal cystic disease is low, with most cysts being asymptomatic. Unlike autosomal dominant polycystic kidney disease, progression to CKD is uncommon. RCC, conversely, is a more serious concern. Present in up to 30%

Table 26.2   von Hippel Lindau Types and Corresponding Tumor Risk

Type	Tumors
Type 1	Low risk of PCC or RCC Retinal and CNS hemangioblastomas, pancreatic and neuroendocrine tumors
Type 2a	PCC, retinal and CNS hemangioblastomas
Type 2b	PCC, RCC, retinal and CNS hemangioblastomas, pancreatic and neuroendocrine tumors
Type 2c	PCC only, often recurrent

CNS, Central nervous system; *PCC*, pheochromocytoma; *RCC*, renal cell carcinoma.

of patients with VHL, metastatic clear cell RCC is the leading cause of death among affected individuals. Renal cysts and tumors typically develop during the third and fourth decades and become more prevalent in older patients. Up to 70% of VHL patients over the age of 60 years have RCC.[36]

Renal disease is rarely the presenting finding in VHL. Clinical signs include flank mass, flank pain, and gross hematuria. Serial imaging with abdominal computed tomography or MRI is recommended to delineate simple cysts (which are usually asymptomatic) from complex cysts that might undergo malignant transformation.

Treatment of RCC in VHL depends on lesion size.[36] No intervention is necessary for lesions smaller than 3 cm. Using a threshold of 3 cm helps distinguish potentially metastatic potential, NSS resection or, more recently, radiofrequency ablation of lesions larger than 3 cm is often performed. Ten-year survival following resection may be as high as 81%.

Genotype-Phenotype Correlations

Germline mutations in the VHL protein (pVHL) is at the root of VHL.[35] The gene is located on the short arm of chromosome 3p.[37] VHL is caused by an inactivation of pVHL and subsequent overproduction of vascular endothelial growth factor (VEGF), platelet-derived growth factor (PDGF), and transforming growth factor (TGF)-α.[37] In vivo, pVHL acts as a tumor suppressor by binding to a hypoxia-inducible factor (HIF). HIF regulates gene expression by oxygen.[38] Loss of pVHL results in high HIF levels and subsequent overproduction of VEGF, PDGF, and TGF-α.[35,39]

Summary

VHL disease is a genetic disorder with autosomal dominant inheritance that results in multiple neoplasms of vascular structures. The most common tumors are CNS hemangioblastomas and retinal tumors, pancreatic islet cell tumors, PCCs, and clear cell renal carcinoma. Early diagnosis and screening for cancers in affected patients is critical to their long-term health.

Key Points

- Wilms tumor is the most common kidney malignancy in childhood.
- Wilms tumor is treated with both surgical resection and chemotherapy, although protocols differ as to the timing of each modality of treatment.
- The survival from Wilms tumor is one of the great success stories of modern medicine, with survival rates rising almost 90% in the past 120 years.
- Patients with von Hippel Lindau disease commonly develop clear cell renal carcinoma along with other malignancies, such as hemangioblastomas, pheochromocytomas, and pancreatic cell tumors.
- Common genetic variants have been strongly associated with both Wilms and von Hippel Lindau disease.

References

1. Irtan S, Ehrlich PF, Pritchard-Jones K. Wilms tumor: "state-of-the-art" update, 2016. *Semin Pediatr Surg.* 2016;25(5):250-256.
10. Al-Hussain T, Ali A, Akhtar M. Wilms tumor: an update. *Adv Anat Pathol.* 2014;21(3):166-173.
21. Kieran K, Ehrlich PF. Current surgical standards of care in Wilms tumor. *Urol Oncol.* 2016;34(1):13-23.
34. Chittiboina P, Lonser RR. Chapter 10 - Von Hippel–Lindau disease. In: Islam MP, Roach ES, eds. *Handbook of Clinical Neurology.* Vol 132. Elsevier: 2015:139-156. https://www.elsevier.com/books/neurocutaneous-syndromes/islam/978-0-444-62702-5

A full list of references is available at Expertconsult.com

Tuberous Sclerosis Complex and the Kidney

JOHN J. BISSLER AND VIJAY S. GORANTLA

Introduction

Tuberous sclerosis complex (TSC) is an often underdiagnosed and misunderstood disease affecting more than one million patients worldwide. Disruptions in the TSC axis lead to cellular abnormalities that result in abnormal development and postpartum cellular growth. TSC affects every organ system and is often thought of as a tumor predisposition syndrome, although the lesions often seem to share characteristics of more benign lesions, and in some ways a dysplastic process. There has been an attribution to "malignant degeneration" of TSC renal lesions, although this seems to be more of a historical footnote rather than a well-studied phenomenon. There is also confusion regarding the true risk of fat-poor renal lesions being malignant. This chapter will address these issues.

Genetics of Tuberous Sclerosis Complex Renal Disease

TSC is an autosomal dominant genetic disorder that has a birth incidence of around 1:5800.[1,2] Proper diagnosis can be certain if the International Guidelines are followed,[3] but diagnosis can be missed if one relies on the Vogt's triad for TSC (facial angiofibromas, developmental delay, and intractable epilepsy) because less than 40% of affected patients have these classic features.[4] Approximately half of the patients demonstrate cognitive impairment, autism, or behavioral disorders.

There are two gene loci associated with TSC: *TSC1*, located on chromosome 9, and *TSC2*, located on chromosome 16. The identification of the *TSC2* gene location was assisted because of an observation in a family with autosomal dominant polycystic kidney disease caused by a balanced translocation in the *PKD1* gene. A child in this family had autosomal dominant polycystic kidney disease and TSC, which helped in the positional cloning of the *TSC2* gene.[5]

TSC may occur by the loss of expression of the nonmutant allele. Both TSC and autosomal dominant polycystic kidney disease are phenotypically expressed because of a second-hit, or somatic mutation mechanism.[6] The kidney disease associated with the *PKD1* and the *TSC2* loci account for a majority of their respective diseases, and both exhibit a more severe phenotype compared with the disease associated with the *PKD2* and *TSC1* loci. This association with more severe disease may have a molecular underpinning. The *PKD1* and *TSC2* loci are immediately adjacent, in a tail-to-tail orientation, on chromosome 16p. The proximity of

the genes may be important because the *PKD1* gene contains an intronic sequence with unique structural properties[7,8] that would predispose to mutation because this tract interferes with deoxyribonucleic acid (DNA) replication and leads to double-strand breaks and an array of somatic mutational effects.[9] This predisposition to DNA double-strand breaks is synergized by the renal microenvironment, which inhibits DNA damage recognition.[10,11] This renal microenvironmental predisposition to disease may also help explain the multifocal and bilateral nature of the TSC cystic disease and the angiomyolipomata.

Tuberous Sclerosis Complex and Renal Function

Premature impairment of glomerular filtration rate (GFR) is reported in up to 40% of patients with TSC.[12,13] This reduction in function occurs in the absence of overt bleeding from angiomyolipomata or interventions, suggesting an intrinsic renal disease,[14] and underscores the need to preserve kidney function by treating hypertension aggressively and avoiding surgical intervention when treating angiomyolipomata preemptively to prevent hemorrhage. Renal function should be assessed at the time of diagnosis and on an annual basis using blood tests to estimate GFR using creatinine[3,15] or cystatin C equations.[16] Renal function in patients with TSC is of critical importance because many of the drugs commonly used to treat epilepsy in patients with TSC are renally cleared.

Biology of Tuberous Sclerosis Complex Renal Disease

ANGIOMYOLIPOMATA

The cell giving rise to the angiomyolipomata, categorized a perivascular epithelial cell tumor (PEComa), has been unknown until recently.[17] Vascular associations with TSC, including aneurysms in the angiomyolipomata,[18] aorta,[19] and brain,[20] along with immunohistochemical staining reveal that angiomyolipomata may arise from vascular mural cells.[21] This origin helps explain the angiomyolipomata propensity to hemorrhage[22] and the proclivity of the cells to home to lung, leading to lymphangioleiomyomatosis.[23,24]

Although the typical TSC-associated angiomyolipoma contains fat, these lesions can also contain spindle cells, epithelioid cells, or a mix of both that express smooth muscle actin and melanocyte markers, such as gp100, a splice variant of Pmel17, and even melanin A (Fig. 27.1). Expression of these melanocyte-associated genes results from *MitF* family transcription factor activity.[25] This increased MITF transcription factor activity has caused confusion between TSC-associated PEComas and those caused by translocations involving *TFE3* or *TFEB*, such as more aggressive renal cell carcinomas (RCCs) and malignant PEComas.[26,27]

Because approximately one-third of TSC-associated angiomyolipomata have fat-poor components (Fig. 27.2), and because at least half of the patients affected with TSC will have cystic disease, it is common for some patients to have a solid mass that is associated with cystic components. These findings should raise concern for RCC in the general population but should not raise the same level of concern in the population with TSC, because RCC is actually very rare in the population of TSC patients. Such lesions can be serially measured and assessed for growth characteristics that can help sort the fat-poor angiomyolipoma from the malignancy.[28] Current research focuses on noninvasive approaches to help better delineate malignancy from fat-poor angiomyolipoma.

CYSTIC DISEASE: INTERSECTION OF CILIAL CYSTOGENIC AND ONCOGENIC SIGNALING PATHWAYS

TSC proteins regulate cell growth and proliferation, which are important for organogenesis, organ maintenance, and malignancy. The mechanistic target of rapamycin complex 1 (mTORC1) signaling pathway integrates intra- and extracellular environmental information to properly regulate metabolism, protein translation, growth, proliferation, autophagy, and survival. The TSC2 protein is reported to interact with cleaved C-terminal tail of polycystin-1 (PC-1) to control the mTORC1 pathway.[29] AKT phosphorylation of TSC2 causes its retention at the cell membrane for this

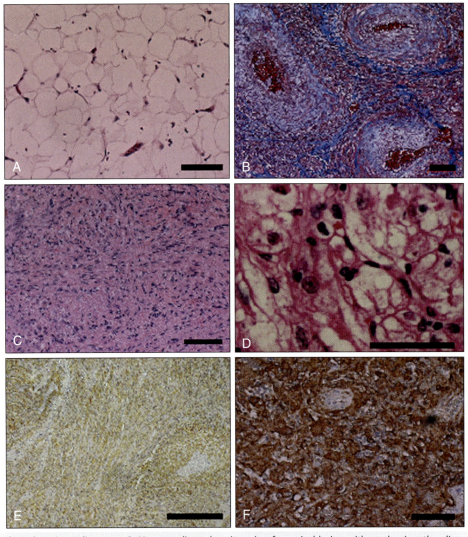

Fig. 27.1 Histology of renal angiomyolipomata. **A.** Hematoxylin and eosin stain of a typical lesion with predominantly adipose tissue. **B.** Masson's trichrome stain of a fat-poor angiomyolipoma, with many vascular structures. **C.** Hematoxylin and eosin stain of a fat-poor angiomyolipoma consisting of smooth muscle-like cells. **D.** Hematoxylin and eosin stain of a fat-poor angiomyolipoma consisting primarily of epithelioid cells. **E.** Fat-poor angiomyolipoma consisting of spindle-shaped cells stain with an antibody to smooth muscle actin. **F.** HMB-45 staining in an angiomyolipoma. *Black bars in each panel represent 100 μm in length.* (From Bissler JJ, Henske E. Renal manifestations of tuberous sclerosis complex. In: Whittemore V, Henske EP, Kwiatkowski D, eds. *Tuberous sclerosis complex: from genes to therapeutics.* New York: Elsevier; 2006, 312.)

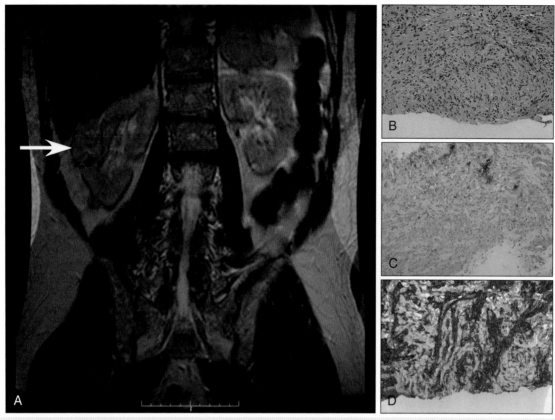

Fig. 27.2 Fat-poor lesions can be smooth muscle predominant. **A.** Fast spin echo T2 magnetic resonance imaging revealing a fat-poor lesion (*arrow*). **B.** Hematoxylin and eosin revealing smooth muscle-like cells. **C.** HMB-45 staining revealing positive cells. **D.** Smooth muscle actin staining. (From Bissler JJ, Henske E. Renal manifestations of tuberous sclerosis complex. In: Whittemore V, Henske EP, Kwiatkowski D, eds. *Tuberous sclerosis complex: from genes to therapeutics.* New York: Elsevier; 2006, 318.)

regulation of mTORC1. This phosphorylation step is inhibited by the uncleaved, membrane bound C-terminal tail of PC-1. Without this phosphorylation, TSC2 complexes with TSC1 to downregulate mTORC1 activity.

The mTORC1 activation also may involve a nuance involving the PC-1 in explaining the cystogenesis that could help explain why the *PKD1/TSC2* contiguous gene syndrome has such a severe phenotype (Fig. 27.3). mTORC1 activity also negatively regulates the biogenesis of PC-1 and proper trafficking of the PC-1/2 complex to cilia. PC-1 is located on the cilia of principal cells, but it is also found on other cell membranes, including intercalated cells,[30–32] and is strongly expressed on extracellular vesicles.[33] Genetic interaction studies have revealed that PC-1 downregulation by mTORC1 leads to cystogenesis in *Tsc1* mutants.[34] These findings may explain the severe renal manifestations of the *PKD1/TSC2* contiguous gene syndrome.

RENAL CELL CARCINOMA

Although RCC has been recognized as part of TSC renal disease for many years,[35] more in-depth analysis of this rare phenomenon is lacking. The literature does contain cases in both children and young adults with what is described as *RCC.* These patients are often reported to have multiple and even bilateral tumors. Histologically there are three main types. Previously reported TSC-associated RCCs have been classified as chromophobe-type or described

resembling chromophobe RCC.[36–38] Guo et al. described this chromophobe morphology in almost 60% of the 57 lesions from eight of the 18 patients (44%) with TSC.[36] They based this designation on the basis of lesions having eosinophilic cytoplasm, nuclear membrane irregularity, and perinuclear halos. They also noted extensive PAX8 nuclear staining that excludes the possibility that the chromophobe-like morphology could represent oncocytoma-like angiomyolipomata, a variant composed of polygonal cells with deeply eosinophilic cytoplasm that mimics oncocytoma or eosinophilic variant of chromophobe RCC.[36] The chromophobe-like RCCs were described as being CK7 positive; however, unlike a prototypical chromophobe RCC that has immunoreactivity for CD117, only one of the six evaluated chromophobe-like morphology tumors in the Guo et al. series had limited staining for CD117.[36]

The second TSC-associated RCC's morphology is the renal angiomyo-adenomatous tumor (RAT).[37] This pattern consists of prominent smooth muscle proliferation with clear neoplastic cells that form predominantly tubules and nests with rare papillae. The Guo et al. series identified this pattern in 39% of patients accounting for 30% of total RCCs.[36] This RAT-like pattern of TSC-associated RCC is reported to be immunohistochemically similar to the RAT and clear cell-papillary RCC spectrum, because they all strongly stain with both CK7 and CA9.

The last TSC-associated tumor histologic morphology is one of a distinct granular eosinophilic-macrocystic

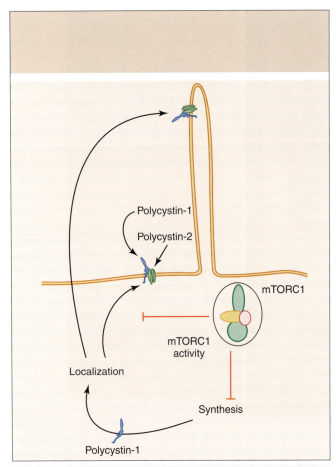

Fig. 27.3 mTORC1 activity negatively regulates the biogenesis of polycystin-1 (PC-1) and proper trafficking of the PC-1/2 complex to cilia.

morphology, and this pattern represented 11% of all the TSC-associated RCCs in the Guo et al. series, but this accounted for one-third of the patients.[36] Schreiner and colleagues identified this as a distinct histologic pattern of RCC in TSC patients.[38] These lesions have neoplastic appearing cells with voluminous granular eosinophilic cytoplasm and frequently have macrocystic architecture with lining epithelial cells showing a "hobnail" pattern that is typical in TSC cysts. The solid areas of these lesions very closely resemble atypical epithelioid angiomyolipomata, but also exhibit strong nuclear PAX8 staining, supporting the classification as a renal carcinoma. These lesions could also resemble the Xp11/TFE3 translocation RCC in large part because they have abundant eosinophilic cytoplasm.[39–41] For these three different patterns, an important missing element is long-term follow-up regarding the patient outcomes. Possibly the histology may be caused by the intrinsic intercalated cell plasticity, and it may turn out that the appearance in these TSC RCC lesions may actually look far more aggressive than they actually are in clinical practice.[42] Embryologically, the collecting duct cells arise from the ureteric bud outpouching of the Wolffian duct and give rise to three types of intercalated cells.[42] There are functional relationships between intercalated cell mTORC1, H1-adenosine triphosphatase, and Wnt signaling pathways that may make TSC renal epithelium uniquely poised to proliferate and develop the appearance of, or actual, malignancy.

Clinical Aspects and Treatment of Tuberous Sclerosis Complex Renal Disease

CHRONIC KIDNEY DISEASE

Some 41% of patients with TSC have an estimated GFR of less than 60 mL/min/1.73 m² (chronic kidney disease [CKD] stage 3 or less) by their mid-50s compared with 3% of the general population.[12,13] However, this percentage may be much higher in those patients with a significant renal angiomyolipomata burden.[29] The risk of end-stage renal failure necessitating renal replacement therapy is reported to be 4% in one study of adults.[43] Patients with reduced renal function experience a high morbidity and mortality from premature cardiovascular disease,[44] with a significant rate of death before developing end-stage renal failure.

Acute kidney injury from renal hemorrhage, loss of normal renal parenchyma following embolization or surgery, hypertension, replacement of normal renal cells with angiomyolipomata or cysts and possibly haploinsufficiency causing mTOR overactivation resulting in premature loss of nephrocytes[45] are thought to contribute to premature loss of GFR. Although TSC patients without identifiable renal tissue on magnetic resonance imaging (MRI) can still have a normal GFR, they most commonly have less renal reserve because of multiple angiomyolipomata or cysts. In this patient group with reduced renal function, special care needs to be taken to prescribe and alter drug doses appropriately for GFR.

Preemptive angiomyolipomata embolization can reduce the risk and consequences of severe hemorrhage but may result in renal impairment. Impaired kidney function was identified in 29% of patients who had undergone embolization compared with 10% for those who had not, although these results may be confounded by the high burden of angiomyolipomata in those who subsequently needed embolization.[43] The use of mTORC1 inhibitors now as the first line of therapy may improve long-term outcome of renal function provided that the mTOR inhibitors do not have an adverse effect. Early work suggests that the use of mTORC1 inhibitors do not interfere with renal function.[46,47]

HYPERTENSION

Hypertension is more common in patients with renal TSC than in the general population.[14,29] We suggest hypertension should be aggressively treated in line with standard recommended targets: 140/80 mm Hg or lower for adults and appropriate age-adjusted targets for children.[48]

Initial guidelines discouraged concurrent use of angiotensin-converting enzyme (ACE) inhibitors in those TSC patients taking mTOR inhibitors because of a possible increase incidence of angioedema.[49] But ACE inhibitors and angiotensin 2 blockers are useful in this patient group. ACE inhibitors may exhibit suppression effects on angiomyolipomata cells[21] and cysts.[50] Angioedema has not been reported in the TSC population as a drug limiting problem; the literature currently advocates the concurrent use of ACE inhibitors and mTOR inhibitors with caution.[51]

NEPHROLITHIASIS

Nephrolithiasis is common in TSC patients because of their renal manifestations and side effects of some anticonvulsant therapies. Topiramate is an effective anticonvulsant for some forms of TSC-associated epilepsy. The drug enhances gamma aminobutyric acid–activated chloride channels and inhibits excitatory neurotransmission to reduce seizure activity. Topiramate also inhibits subtypes II and IV carbonic anhydrase, and thus reduces renal citrate excretion. This reduced citrate excretion increases the risk of nephrolithiasis. The ketogenic diet can also significantly improve seizure control for some patients with TSC, but is associated with hypercalciuria, hypocitraturia, and decreased uric acid solubility caused by the low urine pH. All these factors synergize to increase the nephrolithiasis risk of patients on this treatment.

Significant renal cystic disease can alter acid secretion, causing citrate reclamation and result in hypocitraturia. Identifying nephrolithiasis in a developmentally delayed patient can be challenging, but understanding the risk factors can help guide imaging and diagnosis. Medical therapy for nephrolithiasis in this patient population is relatively straightforward and includes adequate hydration and citrate supplementation when required.

ANGIOMYOLIPOMATA

A major complication of angiomyolipomata is life-threatening hemorrhage, historically reported to occur in 25% to 50% of patients,[52,53] which more recently has been found to average 30% in a larger population-based study of patients not having active surveillance.[54] Angiomyolipomata secrete vasoactive cytokines and can stimulate a robust blood supply.[55] The blood vessels formed enlarge with angiomyolipoma growth but are poorly supported by adventitia and develop aneurysms. Aneurysms larger than 5 mm are at high risk of rupturing.[18]

Patients with *TSC2* mutations seem to develop angiomyolipomata at a younger mean age compared with patients who have *TSC1* mutations (13 vs. 24 years), and more often need intervention (27% vs. 13%).[47] Female gender has been associated with an increased incidence of adverse outcomes from angiomyolipomata based on data from a case series[56] and because of the fact that two-thirds of subjects enrolled in the EXIST-2 (Everolimus for angiomyolipoma associated with tuberous sclerosis complex or lymphangioleiomyomatosis) study were women.[55] However, angiomyolipomata prevalence is not statistically different between males and females in the 2216 Tuberous Sclerosis Registry to Increase Awareness subjects;[47] a relationship between outcome and gender is under investigation in this cohort.

Historically there is an association between the angiomyolipoma size and hemorrhage, with those 30 mm in diameter and still enlarging at greatest risk of bleeding.[45] These data are the basis for the recommendation in the International Guidelines that angiomyolipomata that are 30 mm in diameter and enlarging should be treated preemptively to prevent hemorrhage using an mTORC1 inhibitor.[15]

A proactive monitoring program and preemptive embolization may reduce the high risk of bleeding; but there is still a significant renal morbidity and mortality. In the Eijkemans et al. series of 351 patients,[43] 117 underwent embolization of which 57 needed two or more embolization procedures. Sixteen of these patients required a nephrectomy, seven needed dialysis, and seven went on to transplantation. Of the 29 deaths in this series, nine were caused by renal causes.

With the advent of mTOR inhibitors replacing embolization as first choice for preemptive therapy, hemorrhage has been markedly reduced, being just 5% of 2216 subjects in one large study.[47] A series of phase 2 and phase 3 studies has shown that mTOR inhibitor therapy is highly effective at stabilizing or shrinking angiomyolipomata in both adults[55,57–59] and children[60] in the short term and in preventing bleeding and preserving renal function in the longer term.[46,61,62]

Angiomyolipomata are almost always benign lesions,[63] though non-TSC varieties can be aggressive.[26] Although angiomyolipomata can stop enlarging when the kidney loses its growth and repair potential in mid-adulthood, at least half continue to grow and need eventual intervention.[47] Angiomyolipomata most commonly affect the kidney, but can be found in the liver,[64] local lymphatics, or elsewhere in the abdomen.[65] It is not known if these represent local spread or if they arise in situ. Angiomyolipomata in patients with known TSC showing malignant behavior have been rarely reported,[66] and aggressive angiomyolipomata appear to be associated with mutations in the *MITF/FTE* genes, not the *TSC* genes.[67] The *MITF/FTE* genes have a significant link to malignancy.[68]

Current guidelines for surveillance and treatment of angiomyolipoma in people with TSC are straightforward. Monitoring growth of lesions using MRI, and an mTORC1 inhibitor is the recommended first line of therapy.[15] mTORC1 inhibitors are approved and effective therapy for TSC angiomyolipomata,[55,57] and patients are best followed periodically by TSC centers that follow the guidelines for surveillance and management.[15]

Recognizable Patterns of Tuberous Sclerosis Complex-Associated Renal Cystic Disease

TSC renal cystic disease is detected in approximately 50% of patients by conventional MRI, and it is associated with mutations in either the *TSC1* or *TSC2* genes.[32–34] The TSC renal cysts range in size from the glomerulocystic disease[35] to a polycystic renal phenotype associated with the *TSC2/PKD1* contiguous gene syndrome.[27] To better communicate about TSC renal cystic disease, five basic patterns of cystic disease have been described (Fig. 27.4).[36]

Tuberous Sclerosis Complex Polycystic Kidney Disease

This manifestation involves the contiguous deletion of a portion of the adjacent *TSC2* and *PKD1* genes on chromosome 16p13, and accounts for about 2% of TSC patients.[69] There are rare cases that appear identical to this contiguous gene syndrome that are linked to *TSC1*. Renal cysts in this form of TSC arise from all nephron segments.[35] There is a high frequency of mosaic cases of the polycystic variety,[70] and most have cystic disease in utero or shortly after birth, but quickly develop significant disease by 2 months of age. Hypertension usually develops in the first 2 weeks of life but can be delayed by several months. The hypertension is best

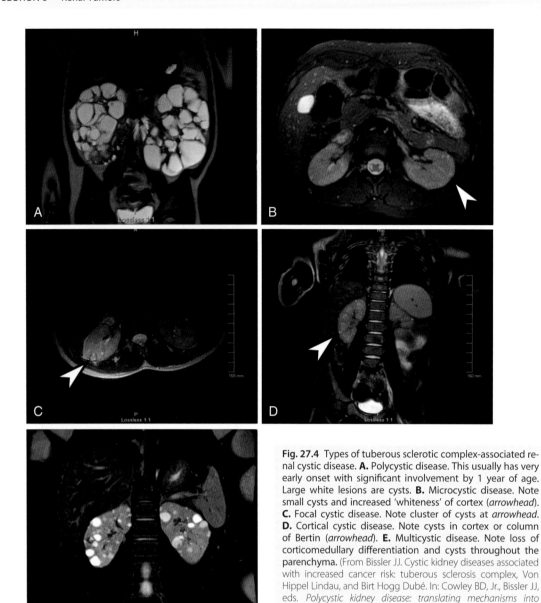

Fig. 27.4 Types of tuberous sclerotic complex-associated renal cystic disease. **A.** Polycystic disease. This usually has very early onset with significant involvement by 1 year of age. Large white lesions are cysts. **B.** Microcystic disease. Note small cysts and increased 'whiteness' of cortex (*arrowhead*). **C.** Focal cystic disease. Note cluster of cysts at *arrowhead*. **D.** Cortical cystic disease. Note cysts in cortex or column of Bertin (*arrowhead*). **E.** Multicystic disease. Note loss of corticomedullary differentiation and cysts throughout the parenchyma. (From Bissler JJ. Cystic kidney diseases associated with increased cancer risk: tuberous sclerosis complex, Von Hippel Lindau, and Birt Hogg Dubé. In: Cowley BD, Jr., Bissler JJ, eds. *Polycystic kidney disease: translating mechanisms into therapy.* New York: Springer; 2018: 51-66; and from Bissler JJ, Kingswood C. Renal manifestation of tuberous sclerosis complex. *Am J Med Genet.* 2018 [Epub ahead of print].)

treated with ACE inhibitors or angiotensin receptor blockers. Because of the renal parenchyma disruption, some of these children develop a urinary concentrating defect, and this may further drive cystogenesis by increasing antidiuretic hormone secretion.[37] There are also practical considerations. Because the kidney mass can be so large, balance can be affected, so the ambulation developmental milestone can be delayed.

Tuberous Sclerosis Complex Cortical Cystic Kidney Disease
Another recognizable pattern of TSC cystic renal disease is that which is limited to the cortex and columns of Bertin. This cystic disease occurs early on and the cysts are remarkably uniform in size, usually about 2 to 4 mm in diameter. This imaging pattern may suggest glomerulocystic

disease, or even dilatation of other tubular segments, and the usual number of cysts is most often less than two dozen.

Tuberous Sclerosis Complex Multicystic Kidney Disease
Cysts can also be distributed throughout the cortical and medullary tissue and exhibit variable sizes. This pattern is also associated with either *TSC1* or *TSC2* mutations and with significant CKD. It can also resemble the polycystic variety, but genetically is different than *TSC2/PKD1* contiguous gene syndrome.

Tuberous Sclerosis Complex Cortical Microcystic Kidney Disease
Cortical microcystic disease can be subtle and is detected by careful inspection of the abdominal MRI. The renal cortex

will exhibit an increased water signal before overt discrete cortical cysts develop. Eventually, the cortex may develop an increased echotexture similar to that which occurs in the medullary pyramids in patients with autosomal recessive polycystic renal disease. Identification of this disease pattern is important because affected patients have a more rapid decline in renal function and develop CKD stage 2 or 3 in their late teens or early 20s. The renal pyramids are spared and the urinary concentration capacity is preserved. Sometimes there is evidence of tubular proteinuria accompanying azotemia, but hypertension is not common until significant CKD develops.

Tuberous Sclerosis Complex Focal Cystic Kidney Disease

Focal cystic disease is thought to be the result of a somatic mutation that occurs during branching of the ureteric bud, such that there is significant cystogenesis in a localized renal pyramid. The developmental timing can be such that a small child can have an isolated renal pyramid with significant cystic disease, although the other pyramids are structurally normal. If the mutation occurs after a critical developmental period, phenotypic expression only will occur after acute kidney injury. Such a renal injury has been postulated to constitute a 'third hit' in autosomal dominant polycystic kidney disease that results in rapid cyst formation in adult research animals.[71] TSC focal cystic kidney disease also appears to follow this same temporal sequence. Risk factors for acute kidney injury in TSC patients include anticonvulsant and nonsteroidal antiinflammatory medications, and rhabdomyolysis and hypoxia induced by status epilepticus.[39]

Key Points

- Patients with TSC experience earlier onset of significant CKD.
- Renal cystic disease is very common and can be severe.
- There are distinct patterns of TSC renal cystic disease.
- There are accepted guidelines for surveillance and management.
- mTORC1 inhibitors are effective treatment for many aspects of TSC.

Key References

1. Crino PB, Nathanson KL, Henske EP. The tuberous sclerosis complex. *N Engl J Med.* 2006;355:1345-1356.
2. Yates JR. Tuberous sclerosis. *Eur J Hum Genet.* 2006;14:1065-1073.
3. Northrup H, Krueger DA, International Tuberous Sclerosis Complex Consensus Group. Tuberous sclerosis complex diagnostic criteria update: recommendations of the 2012 International Tuberous Sclerosis Complex Consensus Conference. *Pediatr Neurol.* 2013;49:243-254.
4. Curatolo P. *Tuberous sclerosis complex: from basic science to clinical phenotypes.* London, UK: Mac Keith Press; 2003.
5. European Chromosome 16 Tuberous Sclerosis Consortium. Identification and characterization of the tuberous sclerosis gene on chromosome 16. *Cell.* 1993;75:1305-1315.
6. Siroky BJ, Yin H, Bissler JJ. Clinical and molecular insights into tuberous sclerosis complex renal disease. *Pediatr Nephrol.* 2011;26:839-852.
8. Blaszak RT, Potaman V, Sinden RR, Bissler JJ. DNA structural transitions within the PKD1 gene. *Nucleic Acids Res.* 1999;27:2610-2617.

10. Dixon BP, Henry J, Siroky BJ, Chu A, Groen PA, Bissler JJ. Cell cycle control and DNA damage response of conditionally immortalized urothelial cells. *PLoS One.* 2011;6:e16595.
12. Kingswood C, Bolton P, Crawford P, et al. The clinical profile of tuberous sclerosis complex (TSC) in the United Kingdom: a retrospective cohort study in the Clinical Practice Research Datalink (CPRD). *Eur J Paediatr Neurol.* 2016;20:296-308.
13. Bissler JJ, Kingswood JC. Optimal treatment of tuberous sclerosis complex associated renal angiomyolipomata: a systematic review. *Ther Adv Urol.* 2016;8:279-290.
14. Janssens P, Van Hoeve K, De Waele L, et al. Renal progression factors in young patients with tuberous sclerosis complex: a retrospective cohort study. *Pediatr Nephrol.* 2018. doi:10.1007/s00467-018-4003-6. [Epub ahead of print].
15. Krueger DA, Northrup H, International Tuberous Sclerosis Complex Consensus Group. Tuberous sclerosis complex surveillance and management: recommendations of the 2012 International Tuberous Sclerosis Complex Consensus Conference. *Pediatr Neurol.* 2013;49:255-265.
17. Hornick JL, Fletcher CD. PEComa: what do we know so far? *Histopathology.* 2006;48:75-82.
18. Yamakado K, Tanaka N, Nakagawa T, Kobayashi S, Yanagawa M, Takeda K. Renal angiomyolipoma: relationships between tumor size, aneurysm formation, and rupture. *Radiology.* 2002;225:78-82.
19. Shepherd CW, Gomez MR, Lie JT, Crowson CS. Causes of death in patients with tuberous sclerosis. *Mayo Clin Proc.* 1991;66:792-796.
20. Beltramello A, Puppini G, Bricolo A, et al. Does the tuberous sclerosis complex include intracranial aneurysms? A case report with a review of the literature. *Pediatr Radiol.* 1999;29:206-211.
21. Siroky BJ, Yin H, Dixon BP, et al. Evidence for pericyte origin of TSC-associated renal angiomyolipomas and implications for angiotensin receptor inhibition therapy. *Am J Physiol Renal Physiol.* 2014;307:F560-F570.
22. Yamamoto S, Nakamura K, Kawanami S, Aoki T, Watanabe H, Nakata H. Renal angiomyolipoma: evolutional changes of its internal structure on CT. *Abdom Imaging.* 2000;25:651-654.
23. Henske EP. Metastasis of benign tumor cells in tuberous sclerosis complex. *Genes Chromosomes Cancer.* 2003;38:376-381.
24. Karbowniczek M, Astrinidis A, Balsara BR, et al. Recurrent lymphangiomyomatosis after transplantation: genetic analyses reveal a metastatic mechanism. *Am J Respir Crit Care Med.* 2003;167:976-982.
26. Argani P, Aulmann S, Illei PB, et al. A distinctive subset of PEComas harbors TFE3 gene fusions. *Am J Surg Pathol.* 2010;34:1395-1406.
28. Patel U, Simpson E, Kingswood JC, Saggar-Malik AK. Tuberose sclerosis complex: analysis of growth rates aids differentiation of renal cell carcinoma from atypical or minimal-fat-containing angiomyolipoma. *Clin Radiol.* 2005;60:665-673, discussion 663-664.
29. Kingswood JC, Nasuti P, Patel K, Myland M, Siva V, Gray E. The economic burden of tuberous sclerosis complex in UK patients with renal manifestations: a retrospective cohort study in the clinical practice research datalink (CPRD). *J Med Econ.* 2016;1-11.
34. Pema M, Drusian L, Chiaravalli M, et al. mTORC1-mediated inhibition of polycystin-1 expression drives renal cyst formation in tuberous sclerosis complex. *Nat Commun.* 2016;7:10786.
35. Weinblatt ME, Kahn E, Kochen J. Renal cell carcinoma in patients with tuberous sclerosis. *Pediatrics.* 1987;80:898-903.
36. Guo J, Tretiakova MS, Troxell ML, et al. Tuberous sclerosis-associated renal cell carcinoma: a clinicopathologic study of 57 separate carcinomas in 18 patients. *Am J Surg Pathol.* 2014;38:1457-1467.
37. Srigley JR, Delahunt B, Eble JN, et al. The International Society of Urological Pathology (ISUP) Vancouver classification of renal neoplasia. *Am J Surg Pathol.* 2013;37:1469-1489.
38. Schreiner A, Daneshmand S, Bayne A, Countryman G, Corless CL, Troxell ML. Distinctive morphology of renal cell carcinomas in tuberous sclerosis. *Int J Surg Pathol.* 2010;18:409-418.
40. Argani P, Ladanyi M. Translocation carcinomas of the kidney. *Clin Lab Med.* 2005;25:363-378.
43. Eijkemans MJ, van der Wal W, Reijnders LJ, et al. Long-term follow-up assessing renal angiomyolipoma treatment patterns, morbidity, and mortality: an observational study in tuberous sclerosis complex patients in the Netherlands. *Am J Kidney Dis.* 2015;66:638-645.
45. Kingswood JC, Bissler JJ, Budde K, et al. Review of the tuberous sclerosis renal guidelines from the 2012 Consensus Conference: current data and future study. *Nephron.* 2016;134(2):51-58.
46. Bissler JJ, Budde K, Sauter M, et al. Effect of everolimus on renal function in patients with tuberous sclerosis complex: evidence from

EXIST-1 and EXIST-2. *Nephrol Dial Transplant.* 2018. doi:10.1093/ndt/gfy132. [Epub ahead of print].

49. Duerr M, Glander P, Diekmann F, Dragun D, Neumayer HH, Budde K. Increased incidence of angioedema with ACE inhibitors in combination with mTOR inhibitors in kidney transplant recipients. *Clin J Am Soc Nephrol.* 2010;5:703-708.

51. Davies M, Saxena A, Kingswood JC. Management of everolimus-associated adverse events in patients with tuberous sclerosis complex: a practical guide. *Orphanet J Rare Dis.* 2017;12:35.

52. Kessler OJ, Gillon G, Neuman M, Engelstein D, Winkler H, Baniel J. Management of renal angiomyolipoma: analysis of 15 cases. *Eur Urol.* 1998;33:572-575.

53. Mouded IM, Tolia BM, Bernie JE, Newman HR. Symptomatic renal angiomyolipoma: report of 8 cases, 2 with spontaneous rupture. *J Urol.* 1978;119:684-688.

54. Kingswood JC, Nasuti P, Patel K, Myland M, Siva V, Gray E. The economic burden of tuberous sclerosis complex in UK patients with renal manifestations: a retrospective cohort study in the clinical practice research datalink (CPRD). *J Med Econ.* 2016;19:1-11.

55. Bissler JJ, Kingswood JC, Radzikowska E, et al. Everolimus for angiomyolipoma associated with tuberous sclerosis complex or sporadic lymphangioleiomyomatosis (EXIST-2): a multicentre, randomised, double-blind, placebo-controlled trial. *Lancet.* 2013;381:817-824.

56. Rakowski SK, Winterkorn EB, Paul E, Steele DJ, Halpern EF, Thiele EA. Renal manifestations of tuberous sclerosis complex: incidence, prognosis, and predictive factors. *Kidney Int.* 2006;70:1777-1782.

57. Bissler JJ, McCormack FX, Young LR, et al. Sirolimus for angiomyolipoma in tuberous sclerosis complex or lymphangioleiomyomatosis. *N Engl J Med.* 2008;358:140-151.

59. Davies DM, de Vries PJ, Johnson SR, et al. Sirolimus therapy for angiomyolipoma in tuberous sclerosis and sporadic lymphangioleiomyomatosis: a phase 2 trial. *Clin Cancer Res.* 2011;17:4071-4081.

60. Kingswood JC, Jozwiak S, Belousova ED, et al. The effect of everolimus on renal angiomyolipoma in patients with tuberous sclerosis complex being treated for subependymal giant cell astrocytoma: subgroup results from the randomized, placebo-controlled, Phase 3 trial EXIST-1. *Nephrol Dial Transplant.* 2014;29:1203-1210.

61. Bissler JJ, Franz DN, Frost MD, et al. The effect of everolimus on renal angiomyolipoma in pediatric patients with tuberous sclerosis being treated for subependymal giant cell astrocytoma. *Pediatr Nephrol.* 2018;33:101-109.

63. Bissler JJ, Kingswood JC. Renal angiomyolipomata. *Kidney Int.* 2004;66:924-934.

64. Jóźwiak S, Sadowski K, Borkowska J, et al. Liver angiomyolipomas in tuberous sclerosis complex-their incidence and course. *Pediatr Neurol.* 2018;78:20-26.

65. Göğüş C, Safak M, Erekul S, Kiliç O, Türkölmez K. Angiomyolipoma of the kidney with lymph node involvement in a 17-year old female mimicking renal cell carcinoma: a case report. *Int Urol Nephrol.* 2001;33:617-618.

66. Al-Saleem T, Wessner LL, Scheithauer BW, et al. Malignant tumors of the kidney, brain, and soft tissues in children and young adults with the tuberous sclerosis complex. *Cancer.* 1998;83:2208-2216.

67. Martignoni G, Pea M, Zampini C, et al. PEComas of the kidney and of the genitourinary tract. *Semin Diagn Pathol.* 2015;32:140-159.

69. Hirokawa M, Miyauchi A, Kihara M, et al. Chromophobe renal cell carcinoma-like thyroid carcinoma: a novel clinicopathologic entity possibly associated with tuberous sclerosis complex. *Endocr J.* 2017;64:843-850.

70. Williamson SR, Hornick JL, Eble JN, et al. Renal cell carcinoma with angioleiomyoma-like stroma and clear cell papillary renal cell carcinoma: exploring SDHB protein immunohistochemistry and the relationship to tuberous sclerosis complex. *Hum Pathol.* 2018;75:10-15.

A full list of references is available at Expertconsult.com

28 *Evaluation of a Renal Cyst/Mass*

PHILLIP M. PIERORAZIO, ANTHONY CHANG, AND SUSIE L. HU

Introduction

EPIDEMIOLOGY AND RISK FACTORS

Renal cell carcinoma (RCC) is the eighth most common malignancy in the world. According to the National Cancer Institute, in 2017 approximately 64,000 diagnoses were made in the United States and more than 330,000 worldwide. The incidence of RCC has been steadily increasing in the United States, but this may be caused by incidental detection from imaging studies. In the 1980s, approximately 40% of renal neoplasms were stage 1 ($\leq$ 7 cm and confined to kidney), but now represent greater than 60% of RCC at presentation.[1,2] If the benign renal masses are included, an estimated 80,000 patients in the United States undergo renal mass evaluation on an annual basis.

Clear cell RCC (ccRCC) comprises greater than 75% of all RCC and papillary RCC is the next most common (predominantly seen in the end-stage renal disease [ESRD] population). The most common hereditary syndrome for RCC (specifically ccRCC) is the von Hippel-Lindau (VHL) disease, which accounts for a small proportion (2%–3%) of patients with RCC. Although only 1.6% of patients with ccRCC have VHL disease, the majority of those with VHL disease will develop ccRCC.[3] The molecular biology and pathogenesis involves loss of VHL tumor suppressor function and persistent hypoxia-inducible factor activity, leading to apparent tissue "hypoxia" and resulting in activation of tumor pathways and promoting tumor growth. This gene mutation is also the most prevalent gene mutation (40%–80%) found in the general (including the sporadic) RCC population.[4,5]

The incidence of RCC is greatest in the sixth to seventh decade with higher risk of RCC among men (1.6:1 male:female ratio) and those of African descent. Potentially modifiable risk factors include tobacco use, obesity, hypertension (HTN), diabetes mellitus (DM), cystic disease, and ESRD.[6–8] Paradoxically, obese patients with RCC have lower mortality. In addition, unlike tobacco exposure, alcohol use is associated with lower risk of RCC, even though it is linked to other cancers.[9,10] Chronic kidney disease (stages 3–4 CKD and ESRD) also appears to increase risk for RCC to some degree and, reciprocally, RCC is associated with increased risk of CKD decline.[8,11] Those with small renal masses and CKD share the same risk factors (tobacco use, obesity, DM, and HTN) partially caused by the high burden of comorbid diseases and may explain this bidirectional relationship.[12]

CHRONIC KIDNEY DISEASE AND RENAL CELL CARCINOMA RISK

RCC risk among CKD patients is high. For the dialysis-dependent ESRD population, the risk of RCC escalates to 100-fold greater than the general population[8] and incidence of RCC among ESRD patients range 1% to 7%.[8,13–16] RCC risk rises with longer duration of dialysis, potentially from dialysis-related inflammatory processes and the link to acquired cystic kidney disease (ACKD).[17] Incidence of ACKD is particularly high among ESRD patients[18] and when progression to RCC occurs, the histologic subtype of papillary RCC is more prominent than in the general population.[19] One Japanese cohort examining the relationship between histologic subtype and dialysis duration found that those with dialysis duration less than 10 years were more likely to have ccRCC, and those on dialysis for longer than 10 years had ACKD-associated RCC (more papillary RCC).[17] The proportion of ESRD patients (22%–37%) with papillary RCC is 4 to 5 times greater than that of the general population (5%–7%).[20,21] Incidence of ccRCC and papillary RCC varies according to population and confers some degree of prognosis, as shown in Table 28.1.[6,22]

Among pre-ESRD CKD patients, risk of RCC is also high and appears to increase with worsening estimated glomerular filtration rate (eGFR). When a cohort of 1 million cancer-free subjects were stratified by CKD stage, RCC risk was 39%, 81% greater for stage 3a and 3b CKD, respectively, than the reference group, then approached twofold greater for those with stage 4 CKD.[11] The potential relationship between RCC and kidney function was further explored among 202,195 transplant recipients. Incidence of RCC rose during periods of graft failure and fell during periods of kidney function.[23] Furthermore, early signs of kidney dysfunction, such as albuminuria, have also been associated with RCC, further supporting the relationship of kidney pathology with RCC.[24]

Despite the adverse relationship between CKD and RCC risk, prognosis of RCC among those with ESRD appears to be better than in the general population,[20,21,25–27] with a 5-year cancer-specific survival of 90.1% for the ESRD population and 69% for the general population.[21] The lower mortality among those with ESRD may be explained by more favorable demographic and tumor characteristics and potentially earlier diagnosis.[20,21,26] A French cohort of ESRD patients was more functional and was diagnosed with RCC at a younger age (fifth vs. sixth decade) than in the general population. Detection appears to be earlier and asymptomatic potentially because of higher frequency of

Table 28.1 Clinical Characteristics of Renal Cell Carcinoma Subtype

Subtype	Incidence (%)	Prognosis	Population
Clear cell carcinoma	70–80	Fair	General
Papillary carcinoma	10–20	Favorable	ESRD, acquired cystic kidney disease
Chromophobe	5	Favorable	

ESRD, End-stage renal disease.

imaging among ESRD patients. The ESRD group had smaller tumor size, lower stage, lower grade, and was less likely to have nodal invasion or metastases. Furthermore, the predominant tumor subtype of papillary RCC tends to have a milder clinical course.[21]

CYSTIC DISEASE

The close association of RCC and ESRD has often been explained by the predominance of ACKD among ESRD patients, with an annual incidence among dialysis patients (0.15%–0.34%) of up to 40 times that of the general population (0.008%).[18] In ESRD, ACKD prevalence ranges 10% to 44% soon after dialysis initiation but exceeds 90% as dialysis vintage reaches 5 to 10 years. In addition to long dialysis duration, male sex and younger age appear to be associated with ACKD. ESRD and male sex are risk factors common to RCC.[28] ACKD is also reported in pre-ESRD CKD (7%–22%) and transplant (23%) populations. Although ACKD prevalence for these groups also far exceeds that of the general population, ACKD remains less common among these groups compared with dialysis patients.[15,19,28,29]

Cysts appear to accumulate because of chronic hypoxia and acid-base dysregulation and possibly in response to growth factors.[13,28,30] The acquired cysts open into the tubules and retain functional capacity to some degree, which is suggested by higher cyst fluid creatinine concentration than serum content and the regression of these cysts after renal transplantation.[28,31]

The cystic lesions of ACKD are thought to be precursors of RCC that progress in the setting of prolonged lack of kidney function.[13] The cystic lesions share common pathologic characteristics with RCC. The most prominent subtype of RCC among ESRD patients is papillary RCC, not the clear cell carcinoma usually seen in the general population. The RCC associated with ESRD has similar immunohistochemical patterns as with ACKD.[19,32]

Cystic diseases other than ACKD have not been closely associated with RCC. The incidence of RCC in polycystic kidney disease is no different from that of the general population.[33–37]

SCREENING FOR RENAL CELL CARCINOMA

Even with the higher incidence of RCC among ESRD patients, routine screening for RCC is not recommended. Decision analysis performed of ACKD screening did not demonstrate a clear benefit to survival in the ESRD population. However, young individuals who are healthy with longer expected lifespan are suggested to be reasonable candidates for screening.[38,39] Debate continues regarding screening among potential transplant recipients who have an equally high rate of RCC as the ESRD population (3.5%).[8,40–42] However, transplant recipients diagnosed with RCC have good prognosis with tumor detection at a younger age, earlier stage, smaller tumor size, and favorable RCC subtype of papillary RCC.[43] Presence of RCC does not adversely affect graft survival.[40] Ten-year cancer-specific survival (~90%) in transplant recipients is higher than for both the general (75%) and ESRD populations (77%).[43,44]

Presentation

Renal cancers present as either solid renal masses or complex cystic renal masses (see Diagnosis later). The majority of renal masses and cancers are diagnosed incidentally and present without overt signs or symptoms. This reflects both the changing epidemiology of renal cancers—in which small, clinically localized renal masses now represent at least 50% of incident tumors—and the widespread use of axial imaging.[1,45] The "classic triad" of symptoms associated with a malignant renal mass include hematuria, flank pain, and abdominal mass. Symptoms associated with RCC are often a result of local tumor growth, hemorrhage, paraneoplastic symptoms, or metastatic disease, and are uncommon in patients with clinically localized disease. In fact, less than 10% of patients in contemporary series present with these symptoms and greater than 50% of renal masses are diagnosed incidentally.[46,47]

Diagnosis

PHYSICAL EXAMINATION

Physical examination has a limited role in the diagnosis of clinically localized disease and is most useful in distinguishing the signs and symptoms of advanced disease. For many years, RCC was known as the *internists' tumor*, reflecting the variety of systemic symptoms and more common presentation at advanced stage. For instance, paraneoplastic syndromes (i.e., hypertension, polycythemia, hypercalcemia, abnormal liver function) are present in approximately 10% to 20% of patients with metastatic RCC.[48,49] In the contemporary era where most patients are diagnosed with clinically localized, early stage disease, physical examination may reveal medical conditions that influence management decisions, including body habitus, prior abdominal scars, stigmata of CKD, and so on.

LABORATORY EVALUATION

There are no biomarkers or routine laboratory tests used to routinely diagnose renal malignancies. As such, laboratory tests are useful in assessment of renal function (glomerular filtration rate) and metastatic evaluation. Routine laboratory tests for renal mass evaluation include complete blood count, basic or complete metabolic panel, and urinalysis.[50] Serum creatinine and urinalysis for protein are recommended before any intervention and, if abnormal, used to classify CKD stage.

IMAGING TECHNIQUES

Contrast-enhanced axial imaging, either computed tomography (CT) or magnetic resonance imaging (MRI), is the ideal imaging technique for the diagnosis and staging of clinically localized renal masses. Masses initially diagnosed by ultrasound or intravenous pyelography should be confirmed with contrast-enhanced imaging. Contrast-enhanced abdominal imaging (CT or MRI) best characterizes the mass, provides information regarding renal morphology (of the affected and unaffected kidney), assesses extrarenal tumor spread (venous invasion or regional lymphadenopathy), and evaluates the adrenal glands and other abdominal organs for visceral metastases.[50] Enhancement of greater than 15 to 20 Houndsfield units on CT or 20% enhancement on MRI is indicative of RCC, but does not preclude benign tumors.[51,52]

Imaging readily distinguishes solid from cystic renal masses. Solid masses are more often presumed malignant whereas cystic renal masses are characterized as simple or complex based on the Bosniak Classification system. The Bosniak system was developed using CT criteria that segregate cystic lesions into categories that define the likelihood of malignancy.[53,54] Bosniak 1 lesions are simple cysts: thin-walled fluid-filled structures with zero risk of malignancy that do not require follow-up. Bosniak 2 lesions are minimally complex with a minimal risk (< 3%) of malignancy. These include nonenhancing septated cysts, cysts with calcifications, infected cysts, and hyperdense cysts. Bosniak 2F cysts include cysts with "perceived" enhancement and hyperdense lesions greater than 3 cm. These cysts have a 3% to 10% risk of malignancy and 15% risk of radiographic progression to a more complex cyst. Complex cystic renal masses that have thickened irregular walls or septa on enhancement are classified as Bosniak 3. Approximately 50% of such lesions prove to be malignant on final pathology. Bosniak 4 complex cystic lesions are very suspicious for malignancy because they contain enhancing nodular soft tissue components and about 75% to 90% of such lesions prove to be RCC on final pathology. Of note, the majority of cystic renal masses are low-grade cystic RCC and behave in an indolent fashion.

Patients with CKD should receive contrast with caution as iodinated contrast agents can transiently or permanently affect GFR (contrast induced nephropathy)[55] and gadolinium-based MRI contrast agents can lead to nephrogenic systemic fibrosis—a devastating and potentially fatal condition.[56] Noncontrast CT or MRI and ultrasound can be used to best characterize renal masses in patients who cannot receive intravenous contrast. Contrast-enhanced ultrasonography (CEUS) uses microbubbles in lieu of contrast agents and early data are promising for the characterization and assessment of enhancement of renal masses. CEUS may play an important role in patients with CKD or those patients who cannot receive typical contrast agents in the future.[57]

In patients with RCC or suspicion of RCC, complete staging is finalized with chest radiography (x-ray). Chest CT scan should be obtained selectively, primarily for patients with pulmonary symptoms or an abnormal chest x-ray.[58,59] Bone scans and brain imaging should be reserved primarily for patients with bone pain, elevated alkaline phosphatase, or neurologic symptoms, respectively.[60–62] Positron emission tomography scan has no role in the routine evaluation or staging of RCC.

CLINICAL DIAGNOSIS AND RISK STRATIFICATION OF RENAL MASSES

Depending on tumor size, 20% to 30% of clinically localized renal masses may be benign.[63,64] As stated earlier, solid renal masses and complex cystic lesions (Bosniak 3 and 4) are considered malignant at diagnosis. However, patient and tumor characteristics can indicate populations more or less likely to harbor benign or malignant disease. For instance, women with smaller tumors have a higher likelihood of having benign tumors.[65–67] However, with the exception of fat-containing angiomyolipoma, none of the current imaging modalities or laboratory tests can reliably distinguish between benign and malignant solid tumors, or between indolent and aggressive tumor biology. A number of predictive clinical models exist for the prediction of RCC; however, these models perform with modest concordance indices of 0.55 to 0.65.[65,68–70] The best predictors of malignancy are male sex and increasing tumor size, where men have a nearly threefold increased risk of malignancy (effect size 2.71, 95% confidence interval [CI], 2.39–3.02) compared with women and likelihood of malignancy increases per cm of tumor diameter (effect size 1.3 per cm increase in diameter, 95% CI, 1.22–1.43).[71]

RENAL MASS BIOPSY

Renal mass biopsy (RMB) currently has an adjunctive role in the diagnosis and risk stratification of patients with renal masses suspicious for RCC and is therefore recommended to be used in a utility-based approach.[50] RMB, or fine needle aspiration (FNA), traditionally was reserved for patients suspected of having metastasis of another primary to the kidney, abscess, or lymphoma, or when needed to establish a pathologic diagnosis of RCC in occasional patients presenting with disseminated metastases or unresectable primary tumors.

The role of RMB for clinically localized RCC has evolved considerably over the past few decades with an increasing use and considerable variance in practice patterns.[72] RMB is demonstrated to be a safe procedure with low rates of hematoma (4.9%), hemorrhage requiring transfusion (0.4%), and no reports of tumor seeding with contemporary techniques.[73] A biopsy indicating RCC is highly reliable with a specificity of 96% and positive predictive value of 99.8%. A significant nondiagnostic rate (14%), negative predictive value (67%), and poor ability to discriminate high-grade cancers (60%–80%) limit the widespread utility in patients in whom a histologic diagnosis would not change management.[50,73] Core biopsy is preferred to FNA, given lower diagnostic yield with the latter; however, the American Society of

Cytopathology endorses rapid on-site evaluation, which can optimize specimen quality for pathologic evaluation by obtaining real-time assessment of FNA or touch imprints of core biopsies to confirm specimen adequacy.[74]

Pathologic Considerations

For the pathologic evaluation of renal mass resection specimens, the College of American Pathologists requires that the following 14 parameters are always reported for RCC (Fig. 28.1): procedure type; laterality; tumor size; tumor focality (single vs. multiple); macroscopic extent of tumor; histologic type and grade; presence/absence of sarcomatoid features; presence/absence of rhabdoid features; tumor necrosis; microscopic tumor extension; margin status; pathologic stage; and nonneoplastic parenchyma. Historically, the evaluation has centered around the RCC, and evaluation of the nonneoplastic parenchyma was optional before 2010 and largely ignored. The importance of nonneoplastic renal diseases and its association with RCC has only been recently recognized. Several studies have observed that nonneoplastic renal diseases, such as diabetic nephropathy (Fig. 28.2) and focal segmental glomerulosclerosis, can be identified in 10% to 15% of specimens.[75–80]

Given that preservation of renal function has become an important objective for low-stage RCC, early detection of a nonneoplastic renal disease, such as diabetic nephropathy, provides an opportunity for medical intervention that can delay the progression of CKD and ESRD. There are many opportunities for improved coordinated care of the kidney cancer patients between urologists, oncologists, nephrologists, and pathologists.

Approximately 25% of renal masses may be benign (e.g., angiomyolipoma, oncocytoma) and synoptic reporting is typically not used for benign neoplasms. In such instances, the proper evaluation of the nonneoplastic parenchyma would be the most important aspect of the pathologic evaluation.

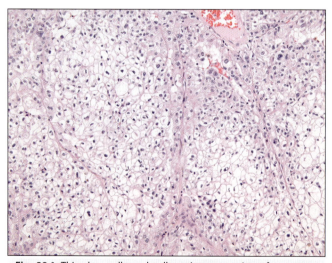

Fig. 28.1 This clear cell renal cell carcinoma consists of numerous neoplastic cells with clear cytoplasm (hematoxylin and eosin).

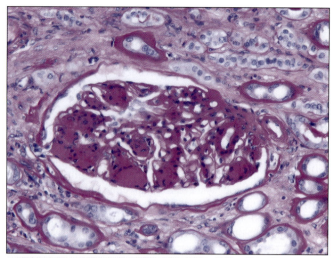

Fig. 28.2 The renal parenchyma, adjacent to and compressed by renal cell carcinoma, also reveals diabetic nephropathy with features of diffuse and frequently nodular mesangial sclerosis (periodic acid-Schiff).

Renal Cell Carcinoma Treatment

PREOPERATIVE MANAGEMENT

Consideration of kidney function given the higher risk of CKD should be made for most patients requiring treatment of RCC with surgical or ablative therapies. Among those with localized RCC, particularly for those with small renal masses (≤ 4 cm), cancer-specific survival approaches nearly 100%; therefore, complications related to CKD and related comorbidities, such as cardiovascular mortality, are more likely to determine morbidity and mortality.

Baseline evaluation of kidney function with measurement of serum creatinine and estimation of GFR will allow for better understanding of the underlying risks of CKD with nephrectomy. A specific creatinine or eGFR threshold for increased postoperative CKD risk has not been clearly defined; however, Lane et al. demonstrated that among those with known CKD (eGFR < 60 mL/min/1.73 m²), postoperative rapid decline (> 50% decline in eGFR or dialysis) in kidney function was 2.33 times more likely than those without CKD. Probability of rapid kidney function decline rose with each increasing CKD stage.[81] A creatinine threshold of greater than 1.5 mg/dL has been associated with higher morbidity and mortality in general, including higher mean postoperative creatinine and risk of dialysis dependence.[82,83] Urinalysis including presence of proteinuria (as measured as albuminuria by urine dipstick analysis, urine albumin to creatinine ratio, or urine protein to creatinine ratio) will identify those with early signs of renal parenchymal damage. Proper blood pressure management and glycemic control before surgery are strategies to reduce risk of eGFR decline. Review and avoidance of nephrotoxic medications, intravenous contrast, and intraoperative hypotension may further lower acute kidney injury (AKI) risk.[84] Nuclear scintigraphy measuring differential kidney function provides some insight to potential postoperative outcomes. These studies tend to underestimate GFR, because they do not account for the usual hypertrophy and hyperfiltration that occurs after nephron mass loss.[85] Surgical factors including larger tumor size ($R^2 = 0.39$) and increased clamp time ($R^2 = 0.17$) were most determinant of the postoperative proportional eGFR decline.[86]

TREATMENT OF SMALL RENAL MASSES

American Urological Association Guidelines and Principles of Management

The American Urological Association (AUA) released updated Guidelines for Renal Mass and Localized Renal Cancer in 2017. The AUA recommends that a urologist lead the counseling process for patients with renal masses and should include nephrologists, pathologists, interventional radiologists, medical oncologists, and genetic counselors when appropriate.[50] This recommendation is based on the familiarity of urologists with the disease process, risk-stratification paradigms (mentioned earlier), surgical management of the disease, the ability to engage other specialists, and to coordinate multidisciplinary care and follow-up.

The data supporting the AUA guidelines were systematically reviewed by the Agency for Healthcare Research and Quality, which made a number of important conclusions regarding the principles of management of renal masses suspicious for RCC.[87] The four, well-recognized management strategies for renal masses suspicious of clinically localized RCC include partial nephrectomy (PN), radical nephrectomy (RN), thermal ablation (TA), and active surveillance (AS). The first principle of management is that oncologic outcomes (cancer-specific and metastasis-free survival) are determined by tumor size and stage regardless of management strategy used. Second, overall survival outcomes are determined by competing risks of death, because most patients with clinically localized RCC die of other causes. Therefore distinguishing features of management strategies include influence on renal functional outcomes, perioperative outcomes, and potential harms, and are discussed later.

Partial Nephrectomy

PN is the preferred management strategy for small renal masses (stage T1a, ≤ 4.0 cm) whenever feasible and is a reasonable option for larger tumors with risk factors for progressive CKD or ESRD.[50] PN is preferred given long-term data demonstrating equivalent oncologic outcomes to RN and a greater appreciation for the deleterious effects of CKD. Surgical principles of PN include preservation of normal renal parenchyma and minimization of prolonged warm ischemia. PN is associated with the highest risk of perioperative complications, including bleeding, urine leak, and other urologic complications (i.e., ureteral injury).[87]

Radical Nephrectomy

RN is recommended if a tumor indicates increased oncologic potential (larger tumor size, infiltrative growth pattern, aggressive histology on RMB, etc.), if PN would be challenging in expert hands, if there is no preexisting CKD, and if the risk of new eGFR less than 45 mL/min/1.73 m² is sufficiently low.[50] RN is associated with low perioperative risks given the high proportion of surgeries performed laparoscopically.[87] RN is associated with the greatest decrease in eGFR (average decrease 10.5 mL/min/1.73 m²) and new onset CKD stage 3 or worse (relative risk, 2.56; 95% CI, 1.97–3.32) compared with all other management strategies.[88]

Of note, the European Organization for Research and Treatment of Cancer (EORTC) 30904 trial randomized 541 patients with 5 cm (or smaller) renal tumors to PN or RN. The trial demonstrated no difference in oncologic outcomes among surgeries and a small but significant worse renal function in patients undergoing RN.[89,90] This trial is discussed in greater detail in the subsequent section, **Renal Cell Carcinoma Treatment Modality and Chronic Kidney Disease Risk**; however, the trial is criticized because most patients were healthy with a normal contralateral kidney and unlikely to see the renal functional detriments of RN in the allotted follow-up.

Thermal Ablation

TA is most commonly achieved through radiofrequency or cryoablation and is considered an established alternative to PN for nephron-sparing surgery.[50] TA has the most favorable perioperative outcome profile (low risk of urologic and nonurologic complications) given the high proportion of patients undergoing percutaneous approaches.[87] TA is associated with the highest rates of local recurrence or persistence after a single treatment; this difference is alleviated when multiple treatment episodes are allowed for TA.[50,87] TA is preferred for peripheral, exophytic masses 3 cm or smaller given decreased oncologic efficacy and higher complication rates for larger, central tumors.[91–93]

Active Surveillance

AS is supported as an initial management strategy for patients with small renal masses (cT1a, ≤ 4 cm), especially those less than 2 cm.[50] This endorsement is based on an improved understanding of the high rate of benign disease, low malignant potential of RCC, slow growth rates, and low rates of metastatic progression while on AS.[63,64,94–97] A large body of retrospective data and growing prospective data indicate growth rates on the order of 1 mm per year and exceedingly low rates of metastatic progression.[95–97] Principles of AS include serial imaging (typically every 6–12 months) to establish growth parameters and facilitate timely intervention to preserve oncologic outcomes and nephron-sparing treatment options. Historically, a growth rate of more than 0.5 cm per year was believed to be indicative of adverse biology;[98] however, more recent data indicate that growth rate may be highly variable and does not reliably predict adverse pathologic features or death from RCC.[97]

CHRONIC KIDNEY DISEASE RISK FACTORS IN RENAL CELL CARCINOMA

Baseline Chronic Kidney Disease Risk in Renal Cell Carcinoma Population

Older age, tobacco exposure, obesity, DM, and HTN are overlapping risk factors for RCC and CKD, which may explain the high prevalence of CKD with RCC (10%–30%) generally,[99–101] and increases to a range of 10% to 52%

among those with small renal masses when compared with controls without cancer.[102–105] Among the most frequent causes of CKD, DM (9%–22%) and HTN (23%–59%) are also commonly seen with RCC.[101,102,104,106,107] DM and HTN in an RCC cohort were double that seen in a case-matched non-RCC control group.[108] Furthermore, when those with RCC were categorized by age, older subgroups had twofold greater CKD than the younger group and those with CKD were more likely to have DM and HTN than those with RCC who did not have CKD.[100,103] The older age and high comorbidity burden predispose the RCC population to kidney function decline after nephron mass loss because of tumor resection.

Postoperative Chronic Kidney Disease Risk

Localized tumors treated with nephrectomy or ablative therapies decrease functional nephron units and therefore can lower GFR, particularly for those with CKD or CKD risk factors who inadequately hypertrophy or lack the capacity for compensatory hyperfiltration. Postnephrectomy CKD risk is dependent on medical factors including preexisting CKD, nutritional factors (hypoalbuminemia), and underlying comorbid diseases (HTN, DM, and obesity).[109–111] For example, those with DM had 20% greater postoperative CKD than the nondiabetic RCC cohort, and only 47% of the diabetic group remained free from CKD after 2 years compared with 76% of their nondiabetic counterpart.[104] Just as importantly, surgical determinants, such as tumor size, warm ischemia time, hypotension, and AKI also influence CKD risk.[103,104,108,112–114] Nephron mass loss from surgical resection results in nearly doubling of CKD prevalence from 10% to 24% to 16% to 52% in observational cohort studies.[102–104] GFR decline after resection was estimated to be 13 mL/min/m^2 (30% reduction) with a corresponding reduction of kidney size of 36% in one RCC cohort undergoing PN.[114]

The United States Renal Data System lists RCC as a cause of ESRD for 0.5% of 360,000 dialysis patients.[110] ESRD incidence rate over 10 years among 2940 RCC patients (4.05%) was 5.6-fold that of a comparative control group (23,520 patients) without RCC (0.68%) in an incident Taiwanese cohort.[108]

RENAL CELL CARCINOMA TREATMENT MODALITY AND CHRONIC KIDNEY DISEASE RISK

RCC treatment can result in eGFR reduction and CKD as discussed previously. For generations, RN has been the primary mode of RCC treatment regardless of tumor size. However, with the recognition that cancer-specific survival approaches 100% among those with small renal masses,[90] less aggressive resection with PN is increasingly performed. PN should be considered standard therapy for T1a tumors according to the AUA guidelines.[50] RN continues to be performed for more advanced stage and surgically complicated tumors.

Preservation of renal parenchyma to minimize loss of kidney function is increasingly being prioritized for small renal masses given the equivalent oncologic outcomes, and comparable overall survival, which may likely be determined by nononcologic factors, such as CKD complications or cardiovascular disease. A systematic review

and metaanalysis of 40,000 patients with localized RCC had 61% lower risk for CKD (hazard ration [HR], 0.39; CI, 0.33–0.47) with PN as compared with RN. All-cause mortality (HR, 0.81; CI, 0.76–0.87) and cancer-specific mortality (HR, 0.71; CI, 0.59–0.85) were also lower for the PN group.[115] Comparable findings were observed in another metaanalysis, with a 2.56-fold greater risk of stage 3 CKD for RN than PN. Pooled eGFR decline was found to be 10.5 mL/min/1.73 m^2 lower for those undergoing PN versus RN. Risk of AKI, however, was no different between the two surgical procedures. However, of those with localized tumors, the subgroup with T1a tumors had slightly higher AKI risk (HR, 1.37; CI, 1.13–1.66) with RN. Nonsurgical nephron-sparing therapies (TA and AS) were additionally considered, revealing similar benefit over RN for preservation of kidney function. However, only two AS studies were included for analysis (one study population with age > 75 years), which may limit the interpretation of these findings. No clear differences were seen between treatment with either TA or PN.[88]

ESRD risk has been found to be similarly higher with RN according to a large systematic review and metaanalysis.[88] ESRD outcomes have also varied according to time period of treatment in a Canadian cohort of 11,937 patients using a multivariable proportional hazards model. During the earlier epoch (1995–2010), ESRD risk was not different between PN and RN groups; however, ESRD was less likely when PN was done rather than RN in a contemporary cohort (2003–2010) (HR, 0.44; 95% CI, 0.25–0.95). Furthermore, those with PN were less likely to develop new CKD (HR, 0.48; 95% CI, 0.41–0.57).[78]

In the one randomized controlled trial, the EORTC study involving 541 patients with small renal masses (≤ 5 cm), risk of CKD was retrospectively examined. Postoperative eGFR was higher with PN (67 mL/min/1.73 m^2) versus RN (53 mL/min/1.73 m^2) even though 10-year survival was not proven to be better with PN. PN was most likely to lower the risk of CKD progression to mild CKD (stage 3) by 21% but did not reduce risk of progression to clinically more meaningful and more advanced stages of CKD (stage 4 and 5).[89]

CKD from surgical resection may not lead to the same degree of progressive CKD decline seen in the corresponding stage of medically induced CKD. In a retrospective study examining patients with CKD from surgical resection, preexisting CKD with also surgically induced CKD, and with CKD caused by medical pathology alone, those with any medically induced CKD were more likely to progress to ESRD. Patients with medically induced CKD were older and had greater comorbidity, which likely explains the more rapid decline of CKD among these groups.[116]

In addition, the lower mortality associated with PN for those with localized renal masses[115] may be mediated by alteration of CKD related cardiovascular disease. Cardiovascular disease risk rises with and is independently associated with falling eGFR.[117] Cardiovascular disease related death was associated with CKD among 1004 case-matched patients with localized tumors (T1b, 4–7 cm). eGFR decline and mortality was greater for those who had RN. For each eGFR decline of 7 mL/min/1.73 m^2, risk of cardiovascular disease rose by 25% and risk of death increased by 17%.[118]

Table 28.2 Modifiable Risk Factors for Chronic Kidney Disease After Treatment for Renal Cell Carcinoma and Potential Interventions

Risk Factors	Potential Intervention	
Diabetes mellitus	Glycemic control	
Hypertension	Blood pressure control	
Preexisting CKD (± proteinuria)	CKD classification including eGFR and proteinuria; antiproteinuric treatment	
Tobacco use	Tobacco cessation	
Obesity	Weight loss and exercise	
Surgical factors	Tumor size	Select most appropriate therapy to maximize GFR preservation without sacrificing oncologic or overall survival
	Surgical modality	Selection of nephron-sparing procedures vs. radical nephrectomy
	Acute kidney injury	Avoidance of nephrotoxic medications, hypotension, and ischemia
	Warm ischemia time	Minimize warm ischemia time

CKD, Chronic kidney disease; *eGFR*, estimated glomerular filtration rate; *GFR*, glomerular filtration rate.

In addition to usual surveillance for RCC after treatment, eGFR and proteinuria assessment and regular blood pressure monitoring may be reasonably performed particularly among those with higher risk of CKD progression (with comorbid diseases) and certainly for those with preexisting CKD (Table 28.2). Like renal transplant donors, initial hyperfiltration and hypertrophy allows for compensatory increase in GFR; but in the RCC population who often have multiple comorbid diseases, these initial responses will often increase risk for proteinuria and nephrosclerosis long-term, leading to decline in kidney function.[119,120] A multidisciplinary team including the nephrologist, urologist, and pathologist would allow for proper diagnosis of CKD pathology and longitudinal management of the kidney cancer and the renal complications related to kidney cancer.

Cancer Follow-Up and Survivorship

The risk of RCC recurrence is stage dependent and postoperative surveillance protocols reflect this risk stratification.[121,122] In general, patients who undergo extirpative surgery (PN or RN) with low-risk RCC, defined as pT1N0M0/X, should undergo serial abdominal and chest imaging for 3 years.[122] Because of the low oncologic potential of these masses, follow-up beyond 3 years is at the discretion of the physician and patient. For patients undergoing extirpative surgery with higher-risk RCC, pT2-4 or N1, abdominal and chest imaging is recommended every 6 months for 3 years and annually until year 5.[122] Follow-up beyond 5 years in these higher-risk patients is at the discretion of the physician and patient. Patients undergoing TA are recommended to undergo serial abdominal imaging at 3 and 6 months given the higher rates of local recurrence and persistence,[87] with annual abdominal and chest imaging to follow based on risk category (see earlier).

Survivorship following surgery for a renal tumor also includes surveillance of renal functional outcomes.

As stated previously, eGFR and proteinuria assessment and regular blood pressure monitoring are recommended with formal nephrology consultation for those patients with preoperative eGFR less than 45 mL/min/1.73 m², postoperative eGFR less than 30 mL/min/1.73 m², confirmed proteinuria, or diabetics with preexisting CKD.[50]

Key Points

- The predictive factors for chronic kidney disease (CKD) among those with small renal masses is not only related to surgical factors, such as acute kidney injury, tumor size, and surgical modality (partial nephrectomy vs. radical nephrectomy) but is also related to common risk factors between renal cell carcinoma (RCC) and CKD (older age, tobacco exposure, obesity, hypertension, and diabetes mellitus), and preexisting CKD (including albuminuria).
- The close link of RCC (papillary) among end-stage renal disease patients on dialysis is attributed to the high prevalence of acquired renal cystic disease observed with prolonged dialysis vintage.
- For solid renal masses, tumor size and male sex predict risk of malignancy and adverse pathology. For cystic renal masses, complex lesions that enhance are more likely to be malignant.
- Partial nephrectomy, radical nephrectomy, thermal ablation, and active surveillance are the well-accepted management strategies for patients with renal masses suspicious for RCC. Choice of management is based on patient and tumor characteristics with consideration of oncologic outcomes, renal functional outcomes, and potential harms of each intervention.
- Concomitant nonneoplastic renal diseases are often present and proper diagnosis and management can result in improved patient outcomes.

Key References

6. Cohen HT, McGovern FJ. Renal-cell carcinoma. *N Engl J Med.* 2005;353:2477-2490.
7. Chow WH, Dong LM, Devesa SS. Epidemiology and risk factors for kidney cancer. *Nat Rev Urol.* 2010;7:245-257.
8. Denton MD, Magee CC, Ovuworie C, et al. Prevalence of renal cell carcinoma in patients with ESRD pre-transplantation: a pathologic analysis. *Kidney Int.* 2002;61:2201-2209.
9. Ljungberg B, Campbell SC, Cho HY, et al. The epidemiology of renal cell carcinoma. *Eur Urol.* 2011;60:615-621.
11. Lowrance WT, Ordoñez J, Udaltsova N, Russo P, Go AS. CKD and the risk of incident cancer. *J Am Soc Nephrol.* 2014;25:2327-2334.
12. Hu SL, Chang A, Perazella MA, Okusa MD, Jaimes EA, Weiss RH. The nephrologist's tumor: basic biology and management of renal cell carcinoma. *J Am Soc Nephrol.* 2016;27:2227-2237.
13. Truong LD, Krishnan B, Cao JT, Barrios R, Suki WN. Renal neoplasm in acquired cystic kidney disease. *Am J Kidney Dis.* 1995;26:1-12.
15. Singanamala S, Brewster UC. Should screening for acquired cystic disease and renal malignancy be undertaken in dialysis patients? *Semin Dial.* 2011;24:365-366.
17. Nouh MA, Kuroda N, Yamashita M, et al. Renal cell carcinoma in patients with end-stage renal disease: relationship between histological type and duration of dialysis. *BJU Int.* 2010;105:620-627.
20. Hashimoto Y, Takagi T, Kondo T, et al. Comparison of prognosis between patients with renal cell carcinoma on hemodialysis and those with renal cell carcinoma in the general population. *Int J Clin Oncol.* 2015;20:1035-1041.
21. Neuzillet Y, Tillou X, Mathieu R, et al. Renal cell carcinoma (RCC) in patients with end-stage renal disease exhibits many favourable clinical, pathologic, and outcome features compared with RCC in the general population. *Eur Urol.* 2011;60:366-373.
23. Yanik EL, Clarke CA, Snyder JJ, Pfeiffer RM, Engels EA. Variation in cancer incidence among patients with ESRD during kidney function and nonfunction intervals. *J Am Soc Nephrol.* 2016;27(5):1495-1504.
24. Jørgensen L, Heuch I, Jenssen T, Jacobsen BK. Association of albuminuria and cancer incidence. *J Am Soc Nephrol.* 2008;19:992-998.
30. Grantham JJ. Acquired cystic kidney disease. *Kidney Int.* 1991;40:143-152.
31. Ishikawa I. Unusual composition of cyst fluid in acquired cystic disease of the end-stage kidney. *Nephron.* 1985;41:373-374.
32. Ahn S, Kwon GY, Cho YM, et al. Acquired cystic disease-associated renal cell carcinoma: further characterization of the morphologic and immunopathologic features. *Med Mol Morphol.* 2013;46:225-232.
38. Sarasin FP, Wong JB, Levey AS, Meyer KB. Screening for acquired cystic kidney disease: a decision analytic perspective. *Kidney Int.* 1995;48:207-219.
39. Aiello FB. Incidental carcinoma of native kidneys in dialyzed and renal transplant patients: do we need new guidelines? *Transpl Int.* 2015;28:790-792.
42. Schwarz A, Vatandaslar S, Merkel S, Haller H. Renal cell carcinoma in transplant recipients with acquired cystic kidney disease. *Clin J Am Soc Nephrol.* 2007;2:750-756.
43. Gigante M, Neuzillet Y, Patard JJ, et al. Renal cell carcinoma (RCC) arising in native kidneys of dialyzed and transplant patients: are they different entities? *BJU Int.* 2012;110:E570-E573.
45. Nguyen MM, Gill IS, Ellison LM. The evolving presentation of renal carcinoma in the United States: trends from the surveillance, epidemiology, and end results program. *J Urol.* 2006;176:2397-2400.
50. Campbell S, Uzzo RG, Allaf ME, et al. Renal mass and localized renal cancer: AUA guideline. *J Urol.* 2017;198:520-529.
53. Bosniak MA. The Bosniak renal cyst classification: 25 years later. *Radiology.* 2012;262:781-785.
54. Israel GM, Bosniak MA. An update of the Bosniak renal cyst classification system. *Urology.* 2005;66:484-488.
64. Johnson DC, Vukina J, Smith AB, et al. Preoperatively misclassified, surgically removed benign renal masses: a systematic review of surgical series and United States population level burden estimate. *J Urol.* 2015;193:30-35.
65. Lane BR, Babineau D, Kattan MW, et al. A preoperative prognostic nomogram for solid enhancing renal tumors 7 cm or less amenable to partial nephrectomy. *J Urol.* 2007;178:429-434.

71. Pierorazio PM, Patel HD, Johnson MH, et al. Distinguishing malignant and benign renal masses with composite models and nomograms: a systematic review and meta-analysis of clinically localized renal masses suspicious for malignancy. *Cancer.* 2016;122:3267-3276.
73. Patel HD, Johnson MH, Pierorazio PM, et al. Diagnostic accuracy and risks of biopsy in the diagnosis of a renal mass suspicious for localized renal cell carcinoma: systematic review of the literature. *J Urol.* 2016;195:1340-1347.
74. Shield PW, Cosier J, Ellerby G, Gartrell M, Papadimos D. Rapid on-site evaluation of fine needle aspiration specimens by cytology scientists: a review of 3032 specimens. *Cytopathology.* 2014;25:322-329.
75. Bijol V, Mendez GP, Hurwitz S, Rennke HG, Nosé V. Evaluation of the non-neoplastic pathology in tumor nephrectomy specimens: predicting the risk of progressive renal failure. *Am J Surg Pathol.* 2006;30:575-584.
76. Henriksen KJ, Meehan SM, Chang A. Non-neoplastic renal diseases are often unrecognized in adult tumor nephrectomy specimens: a review of 246 cases. *Am J Surg Pathol.* 2007;31:1703-1708.
81. Lane BR, Demirjian S, Derweesh IH, et al. Survival and functional stability in chronic kidney disease due to surgical removal of nephrons: importance of the new baseline glomerular filtration rate. *Eur Urol.* 2015;68:996-1003.
83. Fergany AF, Hafez KS, Novick AC. Long-term results of nephron sparing surgery for localized renal cell carcinoma: 10-year followup. *J Urol.* 2000;163:442-445.
84. Thadhani R, Pascual M, Bonventre JV. Acute renal failure. *N Engl J Med.* 1996;334:1448-1460.
87. Pierorazio PM, Johnson MH, Patel HD, et al. Management of renal masses and localized renal cancer: systematic review and meta-analysis. *J Urol.* 2016;196:989-999.
88. Patel HD, Pierorazio PM, Johnson MH, et al. Renal functional outcomes after surgery, ablation, and active surveillance of localized renal tumors: a systematic review and meta-analysis. *Clin J Am Soc Nephrol.* 2017;12:1057-1069.
89. Scosyrev E, Messing EM, Sylvester R, Campbell S, Van Poppel H. Renal function after nephron-sparing surgery versus radical nephrectomy: results from EORTC randomized trial 30904. *Eur Urol.* 2014;65:372-377.
90. Van Poppel H, Da Pozzo L, Albrecht W, et al. A prospective, randomised EORTC intergroup phase 3 study comparing the oncologic outcome of elective nephron-sparing surgery and radical nephrectomy for low-stage renal cell carcinoma. *Eur Urol.* 2011;59:543-552.
99. Kaushik D, Kim SP, Childs MA, et al. Overall survival and development of stage IV chronic kidney disease in patients undergoing partial and radical nephrectomy for benign renal tumors. *Eur Urol.* 2013;64:600-606.
102. Barlow LJ, Korets R, Laudano M, Benson M, McKiernan J. Predicting renal functional outcomes after surgery for renal cortical tumours: a multifactorial analysis. *BJU Int.* 2010;106:489-492.
104. Jeon HG, Jeong IG, Lee JW, Lee SE, Lee E. Prognostic factors for chronic kidney disease after curative surgery in patients with small renal tumors. *Urology.* 2009;74:1064-1068.
107. Takagi T, Kondo T, Iizuka J, et al. Postoperative renal function after partial nephrectomy for renal cell carcinoma in patients with pre-existing chronic kidney disease: a comparison with radical nephrectomy. *Int J Urol.* 2011;18:472-476.
108. Hung PH, Tsai HB, Hung KY, et al. Increased risk of end-stage renal disease in patients with renal cell carcinoma: a 12-year nationwide follow-up study. *Medicine (Baltimore).* 2014;93:e52.
110. Stiles KP, Moffatt MJ, Agodoa LY, Swanson SJ, Abbott KC. Renal cell carcinoma as a cause of end-stage renal disease in the United States: patient characteristics and survival. *Kidney Int.* 2003;64:247-253.
111. Li L, Lau WL, Rhee CM, et al. Risk of chronic kidney disease after cancer nephrectomy. *Nat Rev Nephrol.* 2014;10:135-145.
112. Jeon HG, Choo SH, Sung HH, et al. Small tumour size is associated with new-onset chronic kidney disease after radical nephrectomy in patients with renal cell carcinoma. *Eur J Cancer.* 2014;50:64-69.
113. Cho A, Lee JE, Kwon GY, et al. Post-operative acute kidney injury in patients with renal cell carcinoma is a potent risk factor for new-onset chronic kidney disease after radical nephrectomy. *Nephrol Dial Transplant.* 2011;26:3496-3501.

114. Song C, Bang JK, Park HK, Ahn H. Factors influencing renal function reduction after partial nephrectomy. *J Urol.* 2009;181:48-53, discussion 53-54.
115. Kim SP, Thompson RH, Boorjian SA, et al. Comparative effectiveness for survival and renal function of partial and radical nephrectomy for localized renal tumors: a systematic review and meta-analysis. *J Urol.* 2012;188:51-57.
117. Go AS, Chertow GM, Fan D, McCulloch CE, Hsu CY. Chronic kidney disease and the risks of death, cardiovascular events, and hospitalization. *N Engl J Med.* 2004;351:1296-1305.
118. Weight CJ, Larson BT, Fergany AF, et al. Nephrectomy induced chronic renal insufficiency is associated with increased risk of cardiovascular death and death from any cause in patients with localized cT1b renal masses. *J Urol.* 2010;183:1317-1323.

A full list of references is available at Expertconsult.com

Acute Kidney Injury

29 Acute Kidney Injury Incidence, Pathogenesis, and Outcomes

AMIT LAHOTI AND SHELDON CHEN

Introduction

Advances in therapy, risk stratification, and supportive care have improved survival of patients with cancer over the past 2 decades.[1] Acute kidney injury (AKI) remains a common complication of cancer treatment and entails increased length of stay, cost, and mortality.[2,3] In addition, AKI may also lead to decreased functional status, decreased quality of life, and exclusion from further cancer therapy or trials. The etiology of AKI may be direct injury from the underlying malignancy (e.g., lymphomatous infiltration), drug toxicity (e.g., acute tubular necrosis [ATN]), related to stem cell transplant, or from treatment complications (e.g., tumor lysis syndrome). Patient related risk factors for AKI include older age, female sex, underlying chronic kidney disease (CKD), diabetes mellitus, volume depletion, and renal hypoperfusion.[4] Advances in immunotherapy and targeted therapy have also highlighted the nephrotoxic potential of many of these drugs. Although cancer itself is not a contraindication for starting renal replacement therapy (RRT), the benefits of RRT must be weighed against the overall prognosis of the patient and quality of life.[5] A multidisciplinary discussion between the patient, nephrologist, oncologist, intensivist, and palliative care physician is often necessary to make an informed clinical decision.

Diagnosis

The use of an arbitrary cut-off value of serum creatinine (SCr) for AKI is discouraged because many factors determine a patient's "baseline" creatinine level. Muscle mass, protein intake, volume expansion, and medications all affect SCr levels independent of kidney function. Therefore increases in SCr relative to baseline level are more reflective of AKI. Uniform definitions of AKI, such as RIFLE (Risk, Injury, Failure, Loss of kidney function, and End-stage renal disease [ESRD]) classification, Acute Kidney Injury Network, and the Kidney Disease: Improving Global Outcome, have facilitated the cross-comparison of studies by staging AKI by: (1) relative increases in SCr compared with baseline; or (2) progressive decline in urine output.

Cystatin C, a cysteine protease inhibitor produced by all nucleated cells, is freely filtered by the glomerulus and is neither secreted nor reabsorbed by the tubules. It is almost completely catabolized by the proximal tubular cells. In one particular metaanalysis of 13 studies, cystatin C had a sensitivity and specificity of 0.84 and 0.82, respectively, and an area under the receiver operating characteristic curve of 0.96 to predict AKI.[6] Given that cystatin C is a marker of inflammation, levels correlate with cigarette smoking, steroid use, and C-reactive protein levels. Recent studies have not found a correlation with tumor burden.[7] Given the significant increase in cost with cystatin C versus creatinine measurement, it has not been widely adopted for use in clinical practice.

Novel urinary biomarkers of renal injury, which potentially have better ability in detecting the onset and severity of AKI, are under active investigation. Potential candidate markers include inflammatory biomarkers (NGAL, interleukin [IL]-6, and IL-18), cell injury biomarkers (KIM-1, L-FABP, NHE-3, and netrin 1), and cell cycle markers (TIMP-2 and IGFBP-7). Although some studies have demonstrated benefit of urinary biomarkers for early detection of AKI after chemotherapy, other studies have demonstrated poor diagnostic performance. In addition, no studies have demonstrated improved patient outcomes with earlier detection. At this time, routine use of these newer biomarkers of kidney injury cannot be recommended.

Incidence

The incidence of AKI in cancer varies widely depending on the case mix studied. A large Danish study examined a cohort of 1.2 million people over a 7-year period, of which there were 37,267 incident cases of cancer.[8] As defined by the RIFLE classification, the 1-year risk for the "risk," "injury," and "failure" categories were 17.5%, 8.8%, and 4.5%, respectively. Corresponding 5-year risks for AKI were 27.0%, 14.6%, and 7.6%, respectively. The incidence of AKI was highest in patients with renal cell cancer (44%), multiple myeloma (MM) (33%), liver cancer (32%), and leukemia (28%). Among patients that developed AKI, 5.1% required dialysis within 1 year. In one large single center observational study of 3558 patients, 12% of patients developed AKI after admission.[9] Patients with AKI had increased length of stay, hospital costs, and mortality.

CRITICALLY ILL PATIENTS WITH CANCER

Patients with cancer comprise approximately 20% of all intensive care unit (ICU) admissions.[10] Depending on the case mix, AKI develops in 13% to 42% of critically ill patients with cancer, and 8% to 60% of these patients will require RRT.[11] The need for dialysis is more common in critically ill patients with cancer versus those without cancer. The incidence of RRT for AKI in patients with cancer admitted to the ICU ranges from 9% to 33% and entails a short-term mortality rate of more than 66%.[11] This is likely an underestimate of the actual severity of AKI in this population, given that many patients with cancer choose to forgo life-sustaining treatments. The higher incidence of AKI and RRT in this subgroup of patients is related to a higher incidence of severe sepsis, hypertension, exposure to nephrotoxic antimicrobials and chemotherapy, preexisting CKD, and tumor lysis syndrome. This is especially true for patients with hematologic malignancies who have bone marrow suppression from chemotherapy or complications from hematopoietic stem cell transplantation (HSCT). In the Dutch National Intensive Care Evaluation database, AKI occurred in 19.4% of critically ill patients with hematologic malignancies versus 11% in patients with solid tumors.[12] In addition, Taccone and colleagues reported an increased incidence of RRT in critically ill patients with hematologic malignancies versus patients with solid tumors (21.7% vs. 8%). In a multicenter study of 1753 patients with hematologic tumors who were admitted to the ICU with acute respiratory failure, the incidence of AKI was 33.9%, and 16.3% of patients received RRT. In a single center study of 204 critically ill patients with solid tumors, the incidence of AKI was 59%.[13] Main causes in this study were sepsis (80%), hypovolemia (40%), and urinary outflow tract obstruction (17%). RRT was required in 12% of patients with an associated hospital mortality of 39%.

LEUKEMIA AND LYMPHOMA

AKI may occur in up to 60% of patients with hematologic malignancies at any time during the disease course.[14] Common etiologies include septic and nephrotoxic ATN, hypoperfusion from third spacing and volume depletion, tumor lysis syndrome, and malignant obstruction from lymph nodes. Although leukemic or lymphomatous infiltration of the kidneys may be seen in up to 60% of patients at autopsy, this is an uncommon cause of AKI. Other less common causes of AKI in this subset of patients include hemophagocytic lymphohistiocytosis, vascular occlusion from hyperleukostasis, lysozymuria with direct tubular injury, and intratubular obstruction from medications (e.g., methotrexate). In a single center study looking at 537 patients with acute myelogenous leukemia or high-risk myelodysplastic syndrome undergoing induction chemotherapy, 36% of patients developed AKI as defined by the RIFLE classification.[15] Eight-week mortality was 3.8%, 13.6%, 19.6%, and 61.7% for the non-AKI, risk, injury, and failure categories, respectively. Predictors of AKI in this study were age older than 55 years, mechanical ventilation, vasopressors, intravenous diuretics, administration of vancomycin or amphotericin, and low serum albumin.

HEMATOPOIETIC STEM CELL TRANSPLANT

HSCT is frequently complicated by AKI. Common causes include volume depletion, sepsis, and nephrotoxic antimicrobials. Risk factors for AKI that are rather unique to transplant include marrow infusion toxicity, graft-versus-host disease (GVHD), hepatic sinusoidal obstruction syndrome, thrombotic microangiopathy (TMA), and BK nephritis. The incidence of AKI is 10% after autologous SCT, 50% after reduced-intensity conditioning allogeneic transplant, and 73% after myeloablative allogeneic transplant.[16] The median time to onset of AKI is 33 to 38 days after transplant. Patients that require RRT have a poor prognosis with a reported mortality of 55% to 100%. The greatest decline in kidney function tends to occur within the first year of HSCT and is associated with diabetes mellitus, hypertension, acute GVHD, and cytomegalovirus infection.[17]

MULTIPLE MYELOMA

AKI occurs in up to 40% of patients with MM during the course of their treatment and approximately 10% to 15% will require RRT.[18] Median overall survival is worse for patients with AKI and decreases to 3.5 to 10 months for patients that require RRT. Although there are a variety of pathologic lesions that may be found on kidney biopsy, the most common etiologies include myeloma cast nephropathy (MCN), AL amyloidosis, and monoclonal immunoglobulin deposition disease (MIDD). Less commonly, plasma cells may cause AKI by direct renal infiltration. In one case series of 190 patients with MM who underwent renal biopsy, 33% had MCN, 22% had MIDD, and 21% had AL amyloidosis.[19] However, there may have been some element of detection bias as not all patients with suspected MCN underwent renal biopsy. Autopsy studies have demonstrated MCN in 32% to 48% of patients who died with a diagnosis of MM.[20–22]

RENAL CELL CARCINOMA

Radical nephrectomy is associated with up to a 33.7% risk of AKI and is a strong predictor or CKD at 1 year. In one study examining more than 250,000 patients who underwent nephrectomy over a 22-year period, AKI developed in 5.5% of patients.[23] Radical nephrectomy was associated with a 20% increased risk of AKI versus partial nephrectomy in the multivariate analysis. Predictors of AKI included male sex, radical nephrectomy, older age, black race, CKD stage 3 or greater, and presence of comorbidities. AKI was found to be associated with greater morbidity, mortality, and hospital costs. Although there was a temporal increase in the incidence of AKI over time, this was attributed to the use of a more stringent definition of AKI and an aging population undergoing nephrectomy. A more contemporary analysis from the National Surgical Quality Improvement Program data set of patients undergoing nephrectomy from 2005 to 2011 revealed an incidence of 30-day AKI of only 1.8% within an average of 5.4 days after nephrectomy.[24] The authors note that the improved outcomes may also reflect selection bias towards high-volume and private sector hospitals.

CHEMOTHERAPY

Cisplatin, a platinum-based alkylating agent that inhibits deoxyribonucleic acid (DNA) synthesis, is commonly used to treat solid tumors including sarcomas, small cell lung cancer, ovarian cancer, and germ cell tumors. Renal tubular toxicity generally occurs 7 to 10 days after administration and may lead to hyponatremia, hypomagnesemia, Fanconi syndrome, and AKI. The mechanism of injury may include formation of reactive oxygen molecules, activation of mitochondrial apoptotic pathways, and increased synthesis of tumor necrosis factor alpha.[25] Approximately one-third of patients will experience AKI within days after treatment, and risk increases with repeated dosing. A recent study examined the incidence of AKI (rise in SCr of ≥ 0.3 mg/dL within 14 days of the first cycle of cisplatin) in 2118 patients, of which 13.6% developed AKI. A predictive model consisting of the patient's age, cisplatin dose, hypertension, and serum albumin demonstrated good predictive capability (c statistic = 0.7) of cisplatin associated AKI.[26]

Alkylating agents, such as cyclophosphamide and ifosfamide, cause AKI by multiple mechanisms. Hemorrhagic cystitis may develop with both drugs, leading to obstruction from urinary blood clots. Chloracetaldehyde, a metabolite of ifosfamide, depletes cells of glutathione and other sulfhydryl compounds leading to the proximal tubule injury and AKI.[27] Severe tubular injury may present as Fanconi syndrome, which generally resolves after stopping the drug. Risk of tubular injury is increased with cumulative dosing, younger age patients, and concurrent cisplatin therapy.[28]

Antimetabolite drugs are commonly used to inhibit DNA synthesis. Methotrexate, an antifolate agent, and its metabolite, 7-hydroxymethotrexate, may precipitate as crystals, leading to intratubular obstruction. Risk is increased in patients with volume depletion, acidic urine, or doses in excess of 1 g/m². Methotrexate can also cause a transient decrease in glomerular filtration rate by inducing afferent arteriolar vasoconstriction. Therapy has largely focused on aggressive hydration and alkalinization of the urine to enhance solubility. Glucarpidase, which metabolizes methotrexate into inactive metabolites, was approved by the U.S. Food and Drug Administration in 2012 for the treatment of methotrexate toxicity.

TARGETED THERAPY

Antivascular endothelial growth factor (anti-VEGF) therapy has been successfully used against a variety of tumor types to inhibit angiogenesis and cellular proliferation. VEGF and its receptors are abundantly expressed in the kidney and are vital for glomerular structure and function, repair mechanisms, and maintaining selective permeability of the glomerular basement membrane. Drugs that target the VEGF pathway often lead to hypertension, proteinuria, and less commonly AKI. Renal biopsies of patients with AKI or proteinuria in the setting of anti-VEGF therapy often demonstrate renal-limited TMA, although minimal change disease (MCD), focal segmental glomerulosclerosis (FSGS), and interstitial nephritis have also been described.[29,30] Discontinuation of therapy generally leads to resolution of kidney side effects.

Other targeted therapies are also associated with AKI, although the true incidence is not entirely known for many of these drugs. Inhibitors of the mammalian target of rapamycin pathway may cause AKI, block tubular repair mechanisms, and induce proteinuria. In one study, 15% of patients with renal cell carcinoma developed AKI after everolimus treatment.[31] Crizotinib, an inhibitor of anaplastic lymphoma kinase, may cause a reversible elevation in serum creatinine around 20% to 25%. Whether this is truly reflective of AKI or decreased tubular secretion of creatinine is unclear.[32] v-Raf murine sarcoma viral oncogene homolog B (BRAF) inhibitors, vemurafenib and dabrafenib, are commonly associated with tubulointerstitial nephritis that resolves with discontinuation of the drug.[33]

CANCER IMMUNOTHERAPY

Oncologists have leveraged the ability of the immune system to eradicate cancer since the early 1980s. Interferon-alpha was used in chronic myelogenous leukemia, hairy cell leukemia, metastatic melanoma, and non-Hodgkin lymphoma to promote effector T cell-mediated responses. Podocyte injury may manifest as MCD or FSGS, whereas patients with endothelial damage may present with TMA. IL-2 has also been used to activate T-cells and natural killer cells in the treatment of metastatic renal cell carcinoma and metastatic melanoma. The majority of patients develop capillary leak syndrome and hypotension, leading to prerenal azotemia or ATN.[34,35] However, renal function tends to recover after discontinuation of therapy.

More recently, checkpoint inhibitors (CPI) have been used to activate T-cells via ligand binding to cytotoxic lymphocyte-associated antigen-4 receptor (ipilimumab), programmed cell death protein-1 (PD-1) ligand (atezolizumab), and PD-1 receptor (pembrolizumab and nivolumab). These receptors, which may be activated by tumor cells, negatively regulate T-cell activation and function. Although the overall incidence of CPI-related AKI during clinical trials was 2.2%,[36] the true incidence may be as high as 9.9% to 29%.[37] Renal biopsies generally reveal granulomatous interstitial nephritis, but cases of TMA have also been described. Chimeric antigen receptor (CAR) T-cell therapy uses T-cells modified with lentiviral vector to express receptors that target specific extracellular antigens. In cancer therapy, CAR T-cells may lead to cytokine release syndrome, which may cause AKI. The incidence of AKI is not completely known with these novel therapies.

Outcomes

Although outcomes after development of AKI have been studied extensively, results have been reported only sporadically in patients with cancer. At the University of Texas MD Anderson Cancer Center, over a 3-month period in 2006, approximately 3600 patients were prospectively analyzed.[9]

Among patients admitted to the hospital, the incidence of AKI was 12%. In that group, 45% developed AKI within the first 2 days. The distribution of AKI by RIFLE criteria was risk (68%), injury (21%), and failure (11%). Dialysis was necessary in 4% of patients. The in-hospital mortality rate for the entire cohort was 4.6%. In those who developed AKI, the mortality rate was significantly higher (15.9%) than in those without AKI (2.7%; $p < .001$). Risk factors for mortality included leukemia, diabetes mellitus, hyponatremia, and transfer to the ICU.

Rates of kidney recovery have not been studied in cancer patients per se, but have been studied extensively in many observational trials of AKI. Typically, kidney recovery is defined as a return of SCr to premorbid levels. Among the survivors of AKI, recovery was seen in 50% to 90%,[38–45] even after severe AKI (dialysis requiring) in a critically ill population.[46] Although the majority of survivors eventually recover some kidney function, recovery becomes less likely with more severe grades of AKI. In one study, patients with AKI in the Failure category of the RIFLE criteria had a significantly lower chance of recovery.[47] The recovery rate may also be influenced by the modality of RRT. For those requiring RRT, kidney recovery was less frequent in patients treated with intermittent hemodialysis versus continuous RRT.[44,48–50]

The probability of kidney recovery after AKI is also affected by the kidney function at baseline. Patients with preexisting CKD, as compared with those with normal kidney function, have significantly lower recovery rate when they develop superimposed AKI.[47] Of more recent concern is that a single episode of AKI, even if there is full kidney recovery, increases patients' future risk of progressive CKD. Defined as a sustained reduction in estimated glomerular filtration rate to less than 30 mL/min/1.73 m^2 for at least 3 months during the year after discharge, advanced CKD was independently associated with six variables: older age, female sex, higher baseline creatinine, albuminuria, AKI severity and higher creatinine at time of discharge.[51]

Summary

AKI remains a common complication of cancer treatment and entails increased length of stay, cost, and mortality. The etiology of AKI may be direct injury from the underlying malignancy, drug toxicity, related to stem cell transplant, or from treatment complications. Advances in immunotherapy and targeted therapy have also highlighted the nephrotoxic potential of many of these drugs. Patients with liquid tumors (leukemia, lymphoma, myeloma) have the highest incidence of AKI, especially in the critical care setting. Although AKI does tend to improve in survivors, renal recovery is less likely with more severe grade of AKI. Baseline CKD also confers an increased risk of AKI during cancer treatment. Although cancer itself is not a contraindication for starting RRT, the benefits of RRT must be weighed against the overall prognosis of the patient and quality of life. A multidisciplinary discussion between the patient, nephrologist, oncologist, intensivist, and palliative care physician is often necessary to make an informed clinical decision.

Key Points

- Acute kidney injury occurs commonly in cancer patients.
- Acute kidney injury results from both etiologies common to all hospitalized patients and causes unique to patients with cancer because of the underlying cancer or its treatment.
- Newer biological and immunoregulatory chemotherapeutic agents are associated with unique mechanisms of kidney injury.

References

2. Samuels J, Ng CS, Nates J, et al. Small increases in serum creatinine are associated with prolonged ICU stay and increased hospital mortality in critically ill patients with cancer. *Support Care Cancer.* 2011;19(10):1527-1532.
3. Lahoti A, Nates JL, Wakefield CD, Price KJ, Salahudeen AK. Costs and outcomes of acute kidney injury in critically ill patients with cancer. *J Support Oncol.* 2011;9(4):149-155.
4. Perazella MA. Renal vulnerability to drug toxicity. *Clin J Am Soc Nephrol.* 2009;4(7):1275-1283.
8. Christiansen CF, Johansen MB, Langeberg WJ, Fryzek JP, Sørensen HT. Incidence of acute kidney injury in cancer patients: a Danish population-based cohort study. *Eur J Intern Med.* 2011;22(4):399-406.
9. Salahudeen AK, Doshi SM, Pawar T, Nowshad G, Lahoti A, Shah P. Incidence rate, clinical correlates, and outcomes of AKI in patients admitted to a comprehensive cancer center. *Clin J Am Soc Nephrol.* 2013;8(3):347-354.
11. Benoit DD, Hoste EA. Acute kidney injury in critically ill patients with cancer. *Crit Care Clin.* 2010;26(1):151-179.
12. van Vliet M, Verburg IW, van den Boogaard M, et al. Trends in admission prevalence, illness severity and survival of haematological patients treated in Dutch intensive care units. *Intensive Care Med.* 2014;40(9):1275-1284.
13. Kemlin D, Biard L, Kerhuel L, et al. Acute kidney injury in critically ill patients with solid tumours. *Nephrol Dial Transplant.* 2018;33(11):1997-2005.
14. Darmon M, Vincent F, Canet E, et al. Acute kidney injury in critically ill patients with haematological malignancies: results of a multicentre cohort study from the Groupe de Recherche en Réanimation Respiratoire en Onco-Hématologie. *Nephrol Dial Transplant.* 2015;30(12):2006-2013.
15. Lahoti A, Kantarjian H, Salahudeen AK, et al. Predictors and outcome of acute kidney injury in patients with acute myelogenous leukemia or high-risk myelodysplastic syndrome. *Cancer.* 2010;116(17):4063-4068.
16. Hingorani S. Renal complications of hematopoietic-cell transplantation. *N Engl J Med.* 2016;374(23):2256-2267.
17. Hingorani S, Pao E, Stevenson P, et al. Changes in glomerular filtration rate and impact on long-term survival among adults after hematopoietic cell transplantation: a prospective cohort study. *Clin J Am Soc Nephrol.* 2018;13(6):866-873.
18. Dimopoulos MA, Terpos E, Chanan-Khan A, et al. Renal impairment in patients with multiple myeloma: a consensus statement on behalf of the International Myeloma Working Group. *J Clin Oncol.* 2010;28(33):4976-4984.
23. Schmid M, Krishna N, Ravi P, et al. Trends of acute kidney injury after radical or partial nephrectomy for renal cell carcinoma. *Urol Oncol.* 2016;34(7):293.e1-293.e10.
24. Schmid M, Abd-El-Barr AE, Gandaglia G, et al. Predictors of 30-day acute kidney injury following radical and partial nephrectomy for renal cell carcinoma. *Urol Oncol.* 2014;32(8):1259-1266.
25. Jiang M, Wang CY, Huang S, Yang T, Dong Z. Cisplatin-induced apoptosis in p53-deficient renal cells via the intrinsic mitochondrial pathway. *Am J Physiol Renal Physiol.* 2009;296(5):F983-F993.
29. Izzedine H, Escudier B, Lhomme C, et al. Kidney diseases associated with anti-vascular endothelial growth factor (VEGF): an 8-year observational study at a single center. *Medicine (Baltimore).* 2014;93(24):333-339.

32. Porta C, Cosmai L, Gallieni M, Pedrazzoli P, Malberti F. Renal effects of targeted anticancer therapies. *Nat Rev Nephrol.* 2015;11(6):354-370.

37. Wanchoo R, Karam S, Uppal NN, et al. Adverse renal effects of immune checkpoint inhibitors: a narrative review. *Am J Nephrol.* 2017;45(2):160-169.

44. Goldberg R, Dennen P. Long-term outcomes of acute kidney injury. *Adv Chronic Kidney Dis.* 2008;15(3):297-307.

51. James MT, Pannu N, Hemmelgarn BR, et al. Derivation and external validation of prediction models for advanced chronic kidney disease following acute kidney injury. *JAMA.* 2017;318(18):1787-1797.

A full list of references is available at Expertconsult.com

30 *Tumor Lysis Syndrome*

MANDANA RASTEGAR, ABHIJAT KITCHLU, AND ANUSHREE C. SHIRALI

Introduction

Tumor lysis syndrome (TLS) describes the series of metabolic events that result from the death of rapidly dividing cancer cells. When cancer cells die, either spontaneously or in response to chemotherapy, they lyse and release intracellular contents of electrolytes, nucleic acids, and proteins. These substances accumulate in the systemic circulation and cause multiorgan pathology either directly or via toxic metabolites.

Clinically, patients may experience electrolyte disturbances, such as hyperkalemia, hyperphosphatemia, and hypocalcemia, and end-organ injury, such as acute kidney injury (AKI), seizures, and cardiac arrhythmias. TLS is an oncologic emergency and results in high morbidity and mortality, especially if diagnosis is delayed or prevention and treatment are not quickly instituted. In this chapter, we will focus on the defining characteristics and pathophysiology of TLS, with particular attention to patient- and cancer-specific risk factors that increase susceptibility to TLS. We will also review prevention and treatment strategies that have demonstrated efficacy in reducing the incidence and severity of TLS.

Definition and Classification

Hande and Garrow first systematically defined TLS when, based on a retrospective review of 102 patients with non-Hodgkin lymphoma, they classified TLS as laboratory TLS (LTLS) or clinical TLS (CTLS).[1] LTLS included changes in several electrolytes, whereas CTLS reflected the clinical effect of these changes, including arrhythmia or sudden death. Cairo and Bishop expanded upon these criteria to establish a commonly used classification system for TLS[2] (Table 30.1). With their modifications, Cairo and Bishop define LTLS if two or more of the following biochemical abnormalities are noted in patients who are not volume depleted and who have received prophylactic therapy against hyperuricemia: (1) 25% increase from baseline of serum potassium, phosphorous, or uric acid; (2) 25% decrease from baseline of serum calcium. These criteria must be met within 3 days before or 7 days after starting chemotherapy. If LTLS criteria are accompanied by seizure, arrhythmias, AKI with serum creatinine at or above 1.5 times upper limit of normal, or sudden death, Cairo and Bishop classification designates it as CTLS, if no other causative role (including therapeutic agents) can be found for the clinical manifestations. The severity of TLS is also determined by the Cairo-Bishop criteria by a separate grading scale (see Table 30.1). In addition, a designation of no LTLS or CTLS is given when there are no metabolic or clinical abnormalities.

The Cairo and Bishop classification is used in clinical practice but has been subject to criticism. For example, although it is common for multiple metabolic abnormalities to occur simultaneously in LTLS, some patients may only have one derangement followed by another, which may not be directly related to TLS, for example, hypocalcemia from sepsis. In addition, baseline changes in serum electrolyte levels may not result in values that are outside the range of normal, raising the question whether these patients are truly at risk for concerning clinical sequelae of TLS. Based on this, Howard et al. suggested a modified version of the Cairo-Bishop classification system that proposes simultaneous development of two or more metabolic abnormalities and symptomatic hypocalcemia as a criterion irrespective of the absolute percent change from baseline.[3] Lastly, the AKI criteria used by Cairo and Bishop are not standardized definitions, such as in the Acute Kidney Injury Network (AKIN) or the Risk, Failure, Loss, End-stage (RIFLE) kidney disease classification systems. As such, chronic kidney disease (CKD) patients may be erroneously classified as having AKI, as a result of TLS. Some have proposed that the criteria for AKI should match AKIN Stage I and include an absolute increase in serum creatinine of 0.3 mg/dL within 48 hours or relative increase in creatinine of 150% over 7 days.[4]

Pathogenesis/Pathophysiology

The clinical and biochemical sequelae of TLS occur with the release of intracellular contents when cancer cells lyse. Electrolytes (particularly potassium and phosphate), cytokines, nucleic acids, and their breakdown products enter the extracellular space in excess amounts. This metabolic load can overwhelm the body's homeostatic mechanisms when kidney function is inadequate to allow for urinary excretion. As such, AKI (mediated by acute uric acid nephropathy) plays a central role in the development of TLS.[4]

ACUTE URIC ACID NEPHROPATHY

Released intracellular purines (adenine and guanine) are metabolized to xanthine, and subsequently broken down to uric acid by xanthine oxidase. In humans, uric acid is the final product of purine metabolism (Fig. 30.1). This differs from other mammals that possess the enzyme urate oxidase, which further breaks down uric acid to allantoin (a more soluble substance).[5,6] Uric acid has classically been thought to cause kidney injury via precipitation of crystals in the renal tubules leading to microobstruction.[7] A high concentration of solute, cocrystallizing substances, and slow urine flow predispose to crystal-mediated injury.[8]

More recently, crystal-independent mechanisms for uric acid induced kidney injury have been described. In animal

275

Table 30.1 The Cairo-Bishop Tumor Lysis Syndrome Classification

LABORATORY TUMOR LYSIS SYNDROME: TWO OR MORE ABNORMALITIES WITHIN 3 DAYS PRIOR OR 7 DAYS AFTER INITIATION OF CHEMOTHERAPY		
Metabolic Parameter	Absolute Value	% Change Compared with Baseline
Potassium	> 6 mEq/L	Increase of 25%
Phosphorous	> 4.5 mg/dL (adults), > 6.5 mg/dL (children)	Increase of 25%
Uric Acid	> 8.0 mg/dL	Increase of 25%
Calcium	< 7.0 mg/dL	Decrease of 25%

CLINICAL TUMOR LYSIS SYNDROME: LABORATORY TUMOR LYSIS SYNDROME AND ONE OR MORE OF THE FOLLOWING						
Grade	0 (no LTLS)	1	2	3	4	5
Creatinine	< 1.5 × ULN	< 1.5 × ULN	> 1.5–3 × ULN	> 3–6 × ULN	> 6 × ULN	Death
Cardiac arrhythmia/ sudden death	None	No intervention	Medical intervention (nonurgent)	Uncontrolled medically but controlled with AICD	Life-threatening (shock, syncope)	Death
Seizure	None	—	One brief generalized seizure controlled with AEDs or infrequent focal motor seizures	Seizures with altered consciousness. Poorly controlled with breakthrough despite AEDs	Prolonged, repetitive, or difficult to control	Death

AEDs, anti-epileptic drugs; *AICD,* artificial implantable converter defibrillator; *TLS,* tumor lysis syndrome; *CTLS,* clinical tumor lysis syndrome; *LTLS,* laboratory tumor lysis syndrome; *ULN,* upper limit of normal.

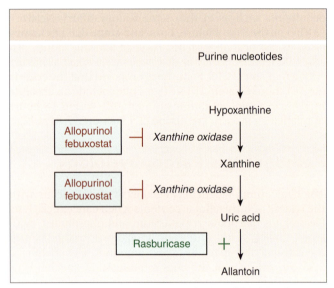

Fig. 30.1 Purine catabolism pathway and targeted drug site of action. Purine catabolism produces hypoxanthine, xanthine, and ultimately the low solubility metabolite uric acid via xanthine oxidase. Allopurinol and febuxostat inhibit xanthine oxidase. Uric acid can be converted to the highly water soluble allantoin with the use of rasburicase, a recombinant urate oxidase.

models, uric acid increases proximal and distal tubular pressures and peritubular capillary vascular resistance.[9] Uric acid may also reduce bioavailable nitric oxide, leading to renal ischemia via vasoconstriction.[10] Soluble uric acid also increases proinflammatory cytokines, such as tumor necrosis factor-α and monocyte chemotactic protein-1, resulting in inflammatory injury.[11,12] These multimodal causes of AKI caused by uric acid in turn impair the kidney's ability to excrete excess electrolytes and nitrogenous waste products.

HYPERKALEMIA, HYPERPHOSPHATEMIA, AND SECONDARY HYPOCALCEMIA

Lysis of tumor cells can lead to a substantially increased extracellular potassium load. Intracellular concentrations of potassium can be as high as 120 mEq/L.[13] This is of particular concern in hematologic malignancies with a large tumor burden. Rapid potassium release may exceed compensatory liver and muscle cell uptake, increasing the risk of hyperkalemia particularly in patients with severe AKI or underlying CKD.[14]

Similar to hyperkalemia, hyperphosphatemia occurs with release of intracellular contents with concomitant impaired renal excretion. Hyperphosphatemia may be more common in therapy-associated versus spontaneous TLS. In the latter, rapidly proliferating tumor cells may consume extracellular phosphate, resulting in a falsely low serum phosphate level (pseudohypophosphatemia).[15,16] Excess phosphorous may chelate with calcium, resulting in calcium-phosphate crystal deposition and hypocalcemia. Intrarenal calcium-phosphate crystal deposition likely also contributes to AKI in this setting.[17,18] These crystals have also been reported to cause dysrhythmia as a result of deposition in the cardiac conducting system.[3] Hypocalcemia secondary to hyperphosphatemia also has potentially severe sequelae, including arrhythmia, seizures, and tetany. Hypocalcemia in TLS may be protracted (even after normalization of phosphate) because of associated acute deficiencies in 1,25-Vitamin-D.[19]

Epidemiology and Risk Factors

INCIDENCE OF TUMOR LYSIS SYNDROME ACROSS HEMATOLOGIC AND NONHEMATOLOGIC MALIGNANCIES

The reported incidence of TLS varies widely among cancers. Hematologic malignancies are at higher risk than solid tumors, with the highest reported incidence in B-cell acute lymphoblastic leukemia (26%), acute myeloid leukemia (AML), particularly with white blood cell (WBC) greater than 75,000 cells/mm³ (18%), and Burkitt lymphoma (15%).[20,21] Intermediate risk hematologic cancers include diffuse large B-cell lymphoma (6%) and AML with WBC 25,000 to 75,000 cells/mm³ (6%).[1,20] More indolent hematologic malignancies are considered to be at lower risk, with incidence of 1% or less, including chronic lymphocytic leukemia and chronic myeloid leukemia and multiple myeloma.[22–24]

TLS has been reported in solid tumors, including breast, colorectal, nonsmall cell lung, and prostate cancers.[25] Although the exact incidence of TLS in solid malignancies is unknown, it is a rare complication, with most cases occurring in patients with a large burden of chemosensitive tumor.

TLS most commonly occurs following cytotoxic therapy; however, it has also been described in response to targeted agents and monoclonal antibodies (e.g., rituximab, bortezomib, imatinib, and other novel agents),[22,26] steroid monotherapy,[27] and radiation treatment.[28]

Spontaneous TLS has been well-documented in high-grade hematologic cancers, including non-Hodgkin lymphoma and acute leukemia,[29] and less so in breast cancer.[30] The incidence and specific precipitants of spontaneous TLS remain unclear.

Risk Assessment and Stratification

Both cancer- and patient-specific risk factors for TLS have been identified. Tumor characteristics, such as a high cellular proliferation rate, high sensitivity to therapy, and large tumor burden, have been associated with increased risk. High tumor burden has been described as bulky disease with diameter greater than 10 cm, WBC greater than 50,000 per μL, lactate dehydrogenase (LDH) more than two times the upper limit of normal, organ infiltration, or bone marrow involvement.

Patient-level risk factors for TLS include pretreatment renal dysfunction (specifically serum creatinine > 1.4 mg/dL), which is associated with a 10-fold increased odds ratio of TLS.[20,31] Similarly, volume depletion, oliguria, and/or acidic urine may predispose patients to TLS as well. Biochemical parameters, such as elevated LDH and pretreatment uric acid levels, have also been observed to predict the development of TLS. In particular, hyperuricemia with serum uric acid in excess of 7.5 mg/dL has been shown to associate with development of TLS.[32] These parameters are incorporated into a number of prediction models for TLS (most often in the setting of acute leukemia).[20,33,34]

Guidelines have sought to combine malignancy type and clinical characteristics to categorize patients into low-, intermediate-, and high-risk strata, with corresponding recommendations as to appropriate prophylaxis (Table 30.2).

Clinical Manifestations

The signs and symptoms of TLS are caused by the metabolic derangements that result from cell lysis. These signs and symptoms range from milder symptoms, such as nausea, vomiting, muscle cramps, and lethargy to severe manifestations, such as tetany, seizure, hematuria, cardiac dysrhythmias, and sudden death.[32] In this section, the clinical manifestations will be described based on the associated laboratory derangement.

Table 30.2 Tumor Lysis Syndrome Risk Stratification

Low Risk	Intermediate Risk	High Risk
LEUKEMIAS		
AML and WBC < 25 × 10⁹/L and LDH < 2 × ULN	AML with WBC 25 to 100 × 10⁹/L AML and WBC < 25 × 10⁹/L and LDH ≥ 2 × ULN	AML and WBC ≥ 100 × 10⁹/L
CLL and WBC < 50 × 10⁹/L treated only with alkylating agents	CLL treated with fludarabine, rituximab, or lenalidomide, or venetoclax and lymph node ≥ 5 cm **or** absolute lymphocyte count ≥ 25 × 10⁹/L, and/or those with high WBC ≥ 50 × 10⁹/L	CLL treated with venetoclax and lymph node ≥ 10 cm, **or** lymph node ≥ 5 cm **and** absolute lymphocyte count ≥ 25 × 10⁹/L and elevated baseline uric acid
	ALL and WBC < 100 × 10⁹/L and LDH < 2 × ULN	Burkitt leukemia Other ALL and WBC ≥ 100 × 10⁹/L and/or LDH ≥ 2 × ULN
CML		
PLASMA CELL DISORDERS		
MM	Plasma cell leukemia	
LYMPHOMAS		
Indolent NHL		
Adult intermediate grade NHL and LDH within normal limits	Adult T-cell leukemia/lymphoma, diffuse large B-cell, transformed, and mantle cell lymphomas with LDH > ULN, nonbulky	Adult T-cell leukemia/lymphoma, diffuse large B-cell, transformed, and mantle cell lymphomas with bulky disease and LDH ≥ 2 × ULN
HL	Childhood intermediate grade NHL stage III/IV with LDH < 2 × ULN	Stage III/IV childhood diffuse large B-cell lymphoma with LDH ≥ 2 × ULN

Continued

Table 30.2   Tumor Lysis Syndrome Risk Stratification—cont'd

Low Risk	Intermediate Risk	High Risk
Adult ALCL	Childhood ALCL stage III/IV	
	Burkitt lymphoma and LDH < 2 × ULN	Burkitt lymphoma stage III/IV and/or LDH ≥ 2 × ULN
	Lymphoblastic lymphoma stage I/II and LDH < 2 × ULN	Lymphoblastic lymphoma stage III/IV and/or LDH ≥ 2 × ULN
SOLID CANCERS		
Most solid cancers	Highly chemosensitive solid cancers with bulky disease (e.g., neuroblastoma, germ cell tumor, small cell lung cancer)	
OTHER		
		Intermediate risk disease with renal dysfunction and/or renal involvement, or uric acid, potassium, and/or phosphate > ULN
SUGGESTED PROPHYLAXIS		
Monitoring	Monitoring	Monitoring
Hydration	Hydration	Hydration
Consider allopurinol	Allopurinol	Rasburicase

ALCL, Anaplastic large cell lymphoma; *ALL,* acute lymphoblastic leukemia; *AML,* acute myeloid leukemia; *CLL,* chronic lymphoid; *CML,* chronic myeloid leukemia; *HL,* Hodgkin lymphoma; leukemia; *LDH,* lactate dehydrogenase; *MM,* multiple myeloma; *NHL,* non-Hodgkin lymphoma; *ULN,* upper limit of normal; *WBC,* white blood cell count.
Modified from Cairo MS, Coiffier B, Reiter A, et al. Recommendations for the evaluation of risk and prophylaxis of tumour lysis syndrome (TLS) in adults and children with malignant diseases: an expert TLS panel consensus. *Br J Haematol.* 2010;149(4):578-586.

HYPERKALEMIA

Patients with hyperkalemia may have neuromuscular complaints, such as muscle cramps, paresthesias, and lethargy, with pronounced hyperkalemia leading to cardiac arrhythmias and sudden death. Electrocardiogram (ECG) findings of hyperkalemia include peaked T-waves, prolongation of the PR and QRS interval, sine waves, or ventricular fibrillation.

HYPERPHOSPHATEMIA AND SECONDARY HYPOCALCEMIA

Hyperphosphatemia occurs with lysis of malignant cells, which can have up to 4 times higher than normal intracellular phosphorus concentrations.[35] This overwhelms the renal capacity for phosphorus excretion, especially when kidney function is impaired. Hyperphosphatemia may cause nausea, vomiting, diarrhea, or lethargy. The critical clinical manifestation of hyperphosphatemia occurs when phosphorus anions complex with calcium cations, leading to secondary hypocalcemia. Together, these insoluble calcium-phosphate complexes can precipitate in the renal interstitium and renal tubules, resulting in nephrocalcinosis, AKI, hematuria, and nephrolithiasis.[17,18,36] The complexes can also deposit in the cardiac conducting system and lead to arrhythmias.[3] Hypocalcemia may manifest as paresthesias, muscle cramps, seizures, hypotension, and widened QRS interval on ECG.

HYPERURICEMIA

When serum uric acid levels are elevated, the reabsorptive and secretory capacity of the kidney to handle the freely filtered uric acid is compromised. Uric acid crystallizes and obstructs the tubular lumen, especially in the setting of acidic urine pH and low urinary volume.[7,8] Patients with uric acid crystals do not usually complain of the renal colic that is associated with uric acid nephrolithiasis. Instead, they typically present with microscopic hematuria or AKI, either from acute urate nephropathy or the crystal-independent hemodynamic changes of hyperuricemia described earlier.[9,10]

ACUTE KIDNEY INJURY

AKI is a critical manifestation of TLS, which may present with oliguria and is detected with elevated serum creatinine and blood urea nitrogen levels above a patient's baseline. As noted previously, AKI in TLS is caused by one or more of the following: nephrocalcinosis causing tubulointerstitial damage, acute urate nephropathy, and/or crystal-independent hemodynamic changes of hyperuricemia.[3,4,9,10] Clinical symptoms vary from asymptomatic azotemia to florid uremia with nausea, vomiting, altered mental status, and seizures.

Prevention

Patients with TLS face increased mortality and higher treatment costs.[20,37,38] Therefore the use of risk stratification guidelines (see Table 30.2) to implement early prophylactic measures is a critical step before cancer treatment initiation. Intravenous (IV) volume expansion and hypouricemic agents are the cornerstone of preventive therapy.

INTRAVENOUS FLUIDS

Patients at any degree of risk for TLS should receive volume expansion with isotonic fluid (0.9% normal saline) to maintain urine output of 2 mL/kg/h, which supports high urine flow rates. This decreases the risk of uric acid or calcium-phosphate precipitation in the renal tubules while maximizing the urinary excretion of potassium, phosphorus, and uric acid.[9,18,32] Furthermore, volume expansion maintains adequate intravascular volume and renal blood flow, thereby reducing risk of prerenal AKI. Aggressive volume expansion demands close monitoring of vital signs and volume status. Urine output should be measured in patients with known AKI, CKD, or cardiac dysfunction. Urinary alkalinization increases uric acid solubility but is not recommended because it promotes urinary precipitation of calcium-phosphate products and exacerbates hypocalcemia. In addition, it has not been shown to be superior to the use of normal saline alone.[9,39]

HYPOURICEMIC AGENTS

Allopurinol

Allopurinol is recommended for patients at low or intermediate risk of developing TLS.[3,32] Allopurinol is converted to oxypurinol, the active metabolite that competitively inhibits xanthine oxidase, blocking the conversion of purines to uric acid (see Fig. 30.1).[32,40] Allopurinol should start 24 to 48 hours before chemotherapy. The recommended oral dose is 100 mg/m^2 every 8 hours, with a maximum daily dose of 800 mg per day in adults.[32] Patients with AKI should have dose reductions to prevent drug and metabolite accumulation. For patients with CKD, there are additional dose recommendations per manufacturer. For some patients, IV allopurinol may be necessary and is given at a single or divided dose of 200 to 400 mg/m^2. The efficacy and safety of IV allopurinol as prophylaxis was studied in 1172 hyperuricemic patients and was shown to prevent an increase in uric acid levels in 93% of adults and 92% of children.[41] Patients of Han Chinese, Thai, and Korean descent are at higher risk of developing a rare hypersensitivity syndrome (fever, rash, eosinophilia) to allopurinol.[42] Rasburicase or febuxostat should be considered as a primary agent in this population.

Rasburicase

Patients with an intermediate or high risk of developing clinical TLS, or with an established treatment uric acid level of greater than 7.5 mg/dL before cancer treatment initiation, should receive rasburicase (see Table 30.2).[31,43] Rasburicase is a recombinant urate-oxidase enzyme that promotes the conversion of uric acid to carbon dioxide, hydrogen peroxide, and water-soluble allantoin (see Fig. 30.1). Various studies have demonstrated that rasburicase significantly reduces uric acid levels within 4 hours of administration and reduces the need for renal replacement therapy.[43–46] The U.S. Food and Drug Administration recommends dosing at 0.15 to 0.2 mg/kg once daily for up to 5 days, with the higher dose recommended for uric acid level of greater than 7.5 mg/dL. Rasburicase does not require dosing adjustment for glomerular filtration rate (GFR). The use of rasburicase is contraindicated in patients with glucose-6-phosphate dehydrogenase deficiency.[43,47]

Febuxostat

Febuxostat, a xanthine oxidase inhibitor, is an alternative to allopurinol as a prophylactic agent for patients who do not have access to rasburicase and are unable to tolerate allopurinol because of hypersensitivity or severely depressed GFR (see Fig. 30.1). Febuxostat dosing is not changed in patients with renal disease and allergic complications have not been reported. The efficacy of febuxostat was compared with allopurinol for the prevention of TLS in 346 patients with intermediate to high risk of TLS.[48] At 24 hours and up to the eighth day of treatment, daily dosing of 120 mg of febuxostat achieved significantly lower uric acid levels compared with allopurinol. However, the primary endpoint of reduction in AKI showed no difference whereas higher liver dysfunction was noted in the febuxostat group.[48] Therefore the routine use of febuxostat is not currently recommended.

In addition to the aforementioned measures, prevention of TLS includes avoiding nephrotoxic agents, removing medications associated with hyperkalemia, and instituting a low potassium and phosphate diet. Individuals with intermediate risk for development of TLS should have laboratory testing every 8 to 12 hours.[3,32] In individuals at high risk for developing TLS, uric acid, phosphorus, potassium, and LDH should be monitored every 6 to 8 hours after the initiation of chemotherapy or radiation therapy.[3,32] Although there are no established guidelines on when to stop prophylactic therapy, it is reasonable to continue until TLS laboratory markers are normal for at least two consecutive measurements in patients who have reduced tumor burden and can maintain adequate oral fluid intake. Patients should be monitored for 24 hours after discontinuation of TLS prophylaxis to confirm stable laboratory values.

Treatment

Patients who present with or develop TLS require intensive care unit admission for supportive care, continuous cardiac and urine output monitoring, and serial blood draws every 4 to 6 hours for potassium, calcium, phosphorus, uric acid, and LDH.[3] The specific treatment of TLS targets the electrolyte and end-organ complications of TLS.

Hyperkalemia carries the highest risk of mortality. Treatment for hyperkalemia promotes transcellular shifts and elimination. Insulin with dextrose and/or inhaled high-dose beta agonist therapy should be used to promote transcellular shifts of potassium from the extracellular space to the intracellular compartment. IV calcium should be provided to all patients with hyperkalemia and ECG changes to prevent cardiac cell membrane depolarization. These measures, however, only temporize critical hyperkalemia. To prevent the inevitable rebound hyperkalemia that occurs once these measures wear off, methods to eliminate potassium from the body must be instituted, either via gastrointestinal or renal excretion. Use of ion exchange resins, such as sodium polystyrene sulfonate, is effective in binding intestinal potassium in exchange for sodium and removing potassium via fecal elimination but should not be used in patients with history of intestinal ischemia. IV loop diuretics can be used to promote renal potassium excretion, but may be ineffective unless higher doses are used if patients have preexisting CKD or AKI related to TLS. Urine output should be monitored to ensure response to loop diuretic therapy is not excessive enough to cause volume depletion. Severe hyperkalemia of 7 mmol/L (or higher) or refractory hyperkalemia will require renal replacement therapy.[32] Early intermittent hemodialysis for the treatment of life-threatening hyperkalemia, followed by a continuous renal replacement therapy (CRRT) to prevent rebound of hyperkalemia, may be required if initial dialysis is insufficient to keep pace with ongoing cell lysis and the resulting metabolic abnormalities, especially in the presence of AKI.[4,49]

Treatment of hyperphosphatemia requires limiting dietary intake and intestinal phosphate absorption with the use of phosphate binders with meals. Several phosphate binders are available, and either a calcium-based binder (calcium acetate, calcium carbonate) or noncalcium-based binder (sevelamer, lanthanum) should be used based on the patient's calcium level. For severe hyperphosphatemia (serum levels $\geq$ 8 mg/dL), aluminum-containing binders can be considered for short-term use. Hypocalcemia should not routinely be treated in TLS caused by the increased risk of calcium phosphate crystallization except in cases of severe symptomatic hypocalcemia in TLS with evidence of cardiac arrhythmias or seizures. Renal replacement therapy, in the form of CRRT, is preferred in patients with refractory hyperphosphatemia, symptomatic hypocalcemia, and an elevated calcium phosphorus product of 70 mg^2/dL or higher.[32,50]

The treatment of severe AKI requiring renal replacement therapy in TLS is similar to other etiologies of AKI, except that a lower threshold for initiation may be required given the ongoing and rapid release of intracellular contents during cancer treatment. In addition, consideration of CRRT must be made if cell lysis is ongoing and results in rebound changes in electrolyte levels.[3,31]

Summary

TLS is a serious complication in patients with malignant diseases, particularly in hematologic malignancies treated with chemotherapy. Because it involves electrolyte and metabolite abnormalities that can cause cardiac and renal toxicity, the negative effect on patient morbidity and mortality is high. Therefore prophylactic measures that focus on volume expansion and antiuric acid agents are critical in preventing development of TLS. If that is not achieved, quick diagnosis of TLS and immediate therapy, including treatment of electrolytes via medical means, and dialysis, are necessary to prevent poor patient outcomes.

Key Points

- Tumor lysis syndrome describes a series of metabolic events that result from the death of rapidly dividing cancer cells that can cause hyperkalemia, hyperphosphatemia, and hypocalcemia, acute kidney injury, seizures, and cardiac arrhythmias.
- Tumor lysis syndrome is an oncologic emergency and results in high morbidity and mortality, especially if diagnosis is delayed or prevention and treatment are not quickly instituted.
- The reported incidence of tumor lysis syndrome varies widely among cancers. Hematologic malignancies are at higher risk than solid tumors, with the highest reported incidence in B-cell acute lymphoblastic leukemia, acute myeloid leukemia, and Burkitt lymphoma.
- Intravenous volume expansion and hypouricemic agents are the cornerstone of preventive therapy.
- Patients with tumor lysis syndrome require intensive care unit admission for supportive care, continuous cardiac and urine output monitoring, and serial blood draws every 4 to 6 hours for potassium, calcium, phosphorus, and uric acid. Specific treatment targets the electrolyte and end-organ complications of tumor lysis syndrome.

References

1. Hande KR, Garrow GC. Acute tumor lysis syndrome in patients with high-grade non-Hodgkin's lymphoma. *Am J Med.* 1993;94(2):133-139.
2. Cairo MS, Bishop M. Tumour lysis syndrome: new therapeutic strategies and classification. *Br J Haematol.* 2004;127(1):3-11.
4. Wilson FP, Berns JS. Onco-nephrology: tumor lysis syndrome. *Clin J Am Soc Nephrol.* 2012;7(10):1730-1739.
6. Wilson FP, Berns JS. Tumor lysis syndrome: new challenges and recent advances. *Adv Chronic Kidney Dis.* 2014;21(1):18-26.
26. Howard SC, Trifilio S, Gregory TK, Baxter N, McBride A. Tumor lysis syndrome in the era of novel and targeted agents in patients with hematologic malignancies: a systematic review. *Ann Hematol.* 2016;95(4):563-573.
31. Cairo MS, Coiffier B, Reiter A, Younes A. Recommendations for the evaluation of risk and prophylaxis of tumour lysis syndrome (TLS) in adults and children with malignant diseases: an expert TLS panel consensus. *Br J Haematol.* 2010;149(4):578-586.
44. Coiffier B, Mounier N, Bologna S, et al. Efficacy and safety of rasburicase (recombinant urate oxidase) for the prevention and treatment of hyperuricemia during induction chemotherapy of aggressive non-Hodgkin's lymphoma: results of the GRAAL1 (Groupe d'Etude des Lymphomes de l'Adulte Trial on Rasburicase Activity in Adult Lymphoma) study. *J Clin Oncol.* 2003;21(23):4402-4406.
45. Jeha S, Kantarjian H, Irwin D, et al. Efficacy and safety of rasburicase, a recombinant urate oxidase (Elitek), in the management of malignancy-associated hyperuricemia in pediatric and adult patients: final results of a multicenter compassionate use trial. *Leukemia.* 2005;19(1):34-38.

A full list of references is available at Expertconsult.com

31 Obstructive Nephropathy in Cancer

INSARA JAFFER SATHICK

Introduction

Acute and chronic renal impairment resulting from urinary tract obstruction is common among patients with cancer and not solely limited to patients with pelvic tumors. Unlike benign causes of urinary tract obstruction, urinary obstruction resulting from malignancies poses several unique clinical challenges. The rate of recurrence of the obstruction and complications from measures undertaken to relieve the obstruction, tends to be higher in the cancer population. The recovery of renal function is related to the severity and duration of obstruction. Hence it is important to diagnose and treat urinary obstruction in cancer patients promptly.

Case Vignette

A 57-year-old woman was evaluated in the onconephrology clinic for elevated creatinine and hypertension. She had a history of stage III ovarian carcinoma treated with debulking surgery, followed by chemotherapy with cisplatin, paclitaxel, and bevacizumab 9 years ago. She was diagnosed with disease progression 7 years after the initial diagnosis and was treated with gemcitabine maintenance therapy. After 2 years of being on gemcitabine therapy, she was found to have schistocytes in the peripheral smear, normal serum creatinine, nonnephrotic range proteinuria, and a new diagnosis of hypertension requiring three antihypertensive agents. Imaging of her abdomen showed incidental finding of new left-sided hydronephrosis and dilatation of the ureter to the level of midpelvis (Fig. 31.1). In addition, peritoneal involvement of malignancy was noted to be stable. She underwent retrograde ureteric stent placement with exchanges every 3 to 4 months. She continued to have difficult to control hypertension and eventually developed acute renal dysfunction for which she was referred to the onconephrologist. Repeat imaging was obtained without contrast and this showed stable peritoneal carcinomatosis and nonobstructed kidneys with left-sided ureteric stent in place. She subsequently underwent a biopsy of the right kidney, which showed features of acute and chronic thrombotic microangiopathy. Gemcitabine was discontinued, and chemotherapy was switched to paclitaxel. Hypertension control and kidney function improved, and she survived another 2 years before succumbing to her cancer.

As illustrated in the aforementioned case vignette, obstructive nephropathy in cancer patients often presents insidiously and in conjunction with other causes of renal dysfunction. This is in stark contrast to benign causes of urinary obstruction, such as nephrolithiasis or benign prostatic hyperplasia, where the clinical presentation is quite straightforward. The clinical team should perform a careful review of the patient's history, current and previous cancer therapies to manage the renal dysfunction, and obstruction to the urinary tract. A high degree of suspicion and vigilance is warranted in managing obstructive nephropathy in the onconephrology world.

Definitions

Hydronephrosis is defined as dilation of the renal pelvis and calyxes proximal to the point of obstruction.[1] Obstructive uropathy refers to blockage of urine flow because of a functional or structural derangement, anywhere from the tip of the urethra back to the renal pelvis that increases pressure proximal to the site of obstruction. Obstructive uropathy may or may not cause renal parenchymal damage. Such functional or pathologic parenchymal damage is referred to as *obstructive nephropathy.* Hydronephrosis and obstructive uropathy are not interchangeable terms—dilation of the renal pelvis and calyces can occur without obstruction and urinary tract obstruction may occur in the absence of hydronephrosis.

Tumors Causing Urinary Tract Obstruction

Urinary obstruction may occur anywhere along the urinary tract, but certain anatomic sites are more prone for obstruction. This is due to the physiologic narrowing of the tract, which increases the risk of obstruction at the uretero pelvic junction, the crossing of the ureter over the common iliac vessels at the pelvic brim and the ureterovesical junction.[2] Ureteric diameter varies along its course: the diameter is 2 to 3 mm at the ureteropelvic junction, it widens to 10 mm until it reaches the pelvic brim and narrows again to 4 to 6 mm, and finally it is narrowest at the ureterovesical junction, about 1 to 5 mm. In women, a fourth area of ureteric narrowing exists at the level of pelvic blood vessels and broad ligament.[3] These are sites of physiologic narrowing of the ureteric diameter and hence prone for obstruction from intrinsic causes, such as calculi. In the setting of malignancy, ureteral obstruction may result from direct tumoral invasion of the ureter or extrinsic compression from lymph nodes or encasement of the ureters in tumoral tissue. Pelvic malignancies, such as prostate, bladder, cervical, uterine, ovarian, and colorectal

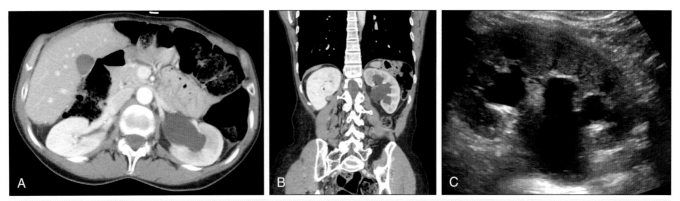

Fig. 31.1 **A.** Computed tomography (CT) abdomen with contrast showing incidental finding of left-sided hydronephrosis. **B.** CT abdomen with contrast, coronal view showing left-sided hydronephrosis. **C.** Ultrasonogram of the same patient demonstrating left-sided hydronephrosis-caliectasis, with interconnected fluid filled areas in the renal pelvis with a branching calyceal pattern.

tumors can cause obstruction by direct metastatic involvement or by external compression.[4]

Given the anatomy of the urinary tract, differences exist in how urinary obstruction affects male and female patients. The commonest malignancies associated with urinary obstruction are cervical cancer in women and prostate cancer in men. Prostate, cervical, and bladder tumors comprise about three-fourths of the tumors causing urinary tract obstruction.[5] The rest are breast cancer, gastrointestinal malignancies, and lymphomas causing urinary obstruction.[6] About 10% of patients with prostate cancer present with or develop symptomatic urinary obstruction during the course of their illness.[7] A significant proportion of patients with colorectal cancer also develop hydronephrosis with renal dysfunction.[8] In fact, any widely metastatic malignancy causing extensive retroperitoneal lymphadenopathy can cause urinary obstruction by extrinsic compression or by causing peritoneal carcinomatosis. In addition, obstruction may also result from radiation therapy and pelvic lymphoceles.[9]

In terms of tumors causing bilateral ureteral obstruction, cervical cancers are the commonest cause followed by stomach cancer and urologic malignancies.[10] Primary tumors of the ureter and urethra are quite uncommon. Ureteric tumors represent only about 2.5% to 5% of transitional cell carcinomas of the urinary tract.[11] Urethral tumors are 4 times more common in women compared with men but are generally uncommon in onconephrology practice.[2]

Pathophysiology of Urinary Obstruction

Acquired obstructive nephropathy in humans results from partial urinary obstruction in most cases and tends to be prolonged in its clinical course. But most physiologic studies of renal function in obstruction are based on models of acute complete obstruction for 24 hours.[12] In the case of cancer patients, the physiology can be altered by numerous other factors, including changes in patients' body weight, nutritional status, and vascular tone. Regardless, the animal models of acute urinary obstruction illustrate several key elements in the underlying pathophysiology.

Urinary obstruction significantly alters renal blood flow, glomerular filtration rate (GFR), and tubular function even before anatomic changes occur in the kidney.[13,14] Within the first 2 to 3 hours of obstruction, there is an early vasodilator response; termed the 'hyperemic phase.'[15] The rise in hydrostatic pressure in the proximal tubule initially results in reduced resistance of the afferent arteriole and increased glomerular hydrostatic pressure to counteract the proximal tubular pressure.[16] Therefore there is afferent arteriolar dilatation. This effect is demonstrably inhibited by nonsteroidal antiinflammatory drugs (NSAIDs) and is also seen in denervated kidneys, indicating that this is an intrarenal autoregulatory response to obstruction.[17] The reduced distal tubular flow contributes to the initial rise in single nephron GFR as part of tubuloglomerular feedback.[18] Thus in the initial phase of obstruction, single nephron GFR is maintained at approximately 80% of the preobstruction values, despite the marked increase in proximal tubular pressure.[15] As obstruction persists in the next 12 to 24 hours, there is a late vasoconstrictor phase, which is characterized by a drop in renal blood flow to about 40% of normal and poor renal perfusion.[12]

Two major vasoconstrictors, angiotensin II and thromboxane A2, play an important role in the markedly reduced renal blood flow and reduction in single nephron GFR in obstruction.[19] After the obstruction is relieved, there is further vasoconstrictor response in the kidney caused by the release of angiotensin II, as the macula densa senses the change in tubular flow. In animal experiments, simultaneous inhibition of thromboxane A2 and angiotensin production normalized GFR in the postobstructed kidney.[19] The administration of atrial natriuretic peptide after release of obstruction in rats also resulted in an increase of GFR, urine flow, and sodium excretion, suggesting a role of atrial natriuretic peptide in the hemodynamic changes of the postobstructed kidney.[19]

Obstruction affects tubular function by reducing the ability of renal tubules to transport sodium (Na+), potassium (K+), and hydrogen (H+), and reduces the ability to concentrate and dilute the urine.[20,21] This contributes to postobstructive diuresis.[22] For example, the apical Na-K-2 chloride (Cl) cotransporter and the basolateral Na+K+ adenosine triphosphatase in fresh suspensions of medullary thick ascending loop cells of obstructed kidneys, show reduced transporter activity.[23] Severe downregulation of aquaporin 2 expression contributes to the impaired urinary concentrating ability.[24] The local increase in prostaglandin E2 synthesis in postobstructed kidney is thought to play a role in aquaporin 2 downregulation.[25] Significant downregulation of apical membrane expression of the distal convoluted tubule Na+ Cl- cotransporter also occurs from obstruction.[20,24] The defect in H+ and K+ secretion in the distal nephron in obstructive uropathy has been shown to be independent of aldosterone.[26]

In the first few days after onset of obstruction, there is interstitial edema and an influx of leukocytes, predominantly macrophages, into the kidneys. If the obstruction is persistent and not relieved, glomerular size decreases, tubular cells lose apical microvilli and basolateral interdigitations and have fewer mitochondria. Nephrons atrophy from reduced renal blood flow and inflammatory responses.[13] If obstruction is maintained for a longer period of time, hydronephrosis eventually develops and there is tissue loss with tubular atrophy, interstitial fibrosis, and interstitial inflammation.[27]

In murine experimental models, interstitial fibrosis has been shown to develop within days in the obstructed kidney with increased renal synthesis of extracellular matrix proteins and transforming growth factor-β.[28] The interstitial fibrosis is also mediated by angiotensin II.[29] Proliferation of interstitial fibroblasts with myofibroblast transformation leads to extracellular matrix deposition. Phenotypic transition of renal tubular cells, endothelial cells, and pericytes has been implicated in this process.[30] The compression of medullary and cortical tissue from the renal calyceal distension results in widespread apoptosis and tubular atrophy as early as 3 days postobstruction.[31] The interstitial response to urinary tract obstruction further intensifies the injury, resulting in renal dysfunction.[31] In patients with malignant urinary obstruction, these changes happen over time and may not manifest as clinically evident renal failure for several days to weeks.

Clinical Presentation

In general, patients with benign acute unilateral ureteric obstruction, from a kidney stone for example, present with acute pain typical of a renal colic. Pain from acute ureteric obstruction is caused by pressure or stretch in the lumen. The ureter is supplied by two distinct types of neurons with different activation thresholds. U1 units are low threshold units activated by peristalsis in the absence of mechanical stimulus and U2 units are activated in response to mechanical stimuli, such as increased pressure. U2 units can activate nociceptive afferent input in the nervous system, even in the absence of inflammation.[32,33]

In the setting of malignant obstruction, the clinical presentation depends on the duration and location of the obstruction. The process is more chronic, with extrinsic obstruction developing over a period of days to weeks, unlike in the setting of acute renal colic. This type of insidious urinary obstruction may be unilateral or bilateral. Most patients with malignant urinary obstruction present with vague symptoms of nonspecific lethargy, flank discomfort, or feeling of fullness or being bloated.[33] These symptoms may be accompanied by varying degrees of nausea or anorexia. It has been postulated that distension of the renal pelvis and ureter from obstruction may cause a reflex change in pyloric sphincter pressure contributing to the nausea and vomiting experienced by patients—the so-called *renogastric reflex*.[34] Urinary tract infection (UTI) may also be a heralding symptom of urinary obstruction.[33] Often, the patient is asymptomatic and the obstruction is identified incidentally on imaging.

Patients with severe renal impairment present with symptoms of renal failure—nausea, vomiting, anorexia, weight loss, edema, and change in mental status. It is important to note that patients with unilateral and even bilateral ureteric obstruction are not necessarily oliguric or anuric. Patients with partial obstruction may continue to have a normal urine output. In some cases polyuria may be noted because of the concentration defect in distal nephron. It is only in cases of complete urinary obstruction that anuria is seen.

Patients with lower urinary obstruction may present with varying degrees of lower urinary tract symptoms including urinary frequency, hesitancy, and sensation of inadequate emptying of the bladder. On physical examination, palpable kidney may be seen only in patients with significant hydronephrosis. Otherwise, examination will show findings of the patients' primary malignancy, such as the presence of pelvic mass, or ascites from peritoneal carcinomatosis.

Though many patients may have a known diagnosis of cancer before presentation, a careful history and physical examination should be performed. In patients with advanced malignancy, more than one cause for renal dysfunction may be present—prerenal injury in the setting of poor oral intake and postrenal failure from obstruction. Most patients with advanced malignancy have poor oral intake and loss of muscle mass may lead to underestimation of the severity of their renal dysfunction. The postrenal component may only reveal itself after the prerenal component is corrected with volume resuscitation. In some patients, urinary obstruction may be the first presentation of malignancy.

Diagnosis

Urine analysis may show microscopic hematuria, pyuria, or mild to moderate proteinuria depending on the duration of obstruction. If leukocyte esterase and nitrites are present, urine cultures should be obtained to rule out UTI.

Early reports of metabolic derangements seen in urinary obstruction detailed the development of hyperkalemia and metabolic acidosis caused by transport defects in the distal nephron, resulting in decreased excretion of K+ and H+.[26]

Varying degrees of renal dysfunction may be seen depending on the duration and severity of urinary obstruction, from asymptomatic urinary obstruction to severe renal failure with life-threatening metabolic derangements. The history, physical examination, and laboratory evaluation will guide further evaluation with imaging.

IMAGING

Imaging modalities for diagnosis of urinary obstruction continue to evolve. Previously, intravenous pyelourography (IVP) was widely used as the gold standard for the diagnosis of urinary obstruction. Functional and anatomic details were provided by this study, but it required both radiation and contrast use.[35] Hence IVP has now been replaced by ultrasonography or computed tomography (CT) in most institutions.

Ultrasonography is the primary screening modality of choice for patients suspected of urinary obstruction. The hallmark of urinary obstruction is dilation of the collecting system of the kidney, which is easily identified on ultrasound as hypoechoic fluid displaces the echogenic parenchyma.[36] In patients with suspected nephrolithiasis, ultrasonography, when performed by a radiologist, resulted in no need for additional CT imaging in most patients in a multicenter comparative effectiveness trial.[37] There were no significant differences between ultrasonography and CT in risk for subsequent serious adverse events, hospitalizations, and return visits to the emergency department.

In the case of patients with suspected malignant obstruction, there are no head to head studies comparing the two modalities. Ultrasonography has several advantages—it is readily available in most institutions, there is no radiation exposure risk, it is noninvasive, no contrast is required, emergency medical professionals can be trained to perform a bedside assessment and, hence, it can be used at point of care.[38,39] In addition to detecting hydronephrosis and pyelectasis in patients with urinary obstruction, ultrasonography is also useful in assessing the kidney size, architecture, and changes in corticomedullary differentiation suggestive of chronic kidney disease. The presence of perinephric abscess and pyonephrosis can also be determined on ultrasound.[40] Because patients with malignant obstruction often present with abnormal renal function, the use of intravenous contrast may be contraindicated. Hence ultrasonography offers several advantages as an initial screening test, given its high sensitivity and specificity for detecting hydronephrosis.

Hydronephrosis may be graded on imaging as: grade I—slight blunting of calyceal fornices; grade II/mild—obvious blunting of calyceal fornices and enlargement of calices, but intruding shadows of papillae easily seen; grade III/moderate—rounding of calices with obliteration of papillae; and grade IV/severe—extreme calyceal ballooning.[36,38] It is important to note that the grading criteria do not correlate with the degree and acuity of obstruction.[38] A patient with grade I hydronephrosis on imaging may have severe obstruction and renal dysfunction, whereas a patient with grade III hydronephrosis may have no clinical signs or symptoms.

There are also disadvantages to the use of ultrasonography alone in the diagnosis of malignant urinary obstruction. To the inexperienced eye, the presence of extrarenal pelvis or renal cysts may simulate hydronephrosis.[40,41] Moreover, in patients with urinary diversion with ileal conduits, hydronephrosis may be a normal finding and not necessarily a sign of urinary obstruction. And importantly, renal ultrasonography may fail to detect early acute urinary obstruction, especially within the first few hours.[35,38,42,43] This is clinically relevant for patients with malignant obstruction, because many of them present with coexisting prerenal injury from dehydration and volume depletion. In some cases, retroperitoneal fibrosis causing early acute urinary obstruction may be missed on ultrasonography.[44] The resistive index (RI) from Doppler assessment has been assessed in the evaluation of urinary obstruction because of the hemodynamic changes that occur in the kidney during obstruction.[45] Although studies have shown a significant difference in the RI values of acutely obstructed versus nonobstructed kidneys, this is not a clinically reliable test because factors other than obstruction may affect the RI.[46]

Noncontrast CT was initially used in patients in whom ultrasonography or IVP did not reveal the cause of urinary obstruction. Now CT is widely used for identifying the cause of urinary obstruction and has replaced IVP for evaluating the upper urinary tract.[47] Older studies have shown CT to be superior to IVP for identifying the cause of obstruction, specifically in patients with cervical cancer.[48] The higher resolution and visualization of the dilated collecting system eliminates the need for contrast. CT can also be performed relatively quickly and can identify all stones, except indinavir stones, which are not visible on CT. In comparison to ultrasonography, CT has the advantage of determining the level of obstruction and the underlying etiology, not just the presence or absence of obstruction.[41]

CT scan can accurately distinguish an intraluminal stone from neoplasm, blood clot, or fungus ball, and characterize secondary signs of obstruction, such as perinephric fat stranding and changes in the renal cortical thickness.[41,49] In patients with malignant obstruction, CT has the advantage of also demonstrating extent of metastases, lymphadenopathy, retroperitoneal fibrosis, and other abdominal pathologies, such as bowel obstruction, diverticulitis, presence of ascites, presence of rectovaginal or colovesical fistulae that may affect patient management.[50] If contrast is given, a delayed nephrogram can be appreciated on the obstructed side as well, similar to IVP, but it is not a requirement.[41]

When compared with standard kidney, ureter, and bladder x-ray with ultrasonography and magnetic resonance urogram (MRU), noncontrast CT was superior to the other two modalities in identifying stone-related obstruction, with a sensitivity of 100% and specificity of 98.2%.[35] However, for other causes of obstruction, MRU had higher sensitivity (89.4%) and specificity (95.9%) compared with CT. T2 weighted sequences can visualize a dilated urinary tract without contrast material and selectively depict urine in the dilated renal collecting system and the ureter. Thus MRU enables accurate diagnosis of the level of obstruction and grade of obstruction, but has limited application in the evaluation of stones as MRI cannot detect calcification. MRU may also miss subtle urothelial abnormalities, such as small malignancies caused by relatively poor spatial resolution and visualization of the anatomic details of renal calyces and infundibula.[51] It is not yet widely available, is expensive, and more time consuming compared with the other modalities. In addition, there is a risk of nephrogenic systemic fibrosis when gadolinium is used in patients with advanced renal impairment.[52] Glomerular filtration rate may be overestimated in patients with cancer due to loss of muscle mass. Because of these reasons, MRU is not the first-line imaging tool in the evaluation of patients with suspected malignant urinary obstruction.

Radionuclide studies can assess the differential function of each kidney. In acute obstruction, the use of technetium 99m pentetate or MAG-3 allows the evaluation of uptake, transit, and elimination of the radionuclide from the kidney. In the setting of unilateral obstruction, parenchymal activity rises at a slower rate and persists for a longer time than the nonobstructed kidney.[41] Disadvantages of radionuclide imaging include lack of precise anatomic detail and delineation of the obstruction and inability to identify the cause. Radionuclide imaging can differentiate a dilated nonobstructed system from a partially obstructed system, with the use of diuretic renogram, by using a dose of furosemide after the radionuclide study. In the former, the collecting system activity will washout within 10 minutes after furosemide, whereas in the latter, there is no response or a slower response to furosemide.[41,53]

The choice of imaging modality will ultimately depend on the availability at a given institution and cost. Ultrasonography can be used as the first screening imaging modality in patients with acute kidney injury and suspected obstructive nephropathy with or without a cancer diagnosis. CT without contrast can be used as the initial imaging modality in patients with a known diagnosis of cancer who present with flank pain or other abdominal symptoms, and if the extent of metastases will affect their clinical course.[49] In most patients with malignant urinary obstruction, CT scan will help establish the extent of their disease and presence of lymphadenopathy, pelvic disease burden, and peritoneal carcinomatosis. This will help the clinician in managing the urinary obstruction and choosing the right intervention for the patient.

Management

The initial management of a patient with malignant urinary obstruction should include correction of hypovolemia. A Foley catheter should be placed, and accurate charting of patient's intake and urine output should be maintained. Consultation with Urology is mandatory. Ideally the Onconephrology team should use a multidisciplinary approach with expertise from Nephrology, Urology, and Interventional Radiology. UTI should be identified and treated. Pain from obstruction should be managed, preferably without the use of NSAIDs, because of their effect on renal perfusion. Patients with advanced malignancies are especially prone to renal failure because of high risk of hypovolemia, and renal vasoconstriction from NSAIDs may tip them over the edge. The use of corticosteroids has been proposed to reduce the risk of edema around obstructing tumors and purported antitumor effect.[54,55] But there is currently no strong evidence for the use of corticosteroids for urinary obstruction in cancer patients.

SURGICAL MANAGEMENT

The decision to proceed to a surgical intervention for a patient with obstructive nephropathy from cancer is a complex one. The median survival of adult patients with malignant obstruction from the time of intervention is reported to be around 96 days (2–1283 days) with 1-, 6-, and 12-month survival rates at 78%, 30%, and 12%, respectively.[56] The procedural risks are low compared with the benefit of avoiding dialysis, even in patients with advanced malignancy. Despite this, there may be a high price to be paid for urinary diversion procedures performed in patients with advanced malignancies. There is a high failure rate associated with ureteric stenting and concern for increased risk of infections and readmissions with percutaneous nephrostomy (PCN) placement.[5,57] Hence the risks and benefits must be considered carefully before recommending urinary diversion for patients with limited treatment options for their primary malignancy.

Once the decision is made, taking into consideration the patient's quality of life, procedural risks, and expected life span, the next step is to choose the best modality to achieve this. Although there have been several retrospective studies published that compare different modalities, few studies have compared modalities in a head to head fashion. Prospective studies and randomized controlled trials are also lacking as most patients' projected life span is short.

Urinary diversion or decompression procedures are generally defined by the approach into the urinary tract—retrograde or antegrade. Retrograde decompression of urinary obstruction is performed by way of cystoscopic ureteric stent placement. The antegrade approach is via PCN placement and insertion of an antegrade ureteric stent at a later stage. Retrograde stenting is usually done under anesthesia, but can be safely performed in patients with deranged coagulation and thrombocytopenia.[9] Nephrostomy placement can be done under local anesthetic but is a high-risk procedure in patients with coagulopathy and thrombocytopenia.[6]

Retrograde Ureteric Stenting

Fluoroscopic guidance is usually used to confirm the stent placement by retrograde approach. The first material used for ureteric stents was silicone in the 1970s; other materials, such as polyethylene, polyurethane, and mesh have been used subsequently.[4,58] There is a high failure rate for urinary decompression with retrograde ureteric stenting, because the lower urinary tract is anatomically challenging to maneuver, given the tortuosity of the obstructed dilated system and obscured ureteric orifices.[4,5] This is especially true in the setting of malignancy; the incidence of stent failure is higher in cases of extrinsic compression compared with intrinsic obstruction, such as stone disease and ureteric strictures.[33] Ureters obstructed by vesical/prostatic/cervical cancers are especially difficult to access.[5] Even when access is obtained into the lower ureter, it may be difficult to advance the guide wire successfully and negotiate the site of rigid lower ureteric obstruction.[5] This imparts a mechanical disadvantage from the lower end, which is much less of a problem during antegrade stenting because of the 'funnel' effect of the dilated proximal ureter.[5] Inability to cannulate the ureteric orifices resulting from trigonal distortion, failure to negotiate the lower ureteric segment, and nonvisualization of the ureteric orifice caused by postoperative scarring, are reported as reasons for retrograde stent failure.[5]

In the context of malignant ureteric obstruction, a wide range of retrograde stent failure rates have been reported from 16% to 58%.[33] A stent failure rate of 35.7% was reported in a study of 157 patients with extrinsic malignant compression.[59] Here, the commonest cancer diagnosis was ovarian, lymphoma, and cervical cancer. In this study, the type of cancer did not predict stent failure and need for PCN.[59] Significant need for PCN was noted among patients who had rectal cancer (seven of 12, 58.3%), sarcoma (five of nine, 55.6%), colon cancer (six of 13, 46.2%), and cervical cancer (six of 16, 37.5%). Invasion into the bladder (55.9% patients), when noted on cystoscopy, significantly predicted the need for PCN ($p = .008$). In another retrospective study of more than 100 patients, the reported stent failure rate was 41%.[60] Here, cancer diagnosis, baseline creatinine over 1.3 mg/dL, and post-stent systemic therapy for metastatic cancer were identified as predictors of stent failure. The diagnosis of cancer, not specific cancer type, was again identified as a strong predictor for stent failure. There was no correlation between the size of the stent and failure rate.

More recent studies continue to show similar stent failure rates, but a trend toward cancer type also influencing stent success rate—in a retrospective study of 53 patients, the stent failure rate was 34%; primary gastrointestinal cancer, poor performance status and severe preoperative hydronephrosis were independent predictors of stent failure.[61] Another notable difference in recent reports is systemic cancer therapy being shown to be a favorable prognostic factor for survival, after retrograde stenting for malignant ureteric obstruction. In a recent study analyzing prognostic factors for overall survival and stent failure in patients treated with retrograde stenting for malignant ureteric obstruction, serum creatinine before stent placement exceeding 1.2 mg/dL and lack of cancer therapy after stent placement were significant unfavorable prognostic factors, whereas gynecologic cancer was a significant favorable predictor of stent-failure free survival.[62] Median survival after stenting in this study was 228 days. These differences may reflect the advances made in cancer therapy in recent times and differences in patient selection and techniques for surgical management of urinary obstruction.

One of the reasons for drainage failure of ureteric stents in advanced pelvic malignancy is postulated to be the lack of long-segment ureteric peristalsis.[6] Stent encrustation with urine and urothelium also develops over time, limiting the duration of stent use, necessitating stent exchanges every 6 to 12 months.[4] Even though overt encrustation may not be present, the lumen of the stents are found to be blocked at the time of routine replacement, hence requiring routine exchange.[5] Complication rates reported after ureteric stenting may be as high as 53%.[59] Early stent-related complications include iatrogenic injury, stent migration, and patient discomfort, whereas late complications include infection, difficulties with stent exchange, hardware malfunction,

infection, and stent encrustation.[63] Stent fragmentation and migration were noted in 8% to 10% of patients. Fever was reported in 31%, and 16% of patients reported flank pain on the stented side on voiding, almost half of those requiring stent removal because of severe pain on voiding.[64] The cause of flank pain during voiding may be secondary to vesicorenal reflux through the stent during periods of increased intravesical pressure. In prospective quality of life questionnaire studies, the patient reported outcomes are worse. Eighty percent of patients experienced bothersome urinary symptoms and stent associated pain.[65] Urinary incontinence and sexual dysfunction also affect patient quality of life.

Percutaneous Nephrostomy

PCNs are tubes placed under sedation and ultrasound or CT guidance by entering the pelvic calyx and using Seldinger technique to dilate the tract. Patients are generally in prone position during procedure.[33] Open nephrostomy tube placements are not favored anymore because of high rate of major complications. PCNs have a high procedural success rate of 90% to 92%.[5] This is offset by the poor quality of life of patients after nephrostomy placement and high rate of complications. Complications following PCN placement include bleeding, tube dislodgement (10%–14% rate), and UTI.[57,66] The UTI rate ranges from 25% to 65%.[57] In a retrospective review of 200 patients with cancer, 19% had PCN-related pyelonephritis and 7.5% had asymptomatic bacteriuria. Eighty-nine percent of infections were with the primary nephrostomy tube, whereas the rest happened after nephrostomy tube exchange. Pyelonephritis developed within the first month in 10% of patients and within 3 months in 20% of patients. Prior UTI and neutropenia were significant risk factors for pyelonephritis. History of diabetes mellitus, chronic kidney disease, and presence of ureteral stents was not associated with increased risk of pyelonephritis. Of note, 99% of patients in this study did receive prophylactic antibiotics before PCN placement. Gram-negative organisms, such as *Escherichia coli*, *Klebsiella*, and *Pseudomonas* caused 40% of UTIs. *Enterococcus* was found in 30%, coagulase-negative *Staphylococci* in 17%, and *Staphylococcus aureus* in 9% of cases. Fungal infections were 12% of the total. Other reported complications from PCN include skin excoriation, urine leak, perirenal abscess formation, perirenal hemorrhage, and high readmission rate related to these events.[66]

A recent study examined the long-term management of malignant urinary obstruction with PCN, including estimation of exchange frequency and the financial impact. The simulation model used suggests that the optimal routine exchange interval for PCN exchanges in patients with malignant urinary obstruction is approximately 60 days.

Comparison of Retrograde and Antegrade Stenting

Based on head to head comparisons of both procedures, albeit retrospectively, some experts recommend a two-staged approach in the context of pelvic malignancies.[5] In a study of 65 patients with predominantly urologic cancer, 24 of 65 patients had an initial attempt at retrograde ureteric stenting as a first-line method of decompression. PCN followed by antegrade ureteric stenting at a later stage within a week of nephrostomy insertion was performed in 41 of 65 patients. If the initial nephrostomy was placed in the lower calyx, a mid-calyceal puncture was performed to facilitate antegrade insertion of stent. Success rate was 21% for endoscopic retrograde stenting, whereas two-stage antegrade ureteric stenting had a success rate of 98% with reported minimal morbidity. Failure of antegrade stenting in one case was caused by an impassable stricture of the lower ureter caused by prostate carcinoma. The high failure rate of retrograde stenting was attributed to inability to cannulate the ureteric orifices, caused by trigonal distortion and failure to negotiate the lower ureteric segment in most patients.[5] Thus PCN, first followed by antegrade stenting approach, allows management to be individualized for the patient and highlights the need for a multidisciplinary approach to managing urinary obstruction in the cancer patient.

Prognostic Model

Some investigators have attempted to predict survival after palliative urinary diversion for malignant ureteric obstruction. In a study of 140 patients undergoing PCN for palliative urinary diversion, in the setting of advanced malignant disease deemed to be incurable, median overall survival was 96 days (2–1283 days) with 1-, 6-, and 12-month survival rates at 78%, 30%, and 12%, respectively.[56] On multivariate analysis, events related to malignant dissemination, degree of hydronephrosis (grade I or II), and serum albumin before nephrostomy (3 g/dL or less) were associated with shorter survival. Patients were divided into three risk groups based on the aforementioned three factors: favorable –0 risk factors, intermediate one risk factor, and poor–two or three risk factors. There were significant differences in survival between the risk groups. The 6-month survival rates for the favorable, intermediate, and poor risk groups were 69%, 24%, and 2%, respectively ($p<$ .0001). Complications after PCN, in this study, included infection (13%), dislodgement (19%), major hemorrhage (2%), and minor hemorrhage (5%). Malignant diagnoses in this study were as follows: gastric, 21%; colorectal, 24%; uterine/cervical, 21%; ovarian, 4%; urothelial, 9%; and breast, 6%. Given the high mortality rate in the first year postprocedure, initial PCN placement with conversion to internal stenting is favored in some patients. Retrograde ureteral stent placement may be attempted first in patients who do not have advanced malignancy, with high tumor burden in the abdomen and pelvis. It is important to identify the patients who would benefit the most from upfront PCN.

Bilateral Obstruction

Few studies have examined long-term outcomes in patients presenting with bilateral ureteral obstruction. In a retrospective study of 87 patients who underwent bilateral ureteral stenting, most common cancer origin was cervical followed by stomach cancer.[10] The mean creatinine at the time of bilateral stenting was 3.3 mg/dL, which did fall to 1.6 mg/dL at 6 months postprocedure, but at 3 years poststenting, there was further deterioration in renal function,

with mean creatinine at 2.3 mg/dL. A percentage of patients (18.3%) developed chronic kidney disease stage 4 or 5 at 6 months and 57.2% at 3 years. Despite the development of chronic kidney disease, ureteral stenting in bilateral malignant ureteral obstruction may be worth pursuing, because dialysis may be avoided for several months to years. About 14% of patients underwent conversion to PCN. Among these patients ($n=12$), eight patients had early conversion to PCN to the dominant kidney or both kidneys less than 1 year after the initial stenting—they showed a trend towards better renal function outcomes compared with patients who had late or no conversion to PCN ($p=.06$). Cancer status was an independent prognostic factor for stent failure. Age older than 55 years, diabetes, and estimated GFR < 60 ml/min before obstructive symptoms or signs developed were significant predictive factors for chronic kidney disease stage 4 or more.

In addition to retrograde ureteric stenting and PCN placement, other surgical approaches have been studied in patients who did not have cancer. These include combined antegrade and retrograde approaches (so-called *rendezvous procedure*), the use of two parallel stents and other methods of ureteric diversion including nephrovesical subcutaneous stent and cutaneous ureterostomy placement.[9,67,68] But these methods have not been studied in patients with cancer and hence cannot be recommended at present.

In the future, antibiotic coated nephrostomy tubes may be developed to reduce the risk of PCN related pyelonephritis.[69] In addition, future management may include urinary proteomes, which are being studied to help identify patients at risk for renal dysfunction from mild obstruction.[70] These innovative approaches may be more relevant in the pediatric population with congenital causes of obstruction rather than adult patients with malignant obstruction.[71]

Palliation

Palliative urinary diversion specifically in the setting of advanced malignancy is a major clinical challenge in onconephrology. The risk and complications from urinary diversion procedures must be balanced against potential benefits for renal function and patient survival. Shekarriz et al. reported outcomes of palliative urinary diversion in the treatment of advanced malignancies in 103 patients treated with either stent or PCN; 92 of 103 patients had bilateral and 11 had unilateral obstruction.[72] Modified Karnofsky performance scale was used for physical performance, range 0 to 4. The median survival reported in this series was 112 days; 15% patients never left the hospital. Fifty-one percent required secondary PCN after initial retrograde stenting, 68.4% had complications, 86% had cancer-related symptoms, despite the urinary diversion. Average survival was 5 months, 50% of which was spent in hospital. Thus it is important to include the patient's quality of life and goals of care in the decision making, before proceeding to urinary diversion for palliation. Pain management and palliation of other symptoms such as nausea should be prioritized while undertaking measures to relieve the obstruction.

In conclusion, the approach to obstructive nephropathy in cancer patients should be individualized taking into consideration patient wishes and predicted survival from the underlying malignancy. Overall survival from the underlying malignancy.

Key Points

- Malignant urinary obstruction often presents with other causes of kidney injury, especially hypovolemia.
- Obstructive nephropathy may not be identified on imaging until hypovolemia is corrected in patients with advanced malignancy.
- Ultrasonography should be used as the initial screening modality for patients with suspected urinary obstruction and acute kidney injury. Computed tomography without contrast may be used as the initial modality in patients with a known cancer diagnosis as the extent of malignancy progression will impact their clinical course.
- Management of malignant urinary obstruction requires a multidisciplinary team approach and should include patients' wishes, quality of life, and goals of care.
- The benefits of relieving urinary obstruction should be balanced by the risks of stent failure, percutaneous nephrostomy tube-associated infections, and readmissions postprocedure.

Key References

5. Chitale SV, Scott-Barrett S, Ho ET, et al. The management of ureteric obstruction secondary to malignant pelvic disease. *Clin Radiol.* 2002;57(12):1118-1121.
6. Sountoulides P, Mykoniatis I, Dimasis N. Palliative management of malignant upper urinary tract obstruction. *Hippokratia.* 2014;18(4):292-297.
9. Liberman D, McCormack M. Renal and urologic problems: management of ureteric obstruction. *Curr Opin Support Palliat Care.* 2012;6(3):316-321.
10. Song SH, Pak S, Jeong IG, et al. Outcomes of stent-change therapy for bilateral malignancy-related ureteral obstruction. *Int Urol Nephrol.* 2015;47(1):19-24.
13. Tanner GA, Evan AP. Glomerular and proximal tubular morphology after single nephron obstruction. *Kidney Int.* 1989;36(6):1050-1060.
14. Tanner GA, Knopp LC. Glomerular blood flow after single nephron obstruction in the rat kidney. *Am J Physiol.* 1986;250(1 Pt 2):F77-F85.
15. Klahr S. New insights into the consequences and mechanisms of renal impairment in obstructive nephropathy. *Am J Kidney Dis.* 1991;18(6):689-699.
16. Harris RH, Gill JM. Changes in glomerular filtration rate during complete ureteral obstruction in rats. *Kidney Int.* 1981;19(4):603-608.
17. Allen JT, Vaughan ED Jr, Gillenwater JY. The effect of indomethacin on renal blood flow and ureteral pressure in unilateral ureteral obstruction in an awake dogs. *Invest Urol.* 1978;15(4):324-327.
18. Wright FS, Briggs JP. Feedback control of glomerular blood flow, pressure, and filtration rate. *Physiol Rev.* 1979;59(4):958-1006.
20. Li C, Wang W, Kwon TH, Knepper MA, Nielsen S, Frøkiaer J. Altered expression of major renal Na transporters in rats with bilateral ureteral obstruction and release of obstruction. *Am J Physiol Renal Physiol.* 2003;285(5):F889-F901.
22. Harris RH, Yarger WE. Renal function after release of unilateral ureteral obstruction in rats. *Am J Physiol.* 1974;227(4):806-815.
23. Hwang SJ, Haas M, Harris HW Jr, et al. Transport defects of rabbit medullary thick ascending limb cells in obstructive nephropathy. *J Clin Invest.* 1993;91(1):21-28.

24. Li C, Wang W, Knepper MA, Nielsen S, Frøkiaer J. Downregulation of renal aquaporins in response to unilateral ureteral obstruction. *Am J Physiol Renal Physiol.* 2003;284(5):F1066-F1079.
26. Batlle DC, Arruda JA, Kurtzman NA. Hyperkalemic distal renal tubular acidosis associated with obstructive uropathy. *N Engl J Med.* 1981;304(7):373-380.
29. Klahr S, Ishidoya S, Morrissey J. Role of angiotensin II in the tubulointerstitial fibrosis of obstructive nephropathy. *Am J Kidney Dis.* 1995;26(1):141-146.
30. Chevalier RL, Forbes MS, Thornhill BA. Ureteral obstruction as a model of renal interstitial fibrosis and obstructive nephropathy. *Kidney Int.* 2009;75(11):1145-1152.
33. Kouba E, Wallen EM, Pruthi RS. Management of ureteral obstruction due to advanced malignancy: optimizing therapeutic and palliative outcomes. *J Urol.* 2008;180(2):444-450.
35. Shokeir AA, El-Diasty T, Eassa W, et al. Diagnosis of ureteral obstruction in patients with compromised renal function: the role of noninvasive imaging modalities. *J Urol.* 2004;171(6 Pt 1):2303-2306.
37. Smith-Bindman R, Aubin C, Bailitz J, et al. Ultrasonography versus computed tomography for suspected nephrolithiasis. *N Engl J Med.* 2014;371(12):1100-1110.
39. Shokeir, AA. The diagnosis of upper urinary tract obstruction. *BJU Int.* 1999;83(8):893-900, quiz 900-901.
42. Gottlieb RH, Weinberg EP, Rubens DJ, Monk RD, Grossman EB. Renal sonography: can it be used more selectively in the setting of an elevated serum creatinine level? *Am J Kidney Dis.* 1997;29(3):362-367.
43. Webb JA. Ultrasonography in the diagnosis of renal obstruction. *BMJ.* 1990;301(6758):944-946.
44. Charasse C, Camus C, Darnault P, et al. Acute nondilated anuric obstructive nephropathy on echography: difficult diagnosis in the intensive care unit. *Intensive Care Med.* 1991;17(7):387-391.
47. Smith RC, Rosenfield AT, Choe KA, et al. Acute flank pain: comparison of non-contrast-enhanced CT and intravenous urography. *Radiology.* 1995;194(3):789-794.
49. Goel RH, Unnikrishnan R, Remer EM. Acute urinary tract disorders. *Radiol Clin North Am.* 2015;53(6):1273-1292.
50. Smith RC, Verga M, McCarthy S, Rosenfield AT. Diagnosis of acute flank pain: value of unenhanced helical CT. *AJR Am J Roentgenol.* 1996;166(1):97-101.
51. Kawashima A, Glockner JF, King BF Jr. CT urography and MR urography. *Radiol Clin North Am.* 2003;41(5):945-961.
56. Ishioka J, Kageyama Y, Inoue M, Higashi Y, Kihara K. Prognostic model for predicting survival after palliative urinary diversion for ureteral obstruction: analysis of 140 cases. *J Urol.* 2008;180(2):618-621, discussion 621.
57. Misra S, Coker C, Richenberg J. Percutaneous nephrostomy for ureteric obstruction due to advanced pelvic malignancy: have we got the balance right? *Int Urol Nephrol.* 2013;45(3):627-632.
59. Ganatra AM, Loughlin KR. The management of malignant ureteral obstruction treated with ureteral stents. *J Urol.* 2005;174(6):2125-2128.
60. Chung SY, Stein RJ, Landsittel D, et al. 15-year experience with the management of extrinsic ureteral obstruction with indwelling ureteral stents. *J Urol.* 2004;172(2):592-595.
61. Kamiyama Y, Matsuura S, Kato M, et al. Stent failure in the management of malignant extrinsic ureteral obstruction: risk factors. *Int J Urol.* 2011;18(5):379-382.
62. Izumi K, Mizokami A, Maeda Y, Koh E, Namiki M. Current outcome of patients with ureteral stents for the management of malignant ureteral obstruction. *J Urol.* 2011;185(2):556-561.
63. Fiuk J, Bao Y, Calleary JG, Schwartz BF, Denstedt JD. The use of internal stents in chronic ureteral obstruction. *J Urol.* 2015;193(4):1092-1100.
64. Richter S, Ringel A, Shalev M, Nissenkorn I. The indwelling ureteric stent: a 'friendly' procedure with unfriendly high morbidity. *BJU Int.* 2000;85(4):408-411.
65. Joshi HB, Stainthorpe A, Keeley FX Jr, MacDonagh R, Timoney AG. Indwelling ureteral stents: evaluation of quality of life to aid outcome analysis. *J Endourol.* 2001;15(2):151-154.
66. Hausegger KA, Portugaller HR. Percutaneous nephrostomy and antegrade ureteral stenting: technique-indications-complications. *Eur Radiol.* 2006;16(9):2016-2030.

67. Yates DR, Mehta SS, Spencer PA, Parys BT. Combined antegrade and retrograde endoscopic retroperitoneal bypass of ureteric strictures: a modification of the 'rendezvous' procedure. *BJU Int.* 2010;105(7):992-997.

68. Rotariu P, Yohannes P, Alexianu M, et al. Management of malignant extrinsic compression of the ureter by simultaneous placement of two ipsilateral ureteral stents. *J Endourol.* 2001;15(10):979-983.

69. Bahu R, Chaftari AM, Hachem RY, et al. Nephrostomy tube related pyelonephritis in patients with cancer: epidemiology, infection rate and risk factors. *J Urol.* 2013;189(1):130-135.

71. Chevalier RL. Obstructive nephropathy: towards biomarker discovery and gene therapy. *Nat Clin Pract Nephrol.* 2006;2(3):157-168.

72. Shekarriz B, Shekarriz H, Upadhyay J, et al. Outcome of palliative urinary diversion in the treatment of advanced malignancies. *Cancer.* 1999;85(4):998-1003.

A full list of references is available at Expertconsult.com

32 Renal Replacement Therapies

KEVIN W. FINKEL AND DIA R. WAGUESPACK

Introduction

Acute kidney injury (AKI) occurs commonly in cancer patients and independently increases morbidity and mortality.[1,2] Despite impressive gains in the understanding of the basic pathophysiologic principles underlying kidney injury, there are no therapeutic options to prevent or ameliorate AKI; treatment consists of supportive care and avoidance of nephrotoxic agents, such as radiocontrast and nonsteroidal antiinflammatory agents.

Patients with cancer are at risk for the development of AKI from causes similar to all hospitalized patients, such as radiocontrast administration, hypotension, antibiotics, infections, and sepsis. Unique causes of AKI in these patients include chemotherapy exposure, tumor lysis syndrome, hematopoietic stem cell transplantation, irradiation, and direct effects of malignancy. In a cross-sectional analysis of prospectively collected data on 3358 patients admitted to a large United States cancer center, 12% developed AKI based on the RIFLE (Risk, Injury, Failure, Loss of kidney function, and End-stage renal disease [ESRD]) creatinine criteria, of whom 4% received dialysis.[3,4] In a multivariate analysis, the development of AKI was associated with a significantly increased odds of death (odds ratio [OR] 4.72; 95% confidence interval [CI], 3.3–6.7).

At a certain point in the course of AKI, use of renal replacement therapy (RRT) may be considered. Although the literature is sparse and somewhat contradictory, most studies show that in patients started on RRT for AKI, survival is significantly lower for those with cancer compared with those without cancer; survival is particularly poor with hematologic malignancies.[5–8] In a retrospective study of 309 cancer patients with AKI (based on criteria proposed by Bellomo et al.), an increased risk of mortality was associated with age greater than 60 years, dysfunction of more than two organs, impaired performance status, and uncontrolled cancer.[9,10] In another analysis, the risk of mortality in 345 patients with hematologic cancer and AKI (based on RIFLE criteria) was significantly associated with septic shock, mechanical ventilation, and allogeneic stem cell transplantation.[8] Patients with all three risk factors had a mortality rate of 86%. Based on such findings, it is somewhat controversial whether initiating RRT in patients with multiple organ dysfunction and uncontrolled cancer is appropriate because RRT is unlikely to change the ultimate outcome.[11] This concern has triggered an interest in "palliative nephrology." For such patients, it may be reasonable to offer a time limited trial of RRT and discontinue treatment if there is no significant improvement in clinical status. Currently, there are no strict guidelines that define what is a reasonable time limit. The Renal Physicians Association, however, has published general guidelines on shared decision making in the appropriate initiation and withdrawal from dialysis.[12]

Although AKI occurs in patients in all hospital units, the highest frequency is in intensive care units (ICUs) and the majority of research described in this chapter relates to critically ill patients. Several critical issues regarding the use of RRT remain controversial and are outlined in Box 32.1.

Initiation of Renal Replacement Therapy (Timing)

The classic "indications" for initiating RRT in a patient with AKI are listed in Box 32.2. It is misleading to refer to these clinical conditions as indications because it implies that RRT should only be started when such criteria are present. Reliance on these criteria could delay appropriate therapy, resulting in serious adverse events in patients. Rather, the conditions listed should necessitate emergent RRT, unless palliative care measures are planned.

In the case of lesser degrees of kidney injury, the timing of RRT remains a contentious issue. On the one hand, early initiation would avoid the development of any serious complication of AKI; however, the early use of RRT could expose patients to the potential harm of RRT, when it might have been unnecessary (Box 32.3).

Two retrospective studies divided patients into "early versus late" groups based on the median blood urea nitrogen (BUN) concentration when RRT was started and found a survival advantage in the early dialysis group.[13,14] In addition, a metaanalysis also reported a benefit to earlier initiation of RRT.[15] Unfortunately, the overall data quality is poor and does not determine when RRT should actually be started.

More recently, two randomized controlled trials on the timing of RRT initiation have been published. In the multicenter trial reported by the AKIKI (Artificial Kidney Initiation in Kidney Injury) study group, 620 patients with Kidney Disease Improving Global Outcomes (KDIGO) stage 3 AKI ($\geq$ threefold increase in baseline serum creatinine or urinary output $<$ 0.3 mL/kg/h for $\geq$ 24 hours) were randomized to early RRT (at enrollment) or delayed RRT (development of hyperkalemia, severe metabolic acidosis, hypervolemia refractory to diuretics, BUN $\geq$ 112 mg/dL, or oliguria $\geq$ 72 hours).[16,17] There was no difference between the early and delayed groups in the primary endpoint of 60 day mortality (48.5% vs. 49.7%, respectively). Importantly, 49% of the delayed group never received RRT, and diuresis, a marker of improved kidney function, occurred significantly earlier. The rate of catheter-related blood

Box 32.1 Prescription of Renal Replacement Therapy

Timing

Early
Delayed

Dose

Conventional
Intensive

Method

Hemofiltration
Hemodialysis
Isolated ultrafiltration

Anticoagulation

Systemic heparin
Regional citrate

Mode

Intermittent
Continuous
Prolonged intermittent

Box 32.2 Indications for Initiation of Renal Replacement Therapy

Severe hyperkalemia
  (≥ 6.5 mEq/L)
Severe acidosis (pH < 7.2)
Hypervolemia refractory
  to diuretics
Uremia
  Encephalopathy
  Bleeding
  Pericarditis

Severe, refractory
  hypercalcemia
Severe tumor lysis syndrome
Severe rhabdomyolysis
Poisonings and intoxications
  Aspirin
  Alcohols

Box 32.3 Complications of Renal Replacement Therapy

Hypotension
Arrhythmias
Air embolism
Hemolysis
Thrombocytopenia
Hypoxia
Blood loss
Dialysis disequilibrium
  Nausea and vomiting

Headache
Seizures
Brain herniation
Dialyzer reactions
Chest pain
Anaphylactoid reaction

stream infections was significantly higher in the early strategy group.

The ELAIN study (Effect of Early vs. Delayed Initiation of Renal Replacement Therapy on Mortality in Critically Ill Patients With Acute Kidney Injury) randomized 231 patients at a single center with KDIGO stage 2 AKI ($\geq$ twofold increase in baseline serum creatinine or urinary output < 0.5 mL/kg/h for ≥ 12 hours) to either early RRT (within 8 hours of diagnosis of KDIGO stage 2 AKI) or delayed RRT (within 12 hours of developing KDIGO stage 3 AKI).[18] Patients in the early group compared with the delayed group had improved survival at 90 days (39.3% vs. 54.7%, respectively). In addition, more patients in the early group recovered kidney function at 90 days compared with the delayed group.

These discordant results are not unexpected. Both studies had a small number of patients, numerous confounders,

enrolled patients at different stages of kidney dysfunction, and relied on arbitrary indications for RRT. The two trials also differed in the population studied, where most patients in AKIKI were medical as opposed to those in ELAIN, who were mainly surgical. Whether this difference makes one trial more applicable to cancer patients than the other is unknown. Therefore initiation of RRT should be individualized to each patient, taking into consideration several factors, including fluid balance, severity of multiple organ dysfunction, urinary output, age, and comorbid conditions.

Discontinuation of Renal Replacement Therapy

Similar to the circumstance of initiating RRT, there are little published data in regards to stopping RRT. Given the complexity of patients with AKI, especially those who are critically ill, it is difficult to imagine devising a generalizable "weaning" plan similar to those used in mechanically ventilated patients. It is also probable that it is easier to determine when RRT can be successfully terminated in patients on intermittent therapy because trends in creatinine levels can be followed.

A retrospective observational case-controlled study was conducted in 304 postoperative patients with AKI receiving intermittent RRT.[19] A total of 94 patients (30.9%) were successfully weaned from RRT for more than 5 days and 64 (21.1%) were free of RRT for at least 30 days. Independent predictors for resuming RRT within 30 days were: (1) longer duration of RRT; (2) higher severity of illness scores on the day of stopping RRT; (3) oliguria (< 100 mL/8 hours) 1 day after stopping RRT; and (4) age over 65 years.

A post-hoc analysis of a prospective observational trial of 529 patients on continuous RRT for AKI was performed to identify variables associated with successful discontinuation.[20] Success was defined as no further RRT for at least 7 days. Multivariate analysis identified increased urine output and decreased creatinine levels as predictors of successful discontinuation. However, the predictability of urine output was significantly reduced by the use of diuretics.

In an anonymous electronic survey of practicing nephrologists treating AKI, the most common criteria used to stop RRT was urine output (51%).[21] Other factors included resolution of hypervolemia (29%), decreased creatinine levels (27%), and correction of hyperkalemia (21%). Overall, however, there was considerable variability in the survey regarding what criteria was used to stop RRT.

It appears that the majority of physicians rely on improvement in urinary output as an indication for stopping dialysis. In those patients with nonoliguric AKI, decreasing creatinine levels and improvement in overall clinical status appears to influence the decision to discontinue RRT.

Modalities

The major objectives of RRT are correction of electrolyte and acid-base disorders, solute clearance, and ultrafiltration (volume removal.) There are two basic methods of solute removal from the blood with RRT: diffusion via dialysis, and convection, or solvent drag, using hemofiltration.

DIALYSIS

Dialysis depends on the diffusion of solute across a semipermeable membrane (dialyzer) based on a concentration gradient. It provides excellent acid-base control and small molecule removal, such as BUN and creatinine. It is also relatively inexpensive because the dialysis solution can be produced in bulk using processed local water and does not need to be ultrapure because bacterial products do not cross most dialyzer membranes. However, as the molecular weight of solute increases, there is a significant decrease in clearance regardless of the concentration gradient because larger molecules move more slowly in an aqueous environment compared with smaller ones. This reduced clearance of so-called *middle molecules*, which includes inflammatory mediators, such as interleukin-6 and tumor necrosis factor alpha, could be an important consideration in critically ill patients with sepsis or shock.

HEMOFILTRATION

Hemofiltration, on the other hand, works by removing large volumes of plasma water across the dialyzer membrane using a pressure gradient, or transmembrane pressure. The lost plasma volume is replenished with concurrent intravenous administration of a physiologic replacement fluid. The removal of plasma water under pressure essentially "drags" solute with it, leading to solute removal and is referred to as *convection*. By this mechanism, middle molecule clearance is superior to dialysis; hence, many clinicians have proposed that hemofiltration is the preferred method of RRT in septic AKI. The major disadvantage of hemofiltration is cost. Replacement fluid, because it is administered intravenously, needs to be ultrapure and is therefore more expensive compared with dialysis fluid.

Despite the hypothetical advantage of hemofiltration over dialysis in septic AKI, there currently are no large, appropriately powered randomized trials demonstrating superiority. In a systematic review of 19 small randomized trials, there was no difference in mortality between the two modalities.[22] In some areas of the world, hemofiltration is used as a treatment for sepsis independent of kidney function, so-called *cytokine dialysis*. However, there is no credible evidence that this practice is beneficial.[23,24] Furthermore, hemofiltration increases middle molecule clearance indiscriminately, as it removes both "good" and "bad" solutes equally.

Based on the foregoing information, there is no evidence favoring the use of one form of clearance over the other. Therefore the choice becomes one of personal opinion considering ease and cost of therapy.

ISOLATED ULTRAFILTRATION

Isolated ultrafiltration (IUF) uses standard RRT equipment that, by applying a transmembrane pressure, removes only volume in either an intermittent or continuous mode.

Fluid overload and positive fluid balance in critically ill patients is associated with increased morbidity and mortality, including an increased risk of AKI (thus dispelling the myth that "the kidneys like to be wet").[25–27] Some authors have suggested that fluid overload be considered "the new AKI."[28] The Fluids and Catheters Treatment Trial showed that a conservative fluid management strategy in critically ill patients with respiratory failure significantly reduced ventilator days without increasing the incidence of AKI.[29] In fact, more patients in the liberal strategy required RRT.

Although diuretics have been the mainstay of the treatment for volume overload, patients often develop diuretic resistance or complications including contraction alkalosis, severe hypokalemia and hypomagnesemia, and worsening kidney function. In patients hospitalized for acute decompensated heart failure (ADHF), close to 50% of patients are discharged to home without any significant weight loss. These factors have led to the consideration of using IUF in place of diuretics. The potential benefits include controlled volume removal, hemodynamic stability, isotonic fluid removal (more sodium removed per liter compared with diuretics), and less activation of adverse neurohumoral mediators (norepinephrine, aldosterone, and renin). Although there are no data comparing IUF with diuretics in cancer patients, studies comparing IUF and diuretics in patients with ADHF provide some useful insights.

Small uncontrolled trials comparing IUF with standard therapy with diuretics suggested superior patient outcomes with IUF.[30,31] In the UNLOAD (Ultrafiltration vs. Intravenous Diuretics for Patients Hospitalized for Acute Decompensated Heart Failure) trial, 200 patients with ADHF were randomized to IUF or standard of care with intravenous diuretics. Those assigned to IUF experienced improved pulmonary decongestion and reduced rehospitalization without an increased risk of AKI.[32] However, this study was relatively small, the routine care group had no prespecified treatment algorithm, and follow-up was not standardized. In the CARRESS (Cardiorenal Rescue Study in Acute Decompensated Heart Failure) trial, 188 patients were randomized to IUF or protocol driven diuretic therapy to achieve urinary output of 3 to 5 L/day.[33] There was no benefit to IUF in terms of decongestion or rehospitalization rates; there was a significantly higher rate of AKI in the IUF group.

Based on the current evidence, diuretics remain the first-line method for volume control in patients with hypervolemia. There is no evidence that IUF is superior to diuretics in patients responding to protocol driven medical therapy. In patients who are refractory to diuretics, IUF should be initiated.

Methods

Once the decision has been made on when to start RRT and what form of clearance will be used, it must be determined what type of delivery method will be used (Table 32.1). Typically, RRT is divided into three major categories: intermittent (IRRT); continuous (CRRT); and prolonged intermittent (PIRRT).

Table 32.1 Comparison of Different Methods of Renal Replacement Therapy

	IRRT	CRRT	PIRRT
Time (hours/day)	3–4	24	8–12
Blood flow rate (mL/min)	300–400	15–300	150–300
Dialysate flow rate (mL/min)	600–800	30–60	100
Replacement fluid flow rate (mL/min)	N/A	30–60	100
Dialysis	Y	Y	Y
Hemofiltration	N	Y	Y
Cost	$	$$$$	$$

CRRT, Continuous renal replacement therapy; *IRRT*, intermittent renal replacement therapy; *PIRRT*, prolonged intermittent replacement therapy.

Peritoneal dialysis (PD), on the other hand, is not routinely prescribed in the acute setting. In the past, PD was widely used because of its easy availability and low cost. With the advent of improved technology in IRRT and CRRT, PD fell out of favor. Decline in the use of PD was also coupled with the concerns of risk of peritonitis, impaired ventilation from abdominal distension, variable volume control, and hyperglycemia from dextrose-based PD fluid. More recently, the use of PD in the treatment of AKI has experienced a renaissance. Renewed interest results from data, mostly reported from countries dependent on PD, as the only method of RRT available to critically ill patients, which demonstrate the effectiveness of acute PD in treating AKI. Several studies in acutely ill patients with AKI have shown that acute PD is not inferior to both daily IRRT and CRRT in terms of metabolic and volume control, and survival.[34–37] However, such studies are small and require verification in larger trials. Nevertheless, these results led to the International Society of Peritoneal Dialysis guideline that PD should be considered as a suitable method of RRT in patients with AKI.[38] Whether the use of PD in the setting of AKI will increase substantially likely depends on the local expertise of treating physicians.

CRRT is performed as either continuous veno-venous hemofiltration or hemodialysis (CVVH and CVVHD, respectively). Although CRRT on a minute by minute basis is less efficient than IRRT because of lower flow rates, it provides excellent volume and solute removal because of its continuous application.

It was thought that CRRT would be superior to IRRT as a modality in critically ill patients because of improved hemodynamic stability, safer volume removal, better acid-base and electrolyte balance, and the ability to give more nutritional supplementation. However, despite these apparent advantages, several randomized controlled trials were unable to demonstrate any benefit to CRRT.[39] It has been argued that this lack of superiority was caused by study design, where the sickest patients were excluded from participation, thereby creating bias. On the other hand, another interpretation is a failure to recognize the potential negative effects from CRRT that could negate its positive attributes as listed in Box 32.4. In a study from the Cleveland Clinic, 27% of patients on CRRT experienced severe hypophosphatemia and its

Box 32.4 Potential Adverse Effects of Continuous and Prolonged Intermittent Renal Replacement Therapy

Enhanced antibiotic removal	Required anticoagulation
Persistent hypophosphatemia	Bleeding
Persistent hypokalemia	Heparin induced
Metabolic alkalosis	thrombocytopenia
Enhanced amino acid and	Citrate toxicity
trace mineral loss	Risk of inadequate dosing
Blood loss from excessive	Competing procedures
clotting	Frequent clotting
Prolonged membrane	Catheter dysfunction
exposure	Morbid obesity

development was associated with a significantly increased risk of respiratory failure necessitating tracheostomy.[40] Furthermore, the most common cause of AKI in critically ill cancer patients is sepsis, and little is currently known about the appropriate dosing of antibiotics in patients receiving CRRT. In a study of 70 patients on CRRT given intravenous vancomycin, drug trough levels were below the recommended threshold in 50% of patients.[41] This finding was independent of location (medical vs. surgical intensive care) and prescriber (physician vs. pharmacist). Because vancomycin levels are easily available, this finding suggests many patients on CRRT may be receiving inadequate doses of other antibiotics where drug levels are not available.

PIRRT, as shown in Table 32.1, is a hybrid therapy of CRRT and intermittent hemodialysis (IHD). The major advantage of PIRRT is freeing the patient for competing procedures, such as imaging studies and surgical interventions, while providing adequate clearance and hemodynamic stability; it also reduces nursing workload. A meta-analysis of seven randomized and 10 observational studies demonstrated that PIRRT is not inferior to CRRT in terms of mortality, fluid removal, and kidney recovery.[42] The choice of PIRRT or CRRT is usually based on local logistics; some view PIRRT as a transition step between CRRT and IHD.

For now, the debate on CRRT/PIRRT versus IRRT continues, although CRRT/PIRRT certainly has a role in the care of a select group of patients. Reasonable guidelines for selecting CRRT/PIRRT are listed in Box 32.5. Patients

Box 32.5 Indications for Continuous and Prolonged Intermittent Renal Replacement Therapy

Shock	Cerebral edema
Cardiac SOFA score > 2	Fulminant hepatic failure
Intraaortic balloon pump (IABP)	Neurotrauma
Left ventricular assist device (LVAD)	Tumor lysis syndrome
	Rhabdomyolysis
	Refractory hypervolemia
Extracorporeal membrane oxygenator (ECMO)	Severe hypercatabolism
	Hyperammonemia

SOFA, Sequential organ failure assessment.
Cardiac SOFA > 2: Use of any vasoactive agent other than low-dose dopamine and/or dobutamine.

especially suited for CRRT/PIRRT are those with cerebral edema associated with hepatic encephalopathy or neurogenic edema.[43,44] Rapid solute removal with IRRT in these situations is associated with increased intracranial pressure and reduced cerebral perfusion.

Intensity of Dialysis

Other than control of metabolic and volume disturbances in patients with AKI, there is the issue of how much dialysis does a patient need, or the concept of dialysis dose. An early study of dialysis intensity in stable outpatient IRRT patients showed that the amount of solute clearance (as measured by the percentage decline in the initial BUN concentration) was more predictive of morbidity and mortality than duration of dialysis.[45] This landmark study led to the concept of urea kinetic modeling as a means to assess "adequate dialysis." In essence, it showed that simply looking at the BUN concentration as a marker of "good" dialysis was severely flawed, because BUN levels are affected by numerous nonkidney factors, such as protein intake, catabolic rate, and medications. What mattered was the percent reduction in the BUN concentration. Adequate dialysis is a greater than 65% reduction in the BUN level at the end of treatment regardless of the initial value. Lesser amounts of reduction in stable outpatient IRRT patients are associated with significantly higher morbidity and mortality rates. In fact, urea reduction ratio (URR) is mandatorily followed in dialysis clinics, as a measure of quality of care.

If the URR is a good measure of adequate dialysis in ESRD patients, what about unstable or critically ill patients with AKI needing RRT? In other words, if "dose" matters in ESRD, does it matter in AKI and how do you measure it? Inherent in the issue is that the URR was only validated in the ESRD population and not patients with AKI.

With this as a background, in the early 2000s, there arose great interest in assessing the "dose" of RRT in critically ill patients with AKI. In a trial by Ronco et al., patients receiving CVVH for ICU acquired AKI were randomized to low-dose (20 mL/kg/h) or high-dose (35–45 mL/kg/h) replacement fluid rates.[46] Patients in the higher-dose group had significantly better survival rates. In another trial of patients receiving IRRT for AKI, Schiffl et al. showed that patients receiving daily dialysis had better survival rates compared with those who received dialysis on an every-other day basis.[47] Based on these findings and other supportive retrospective studies, higher doses of RRT for critically ill patients were strongly encouraged. However, there were several problems with this recommendation: (1) control groups may have been "underdialyzed;" for example, in the Schiffl study, the mean URR during each treatment was below 60%; (2) demographics of the study patients were not reflective of those usually seen in the ICU; in the Ronco trial, 85% of patients were surgical and only 15% had sepsis; (3) volume control was not standardized; and 4) most studies had small numbers of patients and were underpowered.

Based on clinical equipoise, the Veterans Affairs/National Institutes of Health (VA/NIH) Consortium embarked on the ambitious study Acute Renal Failure Trial Network Study (ATN) to address the question of RRT adequacy in ICU patients with AKI.[48] Patients were randomized to either high dose or usual dose dialysis until death, recovery, discharge, or day 30 of hospitalization. Furthermore, modality (CRRT or IRRT) was determined by the cardiac sequential organ failure assessment (SOFA) score. If patients were considered hemodynamically unstable (cardiac SOFA score of 3 or 4), they received CRRT. Otherwise IRRT was performed. Patients switched between modalities as their cardiac SOFA score changed; however, they remained in the same dosing arm. High-dose CRRT was 35 mL/kg/h of dialysate/replacement fluid, whereas usual dose was 20 mL/kg/h. High-dose IRRT was six treatments weekly and usual dose was three weekly treatments. Each treatment was required to achieve a URR of more than 65%. The study randomized more than 1000 patients with a 90% power to detect a 10% absolute reduction in mortality rate with an expected mortality rate of 55%. The study found there was no survival benefit to intensive dialysis in either the entire group or in any predefined subgroup of patients. Note that all patients achieved a URR greater than 65% during IRRT treatments and the CRRT dose (defined as either hours on machine or quantity of used fluids) was achieved in 90% of cases. Therefore "underdosing" of dialysis did not occur.

Likewise, in the RENAL (Randomized Evaluation of Normal vs. Augmented Levels of Renal Replacement) trial with more than 1500 AKI patients in the ICU with similar demographics to the ATN study, randomization to high (40 mL/kg/h) versus usual (25 mL/kg/h) dose CRRT did not confer any survival benefit.[49]

These two trials clearly demonstrate that if an adequate dose of dialysis is delivered to critically ill patients with AKI, higher doses are unnecessary. It is vital to remember that adequate dosing is not what is prescribed but what is achieved. Barriers to achieving the prescribed dose include poor catheter function, filter/blood line clotting, competing procedures (abdominal washouts, radiology procedures), and morbid obesity. Therefore patients with ICU-associated AKI can be safely treated with thrice weekly IRRT (as long as the URR is measured and a target of > 65% is achieved) or CRRT with a dose of 20 to 25 mL/kg/h, as long as they receive at least 22 hours (90% of dose) of therapy per day.

Anticoagulation

Often forgotten in the discussion of RRT is the necessity and complications of anticoagulation. In patients with AKI treated with IRRT, anticoagulation can usually be avoided because of the rapid blood flow rates and relatively short treatment times. However, with more prolonged therapies using slower blood flow rates, especially CRRT, anticoagulation is required to prevent the complications of blood loss from filter clotting and decreased delivery of RRT dose. The need for anticoagulation during CRRT is made more problematic because patients on this mode of RRT tend to be sicker with a higher risk of hemorrhage because of sepsis, disseminated intravascular coagulation, trauma, surgery, and thrombocytopenia. Although various means of achieving anticoagulation in such patients include low-molecular-weight heparins, prostacyclin, thrombin antagonists, and heparin with protamine rescue, the two most common forms of anticoagulation in CRRT are continuous infusion of unfractionated heparin (UFH) and regional anticoagulation with citrate.

UFH is the most frequent anticoagulant used with CRRT. The popularity of UHF is caused by familiarity, low cost, and relative ease of monitoring. Infusion rates of UFH are typically aimed to achieve an activated partial thromboplastin time (aPTT) of 35 to 50 seconds. However, the use of UFH, especially in critically ill patients, is associated with excessive hemorrhage, unpredictable pharmacokinetics, hyperkalemia, and heparin-induced thrombocytopenia with arterial thrombosis. Furthermore, most reports on the effectiveness and safety of UFH in CRRT are small with variable doses of heparin and different aPTT targets.[50]

To avoid the complications of UFH use and provide a means of anticoagulation in patients on CRRT with absolute contraindications to systemic heparinization (patients with trauma, intracranial hemorrhage, burns, recent surgery), regional anticoagulation with citrate (RCA) was developed.[51] Continuous infusion of citrate into the CRRT circuit before entering the filter reduces by chelation the ionized calcium (iCa^{++}) level and thereby inhibits blood coagulation. As blood passes through the filter a certain amount of calcium (Ca^{++}) and citrate is removed. By infusing a constant quantity of Ca^{++} to patients through a central venous catheter to account for the Ca^{++} loss across the filter, a normal serum Ca^{++} level is maintained. In this way, the CRRT circuit has a low iCa^{++} concentration and blood is anticoagulated, and the systemic iCa^{++} level is normal and there is no risk of bleeding. The effectiveness of RCA is verified by a postfilter iCa^{++} level that is 70% lower than normal; safety is confirmed by a normal serum iCa^{++} value. Besides complications caused by prescription errors, the use of RCA can cause hypernatremia (citrate is a trisodium compound) and metabolic alkalosis (citrate delivered to the liver is converted in a 3:1 ratio into bicarbonate); therefore dialysis and replacement fluids used in CRRT with RCA have a lower content of sodium and bicarbonate. In rare instances, patients with severe hepatic failure can develop citrate toxicity. In this circumstance, the liver is unable to metabolize citrate so bicarbonate is not produced and any chelated Ca^{++} is not released to the serum. Subsequently, patients develop metabolic acidosis and an increasing difference between the levels of total Ca^{++} and iCa^{++} (because Ca^{++} bound to citrate is detectable as total Ca^{++}). Toxicity is detected by a total Ca^{++} ratio/iCa^{++} 2.5 or higher.[52]

Several trials have now been reported comparing UFH and RCA with CRRT that demonstrate the superiority of RCA in terms of filter life and hemorrhagic risk.[53] In one trial, compared with UFH, the use of RCA was also associated with a reduced risk of mortality in patients with sepsis.[54] Based on these results, the KDIGO guideline for AKI recommends that in a patient with AKI requiring CRRT that RCA should be used rather than UFH.[55]

Special Considerations

MYELOMA CAST NEPHROPATHY

Multiple myeloma (MM) represents 15% of all hematologic malignancies.[56] Although excessive free light chains (FLC) production can result in AL-amyloidosis and immunoglobulin deposition disease, the most common kidney presentation is AKI from myeloma cast nephropathy.[57] At diagnosis, 20% to 40% of patients with MM will have kidney disease, usually as a result of cast nephropathy, with 10% requiring dialysis.[58]

The key to treating myeloma cast nephropathy is rapid reduction in FLC concentrations.[59] In the past, standard chemotherapy was generally effective in MM patients but the reduction in serum FLCs was gradual and reversal of severe kidney injury was infrequent. Therefore there was great interest in the use of extracorporeal therapies to more rapidly reduce serum FLC levels. Several groups assessed therapeutic plasma exchange (TPE) to accomplish this goal. Despite encouraging results from small observational studies, the only randomized controlled of TPE showed no benefit on the endpoint of kidney recovery.[60]

The modern era of MM treatment was ushered in by the introduction of newer chemotherapeutic agents such as bortezomib, thalidomide, and lenalidomide. In comparison to traditional chemotherapy, bortezomib-based therapy significantly improves clinical response in MM patients including those with myeloma cast nephropathy based on observational analysis.[61–63] The kidney injury response is pronounced enough that bortezomib has been referred to as *renoprotective* chemotherapy.

Along with the introduction of renoprotective chemotherapy, there was a renewed interest in the application of extracorporeal removal of FLCs with newly developed high cut-off hemodialysis (HCO-HD) using a dialysis membrane with a higher molecular weight cut-off pore size compared with conventional high flux (HF) dialyzers. Several small studies demonstrated that HCO-HD was effective in reducing FLC concentrations.[64,65] However, HCO-HD was used in conjunction with bortezomib-based chemotherapy regimens; there were no control groups. Therefore such studies were encouraging, but did not address the fundamental question: does the use of HCO-HD provide additional benefit to bortezomib-based chemotherapy alone? Answering this question requires properly conducted randomized control trials. Two such trials have now been completed.

Studies in Patients with Multiple Myeloma and Renal Failure Due to Myeloma Cast Nephropathy (MYRE) and the European Trial of Free Light Chain Removal by Extended Hemodialysis in Cast Nephropathy (EuLITE) trials both randomized patients with dialysis dependent AKI because of biopsy confirmed myeloma cast nephropathy to bortezomib-based chemotherapy and either conventional HF-HD or HCO-HD with a primary endpoint of discontinuation of

RRT. The MYRE study randomized 98 total patients.[66] In addition to bortezomib-based chemotherapy, patients in the control arm received intensive HF-HD (eight sessions of 5-hour duration over the first 10 days, then thrice weekly). The patients in the HCO-HD arm received a similar treatment regimen using an HCO membrane. There was no difference in the primary endpoint of dialysis independence between the control and HCO-HD groups at 3 months (33.3% vs. 41.3%, respectively; p=.42). However, at 6 months, more patients in the HCO-HD arm than the control group were independent of dialysis (56.5% vs. 34.5%, respectively; p=.04). Although there was no difference between groups in the primary endpoint, the study may have been underpowered to identify a clinically important effect.

In the EuLITE study, 90 patients were randomized to bortezomib-based chemotherapy and either HF-HD or HCO-HD.[67,68] Dialysis regimens used in the study differed significantly from those used in the MYRE trial. In the control arm of EuLITE, patients received standard HF-HD at intervals determined on clinical grounds by a supervising nephrologist (minimum of 4 hours, 3 times per week). Patients in the HCO-HD arm received extended dialysis (8-hour sessions on 8 of the first 10 days followed by 8-hour sessions on alternate days). At 3 months, there was no difference in kidney recovery between the control and HCO-HD groups (55.8% vs. 51.6%, respectively; p= NS.) However, there were significantly more lung infections in the HCO-HD group (12 vs. 3; p=.014).

Bortezomib-based chemotherapy is of considerable benefit in patients with myeloma cast nephropathy compared with conventional agents and the rate of kidney recovery is significantly higher than in the past. Based on the results of randomized controlled trials so far reported, the issue of whether HCO-HD is beneficial in myeloma cast nephropathy remains unanswered. Therefore without more information, the use of HCO-HD should be subjected to more robust clinical trials before the routine use in patients with cast nephropathy can be recommended.

DRUG CLEARANCE

The incidence of cancer in patients with chronic kidney disease (CKD) has been estimated to be as high as 50% to 60%. Given such a high prevalence of CKD in cancer patients and the risk of hospital acquired severe AKI, the question of cytotoxic and biologic drug dosing is a major consideration to optimize therapeutic response without increasing drug toxicity. However, in most oncology clinical trials, patients with CKD are excluded from participation and information about drug dosing for patients with impaired kidney function or receiving dialysis is limited or unknown. What information is available is often outdated or does not consider newer dialysis membranes (higher clearance rates) or techniques (CRRT/PIRRT). In such cases, treatment regimens are often devised based on known pharmacodynamics of an agent, such as molecular weight, volume of distribution, water solubility, and extrarenal clearance. Any metabolites of the particular drug, especially if potentially toxic, must also be taken into account. Drug administration must consider two major factors, reduced kidney function that likely reduces dose, and dialytic clearance that affects timing of therapy.

Dialytic clearance is determined by the reduction of drug concentration across the dialysis membrane and blood flow rate:

$$CL \text{ (mL/min)} = \frac{(C_A - C_V) \times Q_B}{C_A}$$

where C_A is the prefilter drug concentration (mg/mL), C_V is postfilter drug concentration (mg/mL), and Q_B is blood flow rate (mL/min). Clearance measured in this way does not necessarily reflect the efficacy of total body drug removal, because it simply considers free drug present in serum; drugs with large volume of distribution or extensive protein binding are not available for clearance with RRT.

Review of the dialytic clearance of all chemotherapy agents is well beyond the scope of this chapter. Several reviews and monographs are available on this topic keeping the aforementioned caveats in mind.[69–71]

Summary

AKI occurs commonly in cancer patients and independently increases morbidity and mortality rates. Despite increasing understanding of the basic pathophysiologic processes in AKI, there currently are no effective therapies that can reverse or ameliorate renal injury necessitating the use of RRT in some patients. Despite the fact that RRT has been available since the 1950s, several issues related to its use remain controversial. Although the need for dialysis is clear for several life-threatening indications, there is yet a consensus on when RRT should be initiated in less severe circumstances. The proper use of RRT is further shrouded by such topics as means of clearance (diffusion vs. convection) and type of delivery (CRRT/PIRRT vs. IRRT). It is in many ways shocking that RRT has advanced so far technologically, yet we have so many fundamental clinical questions regarding its use.

Key Points

- The need for renal replacement therapy in critically ill patients with cancer is associated with a high mortality rate (50%–70%).
- Although evidence is not rigorous, the consensus is that continuous modes of renal replacement are preferred over intermittent forms in patients with hemodynamic instability.
- Despite the attractiveness of using hemofiltration rather than hemodialysis for better "middle molecule and inflammatory mediator" clearance, there is no evidence that hemofiltration improves patient outcomes.
- Although two randomized controlled trials have been published on the timing of initiation of renal replacement therapy in patients with acute kidney injury, there remains no consensus on the "early versus delayed" initiation debate. Timing of renal replacement initiation must still be based on individual patient characteristics.

■ Two recent trials assessing the benefit of high cut-off hemodialysis in dialysis requiring myeloma cast nephropathy showed no improvement in dialysis independence at 3 months compared with conventional dialysis.

References

1. Zeng X, McMahon GM, Brunelli SM, Bates DW, Waikar SS. Incidence, outcomes, and comparisons across definitions of AKI in hospitalized individuals. *Clin J Am Soc Nephrol.* 2014;9:12-20.
3. Molitoris BA, Levin A, Warnock DG, et al. Improving outcomes of acute kidney injury: report of an initiative. *Nat Clin Pract Nephrol.* 2007;3:439-442.
4. Salahudeen AK, Doshi SM, Pawar T, Nowshad G, Lahoti A, Shah P. Incidence rate, clinical correlates, and outcomes of AKI in patients admitted to a comprehensive cancer center. *Clin J Am Soc Nephrol.* 2013;8:347-354.
5. Rosner MH, Perazella MA. Acute kidney injury in patients with cancer. *N Engl J Med.* 2017;377:500-501.
6. Lam AQ, Humphreys BD. Onco-nephrology: AKI in the cancer patient. *Clin J Am Soc Nephrol.* 2012;7:1692-1700.
7. Lameire N, Vanholder R, Van Biesen W, Benoit D. Acute kidney injury in critically ill cancer patients: an update. *Crit Care.* 2016;20:209.
8. Chuva T, Maximino J, Barbosa J, et al. Haematological malignancies and acute kidney injury requiring nephrology consultation: challenging the worst of the worst. *Clin Kidney J.* 2016;9:418-423.
9. Bellomo R, Kellum J, Ronco C. Acute renal failure: time for consensus. *Intensive Care Med.* 2001;27:1685-1688.
10. Soares M, Salluh JI, Carvalho MS, Darmon M, Rocco JR, Spector N. Prognosis of critically ill patients with cancer and acute renal dysfunction. *J Clin Oncol.* 2006;24:4003-4010.
11. Darmon M, Thiery G, Ciroldi M, Porcher R, Schlemmer B, Azoulay É. Should dialysis be offered to cancer patients with acute kidney injury? *Intensive Care Med.* 2007;33:765-772.
12. Galla JH. Clinical practice guideline on shared decision-making in the appropriate initiation of and withdrawal from dialysis. The Renal Physicians Association and the American Society of Nephrology. *J Am Soc Nephrol.* 2000;11:1340-1342.
14. Liu KD, Himmelfarb J, Paganini E, et al. Timing of initiation of dialysis in critically ill patients with acute kidney injury. *Clin J Am Soc Nephrol.* 2006;1:915-919.
16. Palevsky PM, Liu KD, Brophy PD, et al. KDOQI US commentary on the 2012 KDIGO clinical practice guideline for acute kidney injury. *Am J Kidney Dis.* 2013;61:649-672.
17. Gaudry S, Hajage D, Schortgen F, et al. Initiation strategies for renal-replacement therapy in the intensive care unit. *N Engl J Med.* 2016;375:122-133.
20. Uchino S, Bellomo R, Morimatsu H, et al. Discontinuation of continuous renal replacement therapy: a post hoc analysis of a prospective multicenter observational study. *Crit Care Med.* 2009;37:2576-2582.
21. Mallappallil MC, Mehta R, Yoshiuchi E, Briefel G, Lerma E, Salifu M. Parameters used to discontinue dialysis in acute kidney injury recovery: a survey of United States nephrologists. *Nephron.* 2015;130:41-47.
22. Friedrich JO, Wald R, Bagshaw SM, Burns KE, Adhikari NK. Hemofiltration compared to hemodialysis for acute kidney injury: systematic review and meta-analysis. *Crit Care.* 2012;16:R146.
23. Honore PM, Joannes-Boyau O, Boer W, Collin V. High-volume hemofiltration in sepsis and SIRS: current concepts and future prospects. *Blood Purif.* 2009;28:1-11.
26. Vincent JL, Sakr Y, Sprung CL, et al. Sepsis in European intensive care units: results of the SOAP study. *Crit Care Med.* 2006;34:344-353.
27. Salahuddin N, Sammani M, Hamdan A, et al. Fluid overload is an independent risk factor for acute kidney injury in critically Ill patients: results of a cohort study. *BMC Nephrol.* 2017;18:45.
28. Goldstein SL. Fluid management in acute kidney injury. *J Intensive Care Med.* 2014;29:183-189.
29. National Heart L, Blood Institute Acute Respiratory Distress Syndrome Clinical Trials N, Wiedemann HP, et al. Comparison of two fluid-management strategies in acute lung injury. *N Engl J Med.* 2006;354:2564-2575.
31. Bart BA, Boyle A, Bank AJ, et al. Ultrafiltration versus usual care for hospitalized patients with heart failure: the Relief for Acutely Fluid-Overloaded Patients With Decompensated Congestive Heart Failure (RAPID-CHF) trial. *J Am Coll Cardiol.* 2005;46:2043-2046.
32. Costanzo MR, Guglin ME, Saltzberg MT, et al. Ultrafiltration versus intravenous diuretics for patients hospitalized for acute decompensated heart failure. *J Am Coll Cardiol.* 2007;49:675-683.
33. Bart BA, Goldsmith SR, Lee KL, et al. Ultrafiltration in decompensated heart failure with cardiorenal syndrome. *N Engl J Med.* 2012;367:2296-2304.
35. Ponce D, Berbel MN, Abrão JM, Goes CR, Balbi AL. A randomized clinical trial of high volume peritoneal dialysis versus extended daily hemodialysis for acute kidney injury patients. *Int Urol Nephrol.* 2013;45:869-878.
36. Ponce D, Berbel MN, Regina de Goes C, Almeida CT, Balbi AL. High-volume peritoneal dialysis in acute kidney injury: indications and limitations. *Clin J Am Soc Nephrol.* 2012;7:887-894.
38. Cullis B, Abdelraheem M, Abrahams G, et al. Peritoneal dialysis for acute kidney injury. *Perit Dial Int.* 2014;34:494-517.
39. Bagshaw SM, Berthiaume LR, Delaney A, Bellomo R. Continuous versus intermittent renal replacement therapy for critically ill patients with acute kidney injury: a meta-analysis. *Crit Care Med.* 2008;36:610-617.
40. Demirjian S, Teo BW, Guzman JA, et al. Hypophosphatemia during continuous hemodialysis is associated with prolonged respiratory failure in patients with acute kidney injury. *Nephrol Dial Transplant.* 2011;26:3508-3514.
41. Wilson FP, Berns JS. Vancomycin levels are frequently subtherapeutic during continuous venovenous hemodialysis (CVVHD). *Clin Nephrol.* 2012;77:329-331.
42. Zhang L, Yang J, Eastwood GM, Zhu G, Tanaka A, Bellomo R. Extended daily dialysis versus continuous renal replacement therapy for acute kidney injury: a meta-analysis. *Am J Kidney Dis.* 2015;66:322-330.
43. Davenport A, Will EJ, Davison AM. Early changes in intracranial pressure during haemofiltration treatment in patients with grade 4 hepatic encephalopathy and acute oliguric renal failure. *Nephrol Dial Transplant.* 1990;5:192-198.
44. Davenport A, Will EJ, Davison AM. Continuous vs. intermittent forms of haemofiltration and/or dialysis in the management of acute renal failure in patients with defective cerebral autoregulation at risk of cerebral oedema. *Contrib Nephrol.* 1991;93:225-233.
46. Ronco C, Bellomo R, Homel P, et al. Effects of different doses in continuous veno-venous haemofiltration on outcomes of acute renal failure: a prospective randomised trial. *Lancet.* 2000;356:26-30.
47. Schiffl H, Lang SM, Fischer R. Daily hemodialysis and the outcome of acute renal failure. *N Engl J Med.* 2002;346:305-310.
48. VA/NIH Acute Renal Failure Trial Network, Palevsky PM, Zhang JH, et al. Intensity of renal support in critically ill patients with acute kidney injury. *N Engl J Med.* 2008;359:7-20.
49. RENAL Replacement Therapy Study Investigators, Bellomo R, Cass A, et al. Intensity of continuous renal-replacement therapy in critically ill patients. *N Engl J Med.* 2009;361:1627-1638.
51. Tolwani AJ, Wille KM. Anticoagulation for continuous renal replacement therapy. *Semin Dial.* 2009;22:141-145.
52. Meier-Kriesche HU, Gitomer J, Finkel K, DuBose T. Increased total to ionized calcium ratio during continuous venovenous hemodialysis with regional citrate anticoagulation. *Crit Care Med.* 2001;29:748-752.
53. Morabito S, Pistolesi V, Tritapepe L, Fiaccadori E. Regional citrate anticoagulation for RRTs in critically ill patients with AKI. *Clin J Am Soc Nephrol.* 2014;9:2173-2188.
54. Oudemans-van Straaten HM, Bosman RJ, Koopmans M, et al. Citrate anticoagulation for continuous venovenous hemofiltration. *Crit Care Med.* 2009;37:545-552.
57. Herrera GA, Joseph L, Gu X, Hough A, Barlogie B. Renal pathologic spectrum in an autopsy series of patients with plasma cell dyscrasia. *Arch Pathol Lab Med.* 2004;128:875-879.
59. Hutchison CA, Cockwell P, Stringer S, et al. Early reduction of serum-free light chains associates with renal recovery in myeloma kidney. *J Am Soc Nephrol.* 2011;22:1129-1136.
60. Clark WF, Stewart AK, Rock GA, et al. Plasma exchange when myeloma presents as acute renal failure: a randomized, controlled trial. *Ann Intern Med.* 2005;143:777-784.

61. Dimopoulos MA, Roussou M, Gkotzamanidou M, et al. The role of novel agents on the reversibility of renal impairment in newly diagnosed symptomatic patients with multiple myeloma. *Leukemia.* 2013;27:423-429.

64. Hutchison CA, Cockwell P, Reid S, et al. Efficient removal of immunoglobulin free light chains by hemodialysis for multiple myeloma: in vitro and in vivo studies. *J Am Soc Nephrol.* 2007;18:886-895.

67. Hutchison CA, Cook M, Heyne N, et al. European trial of free light chain removal by extended haemodialysis in cast nephropathy (EuLITE): a randomised control trial. *Trials.* 2008;9:55.

68. Hutchison CA, Cook M, Heyne N, et al. European trial of free light chain removal by extended haemodialysis in cast nephropathy (EuLITE); survival and renal outcomes. *J Am Soc Nephrol.* 2016;27:8A.

71. Aronoff GR, Berns JS, Berns JS, et al. *Drug Prescribing in Renal Failure-Dosing Guidelines for Adults and Children.* 5th ed. Philadelphia, PA: American College of Physicians; 2007.

A full list of references is available at Expertconsult.com

Chronic Kidney Disease and Cancer

33 Chronic Kidney Disease as a Complication of Cancer, With Special Focus on Kidney and Urothelial Tumors

LAURA COSMAI, BEN SPRANGERS, CAMILLO PORTA, AND MAURIZIO GALLIENI

The Prevalence of Chronic Kidney Disease in Cancer Patients

The prevalence of chronic kidney disease (CKD) is reported to be high in patients with malignancy, being 33% and 27% according to Dogan et al.[1] and Launay-Vacher et al., respectively.[2] But the prevalence of CKD stage 3 or more is 20% after age 60 years, and it is 45% after age 70 years; furthermore, cancer is also more common in older people. Thus the percentages reported by Launay-Vacher and colleagues may simply show the coincidence of age, CKD, and cancer. Unfortunately, the Renal Insufficiency and Anticancer Medications (IRMA)-1 lacks any information relative to the timing of CKD prevalence relative to diagnosis and treatment of cancer.

However, the IRMA-1 study provided us with some important findings. It showed that 50% to 60% of the subjects had a reduced glomerular filtration rate (GFR < 90 mL/min/1.73 m^2), whereas serum creatinine (sCr) was normal in most patients.[2] These results emphasize not only that CKD incidence is high in subjects with malignancy, but also that creatinine is not sufficient to monitor such a condition. In France, a prevalence of a GFR below 90 mL/min/1.73 m^2 was 53% in IRMA-1[3] and 50% in IRMA-2,[4] within a cohort of 5000 subjects with different malignancies. According to the Kidney Disease Improving Global Outcomes (KDIGO) definition,[5] the prevalence of CKD stage 3 to 5 (GFR < 60 mL/min), excluding renal replacement therapy, was also high, reaching 12% in IRMA-1 and 12% in IRMA-2, respectively. Huang et al.[6] reported that despite having normal preoperative concentrations of sCr, 87% of renal cancer patients had an estimated GFR (eGFR) less than 90 mL/min/1.73 m^2. This study was performed in a cohort of 662 subjects with a renal cortical tumor, undergoing either partial or radical nephrectomy; in addition, an eGFR less than 60 mL/min/1.73 m^2 was reported in 26% of these patients.[6] Unfortunately, as for the IRMA report, the relative role of age has not been adequately considered as a possible confounding factor. Prevalence of CKD ranged from 16% to 25% in patients with malignancy in Belgium,[7] the United States,[8] and Japan.[9] In the IRMA-1 study, CKD was also highly prevalent, reaching approximately 50%, in breast, colorectal, lung, ovarian, or prostate cancers. The Belgian Renal Insufficiency and Anticancer Medications (BIRMA) study was a large (1218 patients), national, multicenter and retrospective study, performed to evaluate the prevalence of CKD in Belgian patients with malignancy.[7] Differently from the IRMA-1 study, one of the specific aims of BIRMA was also to describe the type and dosage of the antineoplastic agents prescribed according to kidney function.[7] Elevated sCr (≥ 1.2 mg/dL) was found in 15% of patients, but eGFR was below 90 mL/min/1.73 m^2 in 64% of them. Overall, 79% of patients ($n = 1087$) were administered at least one drug requiring dose adjustment because of kidney function, and 78% received at least one drug known to be nephrotoxic. Notably, 56% of CKD patients treated with chemotherapy agents requiring dose adjustment in case of reduced kidney function had no dose reductions.[7] This study proved that prevalence of CKD is high in patients with malignancy and may be underestimated.

CKD is more than just a measurement; it appears to affect survival. Yang et al.[10] reported that 32% of patients with newly diagnosed cancer had CKD; in addition, renal function was inversely related to all-cause mortality. Indeed, eGFR below 60 mL/min/1.73 m^2 was an independent predictor of mortality, as compared with eGFR 60 mL/min/1.73 m^2 or higher, and it was influenced by cancer site. After adjustment for possible confounders, eGFR less than 60 mL/min/1.73 m^2 at the time of diagnosis was associated with a higher mortality risk among patients with both hematologic malignancies and gynecologic cancers.

Wong et al. studied a cohort of 3654 subjects and assessed the relation between eGFR and risk of cancer. They found that in men, but not in women, with an eGFR lower than 55 mL/min/1.73 m^2, the risk for cancer was significantly higher.[11] In particular, lung and urinary tract cancer risk increased by 29% for each 10 mL fall in eGFR. Based on the aforementioned findings, it appears that CKD itself is a risk factor for cancer; in breast, colorectal, lung, ovarian, and skin cancers, the prevalence of CKD was increased. Others have confirmed that breast, cervix, colon, and kidney cancers are more common in CKD patients than in the general population.[12] Thus in addition to the observed increase in CKD prevalence in cancer patients, CKD is a risk factor for several malignancies.[13] However, not all solid tumors appear to be equally represented in this population. A retrospective cohort study of 1,190,538 adults assessed the association between eGFR level and the risk of incident cancer;[12]

Table 33.1   Factors With a Potential Negative Effect on Kidney Function in Cancer Patients

Factors	Proposed Mechanism(s)

Antineoplastic agents
  Cytotoxic agents
  Targeted therapies
  Immunotherapy
	Direct nephrotoxicity (AKI and CKD)
	  ▪ Hypertension and/or proteinuria
	  ▪ TMA
	  ▪ AKI
	Autoimmune nephritis

Other drugs (e.g., NSAIDs, bisphosphonates)	Direct nephrotoxicity
Radiation therapy that includes kidney	Fibrosis, vascular injury
Contrast medium	Direct nephrotoxicity
Paraneoplastic renal manifestations	Immune-mediated mechanisms
Nephrectomy	Loss of nephrons
Obstructions/compressions	Mechanical injury
Tumor infiltration	Kidney infiltration (loss of nephrons)
Comorbidities	▪ Preexisting CKD ▪ Hypertension ▪ Diabetes ▪ Previous episodes of AKI ▪ Previous use of nephrotoxic cancer therapies ▪ Glomerulonephritis

AKI, Acute kidney injury; *CKD*, chronic kidney disease; *NSAIDs*, nonsteroidal antiinflammatory drugs; *TMA*, thrombotic microangiopathy.

during 6,000,420 person years of follow-up, 76,809 incident cancers were identified in 72,875 subjects. After adjustment for time-updated confounders, lower eGFR was associated with an increased risk of renal cancer, with an adjusted hazard ratio (HR) of 2.28 (95% confidence interval [CI], 1.78–2.92) for an eGFR less than 30 mL/min/1.73 m^2.[12] The authors also observed an increased risk of urothelial cancer at an eGFR less than 30 mL/min/1.73 m^2, but no significant associations between eGFR and other cancers. Finally, CKD conferred an increased cancer-specific mortality in patients with kidney and urinary tract cancers.[14] In ESRD patients on dialysis, the observed increased risk for renal parenchymal cancer is related to the development of acquired renal cystic disease, which increases with time on dialysis.[15]

Factors with a potential negative effect on kidney function are summarized in Table 33.1. Thus the relationship between the kidney and cancer appears to be bidirectional.[16] For example, preexisting CKD may impact the bioavailability and/or safety profile of an anticancer drug, potentially leading to different and sometimes suboptimal treatment choices; on the other hand, it is also possible that unexpected renal effects of a novel anticancer drug may lead to progressive kidney injury or to worsening of preexisting CKD.[16]

Assessment of Kidney Function in Patient With Chronic Kidney Disease

The direct measurement of GFR is complex, cumbersome, and time-consuming to perform on an everyday basis. However, sCr may be used to estimate GFR in subjects with stable kidney function,[17] considering that precise GFR measurement is not required in most clinical settings. However, in some clinical situations, measuring GFR may be very useful for adjusting the doses of cancer medications, especially those with a narrow therapeutic index. Inulin clearance is the gold standard for the evaluation of GFR, but it is used only in clinical research settings;[17] alternative methods, radioactive or nonradioactive (iohexol, iothalamate, ethylenediaminetetraacetic acid [EDTA] or diethylenetriaminepentaacetate), represent simpler and less cumbersome methods, as compared with inulin clearance.[5] At present, the most commonly used methods for GFR assessment are the measurement of creatinine clearance (CrCl), and estimation formulas based upon sCr, such as the Cockcroft-Gault formula, the Modification of Diet in Renal Disease study formula, and the Chronic Kidney Disease Epidemiology Collaboration (CKD-EPI) formula.[5] Unfortunately, sCr is an unreliable marker during acute changes in renal function and its use to assess true kidney function has several limitations. A significant decline in GFR can be observed before it is reflected in an increased sCr; indeed, up to 50% of renal function could be lost before significant changes in sCr might be recorded. In addition, sCr does not reflect renal function during acute changes, until a steady state has been reached, which may require several days.

Concerning the different equations available to estimate GFR, the CKD-EPI formula is currently recommended to assess kidney function for screening and diagnosis of CKD, according to the KDIGO guidelines.[5] However, this formula has not been validated in cancer patients. It should also be underscored that people older than 65 years often (but not always) present with a decreased GFR,[18] because other comorbidities may influence kidney function.[19] As reviewed earlier, a reduced GFR is of particular importance in cancer patients for its clinical implications.[20]

A recent publication evaluating GFR estimating equations in cancer patients noted that body surface area (BSA)-adjusted CKD-EPI method appears to be the most accurate published model to estimate GFR in patients with cancer. BSA-adjusted CKD-EPI, based on the analysis of data from 2582 cancer patients using ^{51}Cr-EDTA GFR measurement as the gold standard, was found to be the most accurate and least biased published model to estimate GFR.[21] The authors also developed a new model that further improves the estimation of GFR and allows calculation of predictive confidence intervals for this estimation. The new model has been implemented as an online tool found at the following link: http://tavarelab.cruk.cam.ac.uk/JanowitzWilliamsGFR/. This new model to estimate GFR may represent a new standard of care and should be further examined along with BSA-adjusted CKD-EPI in clinical onconephrology practice.

In the field of cancer pharmacology, until recently, different studies have been performed using different estimation methods for kidney function. This highlights the need for a common language.

Finally, these assessments and adjustments are made on the basis of the apparent GFR. Many drugs are excreted via renal tubular epithelial transporters; measurement of that tubular excretory function is not done in clinical practice or in research. This is a potentially significant gap in our pharmacologic understanding and clinical care.

The Balance Between Toxicity and Efficacy in Chronic Kidney Disease Cancer Patients Treated With Anticancer Agents

Anticancer chemotherapy-related acute kidney injury (AKI) and CKD have been well described over the past decades; despite this, literature suggesting how to modify the doses of these agents in patients with underlying renal dysfunction, and those on dialysis, appears to be controversial, and too often not evidence-based.

Moreover, little is known about the appropriate use of targeted agents and immune checkpoint inhibitors in this population, leading to complex and nonevidence-based decisions in these settings. After decades of use of common cytotoxic drugs, clinicians versed in cancer care and its complications are well aware of the main toxicities of these cytotoxic agents, but less is known for targeted agents, and especially immunotherapy. On the other hand, novel anticancer agents that have recently entered clinical practice have a wide array of previously unrecognized and ill-defined adverse events.[22] Ultimately, these toxicities must be readily recognized and managed by those providing care for patients exposed to these drugs. This includes understanding risk factors for drug-induced kidney injury, appropriate drug dosing for the patient with CKD and those on dialysis, the clinical manifestations of drug nephrotoxicity, and the optimal management of nephrotoxic complications.[22] Whenever oncologists ask their nephrology colleagues to assess the degree of kidney function

to provide insight into dosage adjustment of anticancer therapy, a thorough knowledge of the specific metabolism of each anticancer agent and of its pharmacokinetic and pharmacodynamic properties is mandatory, to decide "if" the drug should be administered, "when" it is appropriate to administer it, and to "what extent" dosage adjustment should be used in the setting of underlying kidney disease.[16] This approach must be accurate, as unnecessary treatment interruptions and drug dose reductions may be associated with suboptimal cancer therapy, thus hampering the clinical benefits of cancer therapy. Optimal management of underlying CKD and its complications, and prevention of further kidney damage from other exogenous nephrotoxins (e.g., contrast medium, nonsteroidal antiinflammatory drugs, and bisphosphonates) in cancer patients with preexisting CKD, is also key to minimize drug-related complications. Patients with CKD and those on dialysis should not be undertreated for their neoplastic disease because of the fear of drug-induced adverse events.[23]

As already discussed, reduced GFR has been reported to be associated with reduced overall survival (HR, 1.27)[12,13] and increased cancer-related mortality,[14,15] with cutoff values for the significance of the effect of 60 (13,14), 70 (12), or 75 mL/min/1.73 m^2.[15] This association has been related to the impact of reduced GFR on the pharmacokinetics of anticancer drugs, leading to overexposure compared with normal renal function and dose-related toxicities.[24] Recently, Chen et al.[25] showed that patients with metastatic colorectal cancer and unrecognized kidney impairment at baseline experienced more toxicities, more often, leading to more treatment discontinuations and reduced time to progression.

The dose of anticancer drugs in CKD patients should be adjusted to avoid severe toxicities. In addition, using chemotherapeutics with potential nephrotoxicity will also require specific monitoring and, when available, specific prevention strategies to reduce the risk of kidney damage, especially in patients with preexisting CKD.[3] Some authorities advise that the noncorrected eGFR be used for adjustment of drug dosages, not the eGFR standardized to 1.73 m^2 BSA. In this perspective, specific and simple guidelines for monitoring each drug should be developed.

To date, only patients with adequate kidney function (sCr < 1.5 × the upper limit of normal) have been included in registered randomized controlled trials. A brief survey of the clinicaltrials.gov website showed that only 25% of active clinical cancer trials allowed subjects with an elevated sCr level. Thus we often lack an evidence base for patients with a CrCl less than 30 mL/min. This leads to limitations on use of some very effective cancer therapies. But this conservative recommendation may sometimes be inappropriate. For example, because large molecular weight monoclonal antibodies are cleared by the reticuloendothelial system and not metabolized or excreted by the kidneys; their clinical use should not be limited to patients with normal kidney function.[26] Although pharmacokinetic studies in patients with impaired renal function are sorely needed, as suggested by a recent European Medicine Agency guideline,[27] it is also clear that harmonization of kidney function assessment is mandatory, not only in early clinical trials, but also within pivotal trials of novel anticancer agents.

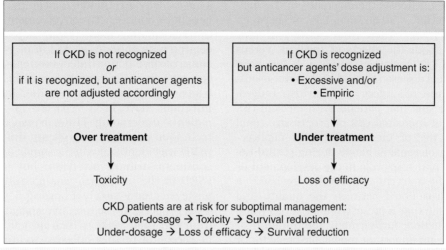

Fig. 33.1 The relationship between chronic kidney disease (CKD) and anticancer agents' dose adjustments. (Courtesy Vincent Launay-Vacher.)

Excluding patients with CKD and ESRD from these trials, especially from those that generate specific pharmacokinetic data, makes the results obtained in these studies not transferrable to the large number of patients with cancer with an underlying kidney disease. For these reasons, nephrologists should be involved in the design of the next generation of oncologic trials, especially when renal toxicity is expected to be an issue. Furthermore, the respective scientific societies should work together to accomplish this goal. Indeed, the full development of onconephrology as a new subspecialty is important because a number of key questions in the field remain not only unanswered, but also never asked.

Finding the right dose of a given anticancer agent in a patient with kidney impairment is key to minimize the risk of increased toxicities and to increase the likelihood of a benefit from the oncologic treatment, either in terms of response or of survival gain (Fig. 33.1).

Chronic Kidney Disease in Renal Cell Carcinoma Patients

Surgical resection remains the gold standard treatment for localized renal cell carcinoma (RCC) and has also been commonly performed for synchronous metastatic disease. Although radical nephrectomy remains the gold standard for many patients, nephron-sparing procedures are increasingly used for the treatment of small renal masses.[29] These two different strategies do not differ in terms of oncologic outcome, but clearly impact differently on the incidence of postoperative CKD and of cardiovascular complications.[30] Less invasive surgical procedures for RCC are associated with improved outcomes with less postoperative AKI and CKD, and less cardiovascular complications.[30] Indeed, 22% of patients with renal tumors had a prenephrectomy stage 3 or greater CKD (eGFR < 60 mL/min/1.73 m^2).[8] In patients 70 years of age and older, this percentage approaches 40%. Furthermore, patients that had postoperative AKI

after radical nephrectomy had a fourfold higher risk of developing new-onset CKD,[31] although others have suggested that most CKD after kidney cancer surgery, is the progression of existing medical renal disease that was present before the diagnosis of cancer. Progression of underlying CKD was also noted in patients undergoing a radical nephrectomy for an RCC.[31] Accordingly, both the American Urological Association[32] and the European Association of Urology[33] endorsed partial nephrectomy as the standard of care for organ-confined tumors smaller than 4 cm (T1a) and suggested that it should be considered for patients with tumors larger than 4 cm but smaller than 7 cm (T1b). Evidence for a relationship between the extent of kidney tissue removal and the risk of CKD comes from single-center retrospective studies, population-based studies, and a single randomized, controlled, phase 3 study.[30] Among the population-based studies available between 1990 and 2011, a metaanalysis of 36 studies, examined 31,729 patients treated with radical nephrectomy and 9281 patients who underwent partial nephrectomy.[34] The results showed that partial nephrectomy was associated with a 19% reduction in the risk of all-cause mortality (HR, 0.81), a 29% reduction in cancer-specific mortality (HR, 0.71), and a 61% reduction in the risk of severe CKD (HR, 0.39), supporting the findings observed in a number of smaller studies.[30] But a randomized controlled trial on the surgical approach to RCC did not show a benefit of partial nephrectomy.[35] This trial reported a 'better' outcome in patients treated with radical nephrectomy compared with those treated with partial nephrectomy. During a median follow-up of more than 9 years, death occurred in 25% of patients treated by partial nephrectomy and in 18% of those undergoing radical nephrectomy. Cardiovascular disease was noted to be the most common cause of death. The intention-to-treat analysis showed a 10-year overall survival rate of 81.1% in the radical nephrectomy group compared with 75.5% in the nephron-sparing surgery group (HR, 1.5; 95% CI, 1.03–2.16). Interestingly, partial nephrectomy was associated with a 21% reduction in the absolute risk of developing moderate CKD (eGFR < 60 mL/min/1.73 m^2) over a median follow-up of 6.7 years, whereas the difference in the incidence of severe CKD (eGFR < 30 mL/min/1.73 m^2) between the two groups was 3.7%.[35] These results have generated various hypotheses about the effects of medical- versus surgical-associated CKD on patient survival. It has been speculated that medical disease-related CKD has worse outcomes than CKD because of surgery (nephron loss). Indeed, a recent report suggested that patients with medical risk factors for CKD are at increased risk of progressive renal impairment, irrespective of the use of partial nephrectomy.[36] The duration of renal ischemia during partial nephrectomy may also play a key role in the development of postoperative CKD. In a recent collaborative review,[37] a strong association was noted between the quality and quantity of renal tissue that is preserved after surgery and long-term kidney function; furthermore, the duration of ischemia proved to be an important modifiable predictor of postoperative kidney function. Prolonged warm ischemia time (WIT) was significantly associated with adverse postoperative kidney function.[37] Indeed, available data suggest a renal benefit of keeping WIT less than 25 minutes. Conversely, cold ischemia appears to safely allow longer durations of ischemia.

Finally, patients with CKD (irrespective of its cause), within the setting of a metastatic cancer, usually tolerate cancer-targeted agents poorly, experiencing higher-grade adverse events compared with patients with normal kidney function.[16] This is another reason to try to preserve as much as possible an adequate renal function from the beginning.

Chronic Kidney Disease in Urothelial Cancer Patients

Renal function loss results from and is an active therapeutic concern for these urinary tract cancers. Despite the good results of two large metaanalyses demonstrating a positive survival impact of either neo-adjuvant[38] or adjuvant[39] chemotherapy in patients with muscle-invasive bladder cancer (MIBC), the percentage of patients treated with perioperative chemotherapy has been astonishingly low until today,[40,41] leaving much room for improvement of clinical care in this patient cohort.

The reasons for such an attitude are diverse and include the fact that many patients affected with MIBC are unsuitable—or else are perceived as such—for cisplatin (CDDP)-based combinations.[42] Such CDDP ineligibility is mainly because of the presence of concomitant illnesses in an often-aging patient population, particularly cardiovascular diseases and more often CKD.[42] Not only is CKD common in patients with MIBC, but it is also an important risk factor for tumor recurrence and progression toward muscle invasive forms and a predictor of poor overall survival.[43] Urothelial cancer is a family of neoplasms characterized by an extremely high incidence of kidney impairment throughout its whole natural history, whereas surgical and medical treatments—the latter including cytotoxic chemotherapy, biological agents, and immune checkpoint inhibitors—often impact on kidney function or cause renal adverse events.

That is why urothelial cancer patients would greatly benefit by a more active involvement of the nephrologists in their management. First, nephrologists could help dealing with episodes of AKI or of worsening of CKD because of obstruction/infections, episodes which are quite common in patients with non-MIBC undergoing several transurethral resections (TURs); indeed, urinary tract infections have been reported in as many as 7% of patients undergoing TURs, irrespective of the specific technique used.[23] No significant difference in the rate of ESRD was identified when comparing ileal conduits with continent urinary diversion, but a significant risk of ESRD in the long term was identified in patients with postcystectomy survival beyond 5 years.[44] If not managed properly, these infective episodes may leave kidney injury in their wake, which may impact on the chance of receiving further effective treatments. In MIBC, the nephrologist could contribute—acting before and during anticancer therapy—to reduce the number of patients unsuitable for CDDP-based neo-adjuvant (or adjuvant) chemotherapy and those who cannot complete the scheduled treatment because of a deterioration in their kidney function.[45,46] In patients receiving nephrectomy (in the case of upper urinary tract neoplasms) or cystectomy, either with neobladder or urinary diversion (in the case of bladder cancers), renal function deterioration is extremely common. Preoperative comorbidities, such as hypertension, diabetes, cardiovascular diseases, preexisting CKD, and postoperative hydronephrosis, pyelonephritis, and ureteroenteric fistulae, represent other potentially modifiable factors associated with a decrease in kidney function.[47] Finally, in the metastatic setting, the nephrologic management of renal toxicities from systemic therapies would be increasingly important. Cis-platinum has well-known toxicity as do other cytotoxic agents (e.g., gemcitabine and vinflunine). To this is added the possible toxicities of immune checkpoint inhibitors that can cause interstitial nephritis and electrolyte disturbances.[48]

It is thus clear that urothelial cancer, which to date has been managed mainly by urologists, and at a lesser extent, by oncologists, should be considered a malignancy where the contribution of the nephrologist is key.

Chronic Kidney Disease Directly Induced by the Tumor

Advanced-stage cancer may be associated with malignant ureteral obstruction, leading to obstructive nephropathy and CKD. Direct ureteral infiltration by tumor or extrinsic ureter compression by bulky tumor masses may cause this.[49] In general, cervical, bladder, and prostate cancers are the most common culprits.[49] However, urinary obstructions can also occur from retroperitoneal fibrosis because of surgery, chemotherapy (especially intraperitoneal), and/or radiotherapy. In these cases, percutaneous nephrostomy tube placement or retrograde ureteral double-J stent placement should be urgently performed, recognizing the associated procedural complications.[49] Recently, a prognostic model for survival after palliative urinary diversion for malignant urinary obstruction has been developed, as reported in this book's chapter on urinary tract obstruction.[50] Even in those patients with the most favorable prognosis, this model showed a 1-year patient survival of only 45%.

Summary

In patients with cancer, estimating renal function with an appropriate and validated method is mandatory to diagnose CKD and improve anticancer drug handling. When a patient has a GFR less than 60 mL/min, nephrotoxic drugs should be avoided whenever possible; when a nephrotoxic drug is mandatory, specific methods to prevent renal toxicity must be used. Dose adjustments according to kidney function may be needed for every anticancer drug, whatever the route of elimination, and whatever the relative risk of renal toxicity.

In conclusion, CKD is highly prevalent in oncologic patients and appears to be a risk factor for the development of cancer. Furthermore, the use of antineoplastic drugs in patients with underlying CKD raises several specific issues: (1) the direct nephrotoxicity of several anticancer agents; (2) the need to adjust antineoplastic doses because of concomitant CKD; (3) the lack of prospective drug dosing data in patients with advanced CKD or those on dialysis; and (4) the nihilistic approach to the treatment of patients with CKD, leading to their frequent undertreatment (or even absence of treatment), ultimately denying them potentially life-prolonging options.

Key Points

- The relationship between chronic kidney disease (CKD) and cancer should be regarded as bidirectional. Preexisting CKD is highly prevalent among cancer patients. Furthermore, cancer patients may present with acute or slowly developing kidney injury because of drug toxicities or other complications.
- The Chronic Kidney Disease Epidemiology Collaboration formula is currently recommended to assess kidney function for screening and diagnosis of CKD, according to the Kidney Disease Improving Global Outcomes guidelines. However, in the field of cancer pharmacology, many studies have been performed using different estimation methods for kidney function. This highlights the need of a common language between oncologists and nephrologists.
- The literature is controversial on how to modify the doses of anticancer agents in patients with underlying renal dysfunction, and those on dialysis. It is often not evidence-based.
- Nephrectomy for kidney cancer is another common cause of CKD, but the use of nephron-sparing surgical techniques may mitigate its severity. Medical disease–related CKD has worse outcomes than CKD because of surgery, taking into account that renal cell carcinoma cancer patients with CKD (irrespective of its cause) usually tolerate cancer treatments poorly, experiencing higher-grade adverse events compared with patients with normal kidney function.

- Urothelial cancer, which to date has been managed mainly by urologists, and at a lesser extent, by oncologists, should be considered a malignancy where the contribution of the nephrologist is key.

References

1. Dogan E, Izmirli M, Ceylan K, et al. Incidence of renal insufficiency in cancer patients. *Adv Ther*. 2005;22:357-362.
2. Launay-Vacher V, Izzedine H, Rey JB, et al. Incidence of renal insufficiency in cancer patients and evaluation of information available on the use of anticancer drugs in renally impaired patients. *Med Sci Monit*. 2004;10:CR209-CR212.
3. Launay-Vacher V, Oudard S, Janus N, et al., for Renal Insufficiency and Cancer Medications (IRMA) Study Group. Prevalence of renal insufficiency in cancer patients and implications for anticancer drug management: the renal insufficiency and anticancer medications (IRMA) study. *Cancer*. 2007;110:1376-1384.
4. Janus N, Oudard S, Beuzeboc P, et al. Prevalence of renal insufficiency in cancer patients: data from the IRMA-2 study. *J Clin Oncol*. 2009;27(suppl 15):e20574.
5. Levey AS, de Jong PE, Coresh J, et al. The definition, classification, and prognosis of chronic kidney disease: a KDIGO Controversies Conference report. *Kidney Int*. 2011;80:17-28.
6. Huang WC, Levey AS, Serio AM, et al. Chronic kidney disease after nephrectomy in patients with renal cortical tumours: a retrospective cohort study. *Lancet Oncol*. 2006;7:735-740.
7. Janus N, Launay-Vacher V, Byloos E, et al. Cancer and renal insufficiency results of the BIRMA study. *Br J Cancer*. 2010;103:1815-1821.
8. Canter D, Kutikov A, Sirohi M, et al. Prevalence of baseline chronic kidney disease in patients presenting with solid renal tumors. *Urology*. 2011;77:781-785.
9. Nakamura Y, Tsuchiya K, Nitta K, Ando M. Prevalence of anemia and chronic kidney disease in cancer patients: clinical significance for 1-year mortality. *Nihon Jinzo Gakkai Shi*. 2011;53:38-45.
10. Yang Y, Li HY, Zhou Q, et al. Renal function and all-cause mortality risk among cancer patients. *Medicine (Baltimore)*. 2016;95(20):e3728.
11. Wong G, Hayen A, Chapman JR, et al. Association of CKD and cancer risk in older people. *J Am Soc Nephrol*. 2009;20:1341-1350.
12. Lowrance WT, Ordoñez J, Udaltsova N, Russo P, Go AS. CKD and the risk of incident cancer. *J Am Soc Nephrol*. 2014;25:2327-2334.
13. Stengel B. Chronic kidney disease and cancer: a troubling connection. *J Nephrol*. 2010;23:253-262.
14. Weng PH, Hung KY, Huang HL, Chen JH, Sung PK, Huang CK. Cancer-specific mortality in chronic kidney disease: longitudinal follow-up of a large cohort. *Clin J Am Soc Nephrol*. 2011;6:1121-1128.
15. Stewart JH, Buccianti G, Agodoa L, et al. Cancers of the kidney and urinary tract in patients on dialysis for end-stage renal disease: analysis of data from the United States, Europe, and Australia and New Zealand. *J Am Soc Nephrol*. 2003;14:197-207.
16. Porta C, Cosmai L, Gallieni M, Pedrazzoli P, Malberti F. Renal effects of targeted anticancer therapies. *Nat Rev Nephrol*. 2015;11:354-370.
17. Rule AD, Bergstralh EJ, Slezak JM, Bergert J, Larson TS. Glomerular filtration rate estimated by cystatin C among different clinical presentation. *Kidney Int*. 2006;69:399-405.
18. Fliser D, Franek E, Joest M, Block S, Mutschler E, Ritz E. Renal function in the elderly: impact of hypertension and cardiac function. *Kidney Int*. 1997;51:1196-1204.
19. Bachorzewska-Gajewska H, Malyszko J, Malyszko JS, Dobrzycki S, Sobkowicz B, Musial W. Estimation of glomerular filtration rate in patients with normal serum creatinine undergoing primary PCI: is it really normal? *Nephrol Dial Transplant*. 2006;21:1736-1738.
20. Iff S, Craig JC, Turner R, et al. Reduced estimated GFR and cancer mortality. *Am J Kidney Dis*. 2014;63:23-30.
21. Janowitz T, Williams EH, Marshall A, et al. New model for estimating glomerular filtration rate in patients with cancer. *J Clin Oncol*. 2017;35(24):2798-2805.
22. Porta C, Paglino C, Imarisio I, Bonomi L. Uncovering Pandora's vase: the growing problem of new toxicities from novel anticancer agents. The case of sorafenib and sunitinib. *Clin Exp Med*. 2007;7:127-134.
23. Cosmai L, Porta C, Gallieni M, Perazzella MA. Onco-nephrology: a decalogue. *Nephrol Dial Transplant*. 2016;4:515-519.

24. Launay-Vacher V. Cancer and the kidney: individualizing dosage according to renal function. *Ann Oncol.* 2013;23:2713-2714.

25. Chen J, Wang XT, Luo PH, He QJ. Effects of unidentified renal insufficiency on the safety and efficacy of chemotherapy for metastatic colorectal cancer patients: a prospective, observational study. *Support Care Cancer.* 2015;23:1043-1048.

26. Porta C, Cosmai L, Gallieni M, Perazella MA. Harmonization of renal function assessment is needed throughout the whole process of anti-cancer drug development. *J Clin Oncol.* 2016;20:2429-2430.

27. European Medicines Agency Committee for medicinal products for human use. *Guideline on the evaluation of the pharmacokinetics of medicinal products in patients with decreased renal function.* 2015. Available at: http://www.ema.europa.eu/docs/en_GB/document_library/Scientific_guideline/2016/02/WC500200841.pdf.

28. Launay-Vacher V. Renal dysfunction has statistically and clinically significant deleterious effects on anticancer drug safety. *J Clin Oncol.* 2016;34(20):2428.

29. Fernando A, Fowler S, O'Brien T; British Association of Urological Surgeons (BAUS). Nephron-sparing surgery across a nation - outcomes from the British Association of Urological Surgeons 2012 national partial nephrectomy audit. *BJU Int.* 2016;177(6):874-882.

30. Li L, Lau WL, Rhee CM, et al. Risk of chronic kidney disease after cancer nephrectomy. *Nat Rev Nephrol.* 2014;10:135-145.

31. Cho A, Lee JE, Kwon GY, et al. Post-operative acute kidney injury in patients with renal cell carcinoma is a potent risk factor for new-onset chronic kidney disease after radical nephrectomy. *Nephrol Dial Transplant.* 2011;26:3496-3501.

32. Campbell SC, Novick AC, Belldegrun A, et al., Practice Guidelines Committee of the American Urological Association. Guideline for management of the clinical T1 renal mass. *J Urol.* 2009;182:1271-1279.

33. Ljungberg B, Bensalah K, Canfield S, et al. EAU guidelines on renal cell carcinoma: 2014 update. *Eur Urol.* 2015;67:913-924.

34. Kim SP, Thompson RH, Boorjian SA, et al. Comparative effectiveness for survival and renal function of partial and radical nephrectomy for localized renal tumors: a systematic review and meta-analysis. *J Urol.* 2012;188:51-57.

35. Van Poppel H, Da Pozzo L, Albrecht W, et al. A prospective, randomised EORTC intergroup phase 3 study comparing the oncologic outcome of elective nephron-sparing surgery and radical nephrectomy for low-stage renal cell carcinoma. *Eur Urol.* 2011;59:543-552.

36. Satasivam P, Reeves F, Rao K, et al. Patients with medical risk factors for chronic kidney disease are at increased risk of renal impairment despite the use of nephron-sparing surgery. *BJU Int.* 2015;116:590-595.

37. Volpe A, Blute ML, Ficarra V, et al. Renal ischemia and function after partial nephrectomy: a collaborative review of the literature. *Eur Urol.* 2015;68:61-74.

38. Leow JJ, Martin-Doyle W, Rajagopal PS, et al. Adjuvant chemotherapy for invasive bladder cancer: a 2013 updated systematic review and meta-analysis of randomized trials. *Eur Urol.* 2014;66(1):42-54.

39. Yin M, Joshi M, Meijer RP, et al. Neoadjuvant chemotherapy for muscle-invasive bladder cancer: a systematic review and two-step meta-analysis. *Oncologist.* 2016;21(6):708-715.

40. Schiffmann J, Sun M, Gandaglia G, et al. Suboptimal use of neoadjuvant chemotherapy in radical cystectomy patients: a population-based study. *Can Urol Assoc J.* 2016;10(3-4):E82-E86.

41. Porter MP, Kerrigan MC, Donato BM, Ramsey SD. Patterns of use of systemic chemotherapy for Medicare beneficiaries with urothelial bladder cancer. *Urol Oncol.* 2011;29:252-258.

42. Cathomas R, De Santis M, Galsky MD. First-line treatment of metastatic disease: cisplatin-ineligible patients. *Hematol Oncol Clin North Am.* 2015;29(2):329-340.

43. Li CE, Chien CS, Chuang YC, Chang YI, Tang HP, Kang CH. Chronic kidney disease as an important risk factor for tumor recurrences, progression and overall survival in primary non-muscle-invasive bladder cancer. *Int Urol Nephrol.* 2016;48(6):993-999.

44. Zabell JR, Adejoro O, Konety BR, Weight CJ. Risk of end stage kidney disease after radical cystectomy according to urinary diversion type. *J Urol.* 2015;193(4):1283-1287.

45. Nicholson S. Chemotherapy for bladder cancer in patients with impaired renal function. *Nat Rev Urol.* 2011;9:52-57.

46. Dash A, Galsky MD, Vickers AJ, et al. Impact of renal impairment on eligibility for adjuvant cisplatin-based chemotherapy in patients with urothelial carcinoma of the bladder. *Cancer.* 2006;3:506-513.

47. Eisenberg MS, Thompson RH, Frank I, et al. Long-term renal function outcomes after radical cystectomy. *J Urol.* 2014;191(3):619-625.

48. Wanchoo R, Karam S, Uppal NN, et al. Adverse renal effects of immune checkpoint inhibitors: a narrative review. *Am J Nephrol.* 2017;45(2):160-169.

49. Russo P. Ureteral obstruction and stents: still a difficult problem for patients and urologists alike. *J Urol.* 2005;174:2088.

50. Cordeiro MD, Coelho RF, Chade DC, et al. A prognostic model for survival after palliative urinary diversion for malignant ureteric obstruction: a prospective study of 208 patients. *BJU Int.* 2016;2:266-271.

34 Incidence of Cancer and Screening Recommendations

GERMAINE WONG AND JEAN L. HOLLEY

Introduction

The purpose of cancer screening is to identify treatable cancers early to improve survival. Effective cancer screening therefore depends on cancer occurrence and risk, the availability and effectiveness of cancer screening tools, and expected survival in a given population. Cancer screening is beneficial if the screening tests used identify early stage, potentially curable cancers in individuals who have long expected survival in the absence of the identified cancer. Ideally, the screening test is sensitive and specific to avoid unnecessary risks and additional testing. Screening tests are also more effective if they are simple to perform and widely available. The best screening tests are also relatively inexpensive. Assuming a screening test detects a cancer at a curable stage, the effectiveness of the screening test can be assessed by calculating quality of life years saved. Implicit in this calculation is an assumption of expected survival and cancer risk in the person to be screened. Using this method, governing bodies and societies make recommendations for cancer screening in populations.

Some recommendations for cancer screening in the adult population are shown in Table 34.1. Most recommendations account for cancer risk factors based on demographics and family history in addition to other underlying factors that are cancer and/or organ-specific. All of the recommendations assume the individual to be screened is healthy with a normal expected survival by gender and age. However, in the case of chronic kidney disease (CKD) or end-stage renal disease (ESRD), survival is lower than the normal population, and thus "routine" cancer screening recommendations require adjustment. This chapter will review the issues affecting cancer screening in those with CKD and ESRD and make recommendations for screening based on these issues.

Cancer Risk in Chronic Kidney Disease and End-Stage Renal Disease

Many retrospective cohort studies have shown an increased incidence of cancer in ESRD patients,[1–3] but the data are less clear among nondialysis CKD patients.[4–10] Table 34.2 summarizes the literature examining cancer incidence among CKD patients not on dialysis. Most of these studies report hazard ratios for cancer. Although cancers of the urinary tract appear to be more common among nondialysis CKD patients,[4,5,7,9,10] overall, the risk for most cancers does not appear to be increased in CKD

patients.[4,8,9] The definition of CKD varies somewhat in these studies, with some reporting specific CKD stages[4] (see Table 34.2) and others relying on billing codes for diagnoses like CKD, chronic glomerulonephritis, hypertensive CKD, and diabetic kidney disease,[10] making comparisons among studies difficult. It should be noted that the higher risk of upper urinary tract urothelial cancers is particularly prominent in studies from Asia, where these cancers also occur more frequently in the general population.[10] The reasons for this are unclear but differences in culture, lifestyle, diet, and drug use are likely.[10] For example, aristocholic acid present in some fruits has been identified as a carcinogenic factor and may represent a risk for this population.[10] In addition, certain causes of CKD, like analgesic abuse (containing phenacetin) and Balkan nephropathy (also related to aristocholic acid) are also associated with an increased risk of urothelial cancers and may be more common among certain populations.

Unlike the CKD population, cancer incidence is usually reported to be higher among ESRD patients.[1–3,11–17] Table 34.3 summarizes the available literature, demonstrating higher standardized incidence ratio (SIR) among ESRD patients for many specific cancers. The SIR is the typical marker for cancer incidence and represents an estimate of the occurrence of cancer in a population relative to what might be expected if the population had the same cancer experience as a larger comparison group. In most of these observational studies, virally mediated cancers are more common in dialysis patients. These cancers include tongue and cervical cancer (associated with human papilloma virus) and liver cancers associated with hepatitis B and C. As in the nondialysis CKD group, cancers of the urinary tract are significantly more common among dialysis patients and include renal cell carcinoma (RCC), bladder cancer, and urothelial cancers of the upper urinary tract.[17–20] Risk factors for these types of cancer in the kidney disease patients include acquired cystic disease in dialysis patients and analgesic abuse and Balkan nephropathy as causes of the ESRD. Most studies do not show an increased SIR for breast, lung, and colorectal cancer in ESRD patients (see Table 34.3). However, thyroid and other endocrine cancers appear to be more common for unclear reasons.[2–4,7]

The stage of cancer at the time of diagnosis is similar in ESRD patients compared with the general population except for colorectal cancers, which tend to be diagnosed earlier in dialysis patients.[21] It is likely that gastrointestinal disorders, such as bleeding, occur commonly in dialysis patients and lead to more frequent investigative procedures that result in a cancer diagnosis. In this study, prostate cancer tended to be diagnosed later in the ESRD patients.[21]

Table 34.1 American Cancer Society Recommendations for Cancer Screening in the Normal Population

Cancer	Recommended Screening
Breast	women age 40–44 years—individualized[a] women age 45–54 years—yearly mammogram women > 55 years—mammogram every 2 years continue as long as expected survival ≥ 10 years

Colon and Rectal	starting at age 50 years:
	  colonoscopy every 10 years or
	  CT colonography every 5 years[b] or
	  flexible-sigmoidoscopy every 5 years[b] or
	  double contrast barium enema every 5 years[b]
	  yearly fecal immunochemical test (FIT)[c]
	  yearly guaiac-based fecal occult blood test[c]
	  stool DNA test every 3 years

Cervical[d]	women age 21–29 years
	  Pap every 3 years, no HPV unless Pap abnormal
	women age 30–65 years
	  Pap + HPV every 5 years or Pap alone every 3 years
	women > 65 years
	  if normal testing past 10 years, no further testing
	  if abnormal testing, continue testing for 20 years
	  Hysterectomy
	  no testing

Lung	for those at high risk
	  annual low-dose CT chest
	high risk = 55–74 years of age in good health;
	  at least 30 pack years smoking and still smoking
	  or quit within the past 15 years

Prostate	men age 50 years—individualized[a] African American or father or brother with prostate cancer ≤ 45 years—individualized* PSA with or without rectal examination

[a]Discuss pros and cons with primary care provider.
[b]If test is positive, colonoscopy should be done.
[c]Multiple stool take home tests required, one office-based test insufficient.
[d]PAP.
CT, Computed tomography; DNA, deoxyribonucleic acid; HPV, human papilloma virus; Pap, Papanicolau smear; PSA, prostate-specific antigen.
Modified from the American Cancer Society website: www.cancer.org/healthy/find-cancer-early/cancer-screening-guidelines.html (Accessed March 10, 2017).

Table 34.2 Cancer Incidence in Chronic Kidney Disease

eGFR, mL/min	Hazard Ratio Overall (CI)	Ref	Hazard Ratio Urinary Tract Cancer	Ref
≥ 60–75	0.98 (0.87–1.10)	4		
≥ 45–60	0.99 (0.88–1.113)	4	1.35–1.39 (1.22–1.58)	4,5
< 45	1.01 (0.84–1.22)	4	1.63–1.81 (1.51–2.17)	4,5
< 30			1.63–2.28 (1.78–2.92)	5,10

CI, Confidence interval; eGFR, estimated glomerular filtration rate.

Cancer Risk in Kidney Transplant Recipients

Kidney transplant recipients experience an increased risk of cancer by at least 2 to 4 times compared with the age and gender-matched general population.[3] The excess risks of cancer among transplant recipients are site specific for virally related cancers, non-melanoma skin cancer, and urothelial cancers. The greatest increased risk is seen in

Table 34.3 Cancer Incidence in End-Stage Renal Disease

Cancer	SIR	Ref
Renal cell	3.6–24.1	1,2,4,12–15,17,20
Bladder & ureter	1.5–16.4	1,213,14–16,17,19,20
Tongue	1.2–1.9	1,2,14
Cervical & uterine	2.7–4.3	1,2
Liver	1.4–4.5	1,2,13,14
Thyroid & other endocrine	2.2–2.3	1,2,4,14
Breast	0.8–1.42	2,14,15
Lung/bronchus	0.5–1.28	2,14,15
Colon, rectum	1.0–1.27	2,14,15,17
Pancreas	1.08	15
Prostate	0.5–1.08	2,14,15

SIR, Standardized incidence ratio

Kaposi sarcoma (up to 300 times), non-NMSC (2–40 times), lip cancer (more than 10 times), and cancers with a suspected viral oncogenesis, such as non-Hodgkin lymphoma/posttransplant lymphoproliferative disorder (4–16 times), and anogenital cancers. RCC is the most common urological malignancy after kidney transplantation. Compared with the general population, the risk of RCC is increased by approximately sixfold. The most common subtypes include papillary and clear cell RCC.[22] There is a modest increased risk for other common cancer types, such as colorectal and lung cancer (by approximately 1.5–3 times), but most observational data show no increased risk for breast and prostate cancer compared with the age- and gender-matched general population.[23]

There is now clear evidence suggesting the increased risk of cancer among transplant recipients is related to the prolonged use of immunosuppression over time. There is also emerging evidence suggesting the pattern of the excess risk may differ by the dose and types of immunosuppression.[24] Transplant recipients who received horse antithymocyte globulin, rabbit antithymocyte globulin (thymoglobulin), or OKT3 as induction therapy had rates of lymphoma more than 20 times that of the age- and gender-matched general population.[25] Use of alemtuzumab for induction therapy is associated with an increased risk of non-Hodgkin lymphoma, colorectal cancer, and thyroid cancer.[26] In the context of maintenance immunosuppression, preclinical evidence has suggested that the oncogenicity of azathioprine and calcineurin inhibitors (CNIs) is associated with impairment in the ability to repair deoxyribonucleic acid (DNA) damage,[27] thus leading to stimulation of prooncogenic cytokines and growth factors, including transforming growth factor β, vascular endothelial growth factor, and their receptors. On the contrary, trial-based evidence of mammalian target of rapamycin (mTOR) inhibitor such as sirolimus, has reported a significant reduction in the overall risk of developing skin cancer, particularly for non-melanoma skin cancer.[28,29] So far, there are three multicentered randomized controlled trials comparing the incidence of non-melanoma skin cancer as the primary outcome between mTOR inhibitors and CNIs, as maintenance immunosuppression after kidney transplantation.[30–32] All found a 20% to 30% reduced risk of squamous cell carcinoma (SCC) among the mTOR inhibitor arms compared with the CNIs arm, after a follow-up time of 12 months. Also, those with a prior history of SCC experienced a longer time to the development of new SCC among the mTOR inhibitors arms.

Efficacy of Cancer Screening Tests

Cancer screening depends on imaging, visual inspection via procedures, and laboratory and histopathologic tests, as described in Table 34.1. The effectiveness of these in ESRD has rarely been assessed and thus the positive and negative predictive value and sensitivity and specificity of these examinations in the ESRD population are not known. Vascular calcification is common in ESRD patients and its presence may complicate interpretation of mammograms in women with ESRD.[33,34] Stool hemoccult testing is a noninvasive means of screening for colon cancer (see Table 34.1) but is subject to high false positive results (positive test caused by noncancer cause) in ESRD patients.[35] Thus positive hemoccult testing in dialysis patients may contribute to higher rates of colonoscopy in this population. We do not have information on the sensitivity and specificity of fecal immunochemical or DNA testing in ESRD patients.

Tumor markers are also used as cancer screening tools but their effectiveness can be affected by kidney dysfunction, primarily caused by reduced clearance. Clearance with dialysis can also influence the use of these proteins in ESRD patients. Table 34.4 shows common tumor markers and their chemical structure and biological function that may be affected by CKD and dialysis.[36] Most tumor markers are unreliable in ESRD patients because they are generally glycoproteins with high molecular weight, rarely removed by dialysis, and rise with hemoconcentration, yielding false-positive results in ESRD. Total prostate specific antigen (PSA) is probably valid in ESRD patients,[37] but free PSA and free/total PSA ratios are less useful, because free PSA

rises with hemoconcentration and high-flux dialysis membranes affect its clearance.[37–39] Controversy continues about screening for prostate cancer in the general population (see Table 34.1). Cancer antigen 125 (CA-125), a tumor marker for ovarian cancer, is produced by mesothelial cells and patients with any serosal fluid (pleural effusion, ascites) will have elevated levels. Thus CA-125 is less useful in ESRD patients, particularly those on peritoneal dialysis. β-human chorionic gonadotropin and α-fetoprotein are probably reliable in ESRD patients.

The performances of cancer screening tests are also likely to be different in kidney transplant recipients. In the case of colorectal cancer screening, transplant recipients receiving immunosuppression with mycophenolate mofetil (MMF) may experience MMF-related enterocolitis and associated occult gastrointestinal bleeding. The use of antiplatelet agents for cardiovascular risk prevention may also affect the false-positive rate of stool hemoccult testing. The development of new breast lesions in patients after renal transplantation on maintenance cyclosporine is not uncommon.[40] Most of these lesions are benign breast disease including fibroadenoma, fibrocystic changes, and dense fibrosis. Many of these lesions may mimic malignant lesion on mammography and ultrasound, and thus influence the overall test specificity. Given the excess risk of RCC in kidney transplant recipients, many transplant centers recommend annual or biennial ultrasonographic screening for both the native and transplanted kidneys in high-risk kidney transplant recipients. Although there has been no trial-based evidence to support or refute routine screening for RCC, modeling analyses report a total of two and one cancer deaths averted in the annually and biennially screened population, with a relative cancer-specific mortality reduction by 25% and 12.5%. However, only an absolute mortality reduction of 0.2% and 0.1% occurred for annual and biannual screening, respectively.[41] Using a series of sensitivity analyses, the benefits from routine screening was most sensitive to the test specificity of ultrasonography, prevalence of disease, and the risk of graft failure in the screened population. The accuracy of ultrasonography is an important determinant of screening efficiency, but it is uncertain in recipients of kidney transplants. Not only is ultrasonography operator-dependent, but its performance also varies with the size and morphology of the patient, the

Table 34.4   Chemical Structure and Biological Function of Tumor Markers and End-Stage Renal Disease/Dialysis

Marker	Weight kDa	Effect of CKD/HD/PD	Chemical Structure	Removed by Dialysis
Carcinoembryonic antigen (CEA)	180	— — —	glycoprotein	no
Alpha fetoprotein (AFP)	65	— — —	glycoprotein	no
Prostate specific antigen (PSA)	33	— — —	protease	yes
Carbohydrate antigen 125 (CA 125)	90	— — ↑	glycoprotein	no
Carbohydrate antigen 19.9 (CA 19.9)	360	? ? ?	glycoprotein	no
Carbohydrate antigen 15.3 (CA 15.3)	300–400	? ? ↑	glycoprotein	no
β-human chorionic gonadotropin	40	↑ ↑	glycoprotein	yes

CKD, Chronic kidney disease; *HD*, hemodialysis; *PD*, peritoneal dialysis.
Modified from Chen JH, Wong G, Chapman JR, Lim WH. Cumulative doses of T-cell depleting antibody and cancer risk after kidney transplantation. *PloS One.* 2015;10(11):e0139479.

kidneys and the tumor. The difficulties associated with ultrasonographic screening in people with CKD include the effect of multicystic diseases and small scarred native kidneys on the overall test accuracy and poor reliability in differentiating small hyperechoic renal cancers from lesions, such as adenomas and angiomyolipomas.

Cost-Effectiveness of Cancer Screening in Chronic Kidney Disease and End-Stage Renal Disease

As discussed earlier, the risk of cancer and expected patient survival play an important role in determining the cost-effectiveness of cancer screening. CKD and ESRD both reduce patient survival and therefore limit the cost-effectiveness of widespread cancer screening in these populations. A hypothetical analysis examining the net gain of life saved and the costs per unit survival for cervical, breast, colorectal, and prostate cancer in dialysis patients found of 5 days of life saved and costs per unit survival benefit 1.6 to 19.3 times higher than the general population.[42] The cancer screening tests modeled in this study included Papanicolaou smears for cervical cancer, mammography for breast cancer, flexible sigmoidoscopy for colorectal cancer, and digital rectal examination coupled with PSA testing for prostate cancer.[42] This theoretical assessment assumed a model in which all screening tests were accurate and all cancers detected were curable, thus biasing the analysis toward cost-effectiveness. Despite this, cancer screening was not cost-effective. Screening for breast cancer in women on dialysis has been examined from a cost-effective standpoint by several investigators using varying models.[43–44] Routine breast cancer screening in women on dialysis was not found to be cost-effective in terms of days of life saved: 12 days for a 60-year-old woman,[45] 1 to 16 days for a 60-year-old white Americans with diabetes mellitus, and 41 to 291 days for a 50-year-old African American;[44] An incremental cost-effectiveness ratio of $109,852/life-years saved was found in one study that also determined the reduction in breast cancer mortality was 0.1% with routine screening of women on dialysis.[43]

The realization that routine cancer screening in dialysis patients is not cost-effective led to the American Society of Nephrology's recommendation against routine cancer screening among asymptomatic nontransplant listed patients.[46] Subsequent studies of cancer screening in dialysis patients found that colon cancer screening was appropriately targeted toward dialysis patients with lower expected mortality and highest likelihood of kidney transplantation.[47] However, absolute rates of colon cancer screening were high: an overall rate of 27.9 colonoscopies per 1000 person-years in the dialysis patients versus 3.4 per 1000 in a subgroup of Medicare beneficiaries with an expected survival less than 5 years, suggesting dialysis patients are screened at a much higher rate relative to life expectancy than those without ESRD.[47] Screening for breast and cervical cancer in women with CKD and ESRD is less common among women with advanced CKD, particularly in older women.[48] However, this study also identified a low rate of cervical cancer screening in transplanted women and younger women on dialysis, groups with higher risk

of cervical cancer,[3] suggesting that appropriate screening for cervical cancer is not being performed in this subgroup.

Recommendations for Cancer Screening in Patients With Chronic Kidney Disease and Potential Transplant Candidates on Dialysis

Early detection through screening and eradication of precancerous lesions is one of the few strategies proven to reduce the risk of cancer-related morbidity and mortality in the general population. Trial-based evidence reports a significant reduction in cancer mortality by at least 20% for solid organ malignancy, such as colorectal cancer, in the screened arms compared with the unscreened arms.[49–51] Despite the increased risk of cancer and cancer-related death in potential transplant candidates, cancer screening uptake in those with ESRD and CKD is much lower than those without kidney disease.[48] The rationale behind the reduced screening uptake is unclear but may reflect patients' preferences for preventive medicine in the context of chronic illness. Also, potential candidates may experience a lower likelihood of benefits from screening even if cancer is diagnosed early because of the reduced life expectancy compared with the general population.

Prior modeling analyses reported the projected gains in life years with screening mammography, colorectal, and cervical cancer screening in patients on dialysis were at least 50% less than expected in the general population, largely because of the risk of competing events in this high risk population, including the risk of death from cardiovascular disease.[52] However, given the increased cancer risk and the lack of quality, primary data to inform cancer screening practices specifically in the ESRD and CKD populations, it may be appropriate for potential transplant candidates to follow the current cancer screening practices for common cancers, such as colorectal, breast, cervical, lung, and prostate cancers, as per the general population[53,54] (see Table 34.1 and Table 34.5; Fig. 34.1).

For other common cancer types that are specific to the ESRD populations, such as cancers of the urinary tract systems, previous research has indicated some benefits of routine ultrasonographic screening for renal cell cancers and urinary cytology/cystoscopies for bladder cancers among high-risk individuals who are listed for kidney transplantation. For potential kidney transplant candidates at risk with underlying liver disease or with high risk conditions such as hepatitis B virus- or hepatitis C virus-infected recipients, the recommendations are to undergo serum alpha-fetoprotein and ultrasound screening every 6 to 12 months. Screening for lung cancer is generally not routinely recommended for average risk individuals. However, those who are long-term current smokers (> 30 years) or who have stopped smoking within the past 15 years should undergo routine screening with chest radiography and low-dose computed tomography[53] (see Tables 34.1 and 34.5).

Table 34.5   Recommendations for Screening in the General Population and Potential Transplant Candidates

Cancer	General Population	Potential Transplant Candidates
Breast	■ Women ages 40 to 49 years should have the choice to start annual breast cancer screening if they wish to do so ■ Biennial mammography is recommended for women age 50 years and above ■ Screening should continue as long as a woman is in good health and is expected to live 10 more years or longer	As per general population
Colorectal	■ Biennial fecal immunochemical testing (FIT) is recommended for all people age 50 years and above. Those with positive FIT should have full examination of the colon, preferably by colonoscopy ■ Flexible sigmoidoscopy (every 5 or 10 years) may also be considered for people age 50 years and above ■ Screening can be stopped for people who are older than 75 years or with life expectancy less than 10 years	As per general population
Cervical	■ Biennial Papanicolaou (Pap) test is recommended for women starting at the age of 18 years, or within two years after becoming sexually active ■ Women older than 69 years should talk to their doctors about whether or not they need to have regular Pap tests. The decision to stop is often based on a woman's history of having normal, or negative, Pap test results ■ Women who had a previous total hysterectomy (removal of the uterus, including the cervix) do not require routine Pap screen	As per general population
Lung	■ Routine screening for lung cancer using chest radiography and low-dose computed tomography (LDCT) **is not recommended** for average risk individuals ■ However, there is some evidence to suggest annual screening for people at high risk of lung cancer using LDCT. Individuals at high risk are adults aged 55 to 80 years who have a smoking history of at least 30 pack-years and currently smoke or have quit within the past 15 years	LDCT of the chest may be recommended for individuals who are at high risk of lung cancer, including a prolonged heavy smoking history
Prostate	■ Routine screening using prostate-specific antigen for prostate cancer is not recommended for average risk individuals	As per general population
Renal	■ Routine screening for renal cell cancer is not recommended for average risk individuals	Ultrasonographic screening for the native kidneys may be recommended for individuals who have a family history of renal cancer, a personal history of acquired cystic disease, analgesic nephropathy, long-term smoking, and/or prolonged waiting time on dialysis
Bladder	■ Routine screening for bladder cancer is not recommended for average risk individuals	Urine cytology and cystoscopies may be recommended for individuals who had been previously exposed to chemotherapeutic agents such as cyclophosphamide or regular users of analgesics

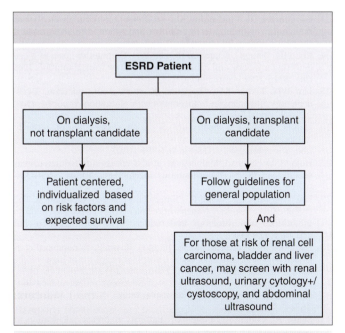

Fig. 34.1 Algorithm for cancer screening in dialysis patients based on transplant candidacy. *ESRD,* End-stage renal disease.

Recommendations for Cancer Screening in Patients on Dialysis Who Are Not Listed for Transplantation

Patients on dialysis who are not suitable for transplantation because of coexisting comorbidities have a much lower expected survival than those who are currently on transplant waiting lists. The median survival for older patients (≥ 60 years) with more than one comorbidity is less than 4.7 years with the major cause of death from cardiovascular related illnesses.[55] Emerging evidence suggests that routine screening in patients with life expectancy less than 5 years is likely futile because these patients may not live long enough to benefit from screening.[56] Even for those who survive, it is often questionable whether the benefits of further testing outweigh the potential harms associated with invasive and unnecessary treatments. General screening guidelines target average-risk individuals, not subsets of patients, such as those with kidney disease who have heterogeneous responses along the care continuum. Therefore a patient-centered and personalized approach that takes into consideration patient preferences, the net gains in both survival and life quality, and additional resources use is needed for decisions in cancer screening in this sub-population of dialysis patients[57,58] (see Fig. 34.1).

Future Research Recommendations

There is a lack of trial-based evidence of cancer screening in the transplant population. Clinicians therefore rely on evidence from observational, registry, and modeling analyses. Given the variations in the accuracy of screening tests in kidney transplant recipients and differing prognoses and life expectancy for individual transplant patients, future research focusing on a personalized approach to shared-decision making for cancer screening is needed. Such an approach will need to take the patients' individual risks of cancer, the competing priorities of other comorbidities and expected survival, and patients' preferences towards cancer screening into consideration.

Key Points

- Overall cancer incidence is higher in dialysis and transplanted patients, especially for virally mediated cancers, like lymphomas (in transplant patients), liver cancer associated with hepatitis, and human papilloma virus associated cancers (tongue and cervical cancers).
- Cancer incidence in chronic kidney disease (CKD) patients is higher only for urothelial cancers of the urinary tract, likely caused by factors increasing the risk of CKD, as well as urothelial cancer (e.g., analgesic abuse).
- Renal cell carcinoma is more common among CKD, dialysis, and transplanted patients.
- Effective cancer screening depends on cancer incidence, risk factors, and overall expected survival, which influences the cost-effectiveness of screening in the end-stage renal disease population because of higher expected mortality than the general population.
- Potential transplant recipients should undergo cancer screening following the guidelines in the general population, with additional screening for renal cell carcinoma. Cancer screening in the nontransplant candidate dialysis patient should be individualized, based on cancer risk and expected survival.

References

1. Buccianti G, Maisonneuve P, Ravasi B, Cresseri D, Locatelli F, Boyle P. Cancer among patients on renal replacement therapy: a population based survey in Lombardy, Italy. *Int J Cancer*. 1996;66:591-593.
2. Maisonneuve P, Agodoa L, Gellert R, et al. Cancer in patients on dialysis for end-stage renal disease: an international collaborative study. *Lancet*. 1999;354:93-99.
3. Vajdic CM, McDonald SP, McCredie MR, et al. Cancer incidence before and after kidney transplantation. *JAMA*. 2006;296:2823-2831.
4. Wong G, Staplin N, Emberson J, et al. Chronic kidney disease and the risk of cancer: an individual data meta-analysis of 32,057 participants from six prospective studies. *BMC Cancer*. 2016;16:488.
5. Christensson A, Savage C, Sjoberg DD, et al. Association of cancer with moderately impaired renal function at baseline in a large, representative, population-based cohort followed for up to 30 years. *Int J Cancer*. 2013;133:1452-1458.
6. Jørgensen L, Heuch I, Jenssen T, Jacobsen BK. Association of albuminuria and cancer incidence. *J Am Soc Nephrol*. 2008;19:992-998.
7. Wong G, Hayen A, Chapman JR, et al. Association of CKD and cancer risk in older people. *J Am Soc Nephrol*. 2009;20:1341-1350.
8. Wong G, Zoungas S, Lo S, et al. The risk of cancer in people with diabetes and chronic kidney disease. *Nephrol Dial Transplant*. 2012; 27:3337-3344.
9. Lowrance WT, Ordoñez J, Udaltsova N, Russo P, Go AS. CKD and the risk of incident cancer. *J Am Soc Nephrol*. 2014;25(10):2327-2334.
10. Chen JS, Lu CL, Huang LC, Shen CH, Chen SC. CKD is associated with upper tract urothelial carcinoma in a nationwide population-based cohort study in Taiwan. *Medicine*. 2016;95(14):e3255.
12. Heidland A, Bahner U, Vamvakas S. Incidence and spectrum of dialysis associated cancer in three continents. *Am J Kidney Dis*. 2000; 35:347-351, discussion 352-353.
13. Chen KS, Lai MK, Huang CC, Chu SH, Leu ML. Urologic cancers in uremic patients. *Am J Kidney Dis*. 1995;25:694-700.
14. Lin HF, Li YH, Wang CH, Chou CL, Kuo DJ, Fang TC. Increased risk of cancer in chronic dialysis patients: a population-based cohort study in Taiwan. *Nephrol Dial Transplant*. 2012;27:1585-1590.
15. Butler AM, Olshan AF, Kshirsagar AV, et al. Cancer incidence among US Medicare ESRD patients receiving hemodialysis,1996-2009. *Am J Kidney Dis*. 2015;65:763-772.
16. Yoo KD, Lee JP, Lee SM, et al. Cancer in Korean patients within end-stage renal disease: a 7-year follow-up. *PLoS One*. 2017;12(7): e0178649.
17. Cheung CY, Chan GC, Chan SK, et al. Cancer incidence and mortality in chronic dialysis population: a multicenter cohort study. *Am J Nephrol*. 2016;43(3):153-159.
18. Farivar-Mohseni H, Perlmutter AE, Wilson S, Shingleton WB, Bigler SA, Fowler JE Jr. Renal cell carcinoma and end stage renal disease. *J Urol*. 2006;175:2018-2020, discussion 2021.
19. Kompotiatis P, Thongprayoon C, Manohar S, et al. Association between urologic malignancies and end-stage renal disease: a meta-analysis. *Nephrology (Carlton)*. 2017. doi:10.1111/nep.13209. [Epub ahead of print].
20. Hsiao PJ, Hsieh PF, Chang CH, Wu HC, Yang CR, Huang CP. Higher risk of urothelial carcinoma in the upper urinary tract than in the urinary bladder in hemodialysis patients. *Ren Fail*. 2016;38(5): 663-670.
21. Taneja S, Mandayam S, Kayani ZZ, Kuo YF, Shahinian VB. Comparison of stage at diagnosis of cancer in patients who are on dialysis versus the general population. *Clin J Am Soc Nephrol*. 2007;2: 1008-1013.
22. Karami S, Yanik EL, Moore LE, et al. Risk of renal cell carcinoma among kidney transplant recipients in the United States. *Am J Transplant*. 2016;16(12):3479-3489.
23. Agraharkar ML, Cinclair RD, Kuo YF, Daller JA, Shahinian VB. Risk of malignancy with long-term immunosuppression in renal transplant recipients. *Kidney Int*. 2004;66(1):383-389.
24. Chen JH, Wong G, Chapman JR, Lim WH. Cumulative doses of T-cell depleting antibody and cancer risk after kidney transplantation. *PloS One*. 2015;10(11):e0139479.
25. Lim WH, Turner RM, Chapman JR, et al. Acute rejection, T-cell-depleting antibodies, and cancer after transplantation. *Transplantation*. 2014;97(8):817-825.
26. Hall EC, Engels EA, Pfeiffer RM, Segev DL. Association of antibody induction immunosuppression with cancer after kidney transplantation. *Transplantation*. 2015;99(5):1051-1027.
27. Hojo M, Morimoto T, Maluccio M, et al. Cyclosporine induces cancer progression by a cell-autonomous mechanism. *Nature*. 1999;397 (6719):530-534.
29. Lim WH, Russ GR, Wong G, Pilmore H, Kanellis J, Chadban SJ. The risk of cancer in kidney transplant recipients may be reduced in those maintained on everolimus and reduced cyclosporine. *Kidney Int*. 2017;91(4):954-963.
30. Campbell SB, Walker R, Tai SS, Jiang Q, Russ GR. Randomized controlled trial of sirolimus for renal transplant recipients at high risk for nonmelanoma skin cancer. *Am J Transplant*. 2012;12(5):1146-1156.
31. Euvrard S, Morelon E, Rostaing L, et al. Sirolimus and secondary skin-cancer prevention in kidney transplantation. *N Engl J Med*. 2012; 367(4):329-339.
33. Evans AJ, Cohen ME, Cohen GF. Patterns of breast calcification in patients on renal dialysis. *Clin Radiol*. 1992;45:343-344.

35. Akmal M, Sawelson S, Karubian F, Gadallah M. The prevalence and significance of occult blood loss in patients with predialysis advanced chronic renal failure (CRF), or receiving dialytic therapy. *Clin Nephrol.* 1994;42:198-202.

36. Coppolino G. Kidney and neoplastic disease: overview with a particular interest to interpretation of cancer biomarkers. In: Patel VB, Preedy VR, eds. *Biomarkers in kidney disease.* Springer Publishing; 2016:249-268.

38. Djavan B, Shariat S, Ghawidel K, et al. Impact of chronic dialysis on serum PSA, free PSA, and free/total PSA ratio: is prostate cancer detection compromised in patients receiving long-term dialysis? *Urology.* 1999;53:1169-1174.

39. Bruun L, Björk T, Lilja H, Becker C, Gustafsson O, Christensson A. Percent-free prostate specific antigen is elevated in men on haemodialysis or peritoneal dialysis treatment. *Nephrol Dial Transplant.* 2003;18:598-603.

40. Sangthawan P, Fox J, Atkins RC, Kerr PG. Increased incidence of benign breast disease in female transplant patients receiving cyclosporin. *ANZ J Surg.* 2002;72(3):222-225.

41. Wong G, Howard K, Webster AC, Chapman JR, Craig JC. Screening for renal cancer in recipients of kidney transplants. *Nephrol Dial Transplant.* 2011;26(5):1729-1739.

42. Chertow GM, Paltiel AD, Owen WF Jr, Lazarus JM. Cost-effectiveness of cancer screening in end-stage renal disease. *Arch Intern Med.* 1996;156:1345-1350.

43. Wong G, Howard K, Chapman JR, Craig JC. Cost-effectiveness of breast cancer screening in women on dialysis. *Am J Kidney Dis.* 2008;52:916-929.

44. LeBrun CJ, Diehl LF, Abbott KC, Welch PG, Yuan CM. Life expectancy benefits of cancer screening in the end-stage renal disease population. *Am J Kidney Dis.* 2000;35:237-243.

45. Kajbaf S, Nichol G, Zimmerman D. Cancer screening and life expectancy of Canadian patients with kidney failure. *Nephrol Dial Transplant.* 2002;17:1786-1789.

46. Williams AW, Dwyer AC, Eddy AA, et al. American Society of Nephrology Quality, and Patient Safety Task Force. Critical and honest conversations: the evidence behind the "Choosing Wisely" campaign recommendations by the American Society of Nephrology. *Clin J Am Soc Nephrol.* 2012;7:1664-1672.

47. Carlos, CA, McCulloch CE, Hsu CY, et al. Colon cancer screening among patients receiving dialysis in the United States: are we choosing wisely? *J Am Soc Nephrol.* 2017;28:2521-2528.

48. Wong G, Hayward JS, McArthur E, et al. Patterns and predictors of screening for breast and cervical cancer in women with CKD. *Clin J Am Soc Nephrol.* 2017;12:95-104.

49. Atkin W, Wooldrage K, Parkin DM, et al. Long term effects of once-only flexible sigmoidoscopy screening after 17 years of follow-up: the UK Flexible Sigmoidoscopy Screening randomized controlled trial. *Lancet.* 2017;389(10076):1299-1311.

51. Robertson DJ, Lee JK, Boland CR, et al. Recommendations on fecal immunochemical testing to screen for colorectal neoplasia: a consensus statement by the US Multi-Society Task Force on Colorectal Cancer. *Gastroenterology.* 2017;152(5):1217-1237.e3.

52. Kiberd BA, Keough-Ryan T, Clase CM. Screening for prostate, breast, and colorectal cancer in renal transplant recipients. *Am J Transplant.* 2003;3(5):619-625.

53. Wong G, Chapman JR, Craig JC. Cancer screening in renal transplant recipients: what is the evidence? *Clin J Am Soc Nephrol.* 2008;3(suppl 2):S87-S100.

54. Batabyal P, Chapman JR, Wong G, Craig JC, Tong A. Clinical practice guidelines on wait-listing for kidney transplantation: consistent and equitable? *Transplantation.* 2012;94(7):703-713.

55. McDonald S. *Chapter 3, 30th report Mortality in End-Stage Kidney Disease.* Australia & New Zealand: ANSDATA Registry; 2016.

56. Royce TJ, Hendrix LH, Stokes WA, Allen IM, Chen RC. Cancer screening rates in individuals with different life expectancies. *JAMA Intern Med.* 2014;174(10):1558-1565.

57. Wong G, Howard K, Tong A, Craig JC. Cancer screening in people who have chronic disease: the example of kidney disease. *Semin Dial.* 2011;24(1):72-78.

58. Holley JL. Screening, diagnosis, and treatment of cancer in long-term dialysis patients. *Clin J Am Soc Nephrol.* 2007;2:604-610.

A full list of references is available at Expertconsult.com

35 Cancer in Renal Transplant Patients

BRAHM VASUDEV AND ERIC P. COHEN

Introduction

Renal transplantation remains the treatment of choice for eligible candidates with end-stage renal disease (ESRD), because it offers improved quality and increased quantity of life to these patients. In the early days of renal transplantation, the lack of potent immunosuppressants resulted in very high acute rejection rates leading to early graft loss and overall poor graft and patient survival. Since the advent of potent immunosuppressants in the 1980s and 1990s, both short-term and long-term graft outcomes have improved. The patient survival also improved, but because of the vascular toxicity and immunosuppressive potency of the immunosuppressive drug combinations used, cardiovascular and infectious disease complications became major concerns. Recognition of these causes of mortality led to the institution of a wide range of pre- and posttransplant screening protocols, better diagnosis and treatment of infectious diseases, aggressive risk factor management, reduction in immunosuppressive medication doses, prophylactic treatments, and early interventional therapies, all of which ultimately led to an increase in the lifespan of these patients.[1]

In addition, the increase in the average age of donors and recipients, use of potent immunosuppressants to decrease acute rejection rates, and an overall improved long-term transplant patient survival has resulted in an increase in the incidence of postrenal transplant cancer. Screening for posttransplant cancer is expensive, and protocols vary from center to center. Unfortunately, the risk factors for posttransplant cancer are often difficult to modify, the treatment options are frequently limited, and prognosis for metastatic disease is overall very poor. In this chapter, we will discuss the incidence, risk factors, potential origins, outcomes, preventive and surveillance strategies, and treatment of postrenal transplant cancer.

Incidence of Postrenal Transplant Cancer

The increased relative risk for cancer in renal transplant recipients (RTRs) compared with the general population has been well established based on data from the Australian and New Zealand Dialysis and Transplant Registry (ANZDATA), Collaborative Transplant Study (CTS), Canadian Transplant Registry, Scientific Registry of Transplant Recipients (SRTR), United Network of Organ Sharing (UNOS), and Israel Penn International Transplant Tumor Registry (IPITTR). The extent of increased risk for different cancer types is consistent in different parts of the world. But the cancer incidence varies among different registries because of the variable reporting of data, different patient demographics, different eras of data measurement, changing and different induction and maintenance immunosuppression protocols across different transplant centers, and methods used for calculating risk. Countries with a single-payer system like Canada, the United Kingdom, and Australia may be able to estimate incidences more accurately compared with countries with multiple payer systems. For example, the estimated sensitivity for identifying cancer using SRTR data was 52.5% and compared with 84.3% for linked central cancer registries.[2] Despite the underreporting of late events, like cancer, or lack of denominators in voluntary registries like IPITTR, it is acknowledged that RTRs incur at least an overall three- to fivefold increased risk of cancer compared with the general population.[3,4,5]

The incidence of cancer postrenal transplantation increases with time. Among RTRs, the average age at diagnosis of cancer is about 40 years and the average time from transplantation to cancer diagnosis is 3 to 5 years. The time between transplantation and development of cancer, however, varies depending on cancer subtype. Cancers such as lymphoma and Kaposi sarcoma occur early after transplantation,[6] whereas epithelial cancers tend to occur later.[7] Excluding skin cancer, data from the United States Renal Data System estimate a cumulative incidence of cancer at 7.5% at 3 years after transplantation.[4] Data from IPITTR estimate the incidence of cancer to be 20% at 10 years after transplantation,[8] and data from ANZDATA estimate the incidence of cancer to be 10% at 10 years and 30% at 20 years after renal transplantation.[9]

Standardized incidence ratio (SIR) can be used to estimate the relative risk of cancer in RTRs relative to the cancer incidence in the general population, after allowing for differences in age, gender, and year of diagnosis. Based on data from ANZDATA, RTRs between 1980 and 2005 had a SIR of 3.56 for all cancers. A study of 175,732 US solid organ transplant recipients (58% of which were RTRs, 21% liver, 10% heart, and 4% lung), during the period of 1987 to 2008, revealed a SIR of 2.1 for all cancers.[10] The increase in SIR was not the same for all types of cancers. The SIRs for nonmelanoma skin cancer and Kaposi sarcoma among the solid organ transplant (SOT) recipients were markedly increased at 14 and 62, respectively. Among the RTRs, the SIR for renal cancer was 7 and for non-Hodgkin lymphoma (NHL), it was 6. These high SIRs for NHL and kidney cancer were particularly increased for the youngest recipients, reflecting large increases relative to the general population.

Data available from Medicare billing claims during the period 1995 to 2001 in the United States showed that

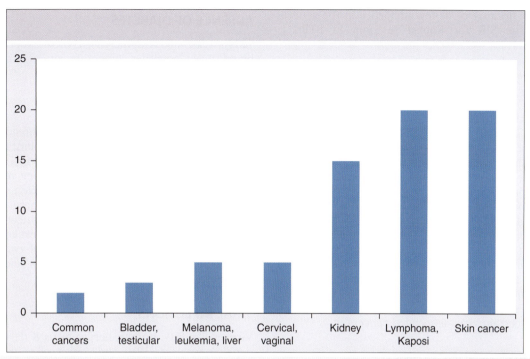

Fig. 35.1 Fold-increase in cancer risk after renal transplantation, for first-time recipients of deceased or living donor kidney transplants. Modified from Kasiske BL, Snyder JJ, Gilbertson DT et al. Cancer after kidney transplantation in the United States. *Am J Transplant.* 2004;4:905-913.

first-time recipients of deceased or living donor kidney transplantations had a twofold increase for common cancers like colon, lung, prostate, stomach, esophagus, pancreas, ovary, and breast, a threefold increase for testicular and bladder cancer, a fivefold increase for melanoma, leukemia, hepatobiliary tumors, cervical, and vaginal cancers, a 15-fold increase for kidney cancer, and a 20-fold increase for Kaposi sarcoma, NHL, and nonmelanoma skin cancer compared with the general population[4] (Fig. 35.1).

Specific Cancer Types

SKIN CANCER

It is the most common cancer in RTRs and its incidence increases with time after transplantation. Its incidence is 50% at 10 years and 61% at 20 years in Great Britain[11] and 82% at 20 years in Australia.[12] The overall risk for basal cell cancer is increased 10-fold, and squamous cell cancer by up to a 100-fold compared with the general population.

POSTTRANSPLANT LYMPHOPROLIFERATIVE DISORDER (LYMPHOMA)

Epstein Barr virus (EBV) seronegative recipients are at increased risk for posttransplant lymphoproliferative disorder (PTLD). It is thus more common in children compared with adults. Among adults, PTLD rates vary from 0.5% to 1.7% for EBV seropositive and seronegative patients, respectively.[13] NHL risk is the highest in the first year after transplant, decreases between 2 to 4 years, and then increases again at 4 to 5 years. Both nodal and extranodal presentation can occur. Among RTRs, there is a slight

predilection for lymphoma to occur in the transplanted kidney.[10] As transplant patients live longer, cases of late (> 10 years posttransplant) lymphoma are also being reported.[14] Data from CTS have shown that central nervous system (CNS) lymphomas are most common in RTRs and use of T-cell depleting therapy increases the risk.[6] CNS lymphomas have also been seen at slightly increased frequency in patients on belatacept. Because of discontinuation of use of OKT-3 and a trend to lesser induction doses of rabbit antithymocyte globulin (rATG), there has been a decrease in the incidence of PTLD in adults.[15] Among children, a decline in PTLD rates has also been observed in recipients transplanted between 2002 to 2012 compared with those transplanted between 2000 to 2009.[13]

RENAL CANCER

Renal cancers in RTRs occur mostly in the native kidneys. There is a greater frequency of papillary cell cancer compared with the general population and the incidence is higher in patients with a history of analgesic abuse or acquired cystic disease in the kidneys. The RTRs have a 15-fold increase in risk for renal cancer.[4]

KAPOSI SARCOMA

Kaposi sarcoma commonly involves the skin but can also involve visceral organs. The incidence of Kaposi sarcoma in RTRs varies with the regimen and intensity of immunosuppression and the risk is less in azathioprine-treated patients compared with cyclosporine-treated patients. Compared with the general population, the rate of Kaposi sarcoma among SOTs and patients with acquired immunodeficiency syndrome (AIDS) is about 500 and 20,000 times, respectively.[16] Because of its low incidence in the general population, the SIR for Kaposi sarcoma in RTRs is increased to 61.[10]

Risk Factors for Postrenal Transplant Cancer

Immunosuppressive medications and viral infections appear to be the most important factors in causing the increased risk of cancer after renal transplant. Immunosuppressive medications have a negative effect on immune surveillance but affect deoxyribonucleic acid (DNA) repair mechanisms as well, leading to irreversible DNA alteration and subsequent carcinogenesis. Transplant patients are at increased risk for new viral infections and for reactivating latent viral infections. Potent immunosuppression used for postrenal transplantation can lead to unchecked viral replication and subsequent viral oncogenesis. Conversely, reducing or stopping immunosuppression can lead to regression of certain virus-associated cancers.[17]

RECIPIENT AGE, GENDER, ETHNICITY, AND POSTTRANSPLANT LIFESPAN

Increasing age, male gender, and Caucasian ethnicity have been identified as risk factors for postrenal transplant cancer.[7,18] This is important given the fact that the average age of RTRs has increased in recent years. The risk for cancer also increases with time posttransplantation because of an accumulation of risk factors like net cumulative immunosuppression, exposure to viruses, sun exposure, and increased age.

GENETIC PREDISPOSITION

Genetic factors are known to predispose to cancer. For example, people with von Hippel–Lindau disease, Wiskott–Aldrich, Lynch, and Drash syndromes are at increased risk of renal cancer.[19] It is possible that as more genetic risk factors for cancer are identified in the future, that immunosuppression after renal transplant may be suitably modified to take this into account.

CHRONIC RENAL DISEASE AND DIALYSIS DURATION

Patients with chronic kidney disease (CKD) and ESRD on dialysis are at increased risk of developing posttransplant cancer.[20] Irrespective of the patient's age, there is a linear relationship between duration of dialysis before transplantation and the risk for developing cancer posttransplantation.[21] The risk is particularly high for Kaposi sarcoma, lip cancer, lymphoma, and genitourinary cancers.

PRESENCE OF CYSTIC KIDNEY DISEASE

In RTRs, renal cancer primarily occurs in native kidneys and not in the transplanted kidney.[4,10] Patients with acquired renal cystic disease are at increased risk of developing renal cancer because of malignant transformation of the cysts.

ABSENCE OF DIABETES

This is associated with increased risk of cancer likely caused by relatively less other competing causes of death, such as cardiovascular disease and infections.

HISTORY OF PRIOR MALIGNANCY

Patients with a history of cancer in remission are a high-risk patient population for renal transplantation, because they have a 30% higher risk of death posttransplantation compared with patients with no history of cancer.[22] A metaanalysis of 32 studies in SOT recipients with history of cancer in remission showed that these patients have increased risk for all-cause mortality, cancer-specific mortality, and are at increased risk for developing de novo malignancies.[23] Patients with history of cancer therefore require personalized screening strategies before placement on waiting list for renal transplantation.

VIRAL INFECTIONS

Viruses like EBV, human herpes virus 8 (HHV 8), human papillomaviruses (HPV), and Merkel cell polyomavirus have a propensity to cause cancer in RTRs.

EBV has been conclusively implicated in the development of Hodgkin disease, NHL, and other manifestations of PTLD.[24] Approximately 90% of adults show serologic evidence of past exposure to EBV.[15] Transplantation from an EBV-positive donor to EBV-negative recipient is associated with a 20-fold increase in risk for PTLD and that is why children are at particularly higher risk. The degree of immunosuppression and use of T-cell depleting therapy also increases the risk.[6] Approximately 80% of PTLD is caused by abnormal B-cell proliferation induced by EBV and the virus can be isolated from the involved tissue. The remaining 20% of PTLD is caused by T-cell proliferation. The manifestation has a bimodal distribution, with the first peak occurring within the first 2 years of transplantation and a second peak after 5 years of transplantation. PTLD can also arise in donor tissue and RTRs particularly may develop lymphoma in the transplanted kidney.

HHV 8 infection is associated with the development of Kaposi sarcoma and has also been implicated in the development of multiple myeloma. In RTRs, Kaposi sarcoma can involve skin and visceral organs.[16] Risk factors include donor to recipient transmission, degree of immunosuppression, geographic area of origin, and male gender.

HPV has multiple genotypes that have been associated with different cancers. Transmission of this infection is through close personal contact, including sexual contact. In RTRs, it is associated with skin cancer, head and neck cancers, and anogenital cancers, including vulvar, vaginal, cervical, penile, and anal cancers.

Merkel cell polyomavirus infection can cause Merkel cell carcinoma. It is an aggressive tumor involving skin and neuroendocrine tissue and has a propensity for lymphatic spread.

CIGARETTE SMOKING

RTRs who smoke are at increased risk of developing lung cancer compared with RTRs who do not smoke. The relative risk of lung cancer increases with prior and current history of smoking. The mortality risk from lung cancer in RTRs is higher in those who continued cigarette smoking compared with those who stopped cigarette smoking after transplantation. Cigarette smoking is also associated with an increased risk of death and graft loss.

SUN EXPOSURE AND GEOGRAPHICAL LOCATION

Sun exposure is a well-established risk factor for the development of skin cancer in RTRs.[7] Sun exposure before transplantation, intensity of immunosuppression, older age, use of calcineurin inhibitors (CNIs) versus mammalian target of rapamycin inhibitor (mTORi) increase the risk. Skin cancer occurs more frequently in sun-exposed areas. Skin pigmentation modifies the risk and African American recipients are at much less risk for skin cancer in sun-exposed areas compared with white Americans.

TYPE OF DONOR

Recipients of living donor kidneys are at reduced risk of cancer, particularly PTLD and genitourinary (GU) cancers, when compared with recipients of expanded criteria donors (ECD). This is independent of their age, gender, and duration on dialysis.[25] Intense inflammatory response posttransplantation among the ECD kidney recipients has been speculated to contribute to the increased cancer risk in this patient population.

DONOR TRANSMITTED CANCER

Many different types have cancers have been reported to be transmitted through donors. In RTRs, the incidence of donor transmitted cancer has been reported to be less than 1 in 3000 (< 0.03%).[26] These events are rare, so that there may be an underestimation of their true incidence. Within the US, the Disease Transmission Advisory Committee (DTAC), in Europe, the Council of Europe and globally, a World Health Organization-sponsored website (www.notifylibrary.org) now actively collect data on donor transmitted cancer and infections.

IMMUNOSUPPRESSIVE DRUG THERAPY

Net cumulative immunosuppression, antibody induction, type of maintenance immunosuppressive medications, number of immunosuppressive medications, rejection treatment, and use of immunosuppressive medications before transplant all contribute to the risk of postrenal transplant cancer.

Immunosuppression may lead to decreased immune surveillance of nascent cancer and may also predispose to viral infections that are oncogenic.[27] The overall risk for postrenal transplant cancer is driven by the duration and intensity of immunosuppression (net immunosuppression). Indirect evidence for this comes from studies showing an increased incidence of cancer in patients treated with intense immunosuppression for treatment of acute rejection[28] and in patients treated with immunosuppression for primary glomerular disease before transplantation. Patients with human immunodeficiency virus/AIDS also have similarly increased rates of oncogenic virus-driven cancers, further supporting that immune deficiency plays a significant role in increased risk. Patients on mTORi have been reported to have reduced risk of cancer; however, this reduced incidence has not been shown to improve the overall survival of RTRs.[29] Although it is possible that small differences exist among the maintenance immunosuppressive drugs, these are likely to be clinically less important given the far greater effect of other known risk factors.[30]

INDUCTION THERAPY

Induction therapy is used in most patients at the time of renal transplant to avoid early rejection. The induction agents include monoclonal antibodies, such as basiliximab (antiinterleukin [IL]-2 receptor antibody) and alemtuzumab (anti-CD52), or polyclonal lymphocyte-depleting antibodies like horse or rATG/thymoglobulin. OKT3/muromonab is more potent than rATG and was associated with increased risk for lymphoma, but it is no longer commercially available. Non-rATG preparations have also been shown to be associated with increased risk for PTLD. rATG is more potent than equine ATG in depleting peripheral blood lymphocytes and is presently the most commonly used polyclonal antibody in the US and worldwide. The risk of infections and cancer increases with increasing dose of T-cell depleting agents and thus over the years, the standard total induction dose of rATG has decreased from 14 to 6 mg/kg. The antibodies against T-cells deplete both CD4+ and CD8+ T-cells, which are crucial in adaptive antiviral immunity, and their depletion increases the risk for diseases caused by uncontrolled virus replication. Polyclonal antibodies also target natural killer (NK) cells, B-cells, and plasma cells, which another mechanism to enable development of EBV-driven PTLD.[6] IL-2 receptor antagonist (IL-2Ra) induction does not appear to be associated with an increase in risk for cancer.[5,6,31]

Maintenance Therapy

PREDNISONE

Because glucocorticoids are mostly used in low doses with other immunosuppressive medications in RTRs, it is not possible to discern the effect of low-dose steroids (5 mg/day) on posttransplant cancer.

CALCINEURIN INHIBITORS

Both cyclosporine and tacrolimus are associated with increased risk of malignancy in RTRs. CNIs promote cancer by aberrant production of cytokines that regulate processes promoting cancer growth, metastasis, and angiogenesis. Lower trough levels of cyclosporine (75–125 ng/dL) are associated with lower risk of cancers compared with standard levels (150–250 ng/dL).[32] Similarly, higher levels of tacrolimus are associated with higher risk of PTLD.[33] Clinical studies such as the European and US multicenter trials comparing maintenance immunosuppression with cyclosporine versus tacrolimus did not show a significant difference in cancer incidence between these two drugs.[34]

AZATHIOPRINE

In addition to blocking proliferation of lymphocyte precursors, this drug promotes carcinogenesis by causing defective DNA repair. Increased risk of nonmelanoma skin cancer, particularly squamous cell cancer in RTRs, is thought to be facilitated by the cumulative dose of azathioprine. It has also been shown to be associated with the development of myelodysplastic syndrome.

MYCOPHENOLATE MOFETIL

Mycophenolate mofetil (MMF) was originally developed as an anticancer drug. It inhibits the maturation of lymphocytes by blocking the isoform of inosine-5'-monophosphate dehydrogenase required for the de novo synthesis of guanine nucleotides. Transplant registry studies show lower rejection rates with MMF containing regimens compared with MMF-free regimens but no difference in cancer rates. A 3-year analysis of MMF versus azathioprine in the Tricontinental Multicenter study[35] and US Randomized Trial[36] showed no difference in cancer between these two drugs. The population analysis performed using the SRTR and UNOS database showed a significantly reduced incidence of any cancer with use of MMF compared with azathioprine in diabetic renal transplant patients.[37] Another study[38] combining 3-year outcome data from the Organ Procurement and Transplant Network and CTS database showed that MMF is not associated with an increased risk of lymphoma or other malignancy postrenal transplant. Lower prevalence of cancer with MMF in RTRs may be related to lower acute rejection rates and therefore lesser use of antibodies to treat acute rejection.

MAMMALIAN TARGET OF RAPAMYCIN INHIBITORS

Sirolimus and everolimus are the two approved mTORi for RTRs. They suppress the immune system by preventing cell cycle progression from G1 to S phase. They also impair vascular endothelial growth factor production, thus blocking angiogenesis. Unlike other immunosuppressants, with mTORi, there is no dose-dependent relationship with malignancy. Many studies have shown reduced incidence of skin cancer and Kaposi sarcoma in patients converted from a CNI to an mTORi. A recent metaanalysis combining 21 randomized control trials demonstrated that sirolimus was associated with 56% reduction in risk for nonmelanoma skin cancer and 40% reduction in risk for cancer compared with controls. These results were only seen in people who were converted to sirolimus from another immunosuppressive regimen and was not seen in de novo sirolimus trials.[29] Moreover, despite the results showing a decrease in cancer rate, there was an overall increase in mortality because of cardiovascular and infection-related deaths.

BELATACEPT

This agent is a novel costimulation blocker that inhibits T-cell proliferation. The Belatacept Evaluation of Nephroprotection and Efficacy as First-line Immunosuppression Trial (BENEFIT) and BENEFIT-EXTended criteria donors (EXT) studies compared the clinical efficacy of belatacept with cyclosporine.[39,40] The studies showed that although the overall malignancy risk among RTRs was similar, there was a slight increase in the incidence of PTLD in patients on belatacept. The risk was higher in EBV-seronegative patients compared with EBV-seropositive patients. That is why belatacept is contraindicated in EBV-seronegative patients.

TREATMENT OF REJECTION

Treatment of acute transplant rejection involves pulse doses of immunosuppressants followed by intensification of maintenance immunosuppression, which increases the risk of cancer. Use of T-cell depleting antibodies for treatment of rejection also leads to increased risk for cancers, particularly PTLD and GU cancers.

Potential Origin of Postrenal Transplant Cancer

POTENTIAL RENAL TRANSPLANT RECIPIENT WITH HISTORY OF A CANCER

The relative risk of developing cancer increases with a decline in glomerular filtration rate.[20] Patients with CKD and patients on chronic dialysis are at increased risk for certain kinds of cancers like Kaposi sarcoma, thyroid cancer, liver cancer, pancreas cancer, GU cancers, and certain oral cancers.[3] Certain cancers, like multiple myeloma and renal cell cancer (RCC), can directly lead to ESRD. Chemotherapeutic agents can be nephrotoxic as well and their use can lead to development of CKD and even ESRD. Transplanting a kidney in a patient with active cancer is likely to increase that patient's immediate mortality; therefore patients with active cancer are excluded from renal transplantation. Patients with history of cancer should undergo a very thorough evaluation to ensure that the patient is cancer-free. Each patient, just like each cancer, is unique and thus it is very difficult to accurately predict the chances of recurrence. The risks however should be very clearly explained to the patient at the beginning of the pretransplant workup because these patients have a higher all-cause mortality postrenal transplantation compared with recipients with no history of cancer.[22,23] Cancers, such as skin cancers, caused by oncogenic viruses have a higher risk of recurrence compared with cancers that may not be influenced by immunosuppression. Longer wait times do not eliminate the risk of cancer occurrence in recipients with a prior history of aggressive cancer. Various societies have published guidelines for the minimum time interval between diagnosis and treatment of various kinds of cancer and renal transplantation.[41] These wait times, however, do not guarantee that there will be no recurrence of cancer after transplantation. These guidelines and recommendations are sometimes discordant among societies and unified recommendations for specific cancers in the renal transplant population are needed. Current guidelines also lack strong evidence because of the absence of large clinical trials. They mainly serve as a guide to establish each patient's risk versus potential benefit from renal transplantation.

Each patient should thus be evaluated on an individual basis and preferably with the involvement of the patient's oncologist to gauge life expectancy, the chances of recurrence, and best surveillance strategies.

POTENTIAL LIVING DONOR WITH HISTORY OF CANCER

Cancer transmission from living donors has been reported. One of the big advantages that living donors have over deceased donors is the availability of time for adequate workup including obtaining a detailed history, examination, imaging, blood tests, biopsies, and appropriate consultations. Age appropriate cancer screening is a part of routine predonation workup. Young donors have a low risk of having cancer and thus a low risk of transmission. Living donors with early-stage cancer cured by surgery, especially in cases of cancer with low metastatic potential, like nonmelanoma skin cancer, can donate. Living donors with a history of metastatic disease are not candidates for donation.

POTENTIAL DECEASED DONOR WITH HISTORY OF CANCER OR INCIDENTAL CANCER FOUND AT THE TIME OF DONATION

The data on cancer transmission from deceased donors mainly come from case reports, but more recently, efforts are being made to collect the data on cancer transmission. Because of lack of an organized approach to assess cancer transmission risk, organs from donors with malignancy are often discarded. The DTAC of the UNOS has published recommendations on this subject.[42] Cancers in the donor, such as basal cell skin cancer, pose little or no risk, small solitary thyroid cancers pose a less than 1% risk, but active breast or colon cancer pose a greater than 10% risk of transmission to the recipient.

LIVING OR DECEASED DONOR WITH UNDETECTED CANCER AT THE TIME OF DONATION OR DISCOVERY OF CANCER IN A DONOR AFTER DONATION

Cancers of many organs including breast, colon, lung, liver, pancreas, ovary, prostate, kidney, lymphoma, melanoma, choriocarcinoma, and glioblastoma multiforme have been known to be transmitted from the donor to the recipient. If multiple organ recipients from a single donor develop the same cancer soon after transplantation, the transmission is classified as proven donor transmitted cancer. If based on the DNA evaluation, the cancer is of donor origin and the time between transplantation and detection of cancer is in weeks, the cancer is classified as donor-transmitted, but if the time difference is in years, then the cancer is classified as donor-derived.[42]

DE NOVO CANCER IN RENAL TRANSPLANT RECIPIENT

RTRs are at increased risk for posttransplant cancer for a multitude of reasons, including duration of chronic renal failure, net immunosuppression, prior or new exposure to oncogenic viruses, sun exposure, age, male gender, presence of cystic renal disease, and other risk factors for cancer as applicable to general population. Because the risk of cancer is lower in the younger population, they have the highest relative increase in risk for posttransplant cancer compared with older transplant patients. Patients with a history of cancer in remission are also at an increased risk of development of de novo cancer posttransplantation.[23]

Outcomes of Renal Transplant Recipients With Cancer After Transplant

Postrenal transplant cancer now accounts for 8% to 10% of all deaths among RTRs in the United States.[43] Cancers in transplant patients tend to be aggressive and the median patient survival after the diagnosis of cancer in RTRs with cancer is 2.1 years from time of diagnosis compared with 8.3 years in matched RTRs without cancer.[44]

Compared with the general population, stage-specific survival for cancers such as breast, bladder, colon, lung, and prostate are considerably lower in posttransplant patients. RTRs with a small solitary RCC detected early and with no invasion of the capsule can be surgically resected and have a good prognosis. In patients with colon cancer, the 5-year patient survival is 27% in posttransplant patients compared with 75% in the general population. The reasons for poor outcomes of posttransplant cancers include aggressiveness of cancer caused by immunocompromised state, late discovery of unsuspected transmission of cancer from the donor to the recipient, perhaps inconsistent cancer screening because of perceived reduced benefit of screening in this population, inability to completely discontinue immunosuppressants because of fear of graft rejection, poor candidacy for surgical options because of comorbid conditions, or limited aggressive chemotherapeutic options because of chronic immunosuppressed state.

Posttransplant recipients older than 60 years of age and with a history of diabetes, cardiovascular disease, and stroke are at increased risk of death from cardiovascular events and have standardized cancer mortality ratio of less than 1, when compared with age- and gender-matched general population. Posttransplant recipients younger than 50 years of age, and without diabetes, have a standardized cancer mortality ratio of more than 1, suggesting that risk of death from cardiovascular causes may be obscuring the effect of immunosuppression on cancer risk in older transplant recipients.[45]

Role of Prevention and Surveillance in Improving Outcomes and Prolonging Survival in Patients With Postrenal Transplant Cancer

RTRs are at increased risk for developing cancers and because late detection of cancer carries a poorer prognosis, preventive strategies and evidence-based cancer surveillance for certain cancers may prolong patient survival.

Preventive strategies include a thorough evaluation of donors and recipients to prevent cancer transmission from the donor or transplanting a recipient with occult malignancy, regular scheduled examination and appropriate tests for patients on the transplant waiting list, quitting smoking before transplantation, avoiding exposure to ultraviolet radiation during peak daylight, use of sun protective clothing and sunscreen, careful selection of induction and maintenance agents based on patients' risk factors for rejection, avoiding overimmunosuppression, improving immunosuppressive medication adherence, so as to prevent acute rejections and subsequent need to use T-cell depleting agents to treat these rejections, and appropriate viral surveillance (for example, EBV) in select patients.

Because of lack of cancer screening trials in RTRs, cancer screening recommendations in this population are extrapolated from the general population. This weakens the evidence base for cancer screening.

Recommendations for Skin Cancer Screening

Skin cancer is by far the most common cancer in RTRs. The incidence increases with time posttransplant. It is more common in the sun-exposed areas of the skin. Monthly self-screening by patients along with annual skin examination by dermatologists is recommended.

Recommendations for Posttransplant Lymphoproliferative Disorder Screening

The incidence of PTLD is highest in the first year after transplantation. Children and adults younger than 25 years of age or older than 60 years of age are at highest risk. Posttransplant EBV surveillance in patients with negative pretransplant EBV serology and high-dose polyclonal antibody induction therapy may be helpful in early detection of PTLD.

Recommendations for Cervical Cancer Screening

The risk for HPV-induced cervical cancer is 2 to 3 times higher in RTRs compared with age- and gender-matched general population. In the general population, HPV vaccines have been shown to reduce the incidence of HPV-16 and -18 cervical dysplasia but data on their safety and efficacy in transplant patients are lacking. Immunosuppression may lead to accelerated viral replication and rapid progression of precancerous lesions. Annual screening is thus recommended and, based on modeled analysis, it has been found to be cost-effective.[46]

Recommendations for Colon Cancer Screening

RTRs are at 2 to 3 times increased risk for colorectal cancer compared with the general population. Modeling studies suggest that screening for colorectal cancer is cost-effective in the transplant population.[47] The American Society of Transplantation (AST) recommends annual fecal occult blood testing and flexible sigmoidoscopy every 5 years for RTRs.[48]

Recommendations for Breast Cancer Screening

AST recommends yearly or every-other-year mammography in all-female transplant recipients between 40 and 49 years and every-other-year screening in those between 50 and 69 years of age.[48]

Recommendations for Renal Cancer Screening

RTRs with a history of analgesic use, previous cancer in a contralateral kidney, or acquired cystic disease of the kidneys are at high risk for developing cancer in the native kidneys. Renal cancer in the transplanted kidney is rare. Screening by ultrasound is operator dependent and presence of polycystic disease or scarred small native kidneys makes the differentiation between small renal cancers and benign lesions, like adenoma or angiomyolipomas, very challenging. Although screening for RCC in native kidneys is not cost-effective in all transplant patients, it may be useful in patients at high risk.

Recommendations for Urothelial Cancer Screening

Routine screening for bladder/urothelial cancer is not recommended. Investigation for diagnosis of these cancers should be guided by signs like hematuria or other GU symptoms.

Treatment of Postrenal Transplant Cancer

Cancers in RTRs tend to be more aggressive and if detected late, they uniformly carry a poor prognosis. Referral to an oncologist should be made as soon as the diagnosis of cancer is confirmed and a referral to a dermatologist should be made for any suspicious skin lesion. A realistic management plan involving the options of surgery, chemotherapy, radiotherapy, cryotherapy, and modification of the patient's immunosuppressive regimen should be discussed with a multidisciplinary treatment team. The patient's wishes, type of cancer and its prognosis, the risk of death from cancer or its treatment, and the risk of graft loss should be taken into consideration when developing a treatment plan.

Surgical resection, cryoablation, and radiotherapy are the best options for local and early-stage cancers. Careful and judicious alteration, reduction or discontinuation of certain immunosuppressants, with close monitoring of graft function, may be warranted especially in cases of oncogenic viruses driven cancers.[27] In some patients receiving chemotherapy, maintenance immunosuppressants may even need to be completely stopped for a variable period of time depending on patient's clinical condition.

mTORi, such as rapamycin, have immunosuppressive and antioncogenic activity. Retrospective studies and prospective clinical trials in RTRs have shown a lower incidence of de novo and recurrent squamous cell skin cancer in patients converted from a CNI to an mTORi.[49] Besides mTORi, retinoid acitretin and low-dose capecitabine have also been shown to be effective for secondary prevention of skin cancers. Switching from a CNI to an mTORi has also been shown to be effective in achieving successful clinical and histologic remission of Kaposi sarcoma.[16] But mTORi have a significant side effect profile and many RTRs are unable to tolerate these medications. mTORi have been used with marginal success for some solid and hematologic cancers, but conversion from a CNI to mTORi to improve outcomes of all cancers or to prevent the development of cancer is not recommended at this time because of lack of sufficient data and also because of the side effect profile of these agents.

New cancer therapies will pose new challenges. Immune checkpoint inhibitors, such as nivolumab or pembrolizumab, may unleash the immune system to attack a patient's cancer, but at the same time provoke acute transplant rejection caused by the disinhibited lymphocytes.[50]

Adroit adjustment of immunosuppression may avert rejection, but this remains an empiric task at present.

Key Points

- Posttransplant cancer is an important cause of death in transplant recipients.
- Intensity of immunosuppression and oncogenic viruses are the major risk factors.
- The value of screening for cancer is extrapolated from the general population but is not proven.
- Better cancer treatments will improve patient survival.

References

1. Sood P, Zhu YR, Cohen EP. Death with functioning kidney transplant: an obituarial analysis. *Int Urol Nephrol*. 2010;42(4):929-934.
2. Yanik EL, Nogueira LM, Koch L, et al. Comparison of cancer diagnoses between the US solid organ transplant registry and linked central cancer registries. *Am J Transplant*. 2016;16:2986-2993.
3. Vajdic CM, McDonald SP, McCredie MR, et al. Cancer incidence before and after kidney transplantation. *JAMA*. 2006;296:2823-2831.
4. Kasiske BL, Snyder JJ, Gilbertson DT, Wang C. Cancer after kidney transplantation in the United States. *Am J Transplant*. 2004;4:905-913.
5. Villeneuve PJ, Schaubel DE, Fenton SS, Shepherd FA, Jiang Y, Mao Y. Cancer incidence among Canadian kidney transplant recipients. *Am J Transplant*. 2007;7:941-948.
6. Opelz G, Döhler B. Lymphomas after solid organ transplantation: a collaborative transplant study report. *Am J Transplant*. 2003;4: 222-230.
7. Euvrard S, Kanitakis J, Claudy A. Skin cancers after organ transplantation. *N Engl J Med*. 2003;348:1681-1691.
8. Buell J, Gross T, Beebe T, et al. Cancer after renal transplantation. In: Cohen EP, ed. *Cancer and the kidney*. New York, NY: Oxford University Press; 2004.
9. Chapman J, Webster AC. *Cancer report: ANZDATA Transplant Registry 2004 report*. Woodville: ANZDATA Registry; Report no. 99, 2004.
10. Engels EA, Pfeiffer RM, Fraumeni JF Jr, et al. Spectrum of cancer risk among US solid organ transplant recipients. *JAMA*. 2011;306: 1891-1901.
11. Bordea C, Wojnarowska F, Millard PR, Doll H, Welsh K, Morris PJ. Skin cancers in renal-transplant recipients occur more frequently than previously recognized in a temperate climate. *Transplantation*. 2004; 77:574-579.
12. Ramsay HM, Fryer AA, Hawley CM, Smith AG, Harden PN. Nonmelanoma skin cancer risk in the Queensland renal transplant population. *Br J Dermatol*. 2002;147:950-956.
13. Kotton CN, Huprikar S, Kumar D. Transplant infectious diseases: a review of the scientific registry of transplant recipients published data. *Am J Transplant*. 2017;17:1439-1446.
14. Morton M, Coupes B, Roberts SA, et al. Epidemiology of posttransplantation lymphoproliferative disorder in adult renal transplant recipients. *Transplantation*. 2013;95(3):470-478.
15. Sprangers B, Nair V, Launay-Vacher V, Riella LV, Jhaveri KD. Risk factors associated with post-kidney transplant malignancies: an article from the Cancer-Kidney International Network. *Clin Kidney J*. 2017; 11(3):315-329.
16. Stallone G, Schena A, Infante B, et al. Sirolimus for Kaposi's sarcoma in renal-transplant recipients. *N Engl J Med*. 2005;352:1317-1323.
17. van Leeuwen MT, Webster AC, McCredie MR, et al. Effect of reduced immunosuppression after kidney transplant failure on risk of cancer: population based retrospective cohort study. *BMJ*. 2010;340:c570.
18. Dantal J, Pohanka E. Malignancies in renal transplantation: an unmet medical need. *Nephrol Dial Transplant*. 2007;22(suppl 1):4-10.
19. Morath C, Mueller M, Goldschmidt H, Schwenger V, Opelz G, Zeier M. Malignancy in renal transplantation. *J Am Soc Nephrol*. 2004;15: 1582-1588.
20. Wong G, Hayen A, Chapman JR, et al. Association of CKD and cancer risk in older people. *J Am Soc Nephrol*. 2009;20:1341-1350.
21. Wong G, Turner RM, Chapman JR, et al. Time on dialysis and cancer risk after kidney transplantation. *Transplantation*. 2013;95:114-121.
22. Brattström C, Granath F, Edgren G, Smedby KE, Wilczek HE. Overall and cause-specific mortality in transplant recipients with a pretransplantation cancer history. *Transplantation*. 2013;96:297-305.
23. Acuna SA, Huang JW, Daly C, Shah PS, Kim SJ, Baxter NN. Outcomes of solid organ transplant recipients with preexisting malignancies in remission: a systematic review and meta-analysis. *Transplantation*. 2017;101:471-481.
24. Young LS, Rickinson AB. Epstein-Barr virus: 40 years on. *Nat Rev Cancer*. 2004;4:757-768.
25. Ma MK, Lim WH, Turner RM, Chapman JR, Craig JC, Wong G. The risk of cancer in recipients of living-donor, standard and expanded criteria deceased donor kidney transplants: a registry analysis. *Transplantation*. 2014;98:1286-1293.
26. Myron Kauffman H, McBride MA, Cherikh WS, Spain PC, Marks WH, Roza AM. Transplant tumor registry: donor related malignancies. *Transplantation*. 2002;74:358-362.
27. Stallone G, Infante B, Grandaliano G. Management and prevention of post-transplant malignancies in kidney transplant recipients. *Clin Kidney J*. 2015;8:637-644.
28. Lim WH, Turner RM, Chapman JR, et al. Acute rejection, T-cell-depleting antibodies, and cancer after transplantation. *Transplantation*. 2014;97:817-825.
29. Knoll GA, Kokolo MB, Mallick R, et al. Effect of sirolimus on malignancy and survival after kidney transplantation: systematic review and meta-analysis of individual patient data. *BMJ*. 2014;349:g6679.
30. Gallagher MP, Kelly PJ, Jardine M, et al. Long-term cancer risk of immunosuppressive regimens after kidney transplantation. *J Am Soc Nephrol*. 2010;21:852-858.
31. Sampaio MS, Cho YW, Qazi Y, et al. Posttransplant malignancies in solid organ adult recipients: an analysis of the U.S. National Transplant Database. *Transplantation*. 2012;94:990-998.

32. Dantal J, Hourmant M, Cantarovich D, et al. Effect of long-term immunosuppression in kidney-graft recipients on cancer incidence: randomised comparison of two cyclosporin regimens. *Lancet.* 1998; 351:623-628.

33. Sampaio MS, Cho YW, Shah T, Bunnapradist S, Hutchinson IV. Association of immunosuppressive maintenance regimens with posttransplant lymphoproliferative disorder in kidney transplant recipients. *Transplantation.* 2012;93:73-81.

34. Pirsch JD, Miller J, Deierhoi MH, Vincenti F, Filo RS. A comparison of tacrolimus (FK506) and cyclosporine for immunosuppression after cadaveric renal transplantation. FK506 Kidney Transplant Study Group. *Transplantation.* 1997;63:977.

35. Mathew TH. A blinded, long-term, randomized multicenter study of mycophenolate mofetil in cadaveric renal transplantation: results at three years. Tricontinental Mycophenolate Mofetil Renal Transplantation Study Group. *Transplantation.* 1998;65:1450.

36. Mycophenolate mofetil in cadaveric renal transplantation. US Renal Transplant Mycophenolate Mofetil Study Group. *Am J Kidney Dis.* 1999; 34:296.

37. David KM, Morris JA, Steffen BJ, Chi-Burris KS, Gotz VP, Gordon RD. Mycophenolate mofetil vs. azathioprine is associated with decreased acute rejection, late acute rejection, and risk for cardiovascular death in renal transplant recipients with pre-transplant diabetes. *Clin Transplant.* 2005;19:279.

38. Robson R, Cecka JM, Opelz G, Budde M, Sacks S. Prospective registry-based observational cohort study of the long-term risk of malignancies in renal transplant patients treated with mycophenolate mofetil. *Am J Transplant.* 2005;5:2954-2960.

39. Vincenti F, Charpentier B, Vanrenterghem Y, et al. A phase III study of belatacept-based immunosuppression regimens versus cyclosporine in renal transplant recipients (BENEFIT study). *Am J Transplant.* 2010;10:535-546.

40. Vincenti F, Rostaing L, Grinyo J, et al. Belatacept and long-term outcomes in kidney transplantation. *N Engl J Med.* 2016;374:333-343.

41. Batabyal P, Chapman JR, Wong G, Craig JC, Tong A. Clinical practice guidelines on wait-listing for kidney transplantation: consistent and equitable? *Transplantation.* 2012;94:703-713.

42. Nalesnik MA, Woodle ES, Dimaio JM, et al. Donor-transmitted malignancies in organ transplantation: assessment of clinical risk. *Am J Transplant.* 2011;11:1140-1147.

43. Collins AJ, Foley RN, Chavers B, et al. United States Renal Data System 2011 annual data report: atlas of chronic kidney disease & end-stage renal disease in the United States. *Am J Kidney Dis.* 2012;59:e1-e420.

44. van de Wetering J, Roodnat JI, Hemke AC, Hoitsma AJ, Weimar W. Patient survival after the diagnosis of cancer in renal transplant recipients: a nested case-control study. *Transplantation.* 2010;90:1542-1546.

45. Kiberd BA, Rose C, Gill JS. Cancer mortality in kidney transplantation. *Am J Transplant.* 2009;9:1868-1875.

46. Wong G, Howard K, Webster A, Chapman JR, Craig JC. The health and economic impact of cervical cancer screening and human papillomavirus vaccination in kidney transplant recipients. *Transplantation.* 2009;87:1078-1091.

47. Wong G, Howard K, Craig JC, Chapman JR. Cost-effectiveness of colorectal cancer screening in renal transplant recipients. *Transplantation.* 2008;85:532-541.

48. Kasiske BL, Vazquez MA, Harmon WE, et al. Recommendations for the outpatient surveillance of renal transplant recipients. American Society of Transplantation. *J Am Soc Nephrol.* 2000;11:S1-S86.

49. Euvrard S, Morelon E, Rostaing L, et al. Sirolimus and secondary skin-cancer prevention in kidney transplantation. *N Engl J Med.* 2012; 367:329-339.

50. Wanchoo R, Riella LV, Uppal NN, et al. Immune checkpoint inhibitors in the cancer patient with an organ transplant. *J Onco-Nephrol.* 2017;1:42-48.

Kidney Infections

36 Renal Infections in Cancer Patients

PRASHANT MALHOTRA, PRANISHA GAUTAM-GOYAL, AND MARCIA E. EPSTEIN

Introduction

EPIDEMIOLOGY

Cancer patients are at a higher risk of infections with a mean annual incidence rate of 1465 cases per 100,000 cancer patients and a relative risk [RR] of 9.77 compared with noncancer patients (95% confidence interval [CI], 9.67–9.88).[1] Bacterial urinary tract infections (UTIs) can commonly be seen both in patients with genitourinary tract cancers and nongenitourinary tract malignancies. Because of their immunosuppression, both hematopoietic stem cell transplant and solid organ transplant patients are at increased risk of viral, fungal, and other atypical bacterial infections, in addition to bacterial infections.[2] Very few studies have described the incidence of kidney infections in cancer patients. In a study among 3355 French patients with primarily hematologic malignancies, 170 UTIs were observed, with an attack rate (number of diagnosed infections/100 patients) of 5.1 and an incidence rate of 2.9 per 1000 patient-days at risk.[3] In this study enterobacteria (60%) were the predominant pathogens. Some 10% of the patients had fungal infections, whereas viruses accounted for only 3%. These rates are higher than the documented UTI rates among hospitalized patients in both the United States of 0.34% (2015) and Europe 1.32% (2010).[4,5]

Although early recognition and management of sepsis in an intensive care setting has improved survival in cancer patients, cancer patients with sepsis continue to have disproportionately higher rates of mortality and morbidity and consequently, incur higher health care costs compared with noncancer patients with sepsis.[6–9]

Infections including UTIs leading to sepsis have been well described in cancer patients and can lead to significant morbidity and mortality. Sepsis is the most common cause of intensive care admissions in cancer patients. In some studies, about 20% of the cancer patients admitted to ICUs had sepsis.[10–12] In a study of 1332 patients that were admitted to an oncology-dedicated ICU, 563 (42%) patients met criteria for sepsis. Of these, 8% of patients had UTIs. Patients with UTIs were shown to have lower mortality rates in this study than those with pneumonias or bacteremias.[10]

Risk Factors for Infections in Cancer Patients

Many factors contribute to a higher risk of infections in cancer patients and involve a complex interplay between the body's natural defenses and microorganisms colonizing the patients.

IMMUNE DYSFUNCTION CAUSED BY CANCER

The innate immune system is the first line of defense of the body and refers to immune responses that are present from birth and are not acquired or adapted as a result of exposure to microorganisms. Host components include mucosal barriers, secretory enzymes, such as lysozyme, certain inflammatory proteins including C-reactive protein, antimicrobial peptides, cell receptors such as Toll-like receptors, phagocytic cells, like neutrophils and macrophages, mast cells and natural killer cells, which release cytokines.[13] On the other hand, the adaptive immune system consists of the T and B lymphocytes, which continually learn, adapt, and help mount immune responses upon recognition of different foreign and tumor antigens. A variety of microorganisms that colonize the skin, respiratory tract, and the gastrointestinal tract constitute the human microbiome and are thought to contribute to the maturation of immune response and controlling the overgrowth of pathogenic microbes.[14]

Cancers can alter both innate and adaptive immune responses. In certain hematologic cancers, like multiple myeloma and chronic lymphocytic leukemia, reduced antibody production and clearance of immune complexes can lead to an increased risk of infections from encapsulated bacteria like *Streptococcus pneumoniae* and *Haemophilus influenzae*. Other malignancies like lymphomas can cause defects in cell-mediated immunity, and lead to increased risk of infections with intracellular organisms, like listeria, salmonella, cryptococcus, and mycobacteria.

CHEMOTHERAPY AND RADIOTHERAPY

Chemotherapy can have several effects on the immune system, leading to infections. The suppression of hematopoiesis by chemotherapy can lead to pancytopenia and functional impairment, thereby decreasing the quantitative and qualitative ability of the immune system to contain infections.

Neutropenia with an absolute neutrophil count (ANC) below 500 cells/microliter increases the risk of bacterial infections in patients. If neutropenia is prolonged, the risk of fungal infections also increases in these patients. In addition to causing neutropenia, chemotherapeutic agents may impair chemotaxis and phagocytosis and decrease the ability of neutrophils to eliminate intracellular pathogens.[15] Other chemotherapeutic agents, such as calcineurin inhibitors, which inhibit T-cell activation, or fludarabine, which affects lymphocyte function, can have severe and longstanding effects on the cell-mediated immunity and can increase the risk for certain infections like *Pneumocystis jiroveci* pneumonia, and viral infections.

Stem cell transplants can have a profound effect on cell-mediated immunity; the use of aggressive chemotherapy and prolonged immunosuppression after stem cell transplants can impair immunity further, leading to increased susceptibility to infection.

Radiotherapy-induced inflammation also contributes to UTIs. In one prospective study, pelvic radiotherapy led to development of UTIs in 17% of the patients studied.[16] Even though patients of both sexes with various pelvic malignancies were included, there was an increased risk of infections in women with bladder and cervical malignancies. In another study of 36 patients with gynecologic malignancies, 25% of patients developed bacteriuria during radiotherapy; a higher risk of infection was associated with advanced stages of cancer.[17] The authors suggested preradiation urine cultures, particularly in patients undergoing cystoscopy and periodic screening in women with advanced cervical cancers, as they were at higher risk.

GLUCOCORTICOIDS AND OTHER MEDICATION-INDUCED IMMUNE DYSFUNCTION

The use of glucocorticoids can impair migration of granulocytes to sites of inflammation and negatively affect phagocytosis and intracellular killing. The opsonization of bacteria and phagocytosis of pathogens by neutrophils and macrophages is also affected adversely by the use of steroids.[2] Furthermore, the introduction of monoclonal antibodies, like alemtuzumab, ibritumomab, and rituximab, has also resulted in an increase in opportunistic infections because of lymphopenia, impaired T-lymphocyte response, and phagocyte dysfunction.[18]

MUCOSITIS

Cachexia and malnutrition are frequently seen in cancer patients and lead to a catabolic state. This is further exacerbated by anorexia because of malignancy and chemotherapy-induced gastrointestinal effects, including nausea and vomiting.[19] All these together cause mucosal atrophy and loss of the epithelial lining, leading to mucositis.

Mucositis results in decreases in secretory defenses, including lysozymes and immunoglobulin (Ig)A, and alterations in the classic and alternative complement pathway.[20] The associated loss of inhibitory substances, such as lactoferrin, lysozyme, defensins, peroxidase, and IgA, can contribute to the impaired clearance of pathogenic organisms and increase the risk of infections.

CHEMOTHERAPY AND RADIOTHERAPY-INDUCED MUCOSITIS

Chemotherapy and radiation therapy can cause mucositis and translocation of the normal microbial flora of the gastrointestinal and genitourinary tract; this in turn leads to invasive infections and bacteremia.[21,22] Chemotherapy-induced hematopoiesis suppression can cause pancytopenia and functional impairment, thereby decreasing the quantitative and qualitative ability of the immune system to contain infections. Various chemotherapeutic agents, including anthracyclines (daunorubicin and doxorubicin), plant alkaloids (vinblastine and vincristine), paclitaxel, cisplatin, melphalan, bleomycin, etoposides, and radiation, have been shown to cause aberrant activation of the immune cascade by activation of nuclear factor (NF)-κβ. Activation of NF-κβ in turn results in macrophages and endothelial cells releasing various proinflammatory cytokines and chemokines like interleukin (IL)-1, IL-6, IL-8, tumor necrosis factor-α, and interferon-gamma.[23] The activation of NF-κβ can lead to apoptosis and both tumor and "innocent bystander" mucosal cell death. As a consequence, ulceration, crypt hypoplasia, and villous atrophy follows, and matrix metalloproteinases are activated, which in turn leads to cleavage of collagen and fibronectin. Mucositis is further amplified by the breaching of natural barriers by bacteria and their proinflammatory cell wall products, such as peptidoglycan and lipopolysaccharides.[24–27] The destruction of residual symbiotic microflora disrupts the microbiome and leads to the overgrowth of pathogenic microorganisms, thereby causing infections.

MECHANICAL FACTORS, DEVICES

Cancer patients have an elevated risk of infections because of the increased use of medical devices, including catheters, stents, and prostheses.[2] The anatomic changes associated with transplantation and various postsurgical complications also predispose these patients to infections. The risk of inflammation is increased in malignancies. UTIs may be caused by invasive gynecologic surgery (for malignancy), associated surgical complications, and invasive instrumentation, which also includes catheterization or cystoscopy.[28] Tumors, by obstructing and invading normal tissue, can cause local organ dysfunction and predispose patients to infections.

Bacterial Infections

Bacterial UTIs are common in cancer patients. In a study of 399 patients with solid tumors, UTIs were significantly more common among patients on glucocorticosteroids and needed a median duration of 11 days to treat. UTIs also led to a 14-day length of hospital stay; a total of 28 patients died in this study.[29]

The microbiology of UTIs is similar in cancer and noncancer patients, although more antimicrobial resistance is seen in cancer patients. In a retrospective study, 100 out of 497 urine samples from cancer patients who were suspected to have UTI had growth on cultures. *Escherichia coli* was the predominant organism in 40% of the cases, followed by *Klebsiella pneumoniae* (25%), *Pseudomonas aeruginosa* (11%), *Enterococcus spp* (11%), and *Proteus mirabilis* (5%). Resistance to antimicrobials was high; 90% of the isolates were resistant to fluoroquinolones, 67% to cephalosporins, 46% to aminoglycosides, and 28% to carbapenems.[30] *E. coli* was also the predominant isolate in another study accounting for 28/66 isolates.[29] Resistance to fluoroquinolones, sulfamethoxazole, and some other antimicrobials and multidrug resistance have also been described and have contributed to a longer length of stay.[31–33] The low yield of cultures could be caused by obtaining them after antimicrobials are started and this makes obtaining cultures before initiating empiric antimicrobials essential. Antimicrobial susceptibility data (local antibiograms) can be used to guide initial antimicrobial therapy. If a patient was on antimicrobials for prophylaxis, a different class of antimicrobial should be chosen for empiric treatment. Also the presence of resistance above 20% to an antimicrobial class in a particular area is thought to preclude its use empirically.[34,35]

In another study of 462 patients hospitalized with *Enterobacteriaceae* bacteremia, *K. pneumoniae* bacteremia (odds ratio [OR], 6.13; $p = .007$), APACHE II score (OR, 1.18; $p = .007$), and exposure to aminopenicillins (OR, 28.84; $p = .015$) were more commonly associated with neoplasms. Among these patients, a genitourinary source of bacteremia was identified in 111 patients (25.5%).[36]

CYSTITIS

The signs and symptoms of UTIs in patients with cancer are similar to those in patients without malignancies. Lower tract UTIs may present with dysuria, urgent or frequent urination, and suprapubic pain or tenderness. In general, the presence of fevers in UTIs is indicative of parenchymal inflammation or upper tract involvement.

Separate guidelines for diagnosis and management of UTIs in cancer patients have not been published. Thus management is mostly based on guidelines in noncancer patients (Table 36.1). For uncomplicated lower tract infections including cystitis, nitrofurantoin, trimethoprim-sulfamethoxazole (160/800 mg [1 double-strength tablet] twice daily for 3 days) or fosfomycin trometamol (3-g single dose) have been recommended in recent guidelines for nonimmunocompromised and noncancer patients.[34] The presence of resistance above 20% to an antimicrobial class in a particular area is thought to preclude its use empirically.[34,35,37] Given the higher prevalence of antimicrobial resistance in cancer patients to fluoroquinolones, cephalosporins, aminoglycosides, and sulfa agents, the use of these agents empirically

is thus not recommended.[30] The higher prevalence of resistance, including to carbapenems, and even multidrug resistance necessitates obtaining urine cultures in these cases essential.[34,38,39]

There is frequent resistance to fluoroquinolones, and they have higher potential for *Clostridium difficile*. Hence alternatives are preferred. There have been studies documenting inferior efficacy of amoxicillin-clavulanate in shorter 3 day courses as compared with fluoroquinolones.[40] However, beta-lactam antibiotics including cephalosporins such as cefdinir, cefaclor, and cefpodoxime-proxetil, and aminopenicillin derivatives including amoxicillin-clavulanate are considered reasonable alternatives in 3- to 7-day regimens, when other agents cannot be used.[41] Other beta-lactams, such as first-generation cephalosporins, including cephalexin, have a narrower gram-negative spectrum, and data supporting their use are scant. However, if susceptibility is confirmed, their use may be reasonable in certain situations.[34,38,39,42]

UPPER URINARY TRACT INFECTIONS INCLUDING PYELONEPHRITIS

Upper tract infections manifest with new onset or worsening of fever, rigors, altered mental status, malaise, or lethargy with no other identified cause, flank pain, costovertebral angle tenderness, acute hematuria, or pelvic discomfort. Catheter-associated UTIs have similar signs.[43]

In patients suspected of having pyelonephritis, a urine culture and susceptibility test should always be performed, and initial empirical therapy should be tailored appropriately based on the infecting pathogen.[41] Guidelines in nonimmunocompromised patients indicate that oral ciprofloxacin is an appropriate therapeutic choice in patients not requiring hospitalization, provided the prevalence of resistance of community-acquired bacteria to fluoroquinolones is known to be below 10% (Table 36.2). The higher resistance and increasing use of fluoroquinolones for prophylaxis in cancer patients makes them unreliable empiric options. In the presence of more than 10% fluoroquinolone resistance, an initial intravenous dose of a

Table 36.1   Treatment of Uncomplicated Cystitis

Antibiotic	Dose & Duration	Adverse Effects	Dose Adjustment for Renal Function
EMPIRIC AGENTS			
Nitrofurantoin	100 mg twice daily × 5–7 days	Nausea, headache	Yes[a]
Trimethoprim-sulfamethoxazole	160/800 mg twice daily × 3 days	Nausea, vomiting, cytopenia, rash	Yes
Fosfomycin	3-g single dose	Nausea, diarrhea, headache	Not defined
ALTERNATE AGENTS			
Ciprofloxacin[b]	500 mg twice a day × 3 days	Nausea, vomiting, headache, diarrhea	Yes
Levofloxacin[b]	250–500 mg daily × 3 days	Nausea, vomiting, headache, diarrhea	Yes
Beta-lactams[c,d]	Dose varies by agent × 3–5 days	Nausea, vomiting, diarrhea, rash	Yes

[a]Contraindicated when creatinine clearance less than 60 mL/min.
[b]High rates of resistance, confirm sensitivity before use. Highly efficacious but also high incidence of adverse effects—considered as alternate agents.
[c]Amoxicillin and ampicillin have high rates of resistance, also relatively poor efficacy; do not use for empiric therapy.
[d]Amoxicillin-clavulanate, cefaclor, cefopodoxime-proxetil, and cefdinir can be used if other agents not available. Lower efficacy and higher adverse effects as compared with other agents.

Table 36.2 Treatment of Upper Tract Infections/Pyelonephritis

Antibiotic	Dose & Duration	Adverse Effects	Dose Adjustment for Renal Function
EMPIRIC AGENTS – OUTPATIENT[a]			
Trimethoprim-sulfamethoxazole[b]	160/800 mg twice daily × 3 days	Nausea, vomiting, cytopenia, rash	Yes
Levofloxacin[c]	250–500 mg daily × 3 days	Nausea, vomiting, headache, diarrhea	Yes
Ciprofloxacin[c]	500 mg twice a day × 3 days	Nausea, vomiting, headache, diarrhea	Yes
INPATIENT REGIMENS[d,e,f]			
Ceftriaxone ± aminoglycoside as later	1 g IV daily	Nausea, vomiting, allergy, neutropenia	Yes
Levofloxacin[b] ± aminoglycoside	250–750 mg IV/po daily	Nausea, vomiting, headache, diarrhea	Yes
Ciprofloxacin[b] ± aminoglycoside as below	200–400 mg IV q 12 hours or 250–750 mg po q 12 hours	Nausea, vomiting, headache, diarrhea	
Piperacillin/tazobactam	3.375 g IV q 6 hours	Allergic reaction, myelosuppression, interstitial nephritis	Yes
Carbapenem Imipenem/cilastatin Meropenem	500 mg IV q 6 hours 500–1000 mg IV q 8 hours	Allergic reactions, seizures, myelosuppression	Yes
AMINOGLYCOSIDES			
Gentamicin	5–7 mg/kg IV daily	Nephrotoxicity, ototoxicity	Yes
Amikacin	7.5 mg/kg IV q 12–24 hours	Nephrotoxicity, ototoxicity	Yes

[a]Urine cultures and susceptibility data should always be obtained.
[b]Only if local resistance rates are less than 10%.
[c]Can be used in a 14-day course if susceptibility is confirmed.
[d]Initial intravenous therapy is recommended. Use based on local antimicrobial resistance data. Modify treatment based on susceptibility data.
[e]7 day regimens of fluoroquinolones may be sufficient.
[f]10–14 day courses of beta-lactams may be needed.
IV, Intravenous; po, by mouth; q, every.

long-acting antimicrobial, such as ceftriaxone or an aminoglycoside, is considered reasonable. If susceptibility is confirmed, oral trimethoprim-sulfamethoxazole for 14 days is considered a reasonable option.

Awaiting susceptibilities, an initial parenteral antimicrobial, like 1-g ceftriaxone or a once-a-day aminoglycoside, is recommended in noncancer patients and would be considered necessary in immunocompromised patients, given the higher probability of resistance. As in cystitis, beta-lactam agents are less effective than other available agents for treatment of pyelonephritis. Efficacy/outcomes for beta-lactams, including cephalosporins, were inferior compared with trimethoprim-sulfamethoxazole and fluoroquinolones.[40,44–46]

Seven-day regimens for fluoroquinolones in noncancer patients have been recommended to treat pyelonephritis. However, most recent guidelines suggest that there are not enough data to treat pyelonephritis with a similar short course of a beta-lactam agent.[34,47,48] Patients with pyelonephritis requiring hospitalization should be initially treated with intravenous antibiotics, such as a fluoroquinolone, an aminoglycoside (with or without ampicillin), an extended-spectrum cephalosporin or extended-spectrum penicillin (with or without an aminoglycoside), or a carbapenem.[49] The choice between these agents should be based on local resistance data, and the regimen should be tailored based on susceptibility results (see Table 36.2).[50,51]

Treatment with agents for longer periods (> 14 days) may result in the development of resistant pathogens by selection pressure.[52] Two weeks of trimethoprim-sulfamethoxazole were shown to be as efficacious as a 6-week course of ampicillin in a study of 60 women with uncomplicated pyelonephritis.[53] The shorter course had fewer adverse effects, lower costs, and also led to the selection of fewer resistant organisms.

CATHETER-ASSOCIATED URINARY TRACT INFECTIONS

Guidelines indicate that if an indwelling catheter has been in place for more than 2 weeks and still needs to be retained, replacement of the catheter helps in treatment of the episode and the prevention of any future recurrences. Urine culture should be obtained from the newly placed catheter before starting antibiotics and used to tailor the antimicrobial choice. However, if the catheter can be removed, a midstream urine sample should be obtained before starting antibiotics and the result used to guide the choice.[34,54]

If symptoms resolve rapidly, 7 days of treatment is considered adequate for most patients with catheter-associated (CA)-UTI. Shorter duration of fluoroquinolones, particularly levofloxacin, has been recommended in patients who are not severely ill.[34] There is some literature supporting a shorter duration (3 days) in nonimmunocompromised patients with no upper tract symptoms in whom the catheter has been removed, although there are no trials to guide therapy in cancer patients.[54,55] In patients with delayed response and immunocompromised patients, a longer (10–14 day) course of treatment may be considered, but data on the optimal duration of therapy are scant, particularly in cancer patients. Given the immunocompromised state, we feel that a 10- to 14-day course would be reasonable in these cases.

PROSTATITIS

In men, the majority of febrile UTIs are associated with prostatitis.[56] The diagnosis of acute prostatitis can be established by urine cultures and prostate examinations. However, the diagnosis of chronic prostatitis may require obtaining prostatic fluid and a urine sample after prostatic massage. Other methods, including the Meares-Stamey four-glass test and the simpler "two-glass" test have been described, but are infrequently used in clinical practice. Prolonged symptoms or refractory cases may require a urologist referral and evaluation. Antimicrobials used to treat UTIs in men should be able to achieve sufficient concentration in the prostatic tissues. Fluoroquinolones and trimethoprim-sulfamethoxazole have excellent penetration, but the increasing resistance may preclude their use.[57] Beta-lactams may result in less optimal outcomes.[58]

Although there is paucity of data on the treatment of UTIs in men, some studies have shown that patients with urologic issues requiring surgical intervention had more recurrences of UTIs (26% vs. 12%).[59] A 2-week antimicrobial course was shown to be adequate in most cases.

MECHANICAL ASPECTS – INFECTIONS CAUSED BY OBSTRUCTION, RECONSTRUCTION

Anatomic obstructions, either via tumor burden or impaired physiology, can lead to inadequate emptying, retention, and reflux, which can lead to development of infections. Surgical procedures can lead to altered anatomy, thereby compromising natural defenses against infection bladder surgeries, for example, reflux.

Obstructive uropathy can also lead to urinary stasis, which encourages bacterial colonization and can further lead to retrograde ascending urinary infections. Complicated infections of this nature will need rapid decompression with placement of stents or percutaneous nephrostomy catheters. Organisms seen in these infections include the expected urinary flora like *E. coli*, klebsiella species, and staphylococci, enterococci, pseudomonas, and candida. Eradication of these infections in the presence of prior foreign bodies often requires removal or replacement of the indwelling devices.[60,61]

Patients with reconstructive surgery and either neobladders or ileoanal conduits have been shown to have persistent bacteriuria after surgery. It can be difficult to distinguish between colonization and infections in these cases and the presence of symptoms is essential in making the distinction between colonization and infections in these cases.[62]

Patients with nephrostomy tubes are at increased risk for development of UTIs. In a tertiary cancer center study, among 200 patients with nephrostomy tubes, 38 (19%) developed pyelonephritis and 15 (7.5%) had asymptomatic bacteriuria. The presence of prior episodes and neutropenia were significant risk factors ($p = .047$ and $p = .03$), respectively.[63]

ASYMPTOMATIC BACTERIURIA IN CANCER PATIENTS

Current guidelines do not support treatment of asymptomatic bacteriuria in cancer patients.[64,65] However, neutropenia, a recent transplant, or other factors causing immunosuppression may necessitate treatment consideration in some patients. Guidelines are not very clear on this, however; an evaluation should be done, and clinical judgment used on a case-by-case basis, especially for indwelling catheters, where catheter-related colonization is common.[66] Urine cultures should be obtained only if there is a clinical suspicion of UTI in these cases.

PROPHYLAXIS

Presently, there are no studies to help guide prophylaxis in patients with cancer and frequent or recurrent UTIs. In nonimmunocompromised patients, prophylactic or suppressive antimicrobials should be considered in case of more than two episodes of lower tract infections in 6 months or more than three episodes in 12 months.[67–69] A workup for reversible anatomic or functional factors including obstruction is required before suppressive therapy. The risk of adverse effects and the development of resistance needs to be considered, as such risks may be higher in cancer patients.[70–73] Emerging data suggest that there may be significant pathologic consequences like the development of antimicrobial resistance, vitamin K deficiency, increased susceptibility to infections, and diarrhea, because of the altered microbiome from suppressive/prophylactic antibiotics.[74,75]

Mycobacterial Infections

BACILLUS CALMETTE-GUÉRIN

Bacillus Calmette-Guérin (BCG) is a live attenuated vaccine obtained from *Mycobacterium bovis*. Use of intravesical BCG for the treatment of superficial bladder cancer was first described in 1976.[76] Its use increased after the U.S. Food and Drug Administration approval in 1990, and currently there are more data on its safety and efficacy with its use over the past quarter of a century. The treatment is usually well tolerated, but rarely, systemic complications, such as fatal BCGosis, occur. Specific side effects involving the kidney are well described.[77] Granulomatous cystitis has been well described after BCG instillation and bladder pathology is useful in establishing diagnosis[78] (Fig. 36.1). Asymptomatic renal granulomas—often detected on follow-up imaging—occur in 1 in 1000 cases. These are thought to likely be related to reflux of the intravesical BCG rather than hematogenous spread. The treatment of these granulomas is not well established; they were commonly treated with antitubercular therapy in the past and some authors still advocate early treatment of renal BCGosis even in asymptomatic patients.[79] However, other studies have demonstrated no progression with no treatment and close observation.[80]

BCG instillation can also lead to interstitial nephritis with or without granuloma. Patients usually present with

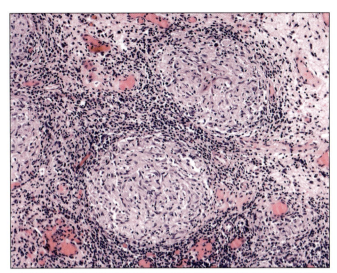

Fig. 36.1 Bladder biopsy showing granulomatous cystitis after intravesical Bacillus Calmette-Guérin (BCG) therapy.

elevated creatinine. A few case reports have described other pathologies, including acute kidney injury with glomerulonephritis,[81] membranous nephropathy,[82] hemolytic uremic syndrome, rhabdomyolysis, and multiorgan failure after BCG treatment.[83] It has been recommended that a decline in renal function, hematuria, or proteinuria during BCG treatment in the absence of other etiologies warrants consideration of renal biopsy.[77]

There are no reliable data available about the incidence of renal toxicity after intravesical BCG; this is in part because of underreporting and in part because other variables influence the occurrence. These other factors include the strain type of BCG used (they have different immunogenicity, virulence, and toxicity), the dose used, repetitive injury, and patient factors.[77]

TUBERCULOSIS

Approximately 1.7 billion individuals are latently infected with *Mycobacterium tuberculosis*.[84] Tuberculosis (TB) is the ninth leading cause of death worldwide, and the leading cause of death from a single infectious agent. In 2016 an estimated 1.7 million people died from TB. It is an infection of major relevance.[85]

Although TB primarily affects the lung, other organs may also be involved. After lymphadenitis, the most common form of nonpulmonary TB is genitourinary disease, accounting for 27% of nonpulmonary cases in the United States, Canada, and the United Kingdom.[84] Respiratory infection with TB can be followed by hematogenous dissemination to the kidneys, epididymis, and the prostate. Implantation usually occurs in the more vascular parts, such as the cortex of the kidney and the globus minor of the epididymis, and is bilateral.[86] Cancer patients are at increased risk for reactivation of their latent tuberculosis, either caused by inherent immunodeficiency from their underlying malignancy or from effects of the cancer treatment—such as fludarabine and glucocorticosteroids that might impair T-cell immunity.[87]

The incidence of TB is 10 to 40 times more common in patients with hematopoietic stem cell transplantation (HSCT) compared with the general population, but the incidence varies depending on geographic location and is directly proportional to the incidence of TB in the general population. Incidences of *M. tuberculosis* in HSCT recipients have been reported to be as low as 0.0014% in the United States and as high as 16% in Pakistan.[88] Risk factors for the development of TB after HSCT include certain leukemias, like acute myeloid leukemia, chronic myeloid leukemia, and myelodysplastic syndrome, the use of certain conditioning therapies, such as busulfan, cyclophosphamide, total body irradiation, corticosteroid therapy, mismatched allografts, graft-versus-host disease (GVHD), or a history of previous TB infection.[89] At least one-third of *M. tuberculosis* infections in HSCT patients are disseminated at presentation.[88]

A high index of suspicion for genitourinary TB is required for timely diagnosis and treatment.[90] Clinical findings are variable, but patients commonly present with dysuria with sterile pyuria or a painless scrotal mass. Diagnosis of genitourinary TB without any systemic involvement can be difficult. Collection of urine, expressed prostatic secretions, postmassage urine and ejaculate for acid fast bacilli smear and mycobacterial culture, and polymerase chain reaction (PCR) may be helpful, although these have a low sensitivity.[91] The gold standard for establishing the diagnosis would be isolation of mycobacteria from the urine. Sterile pyuria may suggest urinary tract TB infection, but a superimposed bacterial infection may delay diagnosis in up to 30% of cases.[90] There is poor sensitivity with traditional staining (Ziehl-Neelsen and auramine stain, being positive in 37%–52% of cases).[90] Furthermore, contamination with *Mycobacterium smegmatis* or fragments of sperm can cause a false positive smear. Nucleic acid amplification can be sensitive and specific, although some urine specimens contain inhibitory substances.[92] Early diagnosis and treatment may prevent the loss of organ function.

Treatment is generally with medical therapy with the standard four drugs (isoniazid, rifampin, pyrazinamide, ethambutol); surgery is rarely required.[93] Special considerations apply to the treatment of TB in patients with renal insufficiency; dose adjustments of some antitubercular drugs, like ethambutol are needed to avoid toxicity, such as optic neuritis (Table 36.3).[92] Aminoglycosides are renally excreted and nephrotoxic and should be avoided in these patients. Rifampin has a number of drug interactions and can increase the metabolism of a wide range of drugs, including steroids, cyclosporine, and tacrolimus. Thus its use may require drug level monitoring and dose adjustment.

Fungal Infections

Fungal infections can be caused by yeasts or molds. Several factors render cancer patients at an increased risk for fungal infections. Prolonged neutropenia, the use of broad-spectrum antibiotics, the presence of indwelling venous catheters, and chemotherapy-associated mucosal injuries put patients at increased risk for invasive candidiasis.[2] GVHD after allogeneic transplantation and prolonged neutropenia pose a risk for mold infections. *Aspergillus* is the most common mold isolated, but other molds, such as

Table 36.3   Antimycobacterial Agents and Dose Adjustments With Renal Impairment

Drug	Major Toxicities	Adjust for Renal Function
Isoniazid	Hepatitis, neuritis, drug-induced lupus, drowsiness, mood changes	No dose adjustment
Rifampin	Multiple drug interactions, hepatitis, flushing, thrombocytopenia, diarrhea, brownish discoloration of skin and secretions, flu-like syndrome	No dose adjustment
Ethambutol	Optic neuritis, rash, abdominal distress	Adjust
Pyrizinamide	Hepatitis rash, arthralgias or arthritis, hyperuricemia	Adjust
Moxifloxacin	Tremors, thrush, diarrhea, interstitial nephritis, Achilles tendon rupture, aneurysm, QTc prolongation, hepatotoxicity	Adjust
Capreomycin	Hearing loss, ataxia, nystagmus, azotemia proteinuria, eosinophilia, serum electrolyte abnormality	Adjust
Amikacin, kanamycin	Hearing loss, ataxia, nystagmus, azotemia proteinuria, eosinophilia, serum electrolyte abnormality	Adjust
Ethionamide	Abdominal pain, nausea, anorexia, dysgeusia, diarrhea, rash, edema, arthralgias, neuropathy, hypothyroidism, temporary alopecia, gynecomastia	Adjust for CrCl < 30 mL/min
Para-aminosalicyclic acid	Abdominal pain, hypothyroid, diarrhea	Adjust
Cycloserine	Mood and cognitive decline, psychosis, tremors, seizures (all concentration dependent)	Use contraindicated in severe renal impairment, some people adjust for severe impairment
Bedaquiline	QTc prolongation, nausea, joint pains, liver dysfunction	No dose adjustment, use with caution for severe renal failure
Linezolid	Bone marrow suppression—especially thrombocytopenia, neuropathy, GI symptoms, serotonin syndrome	No dose adjustment
Clofazamine	Nausea, vomiting, skin discoloration, QTc prolongation	No dose adjustment

CrCl, Creatinine clearance; *GI*, gastrointestinal.

Fusarium, zygomycetes (*Mucor, Rhizopus,* and *Rhizomucor*) and less commonly, *Scedosporium/Pseudoallescheria* and *Trichosporon* can also be seen. Other risk factors for fungal infection include the underlying malignancy, comorbidities, such as diabetes or underlying lung disease, and the types of treatments used.[94]

CANDIDA

The presence of candiduria is a therapeutic challenge. It can represent asymptomatic colonization or be a harbinger of severe sepsis. There are no clear guidelines about treatment. A positive culture often represents colonization, although the distinction between colonization and infection can be difficult to make. Untreated patients also have the risk of progression to disseminated candidiasis. Foley catheters should be removed, and if possible, broad spectrum antibiotics should be discontinued. If there is persistent candiduria, then imaging to look for renal abscess, fungal balls, or evidence of urologic obstruction should be considered.[95]

The significance of candiduria in patients with hematologic malignancies is as confusing as it is in the general population. Neutropenic patients may not have pyuria even with candiduria, and in the presence of indwelling Foley catheters, the diagnosis of candida UTIs becomes very challenging.[96] In a 10-year retrospective study in nonintensive care patients with hematologic malignancies and candiduria, only 4% developed candidemia and the crude mortality was low. The authors concluded that isolated candiduria in patients with hematologic malignancies was not a predictor of subsequent invasive candidiasis. Their conclusion, however, is hard to support, because 88% of the patients in this study were treated with systemic antifungals.[97]

Renal involvement with fungi can be either caused by hematogenous spread or from retrograde extension. Fungi can disseminate to the collecting system and rarely coalesce to form bezoars or fungus balls, which can cause obstructive uropathy. Although candida are the most frequently isolated fungal pathogen species, there are reports of aspergillus bezoar causing bilateral ureteral obstruction. The characteristic radiologic features of fungus balls and intraluminal filling defects are not pathognomonic, and the differential is broad (Fig. 36.2).[98] Fungal infections should always be included in the differential diagnosis of renal obstruction in an immunocompromised patient.

Fluconazole is the drug of choice for candida cystitis because of its favorable pharmacokinetics. Because other azoles and all echinocandins (caspofungin, micafungin, and anidulafungin) are poorly excreted in urine, they have been found to be less effective in candiduric patients. Other options include bladder irrigation with amphotericin B, flucytosine, or parenteral amphotericin B preparations; however, these are more toxic options.[99] Candiduria caused by more resistant non-*Candida albicans* species

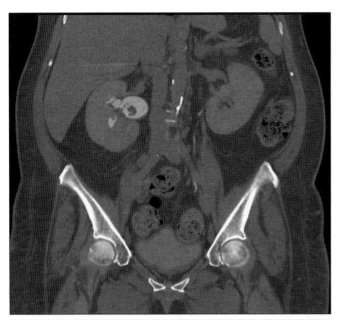

Fig. 36.2 Coronal excretory phase computed tomography with multiple filling defects in the right renal pelvis consistent with a candida fungal ball.

makes treatment even more challenging as few options exist. There have been successful case reports of treating candiduria with echinocandins, but because of their low urinary concentrations, they are not generally recommended. Fungal prostatitis is uncommon, and the collective experience from case reports emphasizes the role of surgical intervention in conjunction with antifungal therapy.[100]

ASPERGILLUS

Aspergillus spp are among the most common mold pathogens in patients with cancer, but they are seen mostly with patients after prolonged neutropenia or in patients with GVHD after allogeneic transplantation. The vast majority of aspergillus infections occur in the lung, the usual portal of entry, but subsequent dissemination to other organs including the kidneys can be seen. The *Aspergillus spp* have angioinvasive properties. The usual presentation of renal aspergillus includes the formation of multiple abscesses (bezoars).[101] Clinically the renal involvement is seen as bezoars in the renal pelvis. Rarely, renal infarcts have also been described.[101] Early diagnosis and bezoar debulking along with systemic antifungal therapy may avert the need for an open resection.[102] Surgical management includes irrigation, lavage, and debulking from either an antegrade or retrograde approach. Refractory cases may end up with partial or complete nephrectomy.[102]

CRYPTOCOCCUS

The incidence of cryptococcal renal disease is not well documented. In 1972, a single center evaluated 32 patients with a serologic or pathologic diagnosis of *Cryptococcus neoformans*. Eight (25%) of the patients had disseminated disease and five had renal involvement. One-third of these patients had lymphoma.[103] The urinary tract can possibly serve as a reservoir for cryptococcus, even after successful treatment for meningitis. It is felt to be sequestered in the prostate and can be found in the urine, or in prostatic secretions after prostatic massage.[104] Unless treated specifically, the patient is at risk for systemic relapse of disease. Transurethral drainage is sometimes needed.[105]

Patients who undergo organ transplantation—either solid or HSCT—are known to be at increased risk of cryptococcal disease. In solid organ transplant recipients, including renal transplants, cryptococcus is one of the most common causes of fungal infection.[106] However, because of the effective fungal prophylaxis, it is not as common in HSCT recipients, representing less than 1% of fungal infections in this population. A rare case of acute kidney injury resulting from disseminated cryptococcal infection in an allogeneic stem cell transplant recipient has been described.[107] The renal failure in this patient was multifactorial and was caused by the acute and evolving thrombotic microangiopathy secondary to the presence of GVHD, tacrolimus, and possibly caused by the cryptococcus infection. The authors were able to document parenchymal invasion by the cryptococcus in this study.

MUCOR

The hallmarks of mucormycosis are vascular invasion and tissue necrosis. The fungi typically appear as broad non-septate hyphae with branches occurring at right angles. Therapy of mucormycosis includes rapid correction of the predisposing factors, surgical debridement of the necrotic tissue when feasible, and antifungal therapy. Adjunctive therapy may include hyperbaric oxygen, granulocyte stimulating factor, and granulocyte transfusion. Lee et al. described two cases of disseminated mucormycosis after HSCT.[108] The first patient had an abscess in the kidney from the mucor and splenic involvement. He was successfully treated with splenectomy, liposomal amphotericin and 5-flucytosine, and discontinuation of cyclosporine and prednisolone.

Viral Infections

Patients with solid tumors are at risk for viral infections. Suppression of cell-mediated immunity is a major risk factor for viral reactivation; the risk correlates with the degree, intensity, and duration of T-cell suppression. Although these patients are much less likely to have prolonged neutropenia in comparison to patients with hematologic malignancies, they have other risk factors as detailed earlier. Solid tumors by themselves, and the traditional chemotherapy used for them, have minimal effects on cell-mediated immunity, and thus the risk of viral reactivation is lower. Hence routine prophylaxis against herpes simplex (HSV), varicella zoster (VZV), Epstein-Barr virus (EBV) or cytomegalovirus (CMV) is not routinely recommended.[109,110] Occasionally, reactivation of certain viral infections (hepatitis B virus [HBV], hepatitis C virus [HCV], and CMV) can be seen and needs to be considered.

The increasing use of monoclonal antibodies, such as alemtuzumab, bortezomib, and immunotherapy agents, predisposes to the reactivation of viral infections. Although there are no specific recommendations in renal cancer patients, prophylaxis with acyclovir and derivatives like valacyclovir against HSV and VZV in patients treated with multiple myeloma and solid tumor patients treated with aforementioned agents have been shown to be highly effective and are recommended.[111]

HEPATITIS

Cancer patients who are hepatitis B surface antigen (HBsAg)-positive and/or anti-HBc–positive are at increased risk of reactivation (pooled incidence, 37%) after immunosuppressive therapy.[112,113] HBV reactivation has been documented in almost 30% to 80% of patients who were seropositive, although it is largely influenced by the chemotherapy regimens. Thus universal screening of individuals before the administration of cytotoxic chemotherapy or immunosuppressive therapy is recommended.[113,114]

The spectrum of infection and reactivation can vary from asymptomatic seropositivity to fulminant transaminitis and development of hepatic failure.

Hepatitis B can have complex renal manifestations.[115] Chronic hepatitis B can lead to many glomerular diseases. Extrahepatic manifestations of hepatitis B can include glomerulonephritis, reactive arthritis, or vasculitis. Glomerular disease is more frequently seen in men than in women and is more common in children than adults. Other manifestations that have been described include membranous nephropathy, membranoproliferative glomerulonephritis, IgA nephropathy, and rarely, focal segmental glomerulosclerosis (FSGS).[116,117] The pathogenic mechanisms are thought to be immune complex-mediated, with the viral antigens eliciting an antibody response.

Lamivudine, entecavir, adefovir, and tenofovir are the agents of choice for prophylaxis in patients who are HepBs Ag and/or HepBc Ab positive and receiving immunosuppressive therapy. The duration of prophylaxis is variable but is usually 6 to 12 months after completion of chemotherapy. Prophylaxis has been shown to result in an 87% RR reduction of reactivation and slows progression to hepatitis and liver failure.[118,119]

The data on HCV reactivation in cancer patients are not as clear as HBV. The overall prevalence of HCV infection in cancer patients has been estimated to be up to 32%.[120,121]

According to recent guidelines from the National Comprehensive Cancer Network, all patients receiving chemotherapy or immunosuppressive therapy should be screened for HCV.[122] Although the data are not definitive, antiviral therapy in HCV-positive patients should also be considered and may lead to improved outcomes.

BK VIRUS

About 60% to 80% of the adult human population is estimated to have infection with BK virus (BKV), a human polyomavirus.[123] Most of the infected individuals are asymptomatic, although seropositivity can be demonstrated. However, in immunosuppressed patients, renal transplant patients in particular, BKV can lead to symptomatic disease and renal failure. Although most of the data regarding BKV reactivation are available in SOT/HSCT patients, BKV can reactivate in cancer patients on heavy immunosuppression.

The mechanisms of infection include reactivation of latent virus and primary infection transmitted from the donor or via blood transfusion.[124] In the setting of severe immunosuppression, reactivation from the urothelial membrane is the most common mechanism.[125,126] Most present within 2 months of transplantation.[127] Rarely, reactivation in native kidneys of patients with hematologic malignancies after monoclonal antibodies like rituximab has been described.[128,129]

Presentations can include asymptomatic hematuria, hemorrhagic cystitis, ureteral stenosis, interstitial nephritis, and renal failure.[130–132]

Various strategies for prevention and treatment of BKV nephropathy have been studied. In most of these, reduction in immunotherapy is thought to be essential in treatment.

Various antipolyomavirus agents, like cidofovir, leflunomide, intravenous Igs, and fluoroquinolones have demonstrated in vitro BKV activity. However, because these agents have been used in conjunction with other modalities, such as immunosuppression reduction, or with other agents, the efficacy of these agents is difficult to assess and is not well established.[133,134]

Interestingly, there is some literature documenting the association between BKV infection and certain genitourinary cancers, including bladder and renal cell cancers. A causative role has not been established; it is unclear whether the BKV is an "innocent bystander" present caused by the cancer-mediated immunosuppression.[135–137]

CYTOMEGALOVIRUS

CMV infection is one of the most common viral infections after renal transplantation (SOT).[138] It can present with a variety of symptoms and is associated with severe morbidity and occasional mortality.[139]

Because CMV reactivation is thought to be uncommon in patients with solid tumors, routine surveillance and testing for CMV disease is not commonly done.[2] However, there are emerging data that CMV disease in these patients may be more common than previously thought. Schlick et al. reported that almost half of the patients with positive CMV PCR eventually developed clinical disease and required treatment.[140]

CMV infection in these patients can present with multi-organ involvement. Gastroenteritis and hepatitis are some of the most common presentations. Development of both early and late disease has been described, although the use of prophylaxis can lead to a shift in the presentation.

Tubulointerstitial nephritis is the most common renal manifestation of CMV in kidney transplant recipients, but others, including glomerulopathy and thrombotic microangiopathy leading to arteriopathy, have been described.[141] The most common histopathologic changes in glomerulopathy are cytopathic changes in glomerular endothelial cells and podocytes with a lack of significant inflammation. On the other hand, CMV-induced arteriopathy usually presents with thrombotic microangiopathy.[142,143]

There is also increasing evidence that even when asymptomatic, CMV itself can facilitate allograft rejection and can be associated with a number of other pathologies, including diabetes, graft loss, and mortality.[144–147]

Various strategies including preemptive CMV therapy or prophylaxis have been used to avert symptomatic CMV infection after HSCT or SOT.[148] Surveillance with serum PCR testing is frequently done, and if any clinical or laboratory evidence of acute infection is seen, therapy with valganciclovir is initiated. However, PCR testing can be nonreproducible between different laboratories, and clear-cut thresholds for initiation of treatment have not been well established. Most centers use a minimum of a fivefold increase over baseline, particularly when low DNA levels are detected. Even though these strategies are well studied in HSCT/SOT, however, there are scant data supporting the use of these strategies in cancer patients.

If PCR testing is not convenient, centers can use prophylaxis with valganciclovir (900 mg/day in patient with normal renal function).[149]

For treatment of active CMV infection, oral valganciclovir is used, but if there is severe disease or gastrointestinal malabsorption, intravenous ganciclovir is used. Foscarnet is an alternative if neutropenia is present.[150] The duration of treatment depends on the severity and the clinical and virologic response. Most centers will treat for 14 to 28 days with full dose, until there is resolution of clinical symptoms and at least two serum CMV PCRs 1 to 2 weeks apart are negative.[150] Subsequent to this, a lower dose for a period of 1 to 3 months, depending on the clinical course and immunosuppression, is used. Use of Igs in CMV infection is controversial.

Although prophylaxis significantly prevents early CMV infection and disease, long-term results did not show a superiority of valganciclovir prophylaxis over preemptive treatment for graft loss and death.[151]

EPSTEIN-BARR VIRUS

Infectious mononucleosis caused by EBV is usually a benign self-limited illness that can cause pharyngitis, fever, hepatosplenomegaly, and lymphadenopathy. Subclinical renal involvement likely occurs in a few patients, but severe renal disease is rare. However, acute renal insufficiency, likely resulting from interstitial nephritis, has been described.

Renal biopsy may show a monocytic interstitial infiltrate. However, minimal glomerular changes have also been documented.[152]

EBV infections are common in certain malignancies and HSCT patients, but there is not much literature documenting an increased incidence of EBV renal disease in cancer patients.

ADENOVIRUS

Adenovirus (ADV) infections most commonly manifest as upper respiratory tract infections, but can also present with gastrointestinal symptoms, hemorrhagic cystitis, and pneumonitis. Most adenovirus infections are self-limiting. Renal infections have occasionally been reported in HSCT patients.[153] ADV nephritis can cause fever, hematuria, and flank pain. In a study, the development of nephritis was associated with renal failure in 90% of the patients.[154] In immunocompromised patients, severe acute necrotizing tubulointerstitial nephritis has been described; this was shown to have poor outcomes and was associated with high mortality.[155] Other reports have described azotemia, gross hematuria (also caused by hemorrhagic cystitis), and occasionally, hydronephrosis.[153,156]

The diagnosis of ADV UTI can be made by isolating the virus in the urine.[154] In immunocompromised patients, shedding of ADV in the urine and stool has been described for months after recovery, and this may lead to difficulty in establishing the diagnosis. Urine or serum PCRs can be done; however, they are not readily available in some institutions. Renal biopsy is indicated if a diagnosis of ADV nephritis is suspected.[157]

In immunosuppressed patients (pediatric HSCT) with severe disease, treatment with cidofovir was found to be safe and efficacious. Other therapies including ribavirin have been described, but no randomized control studies or guidelines exist.[158–161]

HUMAN IMMUNODEFICIENCY VIRUS

The presentation of renal disease in human immunodeficiency virus (HIV) patients with cancer is similar to those with no malignancies. However, cancer patients who have received stem cell transplants are at a higher risk for HSCT-related infectious complications. BKV-associated nephropathy has been described in HIV patients who underwent SCT.[162–166]

Kidney disease in HIV patients can be caused by HIV-associated nephropathy, immune complex kidney disease, thrombotic microangiopathy, and antiretroviral induced injury.[167] Coinfection with hepatitis C is also common in HIV patients and thus HCV-related renal pathologies also need to be considered as part of the differential diagnosis. These include membranoproliferative glomerulonephritis with and without cryoglobulinemia, membranous glomerulopathy, and FSGS.[168–174] Postinfectious glomerulonephritis and fibrillary glomerulonephritis have also been described.[175]

HIV-infected patients may have a higher incidence of BKV viruria as compared with non-HIV patients; the concentration of BKV in the urine was inversely related to the CD-4 cell count.[176–178] HIV patients also shed BKV at higher levels, and immunologic status was shown to influence the amount of viral shedding.[176,177]

Parasitic Infections

SCHISTOSOMIASIS

Schistosomiasis infects about 200 million people and is endemic in more than 70 countries.[167] *Schistosoma haematobium* is associated with cancer of the urinary bladder, and these cancers are usually of the squamous and adenocarcinoma type rather than the transitional type.[179–181] Schistosomes are parasitic blood flukes, which have an intermediate invertebrate host (fresh water snails) and a definitive mammalian host.[167,182] Schistosomiasis has been related to subclinical glomerulonephritis, particularly in the chronic form, although the exact incidence of this complication is not known. Hematuria and dysuria resulting from inflammation and ulceration of the bladder mucosa can be seen 3 to 4 months after the primary infection. Treatment is usually with praziquantel and oxamniquine.

The pathogenesis of schistomiasis is multifactorial. The inflammatory response to the ova deposited in the bladder is associated with the production of oxygen-derived free radicals. Free radicals have been shown to induce genetic mutations and/or promote the production of carcinogenic compounds (such as N-nitrosamines and polycyclic aromatic hydrocarbons) leading to malignant transformation.[183,184] Schistosomiasis can also be associated with chronic bacterial superinfection, which may in itself predispose to squamous cell neoplasia.[185] In epidemiologic studies, the control of schistosomiasis and the subsequent decrease in the intensity of infestation coincided with increase in the number of cancers of urothelial origin, but decrease in the squamous cell types.[186]

STRONGYLOIDIASIS

Strongyloidiasis is a soil-transmitted helminth thought to infect 30 to 100 million people worldwide, mainly in tropical and subtropical countries.[187] The diagnosis of strongyloidiasis should be suspected in cancer patients who are on glucocorticosteroids and present with unusual gastrointestinal or pulmonary findings, or unexplained gram-negative sepsis.[188] The development of clinical manifestations, in many cases, is attributed to a decrease in host resistance caused by debilitating disease, malnutrition, or immunosuppressive drugs. Symptomatic strongyloidiasis is then an often-fatal opportunistic infection for immunocompromised hosts, particularly those receiving corticosteroids. Strongyloides infection is also associated with immune complex−mediated glomerular lesions. Minimal change disease is the most common glomerular disease reported in association with strongyloidiasis, but a few cases of FSGS have been documented in the literature.[189] Treatment includes ivermectin, albendazole, or thiabendazole.[98]

Summary

Renal infections are common in cancer patients. Bacterial infections can be complicated, and the prevalence of antimicrobial resistance is much higher in cancer patients. These patients may require longer and complicated courses of antimicrobials. The management of infections related to indwelling devices, tumor-induced mechanical obstruction, and reconstructive surgeries can be challenging. The distinction between colonization and pathogens in these patients is difficult. Guidelines related to prophylaxis and suppressive regimens remain unclear.

Mycobacterial infections tend to occur either because of the use of BCG in bladder cancer treatment or because of reactivation of tuberculosis. Fungal infections caused by candida and other molds can be complex, although noninfectious candiduria resulting from colonization is common, particularly in patients with catheters. A high index of suspicion and aggressive diagnostic workup and management, including imaging, biopsies, and surgical debridement may be needed.

Viral reactivation is common in both solid organ transplant and HSCT patients. Although upper respiratory viruses have a similar presentation as in noncancer patients, the course may be more aggressive. Hepatitis viruses can have severe renal manifestations. The reactivation of CMV and EBV have myriad presentations, and there are different strategies of management, including preemptive therapy and prophylaxis.

Acknowledgment

The authors would like to acknowledge the role of Smitha Reddy, PhD, for editorial assistance in preparation of the manuscript. We would also like to acknowledge Dr Grimaldi and Dharam Ramnani, MD, at WebPathology.com for their help with the figures.

Key Points

- Cancer patients have a higher risk of renal infections because of their impaired immunity.
- Renal infections cause significant morbidity and mortality in cancer patients.
- There is a higher incidence of antimicrobial resistant infections in cancer patients.
- The presence of foreign bodies, like catheters and surgeries, make management of renal infections in cancer patients complicated.
- There is a paucity of guidelines for management of renal infections in cancer patients.
- Fungal and mycobacterial infections of the kidney can occur in cancer patients and their management is challenging.
- Viral infections, including cytomegalovirus and BK virus, and parasitic renal infections can be seen in selected populations of cancer patients.

References

1. Danai PA, Moss M, Mannino DM, Martin GS. The epidemiology of sepsis in patients with malignancy. *Chest*. 2006;129(6):1432-1440.
2. Rolston KV. Infections in cancer patients with solid tumors: a review. *Infect Dis Ther*. 2017;6(1):69-83.
6. Taccone FS, Artigas AA, Sprung CL, Moreno R, Sakr Y, Vincent JL. Characteristics and outcomes of cancer patients in European ICUs. *Crit Care*. 2009;13(1):R15.
10. Rosolem MM, Rabello LS, Lisboa T, et al. Critically ill patients with cancer and sepsis: clinical course and prognostic factors. *J Crit Care*. 2012;27(3):301-307.
15. Safdar A, Armstrong D. Infections in patients with hematologic neoplasms and hematopoietic stem cell transplantation: neutropenia, humoral, and splenic defects. *Clin Infect Dis*. 2011;53(8):798-806.
28. Foxman B, Somsel P, Tallman P, et al. Urinary tract infection among women aged 40 to 65: behavioral and sexual risk factors. *J Clin Epidemiol*. 2001;54(7):710-718.
29. Homsi J, Walsh D, Panta R, Lagman R, Nelson KA, Longworth DL. Infectious complications of advanced cancer. *Support Care Cancer*. 2000;8(6):487-492.
30. Parikh P, Bhat V. Urinary tract infection in cancer patients in a tertiary cancer setting in India: microbial spectrum and antibiotic susceptibility pattern. *Antimicrob Resist Infect Control*. 2015;4(suppl 1):221.
33. Nicolle LE, SHEA Long-Term-Care-Committee. Urinary tract infections in long-term-care facilities. *Infect Control Hosp Epidemiol*. 2001;22(3):167-175.
34. Hooton TM, Bradley SF, Cardenas DD, et al. Diagnosis, prevention, and treatment of catheter-associated urinary tract infection in adults: 2009 International Clinical Practice Guidelines from the Infectious Diseases Society of America. *Clin Infect Dis*. 2010;50(5):625-663.
37. Kahlmeter G, Eco.Sens. An international survey of the antimicrobial susceptibility of pathogens from uncomplicated urinary tract

infections: the ECO.SENS Project. *J Antimicrob Chemother.* 2003; 51(1):69-76.

41. Gupta K, Hooton TM, Naber KG, et al. International clinical practice guidelines for the treatment of acute uncomplicated cystitis and pyelonephritis in women: a 2010 update by the Infectious Diseases Society of America and the European Society for Microbiology and Infectious Diseases. *Clin Infect Dis.* 2011;52(5):e103-e120.

43. Tambyah PA, Maki DG. Catheter-associated urinary tract infection is rarely symptomatic: a prospective study of 1,497 catheterized patients. *Arch Intern Med.* 2000;160(5):678-682.

49. Sanchez M, Collvinent B, Miró O, et al. Short-term effectiveness of ceftriaxone single dose in the initial treatment of acute uncomplicated pyelonephritis in women. A randomised controlled trial. *Emerg Med J.* 2002;19(1):19-22.

52. Foxman B, Ki M, Brown P. Antibiotic resistance and pyelonephritis. *Clin Infect Dis.* 2007;45(3):281-283.

54. Harding GK, Nicolle LE, Ronald AR, et al. How long should catheter-acquired urinary tract infection in women be treated? A randomized controlled study. *Ann Intern Med.* 1991;114(9):713-719.

58. Lipsky BA. Prostatitis and urinary tract infection in men: what's new; what's true? *Am J Med.* 1999;106(3):327-334.

60. Flukes S, Hayne D, Kuan M, Wallace M, McMillan K, Rukin NJ. Retrograde ureteric stent insertion in the management of infected obstructed kidneys. *BJU Int.* 2015;115(suppl 5):31-34.

62. Gafary M, Bell N, Eagan J, Kamboj M. Catheter associated urinary tract infections (CAUTI) in bladder cancer patients post cystectomy with a neobladder. *Open Forum Infect Dis.* 2015;2(suppl 1):293.

63. Bahu R, Chaftari AM, Hachem RY, et al. Nephrostomy tube related pyelonephritis in patients with cancer: epidemiology, infection rate and risk factors. *J Urol.* 2013;189(1):130-135.

65. Nicolle LE, Bradley S, Colgan R, et al. Infectious Diseases Society of America guidelines for the diagnosis and treatment of asymptomatic bacteriuria in adults. *Clin Infect Dis.* 2005;40(5):643-654.

67. Nicolle LE, Ronald AR. Recurrent urinary tract infection in adult women: diagnosis and treatment. *Infect Dis Clin North Am.* 1987; 1(4):793-806.

74. Langdon A, Crook N, Dantas G. The effects of antibiotics on the microbiome throughout development and alternative approaches for therapeutic modulation. *Genome Med.* 2016;8(1):39.

77. Mohammed A, Arastu Z. Emerging concepts and spectrum of renal injury following intravesical BCG for non-muscle invasive bladder cancer. *BMC Urol.* 2017;17(1):114.

90. Rodrigues NJ, Rodrigues NJ, Viana L, Mansur JB, Tedesco-Silva H, Pestana JOM. Genitourinary tuberculosis - a rare presentation of a still frequent infection in renal transplant recipients. *J Bras Nefrol.* 2017;39(2):224-228.

93. Jacob JT, Nguyen TM, Ray SM. Male genital tuberculosis. *Lancet Infect Dis.* 2008;8(5):335-342.

94. Freifeld AG, Kaul DR. Infection in the patient with cancer. In: *Abeloff's Clinical Oncology.* Niederhuber JE, et al. ed. Philadelphia, PA: Elsevier Inc; 2013:562-580.

95. Fisher JF, Sobel JD, Kauffman CA, Newman CA. Candida urinary tract infections—treatment. *Clin Infect Dis.* 2011;52(suppl 6):S457-S466.

101. Lee JH, Im SA, Cho B. Renal infarction secondary to invasive aspergillosis in a 5-year-old girl with acute lymphoblastic leukemia. *J Pediatr Hematol Oncol.* 2014;36(5):e296-e298.

103. Lewis JL, Rabinovich S. The wide spectrum of cryptococcal infections. *Am J Med.* 1972;53(3):315-322.

106. Pappas PG, Alexander BD, Andes DR, et al. Invasive fungal infections among organ transplant recipients: results of the Transplant-Associated Infection Surveillance Network (TRANSNET). *Clin Infect Dis.* 2010; 50(8):1101-1111.

111. Sandherr M, Hentrich M, von Lilienfeld-Toal M, et al. Antiviral prophylaxis in patients with solid tumours and haematological malignancies—update of the Guidelines of the Infectious Diseases Working Party (AGIHO) of the German Society for Hematology and Medical Oncology (DGHO). *Ann Hematol.* 2015;94(9): 1441-1450.

115. Chan TM. Hepatitis B and renal disease. *Curr Hepat Rep.* 2010; 9(2):99-105.

116. Levy M, Chen N. Worldwide perspective of hepatitis B-associated glomerulonephritis in the 80s. *Kidney Int Suppl.* 1991;35:S24-S33.

124. Fishman JA. BK virus nephropathy—polyomavirus adding insult to injury. *N Engl J Med.* 2002;347(7):527-530.

135. Bulut Y, Ozdemir E, Ozercan HI, et al. Potential relationship between BK virus and renal cell carcinoma. *J Med Virol.* 2013;85(6):1085-1089.

138. Kotton CN, Kumar D, Caliendo AM, et al. Updated international consensus guidelines on the management of cytomegalovirus in solid-organ transplantation. *Transplantation.* 2013;96(4):333-360.

140. Schlick K, Grundbichler M, Auberger J, et al. Cytomegalovirus reactivation and its clinical impact in patients with solid tumors. *Infect Agent Cancer.* 2015;10:45.

143. Richardson WP, Colvin RB, Cheeseman SH, et al. Glomerulopathy associated with cytomegalovirus viremia in renal allografts. *N Engl J Med.* 1981;305(2):57-63.

147. Sagedal S, Hartmann A, Nordal KP, et al. Impact of early cytomegalovirus infection and disease on long-term recipient and kidney graft survival. *Kidney Int.* 2004;66(1):329-337.

177. Knowles WA, Pillay D, Johnson MA, Hand JF, Brown DW. Prevalence of long-term BK and JC excretion in HIV-infected adults and lack of correlation with serological markers. *J Med Virol.* 1999;59(4):474-479.

179. Maguire JH, Douglas M. Trematodes (Schistosomes and Other Flukes). In: Mandell D, ed. *Principles and practice of infectious diseases.* Philadelphia, PA: Churchill Livingstone Elsevier; 2010:3595-3605.

186. Schistosomes, liver flukes and Helicobacter pylori. IARC Working Group on the Evaluation of Carcinogenic Risks to Humans. Lyon, 7-14 June 1994. *IARC Monogr Eval Carcinog Risks Hum.* 1994;61: 1-241.

188. Fardet L, Généreau T, Poirot JL, Guidet B, Kettaneh A, Cabane J. Severe strongyloidiasis in corticosteroid-treated patients: case series and literature review. *J Infect.* 2007;54(1):18-27.

A full list of references is available at Expertconsult.com

Infiltrative Diseases

37 *Kidney Disease in Leukemia*

RANDY L. LUCIANO

Introduction

Leukemia is a group of hematologic malignancies derived from bone marrow cells, respectively. Although not as common as solid organ malignancies, the prevalence is estimated to be greater than 350,000 people with or in remission from leukemia in the United States. Leukemia is the most common cancer diagnosed in children; however, more than 90% of cases are diagnosed in adults. Leukemia can involve almost any organ, including the kidney. Kidney disease manifestations encompass a broad spectrum of disease: prerenal acute kidney injury (AKI), acute tubular necrosis (ATN), renovascular disease, parenchymal infiltration, obstruction, glomerulopathies, and electrolyte and acid-base abnormalities.[1] Kidney injury may result from the underlying malignancy itself or as a secondary complication of therapy. The development of AKI in a patient with leukemia is of concern, as it may delay treatment, which in turn can affect prognosis and mortality. The overlap of the kidney and leukemia will be discussed here; chapters 16, 17, and 18 will discuss chemotherapies that can be used to treat leukemia and the resultant kidney injury that can develop from their use.

Acute Kidney Injury In Leukemia

AKI in patients with leukemia is common. A study examining 349 patients with all forms of hematologic malignancy admitted to the intensive care unit demonstrated some form of AKI in 149 patients (43%). Of patients with AKI, 29% required renal replacement therapy, with a mortality rate of 72%.[2] In 1411 intensive care unit patients, the diagnosis of a hematologic malignancy, leukemia or lymphoma, had the greatest risk for AKI (odds ratio [OR], 2.23), relative to other more common conditions seen in critically ill patients, including infection, cirrhosis, and cardiovascular disease. The presence of hematologic malignancy also had the greatest risk of death (OR 2.31) in all AKI patients.[3] The approach to a patient presenting with AKI in the setting of leukemia involves assessing potential prerenal, intrarenal, and postrenal etiologies (Table 37.1).

PRERENAL ACUTE KIDNEY INJURY

Prerenal AKI is the most common kidney injury in leukemia. Poor oral fluid intake (78%), anorexia (64%), early satiety (50%), emesis (23%), and diarrhea (16%) lead to volume depletion and this can lead to a prerenal AKI.[4] Volume depletion can be exacerbated by insensible losses and decreased effective circulating volume from comorbid conditions, such as cirrhosis or heart failure, or through the use of medications that affect kidney afferent and efferent tone, including renin-angiotensin blockade or nonsteroidal antiinflammatory medications (NSAIDs), or diuretics used for hypertension or to control peripheral edema. Prerenal AKI is often suspected based on the clinical course and history, and supported with physical examination findings that demonstrate signs of volume depletion, including hypotension and orthostatic blood pressure changes, tachycardia, flat neck veins, or poor skin turgor. Laboratory data that can be suggestive of a prerenal AKI include hyponatremia or hypernatremia (depending on the degree of free water loss relative to sodium and water loss) and an elevation in blood urea nitrogen (BUN) and serum creatinine, with the BUN to creatinine ratio generally greater than 20. The urinalysis may show an elevated specific gravity with possible ketonuria; if appetite has been exceedingly poor, urine electrolytes usually reveal a very low urine sodium (< 20 mEq/L) and low fractional excretion of sodium (< 1%), and the urine sediment is usually bland, with occasional hyaline casts or cellular elements. Treatment is supportive, with crystalloid expansion and removal of exacerbating factors that have led to the volume depletion.

POSTRENAL ACUTE KIDNEY INJURY

In patients with leukemia, obstruction is relatively uncommon, but case reports have demonstrated tumor directly impeding ureteral outflow, extramedullary hematopoiesis causing retroperitoneal fibrosis, or more commonly nephrolithiasis from tumor lysis syndrome.[1] In patients with obstructive AKI, hematuria and pyuria may also be present, and kidney ultrasound should demonstrate hydronephrosis, unless collecting system dilatation is prevented by fibrosis or if the patient has severe volume depletion (Fig. 37.1). Treatment is supportive with immediate decompression of the obstruction with nephrostomy tubes to prevent ongoing and permanent injury.

INTRARENAL ACUTE KIDNEY INJURY

Intrarenal causes of kidney injury in leukemia can be grouped into ischemic and nonischemic ATN, tubulointerstitial disorders, renovascular disorders, and glomerulopathies. Hemodynamically mediated injury, caused by severe volume depletion, heart failure, or sepsis, and drug-induced injury are common with leukemia. However, it is critical to separate these processes from AKI directly caused by leukemia, as therapy is targeted towards the malignancy as opposed to general supportive measures, and prognosis depends on successful treatment of the underlying disease. Subsequent sections will focus on intrarenal AKI specific to hematologic malignancy.

Table 37.1 Etiology of Acute Kidney Injury in Leukemia

Prerenal	*Intravascular volume depletion*
	   Nausea, emesis, diarrhea (from chemotherapy or treatment)
	   Hemorrhage
	   Increased insensible losses (fever, tachypnea)
	Reduced renal perfusion
	   Vasoconstriction (hypercalcemia, hyperuricemia)
	   Sepsis
	   Liver disease
	   Medications (RAAS blockers, NSAIDs, diuretics)

Intrarenal	*Acute tubular necrosis*
	   Renal ischemia
	   Lysozymuria
	   Tumor lysis syndrome
	   Medications (antibiotics, chemotherapy)
	Tubulointerstitial disorders
	   Secondary renal infiltration
	   Allergic interstitial nephritis
	Glomerular disorders
	   See Table 37.2 for complete list
	Renovascular disorders
	   Renal vein thrombosis
	   Thrombotic microangiopathy
	   Leukostasis

Postrenal	*Obstruction*
	   External compression (obstructing tumor)
	   Retroperitoneal fibrosis
	   Internal obstruction (nephrolithiasis, crystalluria)

NSAIDs, Nonsteroidal antiinflammatory drugs; *RAAS*, renin-angiotensin-aldosterone system.

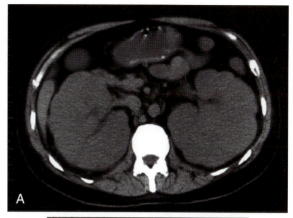

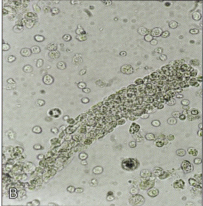

Fig. 37.2 A patient with chronic myeloid leukemia. **A.** Computed tomography showing bilateral enlargement of kidneys. **B.** Urine sediment under light microscopy at 160 ×, showing a white blood cell cast.

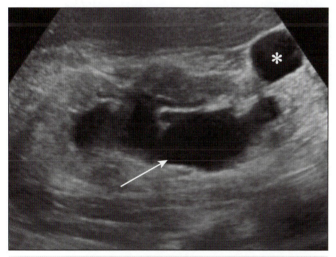

Fig. 37.1 Ultrasound image from a patient with acute myeloid leukemia, with acute kidney injury from obstruction. *White arrow* is pointing to severe hydronephrosis. *White asterisk* is within a benign kidney cyst.

Diagnosis of intrarenal AKI often relies on ancillary tests. Diagnostic imaging, which is involved in staging of leukemia, may be the first insight into kidney involvement. Computed tomography scan may show glomerulomegaly with diffuse bilateral enlargement, pointing to kidney infiltration (Fig. 37.2A). Examination of the urine sediment is critical as its diagnostic potential is significant at a low cost. Renal tubular epithelial cells (RTEC) casts point towards ATN. White cells and white cell casts suggest an underlying malignant infiltration, acute interstitial nephritis, or severe pyelonephritis (Fig. 37.2B). Dysmorphic red cells and red cell casts indicate a glomerular involvement. Kidney biopsy remains the gold standard in diagnosis and can help delineate all forms of intrarenal injury. Light microscopy with hematoxylin and eosin staining can demonstrate glomerular, tubulointerstitial, or vascular disorders. Special clonal cellular immunohistochemistry can elucidate the nature of the cells on the specimen. Immunofluorescence and electron microscopy can provide additional information on glomerular involvement. However, biopsy may be difficult in a patient with leukemia because of thrombocytopenia, which increases the risk of bleeding.

ACUTE TUBULAR NECROSIS

ATN is the most common cause of intrinsic AKI in leukemia. In a single center study, out of all patients with hematologic malignancy with AKI, 83% had ATN, with 96% of those patients experiencing sepsis and 88% receiving nephrotoxic medications.[5] ATN can be detected through evaluation of the urinary sediment with the presence of granular casts or RTEC (Fig. 37.3A). If the diagnosis is ambiguous, biopsy can be performed and would demonstrate acute tubular injury, as manifested as renal tubular cells with nuclear dropout, loss of brush border, and cytoplasmic vacuolization (Fig. 37.3B). Disease specific etiologies of ATN are discussed later.

Lysozyme-induced tubular necrosis is a rare but documented cause of kidney injury in patients with leukemia.[6]

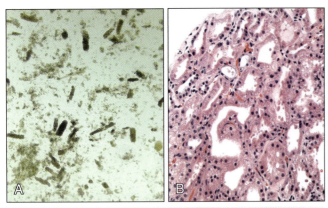

Fig. 37.3 Acute tubular necrosis in a patient with acute kidney injury from severe volume depletion and hypotension in the setting of chronic lymphocytic leukemia. **A.** 16× light microscopy showing many dense granular casts. **B.** 40× specimen from a kidney biopsy (stained with hematoxylin and eosin), showing dilated renal tubules, renal tubular cell cytoplasmic vacuolization, and nuclear dropout.

Lysozyme is a cationic enzyme stored in macrophages and monocytes that may be released to lyse bacterial cell walls. In certain leukemias, clonal expansion increases lysozyme production, which is freely filtered by the glomerulus and then reabsorbed by the proximal tubule cells. At high concentrations, as seen in leukemia, lysozyme induces direct tubular damage causing kaliuresis and proteinuria. High concentrations of urinary lysozyme, exacerbated by proximal tubule injury, which prevents reabsorption, can present as nephrotic range proteinuria, leading to a pseudo-nephrotic syndrome.[6] When suspected, the protein can be measured with serum and urine protein electrophoresis revealing increased γ globulin levels, and confirmed with immunofixation to exclude monoclonal paraproteins.[7] Treatment of the underlying malignancy will decrease lysozyme and improve kidney function.

Tumor lysis syndrome results from the release of intracellular potassium, phosphate, and nucleic acids from rapidly growing cancer cells. This can be spontaneous or the direct effect of chemotherapy. Purine nucleic acids are converted to xanthine and then to uric acid by xanthine oxidase.[8] At high levels, uric acid crystals can precipitate in renal tubules, leading to direct tubular injury. This can be seen through evaluation of the urinary sediment demonstrating uric acid crystals in isolation or incorporated in casts (Fig. 37.4A and B). In addition, uric acid is a vasoconstrictor that may exacerbate renal tubular damage, recruit proinflammatory cytokines to the renal interstitium, and delay recovery.[9] Direct tubular injury can be seen by the presence of RTEC or granular casts in the urine sediment (Fig. 37.4C and D). Prevention of tumor lysis syndrome with adequate hydration or direct xanthine oxidase inhibitors, such as allopurinol or febuxostat, is ideal. If uric acid

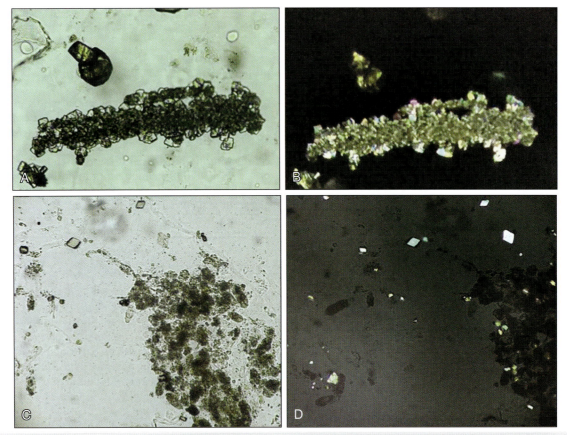

Fig. 37.4 Urine sediment from a patient with tumor lysis syndrome and hyperuricemia. **A.** 160× light microscopy showing urate crystal cast. **B.** 160× light microscopy with polarization showing birefringence of urate crystal cast. **C.** 40× light microscopy showing urate crystals and granular casts urate crystals. **D.** 40× light microscopy with polarization demonstrating birefringence of urate crystals.

levels increase despite these efforts, rasburicase, a recombinant urate oxidase that converts uric acid to allantoin, can be used.[8]

ACUTE KIDNEY INJURY FROM KIDNEY INFILTRATION

The kidney is the most common extrareticular and extrahematopoietic organ infiltrated by leukemia, with infiltration seen in 60% to 90% of patients with hematologic malignancy.[10] Kidney dysfunction varies from asymptomatic increases in serum creatinine to severe AKI requiring dialytic support. The rate of infiltration parallels stage and grade of disease. In a series of 1200 autopsy cases, the prevalence of renal infiltration was 63% in chronic lymphocytic leukemia (CLL), 54% in acute lymphoblastic leukemia (ALL), 34% in chronic myeloid leukemia (CML), and 33% in acute myeloid leukemia (AML);[11] however, the association with elevated serum creatinine and AKI was not reported. Although infiltration is possible, kidney failure primarily caused by leukemic infiltration is rare. AKI from infiltration is seen in only 1% of cases of all patients with acute leukemias and even less commonly in chronic leukemia.[12]

Symptoms and signs that may be associated with infiltration include flank pain, hematuria, abdominal distension, or hypertension.[1] Infiltration has to be bilateral in nature, as circulating cells have access to both kidneys, and enlargement is usually uniform throughout the superior, inferior, and mid-pole regions of the kidney. Renal biopsy is often useful in patients with leukemia who present with AKI in the setting of enlarged kidneys. Biopsy will reveal the extent of infiltration and underlying fibrosis both of which tend to influence prognosis (Fig. 37.5A). Kidney injury resulting from infiltration is thought to be secondary to acute tubular compression and disruption of the renal microvasculature, from increased interstitial pressure leading to ATN. Biopsy may also help differentiate subtypes of leukemia and alter disease treatment (Fig. 37.5B). Specific stains can be used to identify cellular markers of differentiation leading to targeted chemotherapy. Regression and improvement in kidney function should be prompt once therapy is initiated, even occurring within 2 to 3 days of therapy.[1]

ACUTE KIDNEY INJURY FROM RENOVASCULAR DISORDERS

Renovascular-mediated kidney injury includes disorders that lead to the thrombosis of large vessels that perfuse (arteries) or drain (veins) the kidneys or endothelial damage and injury to the microvasculature of the kidney. In these diseases, several factors contribute to thrombosis of the renal vasculature, including leukostasis, malignancy-associated nephrotic syndrome leading to loss of procoagulant molecules, and comorbid conditions or treatments that can lead to activation of the clotting cascade. Both renal artery and renal vein thrombosis have been described in leukemia.[13] Thrombotic microangiopathies have also been reported in both acute and chronic leukemias, resulting in AKI.[14]

Although quite rare, AKI from leukostasis has been reported. In an autopsy study consisting of patients with AML, 6% of patients had intravascular leukocyte thrombi and fibrin strands in the renal vasculature.[15] Leukocytosis causing AKI is more commonly seen in myeloid leukemias when white blood cell (WBC) counts exceed 100 × 1000 cells/µL. This is thought to be secondary to the morphology and poor distensibility of rigid myeloblasts in hyperviscous plasma. Despite the predominance of leukostasis-associated AKI in myeloid leukemia, cases of similar AKI in lymphocytic leukemia have also been reported.[16] Treatment of the underlying malignancy and subsequent improvement in leukocyte count usually resolves the injury. Failure of the kidney injury to improve may be suggestive of either prolonged injury leading to interstitial fibrosis and tubular atrophy or a concomitant injury that has not been treated.

Glomerular Disease With Hematologic Malignancies

Glomerulopathies have been described in all forms of leukemia. The following section outlines specific glomerular lesions based on underlying malignancy (Table 37.2).[17] When urinalysis suggests glomerular pathology, with the presence of hematuria, with acanthocytes or red cell casts, proteinuria, with a predominance of albuminuria relative

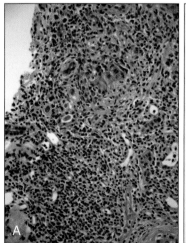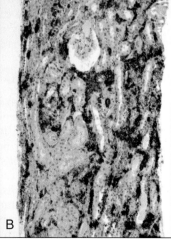

Fig. 37.5 Kidney biopsy from a patient with chronic lymphocytic leukemia and acute kidney injury. **A.** 160× light microscopy image of kidney biopsy specimen (stained with hematoxylin and eosin) showing extensive interstitial inflammation and renal tubule compression. **B.** 160× light microscopy image of kidney biopsy specimen (stained with anti-CD3 T-cell marker) showing a significant infiltrate of CD3 positive T-cells.

Table 37.2 Summary of Glomerulopathies Seen in Leukemia

Malignancy	Glomerular Lesions	Important Points
ALL	MCD FSGS	▪ Proteinuria can be caused by lysozymuria-induced tubular damage ▪ More often glomerular damage precedes malignancy ▪ Predominantly seen in children
AML	MCD FSGS MPGN Mesangioproliferative GN	▪ Proteinuria can be caused by lysozymuria-induced tubular damage ▪ Possible association with oncornavirus antigens
CLL	MCD FSGS Membranous nephropathy MPGN IgG kappa and lambda Amyloidosis (AA) Crescentic GN Immunotactoid GN Mesangioproliferative GN	▪ Associated with autoimmune disease ▪ Infiltration in 90% of patients (asymptomatic and symptomatic)
CML	MCD Membranous nephropathy MPGN	▪ Very rare with primary disease ▪ Associated with interferon-alpha therapy and posthematopoietic stem cell transplantation

ALL, Acute lymphoblastic leukemia; *AML,* acute myeloid leukemia; *CLL,* chronic lymphocytic leukemia; *CML,* chronic myeloid leukemia; *MCD,* minimal change disease; *FSGS,* focal segmental glomerulosclerosis; *MPGN,* membranoproliferative glomerulonephritis; *GN,* glomerulonephritis.

to total proteinuria, or both, kidney biopsy should be performed. As with other forms of kidney injury directly related to leukemia, glomerulopathies require successful treatment of the underlying disease.

ACUTE LYMPHOBLASTIC LEUKEMIA

Proteinuria in ALL is usually pseudonephrotic syndrome, associated with lysozymuria.[6] However, in children, nephrotic syndrome may portend a future diagnosis of ALL. In eight pediatric cases, focal segmental glomerulosclerosis (FSGS) or minimal change disease (MCD) preceded the diagnosis of ALL by less than 1 year.[18-20] At presentation, these patients demonstrated abnormal leukocyte profiles and were treated with glucocorticoids. It is unclear whether nephrotic syndrome is an early manifestation of ALL or whether immunosuppressive treatment causes proliferation of an abnormal WBC clone. MCD has been diagnosed during induction chemotherapy for known ALL, suggesting that an immune cell dysregulation is common between the two disease entities. However, given the paucity of cases, mechanisms are purely speculative. As ALL is mostly a disease of childhood, glomerular lesions have not been reported in adults.

ACUTE MYELOID LEUKEMIA

Proteinuria in AML can also be related to lysozymuria. Biopsies from patients with nephrotic range proteinuria, in the absence of lysozymuria, have identified FSGS, MCD, mesangioproliferative glomerulonephritis, and membranoproliferative glomerulonephritis (MPGN)[21,22] (Fig. 37.6). In two of these cases, nephrotic range proteinuria was present at the time of disease diagnosis, with a positive correlation between the degree of proteinuria and leukemic burden. In other cases, nephrotic syndrome developed months after diagnosis or in association with chemotherapy. The etiology of glomerulonephritis (GN) and nephrotic syndrome in

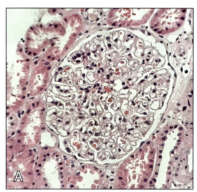

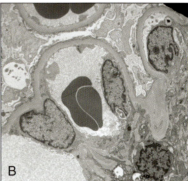

Fig. 37.6 Patient with minimal change disease in the setting of acute myeloid leukemia. **A.** 160× light microscopy image of kidney biopsy specimen (stained with hematoxylin and eosin) of a patient with minimal change disease showing a glomerulus with normal cellularity and patent capillary loops. **B.** Electron micrograph at 8000× of patient with minimal change disease showing complete foot process effacement.

AML is currently unclear and likely multifactorial. Studies of subclinical immune complexes in kidneys of patients with AML have identified antigens related to oncornaviruses, suggesting a possible viral related etiology to the immune mediated glomerular lesions.[23]

CHRONIC LYMPHOCYTIC LEUKEMIA

CLL infiltrates the kidney interstitium of approximately 90% of patients at the time of autopsy, yet clinical kidney disease is uncommon.[24] Although many glomerular lesions have been reported, MPGN is the most common followed by membranous nephropathy[24] (Fig. 37.7). Other reported causes are presented in detail in Table 37.2. The pathophysiology of GN is thought to be multifactorial. CLL is characterized by aberrant proliferation of a monoclonal B-cell clone and it is the deposition of the monoclonal immune complexes in the glomerulus that is thought to be pathologic.[25] CLL is also associated with various autoimmune disorders, which may predispose patients to cryoglobulin production and subsequent immune complex deposition.[26] Lastly, CLL patients are prone to infection, from either immunosuppression because of clonal expansion or functional asplenism, both of which may contribute to infection related GN.

CHRONIC MYELOID LEUKEMIA

Glomerular disease associated with CML is rare. Reports of nephrotic syndrome have been primarily the result of interferon-α therapy or hematopoietic stem cell transplants.[27] However, cases of MPGN, membranous nephropathy, and MCD associated with CML have also been reported[28,29] (Fig. 37.8). Glomerular injury in CML has occurred in both

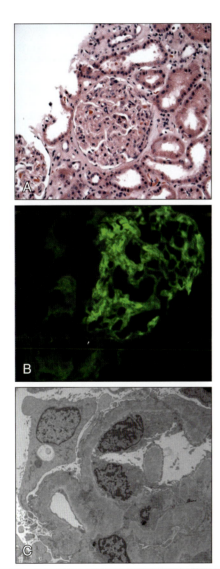

Fig. 37.7 Patient with a membranoproliferative glomerulonephritis (MPGN) in the setting of chronic lymphocytic leukemia. **A.** 40× light microscopy image of kidney biopsy specimen (stained with hematoxylin and eosin) showing a glomerulus with hypercellularity, lobulation and endocapillary proliferation. **B.** Immunofluorescence at 160× stained with immunoglobulin G showing granular subendothelial staining. **C.** Electron micrograph at 8000× of patient with MPGN showing a predominance of subendothelial electron dense deposits.

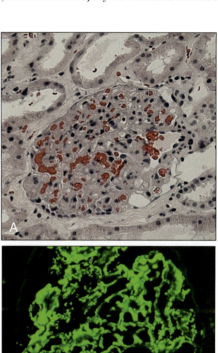
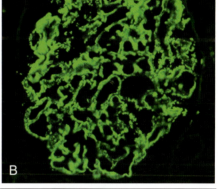
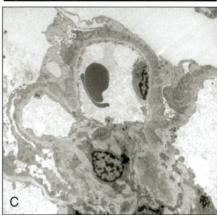

Fig. 37.8 Patient with a membranous nephropathy (MN) in the setting of chronic myeloid leukemia. **A.** 160× light microscopy image of kidney biopsy specimen (stained with hematoxylin and eosin) showing a glomerulus with thickened capillary loops. **B.** Immunofluorescence at 160× stained with immunoglobulin G showing granular pericapillary loop staining. **C.** Electron micrograph at 8000× of patient with MN showing a predominance of subepithelial electron dense deposits.

blast crisis and the chronic phase of malignancy, making an association with disease state difficult. Speculation on the cause of these glomerular lesions in CML includes infection-related processes in the setting of splenomegaly-induced immunosuppression, autoimmune dysregulation, or deposition of disease-mediated immune complexes. However, given the very low incidence, etiology remains poorly understood.

Electrolyte and Acid-Base Disorders

A variety of electrolyte and acid-base abnormalities have been described in the setting of leukemia (Table 37.3). These disorders are caused by the malignancy, direct infiltration of organs, cell lysis, or chemotherapeutic agents leading to AKI. Hypokalemia is the most prevalent abnormality (43%–64%), followed by hypomagnesemia (25%–32%) and hypophosphatemia (16%–30%).[30]

POTASSIUM DISORDERS

In a case series of 22 patients with acute leukemia, total body potassium per kilogram of body weight was significantly lower in leukemic patients relative to healthy subjects.[31] Patients with malignancy may have a reduction in caloric intake, but this rarely results in hypokalemia unless potassium intake is less than 20 mEq/day.[32] Emesis and the loss of hydrogen ions may result in metabolic alkalosis, with the increased serum bicarbonate levels, eventually overwhelming the proximal tubular reabsorptive capacity of bicarbonate. As a result, increased distal delivery of sodium bicarbonate (bicarbonaturia) promotes enhanced potassium excretion by the principal cell in the setting concomitant secondary hyperaldosteronism.

In addition, the ability of the kidney to handle potassium appropriately may also be affected by medications commonly prescribed to patients with leukemia, such as penicillins, aminoglycosides, and amphotericin, used in the setting of infections. These medications can be directly toxic to tubular cells, disrupting apical potassium channel function or by impairing the luminal electrochemical gradient, enhancing potassium secretion. A less common cause of hypokalemia that has been reported in AML is through paraneoplastic activation of the renin-angiotensin-aldosterone system by the production of renin.[33]

A hypothesized nonrenal cause of hypokalemia in hematologic malignancy is the possibility that increased cellular uptake of potassium into metabolically active leukemic cells via active Na^+/K^+ adenosine triphosphatase will lead to a deficiency of extracellular potassium.

Hyperkalemia in leukemia is less common. It is most often caused by potassium release from leukemic cell lysis, either from spontaneous destruction of rapidly growing cells or as a desired consequence of chemotherapy.[8] Because these patients tend to have very elevated WBC counts, pseudohyperkalemia from postphlebotomy cell destruction must also be considered.[34] In patients with severe hyperkalemia, plasma potassium can be compared with serum potassium to confirm true versus pseudohyperkalemia. It is important to recognize this phenomenon to avoid unnecessary

Table 37.3   Electrolyte and Acid-Base Disorders in Leukemia

Electrolyte Disorder	Etiology

Hypokalemia	*Gastrointestinal loss (diarrhea, emesis)*
	Kaliuresis
	    Tubular dysfunction (medications, lysozymuria)
	    Hypomagnesemia
	Renin-angiotensin-aldosterone system activation
	    Volume depletion
	    Paraneoplastic renin release
	Intracellular shift
	    Potassium entry into actively proliferating cells

Hyperkalemia	*Cellular lysis* (tumor lysis syndrome) *Reduced GFR* (acute kidney injury) *Pseudohyperkalemia* (cell lysis associated with blood collection)
Hypomagnesemia	*Gastrointestinal losses* *Magnesuria* Tubular dysfunction (lysozyme, medications) *Intracellular magnesium shift*
Hypophosphatemia	*Gastrointestinal loss* *Phosphaturia* (tubular dysfunction) *Intracellular phosphate shift*
Hyperphosphatemia	*Cellular lysis* (tumor lysis syndrome) *Reduced GFR* (acute kidney injury)
Hyponatremia	*Hypovolemic hyponatremia* *SIADH*
Hypernatremia	*Central diabetes insipidus*
Hypocalcemia	*Calcium-phosphate precipitation in tumor lysis syndrome* *Low vitamin D* *Chronic respiratory alkalosis* *Hypoalbuminemia* *Hypomagnesemia*
Hypercalcemia	*PTHrp expression* *Upregulation of RANK-L by cytokines*
Metabolic acidosis	*Type B lactic acidosis*

GFR, Glomerular filtration rate; *PTHrp*, serum parathyroid hormone-related protein; *RANK-L*, receptor activator of nuclear factor kappa-B ligand; *SIADH*, syndrome of inappropriate antidiuretic hormone.

treatment of normal potassium levels that can lead to potentially dangerous hypokalemia.

MAGNESIUM DISORDERS

Magnesium balance is influenced by gastrointestinal, hematologic, and renal mechanisms. Diarrhea or poor oral intake may contribute to hypomagnesemia in patients with leukemia. As with potassium, cellular uptake of magnesium occurs in patients with leukocytosis and high cellular metabolic activity.[30] Hypomagnesemia can also be caused by defects in renal magnesium handling. Hypermagnesuria occurs in approximately 15% of acute leukemic patients.[35] Lysozymuria through direct tubular toxicity has been shown to lead to magnesuria.[6] Many pharmacologic agents, such as aminoglycosides, amphotericin, and pentamidine, used in infectious complications in immunosuppressed patients have been implicated in decreased magnesium absorption through paracellular or active transport.

PHOSPHATE DISORDERS

As with potassium and magnesium, hypophosphatemia may be multifactorial in patients with a hematologic malignancy. Acute diarrhea leads to significant phosphate loss, as can acute antacid ingestion. Dietary phosphate complexes with calcium or other metals in the antacid preparations, which impedes phosphate absorption. Hypophosphatemia can occur from acute shifts of phosphate into metabolically active leukemic cells.[36] As with magnesium and potassium, direct tubular damage, through lysozyme or medication, can lead to tubular dysfunction and Fanconi syndrome, resulting in increased urinary phosphate loss. Hyperphosphatemia is most commonly seen in the setting of AKI, leading to decreased renal phosphate excretion, and in tumor lysis syndrome through the release of intracellular phosphate.

SODIUM DISORDERS

Hyponatremia has been estimated to occur in approximately 10% of patients with acute hematologic malignancies.[30] The most common cause of hyponatremia in these patients is hypovolemic hyponatremia from volume depletion in the setting of poor oral intake, emesis, and diarrhea. Euvolemic hyponatremia from syndrome of inappropriate antidiuretic hormone (SIADH) secretion is uncommon. However, SIADH may be present in the setting of an underlying lung infection or central nervous system (CNS) involvement with leukemia. Hypernatremia is extremely rare in hematologic malignancies but can be associated with poor access to free water, or rarely has been associated with CNS leukemic or infiltration producing a central diabetes insipidus state.[37] Interestingly, the presence of certain cytogenetic abnormalities with AML have been linked to the development of diabetes insipidus.[38]

CALCIUM DISORDERS

Hypercalcemia is the most common disturbance of calcium homeostasis in hematologic malignancies. In leukemia, hypercalcemia can occur in both the acute and chronic phases. In CML, it usually presents with blast crisis or an accelerated phase of leukemia. Inflammatory mediators such as transforming growth factor (TGF)-α, TGF-β, prostaglandin E2, and interleukin-6 are elevated in CML blast crisis and acute leukemia and these mediators may cause upregulation of receptor activator of nuclear factor kappa-β ligand (RANK-L) expression and 1,25-$(OH)_2D_3$.[39] RANK-L leads to increased osteoclast activity, thereby contributing to increased serum calcium levels, whereas activated vitamin D leads to increased bone turnover and increased intestinal absorption of calcium. Elevations of serum parathyroid hormone-related protein (PTHrP) have been described in a few cases of CML.[40] PTHrP leads to increased levels of calcium by increasing bone resorption and increased distal tubule calcium reabsorption.

Hypocalcemia is rare in hematologic malignancy. It can result from various factors including hypoalbuminemia, malnutrition, malabsorption, vitamin D deficiency, coexisting hypomagnesaemia or chronic respiratory alkalosis. Tumor lysis resulting in high serum phosphorous concentrations can lead to calcium-phosphate deposition, thereby lowering serum calcium levels.

ACID-BASE DISORDERS

Acid-base disorders are quite common in hematologic malignancies, with the prevalence of metabolic alkalosis up to 30% and metabolic acidosis up to 10% of patients with acute leukemia.[41] However, the complexity of patients with acute hematologic malignancies makes interpretation of acid-base disorders somewhat challenging; rarely is there one explanation for the underlying disorder and often there is a mixed acid-base disorder.

Summary

With the increased incidence of hematologic malignancy and new therapies that are prolonging survival in patients with leukemia, AKI and chronic kidney injury and other complications will undoubtedly become more prevalent. As the differential is broad for AKI in these patients, the nephrologist must be thorough to correctly diagnose cause of injury. Therapy for AKI, glomerulopathies, or electrolyte disorders is largely supportive with treatment of the underlying malignancy is the mainstay.

Key Points

- Acute kidney injury (AKI) is quite common in patients with leukemia contributing to increased morbidity and mortality.
- Diagnosing AKI in patients with leukemia is similar to other forms of AKI, but there are certain disease-specific entities (such as lysozyme-induce kidney injury, tumor lysis syndrome, direct kidney infiltration, and hematologic mediated obstruction).
- Acute and chronic leukemias are associated with nephrotic syndrome and glomerulonephritis.
- Disorders of potassium, magnesium, phosphate, sodium, and calcium, and lactic acidosis are common in patients with leukemia.

References

1. Luciano RL, Brewster UC. Kidney involvement in leukemia and lymphoma. *Adv Chronic Kidney Dis.* 2014;21:27-35.
2. Lanore JJ, Brunet F, Pochard F, et al. Hemodialysis for acute renal failure in patients with hematologic malignancies. *Crit Care Med.* 1991;19:346-351.
3. de Mendonça A, Vincent JL, Suter PM, et al. Acute renal failure in the ICU: risk factors and outcome evaluated by the SOFA score. *Intensive Care Med.* 2000;26:915-921.
4. Sarhill N, Walsh D, Nelson K, Davis M. Evaluation and treatment of cancer-related fluid deficits: volume depletion and dehydration. *Support Care Cancer.* 2001;9:408-419.

5. Harris KP, Hattersley JM, Feehally J, Walls J. Acute renal failure associated with haematological malignancies: a review of 10 years experience. *Eur J Haematol.* 1991;47:119-122.

6. Patel TV, Rennke HG, Sloan JM, DeAngelo DJ, Charytan DM. A forgotten cause of kidney injury in chronic myelomonocytic leukemia. *Am J Kidney Dis.* 2009;54:159-164.

7. Levinson SS, Elin RJ, Yam L. Light chain proteinuria and lysozymuria in a patient with acute monocytic leukemia. *Clin Chem.* 2002;48: 1131-1132.

8. Wilson FP, Berns JS. Onco-nephrology: tumor lysis syndrome. *Clin J Am Soc Nephrol.* 2012;7:1730-1739.

9. Cirillo P, Gersch MS, Mu W, et al. Ketohexokinase-dependent metabolism of fructose induces proinflammatory mediators in proximal tubular cells. *J Am Soc Nephrol.* 2009;20:545-553.

10. Richmond J, Sherman RS, Diamond HD, Craver LF. Renal lesions associated with malignant lymphomas. *Am J Med.* 1962;32:184-207.

11. Barcos M, Lane W, Gomez GA, et al. An autopsy study of 1206 acute and chronic leukemias (1958 to 1982). *Cancer.* 1987;60:827-837.

12. Lundberg WB, Cadman ED, Finch SC, Capizzi RL. Renal failure secondary to leukemic infiltration of the kidneys. *Am J Med.* 1977;62:636-642.

13. Levin MD, Betjes MG, Kwast TH, Wenberg BL, Leebeek FW. Acute renal cortex necrosis caused by arterial thrombosis during treatment for acute promyelocytic leukemia. *Haematologica.* 2003;88:ECR21.

14. Clarke RT, Mitchell C. Haemolytic uraemic syndrome in a patient with acute lymphoblastic leukaemia. *Pediatr Blood Cancer.* 2010;55: 1402-1405.

15. McKee LC Jr, Collins RD. Intravascular leukocyte thrombi and aggregates as a cause of morbidity and mortality in leukemia. *Medicine (Baltimore).* 1974;53:463-478.

16. Dietrich PY, Pedraza E, Casiraghi O, Bayle C, Hayat M, Pico JL. Cardiac arrest due to leucostasis in a case of prolymphocytic leukaemia. *Br J Haematol.* 1991;78:122-123.

17. Poitou-Verkinder AL, Francois A, Drieux F, et al. The spectrum of kidney pathology in B-cell chronic lymphocytic leukemia/small lymphocytic lymphoma: a 25 year multicenter experience. *PLoS One.* 2015;10:e0119156.

18. Bhatia M, Kher K, Minniti CP. Acute lymphoblastic leukemia in a child with nephrotic syndrome. *Pediatr Nephrol.* 2004;19:1290-1293.

19. Müller W, Brandis M. Acute leukemia after cytotoxic treatment for nonmalignant disease in childhood. A case report and review of the literature. *Eur J Pediatr.* 1981;136:105-108.

20. Sathiapalan RK, Velez MC, McWhorter ME, et al. Focal segmental glomerulosclerosis in children with acute lymphocytic leukemia: case reports and review of literature. *J Pediatr Hematol Oncol.* 1998;20: 482-485.

21. Dosa S, Phillips TM, Antonovych TT, Segal A, Guha A, Thompson AM. Acute myelomonocytic leukemia associated with nephrotic syndrome. A case report with immunological studies. *Nephron.* 1983;34:125-129.

22. Omura K, Kawamura T, Utsunomiya Y, Abe A, Joh K, Sakai O. Development of nephrotic syndrome in a patient with acute myeloblastic leukemia after treatment with macrophage-colony-stimulating factor. *Am J Kidney Dis.* 1996;27:883-887.

23. Sutherland JC, Mardiney MR Jr. Immune complex disease in the kidneys of lymphoma-leukemia patients: the presence of an oncornavirus-related antigen. *J Natl Cancer Inst.* 1973;50:633-644.

24. Da'as N, Polliack A, Cohen Y, et al. Kidney involvement and renal manifestations in non-Hodgkin's lymphoma and lymphocytic leukemia: a retrospective study in 700 patients. *Eur J Haematol.* 2001; 67:158-164.

25. Seney FD Jr, Federgreen WR, Stein H, Kashgarian M. A review of nephrotic syndrome associated with chronic lymphocytic leukemia. *Arch Intern Med.* 1986;146:137-141.

26. Gale RP, Foon KA. Biology of chronic lymphocytic leukemia. *Semin Hematol.* 1987;24:209-229.

27. Budak-Alpdoğan T, Lawrence RA, Bayik M, Akoğlu E. Nephrotic syndrome associated with alpha interferon therapy in chronic myeloid leukemia. *Clin Nephrol.* 1997;48:59-60.

28. Agarwal RG, Gupta KD, Bharadwaj TP. Nephrotic syndrome in the possible terminal blast-cell crisis in myeloid leukaemia (a case report). *J Assoc Physicians India.* 1972;20:799-801.

29. Talwar R, Dash SC, Kucheria K. A case of chronic myeloid leukemia complicated with minimal change nephrotic syndrome. *Acta Haematol.* 2003;109:101-103.

30. Filippatos TD, Milionis HJ, Elisaf MS. Alterations in electrolyte equilibrium in patients with acute leukemia. *Eur J Haematol.* 2005;75: 449-460.

31. Lantz B, Carlmark B, Reizenstein P. Electrolytes and whole body potassium in acute leukemia. *Acta Med Scand.* 1979;206:45-50.

32. Gallen IW, Rosa RM, Esparaz DY, et al. On the mechanism of the effects of potassium restriction on blood pressure and renal sodium retention. *Am J Kidney Dis.* 1998;31:19-27.

33. Wulf GG, Jahns-Streubel G, Strutz F, et al. Paraneoplastic hypokalemia in acute myeloid leukemia: a case of renin activity in AML blast cells. *Ann Hematol.* 1996;73:139-141.

34. Bronson WR, DeVita VT, Carbone PP, Cotlove E. Pseudohyperkalemia due to release of potassium from white blood cells during clotting. *N Engl J Med.* 1966;274:369-375.

35. Milionis HJ, Bourantas CL, Siamopoulos KC, Elisaf MS. Acid-base and electrolyte abnormalities in patients with acute leukemia. *Am J Hematol.* 1999;62:201-207.

36. Zamkoff KW, Kirshner JJ. Marked hypophosphatemia associated with acute myelomonocytic leukemia. Indirect evidence of phosphorus uptake by leukemic cells. *Arch Intern Med.* 1980;140:1523-1524.

37. Miller VI, Campbell WG Jr. Diabetes insipidus as a complication of leukemia. A case report with a literature review. *Cancer.* 1971;28: 666-673.

38. Dy P, Chua P, Kelly J, Liebman S. Central diabetes insipidus in the setting of acute myelogenous leukemia. *Am J Kidney Dis.* 2012;60: 998-1001.

39. Noguchi M, Oshimi K. Extensive bone marrow necrosis and symptomatic hypercalcemia in B cell blastic transformation of chronic myeloid leukemia: report of a case and review of the literature. *Acta Haematol.* 2007;118:111-116.

40. Miyoshi N, Tanaka H, Ito T, et al. Use of imatinib mesylate for favorable control of hypercalcemia mediated by parathyroid hormone-related protein in a patient with chronic myelogenous leukemia at blast phase. *Int J Hematol.* 2005;82:333-337.

41. Mir MA, Delamore IW. Metabolic disorders in acute myeloid leukaemia. *Br J Haematol.* 1978;40:79-92.

38 *Kidney Disease in Lymphoma*

RANDY L. LUCIANO

Introduction

Lymphoma is a hematologic malignancy caused by the abnormal proliferation of lymphoid cells. An estimated 80,000 people will be diagnosed with lymphoma in the United States in 2018. Because of more targeted therapies, patients with lymphoma are living longer. Lymphoma can broadly be divided into Hodgkin and non-Hodgkin lymphoma, based on cellular characteristics. Lymphoma can involve organs other than the lymph nodes, including the kidney and kidney-associated lymph tissue. Patients can develop kidney injury as a result of the lymphoma itself either through primary or secondary interactions with the kidney, a consequence of the comorbid illness or conditions brought on by either treatment of lymphoma or the malignancy itself. In addition, medications used to treat the lymphoma or associated side effects from treatment may also cause kidney injury. As with leukemia, kidney manifestations encompass a broad spectrum of disease: prerenal acute kidney injury (AKI), acute tubular necrosis (ATN), renovascular disease, parenchymal infiltration, urinary obstruction, glomerulopathies, and electrolyte and acid-base abnormalities.[1] Recognizing and addressing kidney injury in patients with lymphoma is crucial to halt progressive injury and avoid a delay in chemotherapy. This chapter will focus on kidney injury in patients with lymphoma as it pertains to the malignancy and complications from treatment. Chapters 16, 17, and 18 address kidney injury associated with therapeutic agents used to treat lymphoma and other malignancies. Because many of the concepts are similar to those presented in the prior chapter on kidney injury and leukemia, this chapter will provide an overview on shared mechanisms, while focusing more on lymphoma-specific causes of kidney injury.

Acute Kidney Injury in Lymphoma

AKI in patients with hematologic malignancies is common with upwards of 43% of patients in the intensive care unit with leukemia or lymphoma having some form of AKI. The presence of AKI in patients with lymphoma has therapeutic and prognostic implications, with 29% of those patients requiring renal replacement therapy and a mortality rate of upwards of 72%, the latter being higher than those patients with hematologic malignancies that do not develop AKI.[2] As with leukemia, the presence of lymphoma portends a much higher rate of AKI than patients with other diseases, including cirrhosis or cardiovascular disease. The diagnostic approach to a patient presenting with AKI in the setting of lymphoma involves elucidation of prerenal, intrarenal, and postrenal etiologies (Table 38.1).

PRERENAL ACUTE KIDNEY INJURY

Prerenal AKI is the most common kidney injury in patients with lymphoma. Prerenal AKI is most often caused by volume depletion from poor oral fluid intake (78%), anorexia (64%), early satiety (50%), emesis (23%), or diarrhea (16%).[3] In addition, the use of certain medications in the setting of volume depletion may exacerbate or magnify the severity of prerenal AKI in a patient with lymphoma. Medications that affect kidney afferent and efferent tone, including renin-angiotensin blockade or nonsteroidal antiinflammatory medications, or diuretics may worsen the kidney injury. Prerenal AKI is often suspected based on clinical context and history, and supported with physical examination demonstrating orthostatic hypotension or tachycardia, and laboratory data demonstrating an elevated blood urea nitrogen (BUN) and creatinine, often with a BUN to creatinine ratio greater than 20. Urine studies usually show and elevated specific gravity, a low urine sodium (often less than 20 mEq/L), low fractional excretion of sodium (< 1%), and bland urine sediment with occasional hyaline casts or renal tubular epithelial cells. Treatment of prerenal AKI is supportive, with intravenous crystalloid expansion and removal of exacerbating factors that lead to injury.

POSTRENAL ACUTE KIDNEY INJURY

In patients with lymphoma, obstruction may result from direct compression or encasement of ureteral outflow by tumor or lymph nodes, retroperitoneal fibrosis, or nephrolithiasis from tumor lysis syndrome.[4,5] The retroperitoneum has many lymph nodes that can become affected by systemic disease. Anuric kidney failure should raise the concern for bilateral urinary tract obstruction, which is possible with lymphoma and extensive disease burden. Kidney ultrasound or CT scan should demonstrate varying degrees of hydronephrosis depending on the extent of obstruction (Fig. 38.1). Treatment should happen quickly with immediate decompression with nephrostomy tubes to prevent permanent tubular atrophy and interstitial fibrosis.

Table 38.1 Etiology of Acute Kidney Injury in Lymphoma

Prerenal	*Intravascular volume depletion*
	Nausea, emesis, diarrhea (from chemotherapy or treatment)
	Hemorrhage
	Increased insensible losses (fever, tachypnea)
	Reduced renal perfusion
	Vasoconstriction (hypercalcemia, hyperuricemia)
	Sepsis
	Liver disease
	Medications (RAAS blockers, NSAIDs, diuretics)
Intrarenal	*Acute tubular necrosis*
	Renal ischemia
	Tumor lysis syndrome
	Medications (antibiotics, chemotherapy)
	Tubulointerstitial disorders
	Secondary renal infiltration
	Primary renal lymphoma
	Allergic interstitial nephritis
	Glomerular disorders
	See Table 38.2 for complete list
	Renovascular disorders
	Renal vein thrombosis
	Thrombotic microangiopathy
Postrenal	*Obstruction*
	Exterior compression (lymphadenopathy)
	Retroperitoneal fibrosis
	Internal obstruction (nephrolithiasis, crystalluria)

NSAIDs, Nonsteroidal antiinflammatory drugs; *RAAS*, renin-angiotensin-aldosterone system.

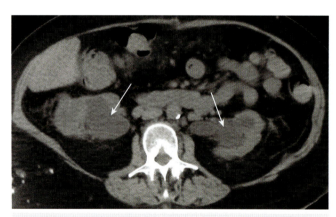

Fig. 38.1 A computed tomography scan from a patient with non-Hodgkin lymphoma with significant retroperitoneal lymph node involvement causing bilateral ureteral compression. The kidneys show severe hydronephrosis. The *white arrows* are pointing to severely dilated collecting system.

INTRARENAL ACUTE KIDNEY INJURY

Intrarenal causes of kidney injury in hematologic malignancy can be grouped into ischemic and non-ischemic ATN, tubulointerstitial disorders, renovascular disorders, and glomerulopathies. Hemodynamically mediated injury from severe volume depletion, heart failure, or sepsis, and drug-induced injury are common with hematologic malignancy. However, kidney injury directly caused by hematologic malignancy is possible and should be distinguished from other forms of tubular injury, as prognosis is dependent on treatment of the underlying disease.

Diagnosis of intrarenal AKI often relies on diagnostic imaging, urinary sediment analysis, or kidney biopsy. Diagnostic imaging with either renal ultrasound or computed tomography (CT) imaging may demonstrate diffuse bilateral kidney enlargement, suggesting kidney infiltration. Urine sediment analysis can reveal cells or casts that can help distinguish between tubulointerstitial disease or glomerular disease. Biopsy remains the gold standard in diagnosis, and can help identify glomerular, tubulointerstitial, or vascular disorders. Because kidney biopsy does have some risk, it may not possible in a patient with complicated hematologic malignancy, and coagulopathy.

ACUTE TUBULAR NECROSIS

ATN is the most common cause of intrinsic AKI in lymphoma, with more than 75% of patients with AKI having ATN.[6] ATN can often be diagnosed through clinical history and urinary sediment, which will show renal tubular epithelial cells or granular casts, but at times a biopsy may be necessary to exclude other causes of intrinsic AKI (Fig. 38.2A and B). Although the majority of patients with ATN will have ischemia-induced tubular injury, other causes of AKI exist, including drug-related nephrotoxicity and tumor lysis syndrome.

Tumor lysis syndrome occurs when intracellular potassium, phosphate, and nucleic acids are released into the serum from cancer cells. This can be spontaneous release from the death of rapidly growing cancer cells or the direct effect of chemotherapy. Purine nucleic acids that are released are converted to xanthine and then to uric acid by xanthine oxidase.[7] At high levels uric acid crystals can precipitate within the renal tubules and directly injure renal tubule epithelial cells from an associated inflammatory response. This can be detected on the urine sediment by the presence of uric acid crystals that polarize brightly under a polarization filter (Fig. 38.3A and B). In addition, uric acid can also function as a vasoconstrictor, leading to ischemic renal tubular damage through the recruitment of proinflammatory cytokines to the renal interstitium. The risk of tumor lysis syndrome can be mitigated with adequate hydration with nonbicarbonate-containing fluids or xanthine oxidase inhibitors,

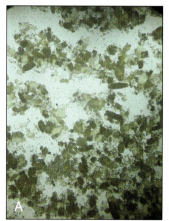
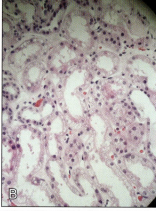

Fig. 38.2 Acute tubular necrosis in a patient with septic shock in the setting of Hodgkin lymphoma. **A.** 16× light microscopy showing many dense granular casts. **B.** 40× specimen from a kidney biopsy (stained with hematoxylin and eosin), showing dilated renal tubules, nuclear dropout, and renal tubular cytoplasmic vacuolization.

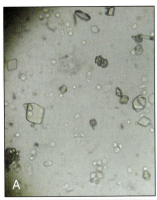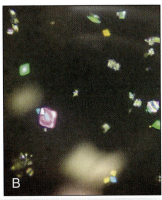

Fig. 38.3 Urine sediment from a patient with tumor lysis syndrome and hyperuricemia. **A.** 160× light microscopy showing urate crystals and white blood cells. **B.** 160× light microscopy with polarization demonstrating birefringence of urate crystals.

such as allopurinol or febuxostat, in at risk patients. However, if uric acid levels increase substantially (upwards of 10 mg/dL), rasburicase, a recombinant urate oxidase, can be used to convert uric acid to allantoin, a nonnephrotoxic metabolite that is highly soluble in the urine.

ACUTE KIDNEY INJURY FROM KIDNEY INFILTRATION

The kidney is the most common extrareticular and extrahematopoietic organ infiltrated by lymphoma.[8] The

consequence is either asymptomatic infiltration with no serologic evidence of a reduced glomerular filtration rate (GFR) or severe dysfunction requiring renal replacement therapy. The degree of infiltration and subsequent severity of kidney injury parallels stage and grade of disease. In an autopsy study in 700 patients with lymphoma, kidney infiltration was present in 34% of patients with Hodgkin (HL) and non-Hodgkin lymphoma (NHL).[8]

Severe kidney injury and subsequent kidney failure primarily caused by lymphomatous infiltration is rare. AKI from infiltration is seen in less than 1% of cases of all patients with lymphomas. Symptoms and signs associated with infiltration include flank pain, hematuria, abdominal distension, or hypertension.[9] Infiltration is bilateral in nature, and enlargement of the kidneys is usually uniform, unless there was an appreciable size differential before infiltration. Kidney biopsy may be required to separate lymphomatous infiltration from nonmalignant acute interstitial nephritis, most often caused by medications or infections. Biopsy demonstrates a dense interstitial infiltrate with immunohistochemistry revealing a predominance of lymphocytes (Fig. 38.4). The extent and location of infiltration tends to influence prognosis, with interstitial infiltration associated with AKI, and glomerular infiltration, associated with glomerular disease.[10] Kidney failure resulting from infiltration is thought to be secondary to compression of renal tubular epithelial cells and disruption of the renal microvasculature, both of which lead to ATN. Targeting lymphocytes with chemotherapy or radiotherapy is important, as

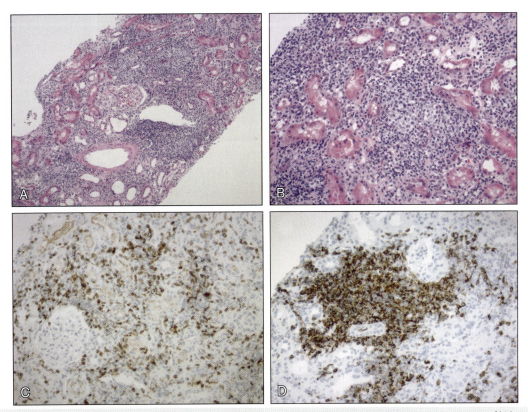

Fig. 38.4 Kidney biopsy from a patient with non-Hodgkin lymphoma and acute kidney injury. **A.** 40× light microscopy image of kidney biopsy specimen (stained with hematoxylin and eosin) showing extensive interstitial inflammation and renal tubule compression. **B.** 160× light microscopy image of kidney biopsy specimen (stained with hematoxylin and eosin) showing interstitial inflammation and renal tubule injury with nuclear dropout and vacuolization. **C.** 160× light microscopy image of kidney biopsy specimen (stained with anti-CD3 T-cell marker) showing a mild infiltrate of CD3 positive T-cells. **D.** 160× light microscopy image of kidney biopsy specimen (stained anti-CD20 B-cell marker) showing extensive B-cell infiltration.

improvement of kidney function is solely dependent on treatment of underlying disease and resolution of infiltration. Kidney function can improve in as little as 2 to 3 days of initiation of therapy.[9]

Primary renal lymphoma (PRL), characterized by primary localization of the lymphoma to the kidney, is extremely rare, with an incidence of 0.7% of all extranodal lymphomas.[11] Because the kidney itself is devoid of any significant lymphoid tissue, the small amount of lymphoid tissue in the renal capsule and renal sinus lymph nodes is thought to be the source of the malignancy. However, chronic inflammation in the kidney is likely necessary to stimulate lymphoid transformation, similar to the transformation of chronic inflammatory processes in other organs (for example, the association of Hashimoto thyroiditis with thyroid lymphoma). PRL usually presents with AKI and hypertension. Histology demonstrates interstitial infiltration with minimal fibrosis. Prognosis of PRL is exceedingly poor.[11]

ACUTE KIDNEY INJURY FROM RENOVASCULAR DISORDERS

Renovascular kidney injury can be associated with lymphoma. Various factors can contribute to thrombosis of the renal vasculature, including leukostasis, malignancy-associated nephrotic syndrome leading to loss of anticoagulant molecules, and comorbid conditions or treatments that activate the clotting cascade. Antiphospholipid syndrome, acquired through antiphospholipid antibody production in malignant states, has been seen with lymphomas. This can increase the risk of venous and arterial thrombus formation, with resultant kidney infarcts.[12] Thrombotic microangiopathies have also been reported in lymphomas, resulting in AKI.[13]

Glomerular Disease With Hematologic Malignancies

Glomerulopathies have been described in all hematologic malignancies. The following section outlines specific glomerular lesions based on underlying malignancy (Table 38.2). When urinalysis suggests glomerular pathology, kidney biopsy should be performed. As with other forms of kidney injury in hematologic malignancy, glomerulopathies require successful treatment of the underlying disease.

HODGKIN LYMPHOMA

The most common glomerular lesion associated with HL is minimal change disease (MCD), although focal segmental glomerulosclerosis (FSGS) has also been reported.[14] In these patients with nephrotic syndrome, diagnosis is usually made with biopsy; urine sediment may reveal lipiduria (Fig. 38.5). Amyloidosis (in particular AA amyloid) has been described in HL; however, its prevalence has decreased with improved treatment.[14] Antiglomerular basement membrane disease, which occurs with a frequency several fold higher than in patients without malignancy, and

Table 38.2 Summary of Glomerulopathies Seen in Lymphoma

Malignancy	Glomerular Lesions	Important Points
HL	MCD FSGS Amyloidosis (AA) Crescentic GN	Occur late in disease No correlation with disease progression or severity Associated with elevated VEGF-25, TGF-β expression in models
NHL	MCD FSGS Membranous nephropathy MPGN Mesangioproliferative GN Crescentic GN Amyloidosis (AL) IgA nephropathy Immunotactoid GN Fibrillary GN	Occur early in disease Severity mirrors disease progression Associated with hepatitis C and Epstein-Barr viral infections

FSGS, Focal segmental glomerulosclerosis; *GN*, glomerulonephritis; *HL*, Hodgkin lymphoma; *MCD*, minimal change disease; *MPGN*, membranoproliferative glomerulonephritis; *NHL*, non-Hodgkin lymphoma; *TGF-β*, transforming growth factor β; *VEGF-25*, vascular endothelial growth factor 25.

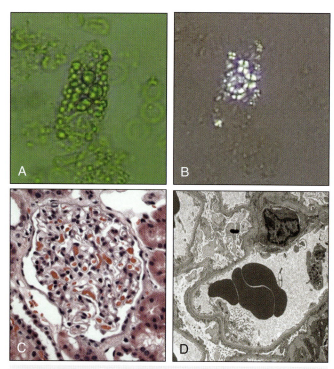

Fig. 38.5 Patient with nephrotic syndrome in the setting of Hodgkin lymphoma. **A.** Urine sediment at 160× under light microscopy showing lipid droplets in a hyaline cast. **B.** Urine sediment at 160× under light microscopy, with polarization, showing Maltese cross appearance of lipid droplets. **C.** 160× light microscopy image of kidney biopsy specimen (stained with hematoxylin and eosin) of a patient with minimal change disease showing a glomerulus with normal cellularity and patent capillary loops. **D.** Electron micrograph at 8000× of patient with minimal change disease showing complete foot process effacement.

pauci-immune crescentic glomerulonephritis (GN) have been reported.[15] The development of a glomerulopathy in HL is likely secondary to abnormal cytokine production and secretion by affected T-cells. This leads to alterations in glomerular permeability and thereby proteinuria. In particular, Reed Sternberg cells express vascular endothelial growth factor and transforming growth factor-β_1, cytokines linked to the pathogenesis of FSGS.[16] The association of MCD or FSGS with HL may ultimately depend on the specific cytokines and growth factors secreted and protooncogenes expressed by affected T-cells.

NON-HODGKIN LYMPHOMA

Glomerular lesions in patients with NHL vary widely and depend on the stage of lymphoma. In contrast to HL, where glomerular involvement occurs later in disease without correlation to progression or aggressiveness, glomerulopathies in NHL occur earlier and progress with disease. Proliferative lesions are more common in NHL, compared with HL, and may account for up to 30% of glomerular diseases.[11] Membranoproliferative glomerulonephritis, with or without immune complex deposition, has been reported (Fig. 38.6).[17] In a series of 37 patients with NHL, crescentic GN was seen in five cases, immunoglobulin A nephropathy in four cases, and fibrillary glomerulonephritis in one case.[11] Amyloidosis, as with HL, is less common with current chemotherapeutic options, but unlike HL tends to be the AL amyloid subtype.[17] Other lesions are reported in Table 38.2. NHL is thought to cause GN through dysfunctional cytokine production leading to immune complex deposition and cellular proliferation. A subset of patients with NHL may develop kidney lesions in association with concurrent hepatitis C virus infection with or without cryoglobulinemia. Other viral infections, such as Epstein–Barr virus, have been implicated in immune complex deposition causing glomerulopathies in NHL.

Electrolyte and Acid-Base Disorders

A variety of electrolyte and acid-base abnormalities have been described in lymphomas (Table 38.3). These disorders are caused by the malignancy, direct infiltration of organs, cell lysis, or chemotherapeutic agents leading to AKI. Hypokalemia is the most common disorder (estimated between 43%–64% of all hematologic malignancies), followed by hypomagnesemia (estimated between 25%–32% of all hematologic malignancies) and hypophosphatemia (estimated between 16%–30% of all hematologic malignancies).[18]

POTASSIUM DISORDERS

Hypokalemia can be seen in patients with lymphoma, with the etiology being multifactorial. Reduced caloric intake may contribute slightly to hypokalemia, but the calorie restriction has to be significant, with total daily potassium intake as low as 20 mEq/day.[19] Chemotherapeutic agents and disease itself can lead to persistent emesis, resulting in the loss of H+ ions and associated metabolic alkalosis, leading to increased kaliuresis. This process creates metabolic alkalosis, resulting in increased serum bicarbonate levels, eventually overwhelming the tubular reabsorptive capacity of bicarbonate. This results in increased distal delivery of sodium bicarbonate in the setting of secondary hyperaldosteronism, which promotes enhanced potassium excretion by the principal cell. Renal potassium wasting can also be exacerbated by medications commonly used in patients with lymphoma, such as penicillins, aminoglycosides, and amphotericin, which can be directly toxic to renal tubules or potassium channels, thereby disrupting the net charge in the tubule lumen. A hypothesized cause of hypokalemia in hematologic malignancy is the increased uptake of potassium into metabolically active lymphoma cells via active Na^+/K^+ adenosine triphosphatase.

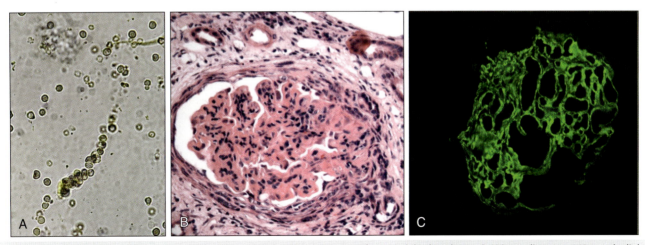

Fig. 38.6 Patient with a membranoproliferative glomerulonephritis in the setting of non-Hodgkin lymphoma. **A.** Urine sediment at 160× under light microscopy showing a red cell cast. **B.** 160× light microscopy image of kidney biopsy specimen (stained with hematoxylin and eosin) showing a glomerulus with hypercellularity, lobulation, and endocapillary proliferation. **C.** Immunofluorescence at 160× stained with immunoglobulin G showing granular subendothelial staining.

Table 38.3 Electrolyte and Acid-Base Disorders in Lymphoma

Electrolyte Disorder	Etiology

Hypokalemia	Gastrointestinal loss (diarrhea, emesis)
	Kaliuresis
	  Tubular dysfunction (medications)
	  Hypomagnesemia
	Renin-angiotensin-aldosterone system activation
	  Volume depletion
	Intracellular shift
	  Potassium entry into actively proliferating cells

Hyperkalemia	Cellular lysis (tumor lysis syndrome) Reduced GFR (acute kidney injury) Pseudohyperkalemia (cell lysis associated with collection)
Hypomagnesemia	Gastrointestinal losses Magnesuria Tubular dysfunction (lysozyme, medications) Intracellular magnesium shifts
Hypophosphatemia	Gastrointestinal loss Phosphaturia (tubular dysfunction) Intracellular phosphate shift
Hyperphosphatemia	Cellular lysis (tumor lysis syndrome) Reduced GFR (acute kidney injury)
Hyponatremia	Hypovolemic hyponatremia SIADH
Hypernatremia	Central diabetes insipidus
Hypocalcemia	Calcium-phosphate precipitation in tumor lysis syndrome Low vitamin D Chronic respiratory alkalosis Hypoalbuminemia Hypomagnesemia
Hypercalcemia	from calcitriol production
Metabolic acidosis	Type B lactic acidosis

GFR, Glomerular filtration rate; *SIADH*, syndrome of inappropriate antidiuretic hormone.

Hyperkalemia in lymphoma is less common than hypokalemia. It is most often caused by potassium release from cell lysis, either from spontaneous destruction of rapidly growing cells or as a direct effect of chemotherapy.[7]

MAGNESIUM DISORDERS

Magnesium balance is influenced by gastrointestinal, hematologic, and renal mechanisms. Diarrhea or poor oral intake may contribute with the latter being relatively uncommon. In patients with dyspepsia or acid reflux secondary to chemotherapy agents, the use of proton pump inhibitors (PPI) has been associated with hypomagnesemia, and therefore a temporal relationship of serum magnesium levels with the initiation of a PPI can occur. As with potassium, magnesium can shift into cells with high metabolic activity, contributing to hypomagnesemia.[18] Many pharmacologic agents, such as aminoglycosides, amphotericin, and pentamidine, are used to treat infectious complications in immunosuppressed patients. These drugs can lead to decreased magnesium absorption through paracellular or active transport, creating renal magnesium wasting and hypomagnesemia.

PHOSPHATE DISORDERS

As with potassium and magnesium, hypophosphatemia is multifactorial in patients with a hematologic malignancy. One common gastrointestinal cause of hypophosphatemia is acute diarrhea, often from chemotherapy or infection, leading to significant intestinal phosphate. In addition, patients who use antacids to control acid reflux or dyspepsia, can develop hypophosphatemia. Dietary phosphate can complex with calcium or other metals in the antacid preparations, which can impede intestinal phosphate absorption. Hypophosphatemia, as with the aforementioned electrolytes, can occur from acute shifts of phosphate into metabolically active cells.[20] Direct tubular damage, from hyperuricemia that develops with tumor lysis, or from medications that have nephrotoxic effects on kidney tubules, can lead to tubular dysfunction and Fanconi syndrome, resulting in increased urinary phosphate loss.

Hyperphosphatemia is most commonly seen in the setting of AKI from prerenal, obstructive, or acute ischemic insults resulting in ATN. Kidney injury reduces GFR, which leads to decreased renal phosphate excretion. Hyperphosphatemia is also commonly seen in tumor lysis syndrome and may also cause renal tubular calcium-phosphate deposition. Patients with acute hematologic malignancies may be predisposed to hyperphosphatemia as lymphoblasts have been shown to have a fourfold higher concentration of phosphate as opposed to a normal lymphocyte.

SODIUM DISORDERS

Hyponatremia may occur in approximately 10% of patients with acute hematologic malignancies.[19] Hypovolemic hyponatremia caused by volume depletion from poor oral intake, emesis, or diarrhea is the most common cause of hyponatremia in patients with lymphoma. Euvolemic hyponatremia from inappropriate antidiuretic hormone secretion is uncommon in lymphoma but may be seen in lung involvement or a lung infection or central nervous system (CNS) involvement. Hypernatremia is extremely rare in hematologic malignancy but can be associated with poor access to free water, and from CNS lymphomatous infiltration causing central diabetes insipidus.[21]

CALCIUM DISORDERS

Hypercalcemia is the most common disturbance of calcium homeostasis in hematologic malignancies. Hypercalcemia occurs in approximately 13% of patients with NHL and in 5.4% of patients with HL.[22] In NHL, hypercalcemia correlates with more advanced disease and median survival is significantly shorter, at 10 months compared with 21 months, relative to those patients with normal calcium levels. Calcitriol [1,25-(OH)2D3] has been implicated as a key mediator of hypercalcemia in almost all cases of HL and in 30% to 40% of cases of NHL.[23] Local osteolysis with increased expression of osteoclast-activating factors, including macrophage inflammatory protein (MIP)-1a, MIP-1b, and receptor activator of nuclear factor kappa-β ligand, in diffuse large B-cell lymphoma cells causes hypercalcemia.[24] Parathyroid hormone-related protein has also been reported as proposed factor for hypercalcemia in some cases with B-cell NHL, especially in cases with Richter's transformation.[25]

Hypocalcemia is rare in hematologic malignancy. It can result from various factors, including hypoalbuminemia, malnutrition, malabsorption, vitamin D deficiency, coexisting hypomagnesemia, or chronic respiratory alkalosis. Tumor lysis with resulting high serum phosphorous concentrations can lead to calcium-phosphate deposition, thereby lowering serum calcium levels.

ACID-BASE DISORDERS

Acid-base disorders are quite common in hematologic malignancies; and the complexity of patients with these malignancies makes interpretation of acid-base disorders somewhat challenging. Disorders of acid-base regulation are usually caused by more than one factor and most often there is a mixed acid-base disorder. Specific to lymphoma, a type B lactic acidosis may occur as well with lactate generation in the absence of tissue hypoperfusion or severe hypoxemia.[26] There may be deficient conversion of lactate to pyruvate and glucose by dysfunctional kidneys and liver in the state of active tumor growth that largely uses anaerobic metabolism. Also malnutrition, causing a relative thiamine deficiency, may reduce pyruvate dehydrogenase activity and result in lactate production from pyruvate.

Conclusion

The increased incidence of lymphoma and the new therapies that prolong survival in these patients are commonly complicated by AKI and chronic kidney injury or glomerular disease. Nephrologists, hematologists, oncologists, and internists who care for these patients must be aware of all the factors that can lead to AKI and other renal complications. Therapy for AKI, glomerulopathies, or electrolyte disorders is largely supportive with treatment of the underlying malignancy remaining essential.

Key Points

- Acute kidney injury (AKI) is common in patients with lymphoma, leading to increased morbidity and mortality and delays in life-saving treatment.
- Diagnosing AKI in patients with lymphoma is similar to other forms of AKI with certain disease-specific entities (such as tumor lysis syndrome, direct kidney infiltration, and retroperitoneal obstruction).
- Both Hodgkin lymphoma and non-Hodgkin lymphoma are associated with nephrotic syndrome and glomerulonephritis.

- Disorders of potassium, magnesium, phosphate, sodium, and calcium, and type B lactic acidosis are common in patients with lymphoma.

References

1. Luciano RL, Brewster UC. Kidney involvement in leukemia and lymphoma. *Adv Chronic Kidney Dis.* 2014;21:27-35.
2. Lanore JJ, Brunet F, Pochard F, et al. Hemodialysis for acute renal failure in patients with hematologic malignancies. *Crit Care Med.* 1991;19:346-351.
3. Sarhill N, Walsh D, Nelson K, Davis M. Evaluation and treatment of cancer-related fluid deficits: volume depletion and dehydration. *Support Care Cancer.* 2001;9:408-419.
4. Chong BH, Trew P, Meng L, et al. Anuric renal failure due to encasement of the ureters by lymphoma—ureteric obstruction without dilatation. *AUZ J Med.* 1981;11:542-544.
5. Mekori YA, Steiner ZP, Bernheim J, Manor Y, Klajman A. Acute anuric bilateral ureteral obstruction in malignant lymphoma. *Am J Med Sci.* 1984;287:70-73.
6. Harris KP, Hattersley JM, Feehally J, Walls J. Acute renal failure associated with haematological malignancies: a review of 10 years experience. *Eur J Haematol.* 1991;47:119-122.
7. Wilson FP, Berns JS. Onco-nephrology: tumor lysis syndrome. *Clin J Am Soc Nephrol.* 2012;7:1730-1739.
8. Richmond J, Sherman RS, Diamond HD, Craver LF. Renal lesions associated with malignant lymphomas. *Am J Med.* 1962;32:184-207.
9. Obrador GT, Price B, O'Meara Y, Salant DJ. Acute renal failure due to lymphomatous infiltration of the kidneys. *J Am Soc Nephrol.* 1997;8:1348-1354.
10. Törnroth T, Heiro M, Marcussen N, Franssila K. Lymphomas diagnosed by percutaneous kidney biopsy. *Am J Kidney Dis.* 2003;42:960-971.
11. Da'as N, Polliack A, Cohen Y, et al. Kidney involvement and renal manifestations in non-Hodgkin's lymphoma and lymphocytic leukemia: a retrospective study in 700 patients. *Eur J Haematol.* 2001;67:158-164.
12. Gómez-Puerta JA, Cervera R, Espinosa G, et al. Antiphospholipid antibodies associated with malignancies: clinical and pathological characteristics of 120 patients. *Semin Arthritis Rheum.* 2006;35:322-332.
13. Clarke RT, Mitchell C. Haemolytic uraemic syndrome in a patient with acute lymphoblastic leukaemia. *Pediatr Blood Cancer.* 2010;55:1402-1405.
14. Mallouk A, Pham PT, Pham PC. Concurrent FSGS and Hodgkin's lymphoma: case report and literature review on the link between nephrotic glomerulopathies and hematological malignancies. *Clin Exp Nephrol.* 2006;10:284-289.
15. Cil T, Altintas A, Isikdogan A, Batun S. Prevalence of antineutrophil cytoplasmic antibody positivity in patients with Hodgkin's and non-Hodgkin lymphoma: a single center experience. *Int J Hematol.* 2009;90:52-57.
16. Doussis-Anagnostopoulou IA, Talks KL, Turley H, et al. Vascular endothelial growth factor (VEGF) is expressed by neoplastic Hodgkin-Reed-Sternberg cells in Hodgkin's disease. *J Pathol.* 2002;197:677-683.
17. Audard V, Larousserie F, Grimbert P, et al. Minimal change nephrotic syndrome and classical Hodgkin's lymphoma: report of 21 cases and review of the literature. *Kidney Int.* 2006;69:2251-2260.
18. Filippatos TD, Milionis HJ, Elisaf MS. Alterations in electrolyte equilibrium in patients with acute leukemia. *Eur J Haematol.* 2005;75:449-460.
19. Gallen IW, Rosa RM, Esparaz DY, et al. On the mechanism of the effects of potassium restriction on blood pressure and renal sodium retention. *Am J Kidney Dis.* 1998;31:19-27.
20. Zamkoff KW, Kirshner JJ. Marked hypophosphatemia associated with acute myelomonocytic leukemia. Indirect evidence of phosphorus uptake by leukemic cells. *Arch Intern Med.* 1980;140:1523-1524.
21. Zheng WL, Zhang GS, Tan CL, Shen JK, Yang JJ, Zhong HY. Diabetes insipidus as main presentation of non-Hodgkin's lymphoma with hypophyseal involvement: two case reports. *Leuk Res.* 2010;34:e32-e34.
22. Burt ME, Brennan MF. Incidence of hypercalcemia and malignant neoplasm. *Arch Surg.* 1980;115:704-707.
23. Seymour JF, Gagel RF. Calcitriol: the major humoral mediator of hypercalcemia in Hodgkin's disease and non-Hodgkin's lymphomas. *Blood.* 1993;82:1383-1394.

24. Matsuhashi Y, Tasaka T, Uehara E, et al. Diffuse large B-cell lymphoma presenting with hypercalcemia and multiple osteolysis. *Leuk Lymphoma*. 2004;45:397-400.

25. Beaudreuil J, Lortholary O, Martin A, et al. Hypercalcemia may indicate Richter's syndrome: report of four cases and review. *Cancer*. 1997;79:1211-1215.

26. Ruiz JP, Singh AK, Hart P. Type B lactic acidosis secondary to malignancy: case report, review of published cases, insights into pathogenesis, and prospects for therapy. *Sci World J*. 2011;11:1316-1324.

Index

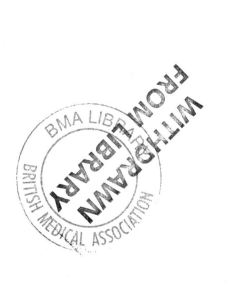